P9-DED-827

Clinical
Neurology
fifth edition

David A. Greenberg, MD, PhD
Professor and Vice-President for Special Research Programs
Buck Institute for Age Research
Novato, California

Michael J. Aminoff, MD, DSc, FRCP
Professor of Neurology
Department of Neurology
School of Medicine
University of California, San Francisco

Roger P. Simon, MD
Robert Stone Dow Chair of Neurology
Director of Neurobiology Research
Legacy Health Systems
Portland, Oregon

Lange Medical Books/McGraw-Hill
Medical Publishing Division

New York   Chicago   San Francisco   Lisbon   London   Madrid   Mexico City
Milan   New Delhi   San Juan   Seoul   Singapore   Sydney   Toronto

McGraw-Hill

A Division of The McGraw·Hill Companies

Clinical Neurology, Fifth Edition

Copyright © 2002 by The **McGraw-Hill** Companies, Inc. All rights reserved. Printed in The United States of America. Except as permitted under the United States Copyright Act of 1976, no part of this publication may be reproduced or distributed in any form or by any means, or stored in a data base or retrieval system, without prior written permission of the publisher.

Previous editions copyright © 1999, 1996, 1993, 1989 by Appleton & Lange.

2345678910   DOC/DOC   098765432

ISBN: 0-07-137543-0

ISSN: 1522-6875

Notice

This book was set in Adobe Garamond by Rainbow Graphics.
The editors were Janet Foltin, Harriet Liebowitz, Scott Kurtz, and Nicky Panton.
The production supervisor was Philip Galea.
The cover designer was Mary McKeon.
The index was prepared by Steve Shimer.

R. R. Donnelley & Sons was printer and binder.

This book is printed on acid-free paper.

INTERNATIONAL EDITION ISBN 0-07-121225-6
Copyright © 2002. Exclusive rights by The McGraw-Hill Companies, Inc., for manufacture and export. This book cannot be re-exported from the country to which it is consigned by McGraw-Hill. The International Edition is not available in North America.

To Our Families

Contents

Preface

The fifth edition of *Clinical Neurology*, like its predecessors, offers a problem-oriented approach to neurology based on the authors' experience in teaching medical students and house staff at the University of California, San Francisco. Chapters are organized according to problems such as headache, seizures, stroke, and coma, because these are the conditions for which patients usually seek medical care. Careful history taking and neurologic examination are emphasized, as these remain the cornerstones of neurologic diagnosis, even in an era of technologic diagnostic advances.

The need to update this book arises from two main sources: rapid expansion of knowledge about the molecular basis of neurologic diseases and recent innovations in the treatment of disorders such as headache, epilepsy, stroke, Parkinson's disease, and multiple sclerosis. Accordingly, increased prominence has been given to molecular mechanisms of diseases—for example, Alzheimer's disease and the polyglutamine disorders, including Huntington's disease. Sections on treatment have been updated and expanded to reflect the introduction of new therapies for neurological disorders. The summary tables of therapeutic drugs and genetic disorders inside the front and back covers, which were introduced in the last edition, have been revised to maintain currency.

Key Concepts is a new feature that has been introduced in this issue. In the beginning of each chapter, some of the major concepts are presented with numbered icons. These same numbered icons appear within the text to indicate where these specific points are discussed in the chapter.

We thank our colleagues, who have contributed their expert advice to the preparation of this new edition of *Clinical Neurology*, especially Lydia Bayne, Megan Burns, Chadwick Christine, Paul Garcia, Alisa Gean, Cheryl Jay, Catherine Lomen-Hoerth, Neil Raskin, Tom Shults, and Norman So. The staff at McGraw-Hill have been enormously helpful in moving this book through editing and production. We hope our efforts will help to demystify clinical neurology for students and practitioners and contribute to providing patients better and more focused diagnosis and treatment.

David A. Greenberg
Michael J. Aminoff
Roger P. Simon

Novato, San Francisco, and Portland
February 2002

Disorders of Consciousness

1

CONTENTS

KEY CONCEPTS

 Disorders of consciousness include disorders in which the level of consciousness (arousal or wakefulness) is impaired, such as acute confusional states and coma, and those in which the level of consciousness is normal but the content of consciousness (cognitive function) is altered, such as dementia and amnestic disorders.

 An acute confusional state can be most readily distinguished from dementia by the time course of the impairment: acute confusional states are acute or subacute in onset, typically developing over hours to days, whereas dementia is a chronic disorder that evolves over months or years.

 Certain causes of acute confusional state must be identified urgently because they may lead rapidly to severe structural brain damage or death, and prompt treatment can prevent these complications: hypoglycemia, bacterial meningitis, subarachnoid hemorrhage, and traumatic intracranial hemorrhage.

 The most common causes of dementia are Alzheimer's disease, dementia with Lewy bodies, and vascular dementia; treatable causes of dementia are rare, but are important to diagnose.

Consciousness is awareness of the internal or external world, and disorders of consciousness can affect either the level of consciousness or the content of consciousness.

Disturbances of the Level of Consciousness

 Abnormalities of the level of consciousness are characterized by impaired arousal or wakefulness, and they result from acute lesions of the ascending reticular activating system (Figure 1–1) or

both cerebral hemispheres. The most severe degree of depressed consciousness is **coma,** in which the patient is unresponsive and unarousable. Less severe depression of consciousness results in an **acute confusional state** or **delirium,** in which the patient responds to at least some stimuli in a purposeful manner but is sleepy, disoriented, and inattentive. In some acute confusional states, agitation predominates or alternates with drowsiness, and may be accompanied by autonomic changes (fever, tachycardia, hypertension, sweating, pallor, or flushing), hallucinations, and motor abnormalities (tremor, asterixis, or myoclonus).

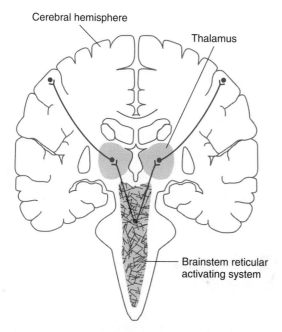

Figure 1–1. Brainstem reticular activating system and its ascending projections to the thalamus and cerebral hemispheres.

Disturbances of the Content of Consciousness

(1) Many pathologic conditions can impair the content of consciousness without altering the level of consciousness. Examples include isolated disorders of language or memory due to focal brain lesions and widespread deterioration of mental function (**dementia**) from more diffuse, chronic pathologic processes. Dementia differs from acute confusional states in several respects (Table 1–1), and distinguishing between between these two syndromes is the pivotal step in evaluating a patient with altered consciousness.

(2) *The time course of the disorder—acute or subacute in acute confusional states and chronic in*

dementia—is the single most helpful differentiating feature.

Confusional states, dementia, and circumscribed memory disorders are discussed in this chapter. Coma is discussed in Chapter 10.

■ I. APPROACH TO DIAGNOSIS

Evaluation of the patient with a suspected disorder of consciousness is aimed first at characterizing the nature of the disorder (eg, acute confusional state, coma, dementia, amnestic syndrome) and second at determining the cause. The approach used is outlined below.

HISTORY

History of Present Illness

The history should establish the time course of the disorder and provide clues to its nature and cause. Confusional states are acute to subacute in onset, whereas dementias are chronic disorders. In an acute confusional state, the observations of others may be the only historical information available. When dementia is suspected, it is useful to have access to a relative or close acquaintance who can furnish details about the patient's previous level of functioning; the time when dysfunction became evident; and the nature of any changes in personality, behavior, mood, intellect, judgment, memory, or facility with language. Associated problems such as gait disorders, incontinence, and headaches should also be explored.

Prior Medical History

A. CARDIOVASCULAR SYSTEM

A history of stroke, hypertension, vasculitis, or cardiac disease may suggest a vascular cause of a confusional state or multiinfarct dementia.

Table 1–1. Differences between acute confusional states and dementia.

	Acute Confusional State	Dementia
Level of consciousness	Impaired	Not impaired, except occasionally late in course
Course	Acute to subacute; fluctuating	Chronic; steadily progressive
Autonomic hyperactivity	Often present	Absent
Prognosis	Usually reversible	Usually irreversible

B. DIABETES

Cognitive disturbance in diabetic patients may result from a hyperosmolar nonketotic state or insulin-induced hypoglycemia.

C. SEIZURE DISORDER

A history of epilepsy suggests ongoing seizures, a postictal state, or head trauma in a confused patient.

D. HEAD TRAUMA

Recent head trauma suggests intracranial hemorrhage. Remote head trauma may produce amnestic syndrome or chronic subdural hematoma with dementia.

E. ALCOHOLISM

Alcoholism predisposes patients to acute confusional states from intoxication, withdrawal, postictal state, head trauma, hepatic encephalopathy, and Wernicke's encephalopathy. Chronic memory disturbance in an alcoholic is likely due to Korsakoff's syndrome.

F. DRUG HISTORY

A confusional state can result from overdose with insulin, sedative-hypnotics, opioids, antidepressants, antipsychotic agents, or hallucinogens, or from sedative drug withdrawal. Elderly patients may be more sensitive to the cognitive side effects of drugs that are well tolerated by younger patients.

G. PSYCHIATRIC HISTORY

A history of psychiatric illness may suggest overdose with psychotherapeutic drugs such as benzodiazepines, antidepressants, or antipsychotic agents; a previously undiagnosed medical disorder capable of producing organic psychosis (hypothyroidism, vitamin B_{12} deficiency); or a functional disorder masquerading as an acute confusional state or dementia.

H. OTHER

Individuals who engage in unprotected sexual intercourse, intravenous drug users, recipients of contaminated blood or clotting factor transfusions, the sexual partners of all these persons, and infants of infected mothers are at particular risk for developing acquired immunodeficiency syndrome (AIDS).

Family History

The family history can point to a heredodegenerative disorder, such as Huntington's disease, as the cause of dementia.

GENERAL PHYSICAL EXAMINATION

A general physical examination helps to classify the disorder as either an acute confusional state or dementia and may suggest a systemic disease as its cause (Tables 1–2 and 1–3).

Vital Signs & General Appearance

Fever, tachycardia, hypertension, and sweating occur in many confusional states, but meningitis or sepsis must receive early consideration in the febrile patient. Hypertension should raise the possibility of hypertensive encephalopathy, intracranial hemorrhage, renal disease, or Cushing's syndrome. Hypothermia occurs with exposure to cold, ethanol or sedative drug intoxication, hypoglycemia, hepatic encephalopathy, Wernicke's encephalopathy, hypothyroidism, or shock. In most dementias, the patient does not appear acutely ill unless a systemic disorder is also present.

Skin & Mucous Membranes

Jaundice suggests hepatic disease, and lemon-yellow coloration of the skin may occur in vitamin B_{12} deficiency. Coarse dry skin, dry brittle hair, and subcutaneous edema are characteristic of hypothyroidism. Petechiae are seen in meningococcemia, and petechiae or ecchymoses may reflect coagulopathy caused by liver disease, disseminated intravascular coagulation, or thrombotic thrombocytopenia purpura. Hot, dry skin is characteristic of intoxication with anticholinergic drugs. Cushing's syndrome may be associated with acne. Hyperpigmentation of the skin may be evidence of Addison's disease. Needle tracks associated with intravenous drug use suggest drug overdose, AIDS, or infective endocarditis.

Head & Neck

Examination of the head may reveal signs of trauma, such as scalp lacerations or contusions, postauricular hematoma (Battle's sign), periorbital hematoma (raccoon eyes), hemotympanum, or cerebrospinal fluid (CSF) otorrhea or rhinorrhea. Percussion of the skull over a subdural hematoma may cause pain. Meningeal signs, such as neck stiffness on passive flexion, thigh flexion upon flexion of the neck (Brudzinski's sign), or resistance to passive extension of the knee with the hip flexed (Kernig's sign), are seen in meningitis and subarachnoid hemorrhage.

Chest & Abdomen

Cardiac murmurs may be associated with infective endocarditis and its neurologic sequelae. Abdominal examination may reveal a source of systemic infection or suggest liver disease. Rectal examination may provide evidence of gastrointestinal bleeding, which often precipitates hepatic encephalopathy.

Table 1–2. Clinical features helpful in the differential diagnosis of acute confusional states.

Feature	Most Suggestive of	Feature	Most Suggestive of
Headache	Head trauma, meningitis, subarachnoid hemorrhage	**Cranial nerves** Papilledema	Hypertensive encephalopathy, intracranial mass
Vital signs Fever	Infectious meningitis, anticholinergic intoxication, withdrawal from ethanol or sedative drugs, sepsis	Dilated pupils	Head trauma, anticholinergic intoxication, withdrawal from ethanol or sedative drugs, sympathomimetic intoxication
Hypothermia	Intoxication with ethanol or sedative drugs, hepatic encephalopathy, hypoglycemia, hypothyroidism, sepsis	Constricted pupils	Opioid intoxication
Hypertension	Anticholinergic intoxication, withdrawal from ethanol or sedative drugs, hypertensive encephalopathy, subarachnoid hemorrhage, sympathomimetic intoxication	Nystagmus/ ophthalmoplegia	Intoxication with ethanol, sedative drugs, or phencyclidine, vertebrobasilar ischemia, Wernicke's encephalopathy
Tachycardia	Anticholinergic intoxication, withdrawal from ethanol or sedative drugs, thyrotoxicosis, sepsis	**Motor** Tremor	Withdrawal from ethanol or sedative drugs, sympathomimetic intoxication, thyrotoxicosis
Bradycardia	Hypothyroidism	Asterixis	Metabolic encephalopathy
Hyperventilation	Hepatic encephalopathy, hyperglycemia, sepsis	Hemiparesis	Cerebral infarction, head trauma, hyperglycemia, hypoglycemia
Hypoventilation	Intoxication with ethanol or sedative drugs, opioid intoxication, pulmonary encephalopathy	**Other** Seizures	Withdrawal from ethanol or sedative drugs, head trauma, hyperglycemia, hypoglycemia
General examination Meningismus	Meningitis, subarachnoid hemorrhage	Ataxia	Intoxication with ethanol or sedative drugs, Wernicke's encephalopathy
Skin rash	Meningococcal meningitis		
Tetany	Hypocalcemia		

NEUROLOGIC EXAMINATION

Mental Status Examination

Evaluation of mental status (Table 1–4) helps to classify a disorder as a confusional state, dementia, a circumscribed cognitive disturbance (aphasia, amnesia), or a psychiatric illness. The mental status examination is most useful if performed in a standardized fashion, and complex functions can be adequately evaluated only when the basic processes upon which they depend are preserved. Thus, memory, language, calculation, or abstraction cannot be reliably assessed in a patient who is poorly arousable or inattentive. The Minimental Status Examination (Table 1–5) is often used as a rapid bedside screening test for dementia.

In performing the mental status examination, the level of consciousness and attention are evaluated first. If these are impaired, an acute confusional state exists, and it may be difficult or impossible to conduct the remainder of the mental status examination. If the level of consciousness and attention are adequate, more complex cortical functions are examined next to determine whether there is global cortical dysfunction, which indicates dementia.

A. LEVEL OF CONSCIOUSNESS

The level of consciousness is described in terms of the patient's apparent state of wakefulness and response to stimuli. Impairment of the level of consciousness should always be documented by a written description of the patient's responses to specific stimuli rather than by the use of nonspecific and imprecise terms such as "lethargy," "stupor," or "semicoma."

1. Normal—The patient with a normal level of consciousness appears awake and alert, with eyes open at rest. Unless there is deafness or a language disorder, verbal stimulation results in appropriate verbal responses.

Table 1–3. Clinical features helpful in the differential diagnosis of dementia.

Feature	Most Suggestive of	Feature	Most Suggestive of

History
  Unprotected sexual intercourse, intravenous drug abuse, hemophilia, or blood transfusions
	AIDS dementia complex	**Motor**
		  Tremor
			Dementia with Lewy bodies, corticobasal ganglionic degeneration, acquired hepatocerebral degeneration, Wilson's disease, AIDS dementia complex

Family history	Huntington's disease, Wilson's disease	Asterixis	Acquired hepatocerebral degeneration
Headache	Brain tumor, chronic subdural hematoma	Myoclonus	Creutzfeldt-Jakob disease, AIDS dementia complex
Vital signs Hypothemia	Hypothyroidism	Rigidity	Dementia with Lewy bodies, corticobasal ganglionic degeneration, acquired hepatocerebral degeneration, Creutzfeldt-Jakob disease, progressive supranuclear palsy, Wilson's disease
Hypertension	Multiinfarct dementia		
Hypotension	Hypothyroidism		
Bradycardia	Hypothyroidism	Chorea	Huntington's disease, Wilson's disease

General examination
  Meningismus
	Chronic meningitis	**Other**
		  Gait apraxia
			Normal pressure hydrocephalus

Jaundice	Acquired hepatocerebral degeneration	Polyneuropathy with hyporeflexia	Neurosyphilis, vitamin B_{12} deficiency, AIDS dementia complex
Kayser-Fleisher rings	Wilson's disease		
Cranial nerves Papilledema	Brain tumor, chronic subdural hematoma		
Argyll Robertson pupils	Neurosyphilis		
Ophthalmoplegia	Progressive supranuclear palsy		
Pseudobulbar palsy	Multiinfarct dementia, progressive supranuclear palsy		

2. Impaired—Mild impairment of consciousness may be manifested by sleepiness from which the patient is easily aroused when spoken to. As consciousness is further impaired, the intensity of stimulation required for arousal increases, the duration of arousal declines, and the responses elicited become less purposeful.

B. ATTENTION

Attention is the ability to focus on a particular sensory stimulus to the exclusion of others; **concentration** is sustained attention. These processes are grossly impaired in acute confusional states, usually less impaired in dementia, and unaffected by focal brain lesions. Attention can be tested by asking the patient to repeat a series of digits or to indicate when a given letter appears in a random series. A normal person can repeat five to seven digits correctly and identify a letter in a series without error.

C. LANGUAGE AND SPEECH

The essential elements of language are comprehension, repetition, fluency, naming, reading, and writing, all of which should be tested when a language disorder (**aphasia**) is suspected. Calculation disorders (**acalculia**) are probably closely related to aphasia. Speech, the motor activity that is the final step in the expression of language, is mediated by the lower cranial nerves and their supranuclear connections. **Dysarthria,** a disorder of articulation, is sometimes difficult to distinguish from aphasia, but it always spares oral and written language comprehension and written expression.

Table 1–4. Comprehensive mental status examination.

Level of consciousness
Attention and concentration
Language and speech
  Comprehension
  Repetition
  Fluency
  Naming
  Reading
  Writing
  Calculation
  Speech

Mood and behavior
Content of thought
  Hallucinations
  Delusions
  Abstraction
  Judgment

Memory
  Immediate recall
  Recent memory
  Remote memory

Integrative sensory function
  Astereognosis
  Agraphesthesia
  Two-point discrimination
  Allesthesia
  Extinction
  Unilateral neglect and anosognosia
  Disorders of spatial thought

Integrative motor function
  Apraxia

Table 1–5. Minimental status examination.

Item	Points[1]
Orientation	
Time (1 point each for year, season, month, date, and day of the week)	5
Place (1 point each for state, county, city, building, and floor or room)	5
Registration	
Repeat names of three objects (1 point per object)	3
Attention and calculation	
Serial 7s or spell "world" backward (1 point per subtraction or letter)	5
Recall	
Recall names of three objects repeated previously (1 point per object)	3
Language	
Name pencil and watch (1 point each)	2
Repeat "no ifs, ands or buts"	1
Follow three-step command (1 point per step)	3
Read and follow: "close your eyes"	1
Write a complete sentence	1
Construction	
Copy two intersecting pentagons	1
Total	30

[1] A total score of <24 should generally lead to more detailed investigation of the possibility of dementia, although norms vary to some extent with age and education.

Adapted from Greenberg DA: Dementia. In: *Geriatrics.* Lonergan ET (editor). Appleton & Lange, 1996.

Aphasia may be a feature of diffuse cortical disease, as it is in certain dementias, but language impairment with otherwise normal cognitive function should suggest a focal lesion in the dominant hemisphere. A disorder of comprehension (**receptive, or Wernicke's, aphasia**) commonly leads to a false impression of a confusional state or psychiatric disturbance.

There are a variety of aphasic syndromes, each characterized by a particular pattern of language impairment; several have fairly precise pathoanatomic correlations (Figure 1–2).

D. Mood and Behavior

Demented patients may be apathetic, inappropriately elated, or depressed, and their moods can fluctuate. If the examination is otherwise normal, early dementia can easily be confused with depression. Delirious patients are agitated, noisy, and easily provoked to anger.

E. Content of Thought

Abnormalities of thought content can help to distinguish organic from psychiatric disease. **Visual hallucinations** are common in acute confusional states, whereas **auditory hallucinations** and **fixed delusions** are most common with psychiatric disorders. **Impairment of abstraction** may be revealed by the patient's concrete (literal) interpretation of proverbs or inability to recognize conceptual differences and similarities. **Judgment** is commonly tested by asking what the patient would do in a hypothetic situation, such as finding a stamped, addressed letter on the sidewalk.

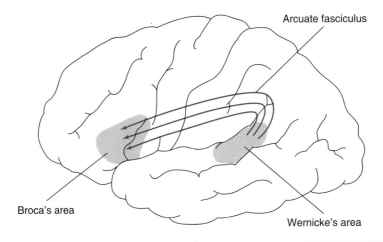

Figure 1–2. Anatomic basis and clinical features of aphasias.

Pathologic Site	Type of Aphasia	Language Functions Preserved		
		Comprehension	Repetition	Fluency
Wernicke's area	Receptive	–	–	+
Arcuate fasciculus	Conductive	+	–	+
Broca's area	Expressive	+	–	–

F. MEMORY

1. Functional components of memory—Memory is the ability to register, store, and ultimately retrieve information. Storage and retrieval of memories can be impaired by either diffuse cortical disease or focal bilateral dysfunction of the medial temporal lobes or their connections.

a. Registration—The ability to receive information through the various sensory modalities is largely a function of attention.

b. Storage—The process whereby selected new information is learned, or memorized, may be mediated by limbic structures, including the hippocampus. Stored memories are reinforced by repetition and by emotional significance; they are thought to be diffusely distributed in association areas of the cerebral cortex.

c. Retrieval—Retrieval is the ability to access previously learned information.

2. Amnesia—Memory disorder (amnesia) may be an isolated deficit or one feature of global cognitive dysfunction. In acute confusional states, attention is impaired, resulting in defective registration and an inability to learn new material. In dementia, attention is typically normal and problems with recent and—to a lesser extent—remote memory usually predominate.

In **psychogenic amnesia,** subjective and emotionally charged memories are affected more than retention of objective facts and events; in **organic amnesia,** the reverse is true. Isolated loss of memory for personal identity (the inability to remember one's own name) in an awake and alert patient is virtually pathognomonic of a psychogenic disorder.

Additional terms sometimes used to denote aspects of acute-onset amnesia (eg, following head trauma) include **retrograde amnesia,** loss of memory for events immediately prior to the onset of the disorder, and **anterograde** or **posttraumatic amnesia,** impairment of memory in the period following the insult.

3. Testing of memory—Memory is assessed clinically by testing **immediate recall, recent memory,** and **remote memory,** which correspond roughly to registration, storage, and retrieval, respectively.

a. Immediate recall—Tests of immediate recall are similar to tests of attention and include having the patient repeat a random series of numbers or other information that has not been previously learned. The ability to repeat implies that the material has been registered. Most normal adults can repeat a series of seven numbers forward and five backward without difficulty.

b. Recent memory—Tests of recent memory assess the ability to learn new material. Typically, the patient is given three or four items to remember and asked to recall them 3 minutes later. Nonverbal tests, in which an object previously shown to the patient is selected from a group of objects, may be useful, especially for patients with expressive aphasia. Orientation to place and time, which requires newly learned information, is another important test of recent memory.

c. Remote memory—The practical distinction between recent and remote memory is that only recent memory requires an ongoing ability to learn new information. Remote memory is tested by asking the patient to recall material that someone of comparable cultural and educational background can be assumed to know. Common examples are personal, historical, or geographic data, but the questions selected must be appropriate for the patient, and personal items must be verifiable.

G. Integrative Sensory Function

Sensory integration disorders from parietal lobe lesions are manifested by misperception of or inattention to sensory stimuli on the contralateral side of the body, when the primary sensory modalities are intact.

Patients with parietal lesions may exhibit the following signs:

1. Astereognosis—The patient cannot identify, by touch, an object placed in the hand.

2. Agraphesthesia—The patient is unable to identify a number written on the hand.

3. Absence of two-point discrimination—This is an inability to differentiate between a single stimulus and two simultaneously applied adjacent, but separated, stimuli that can be distinguished by a normal person.

4. Allesthesia—This is misplaced localization of a tactile stimulus.

5. Extinction—A visual or tactile stimulus is perceived when applied alone to the side contralateral to the lesion but not when stimuli are applied bilaterally.

6. Unilateral neglect and anosognosia—Body image disorders caused by parietal lobe lesions take the form of unilateral neglect. The patient tends not to use the contralateral limbs, may deny that there is anything wrong with them (anosognosia), and may even fail to recognize them.

7. Disorders of spatial thought—These include **constructional apraxia, right/left disorientation, and neglect of external space** on the side opposite the affected parietal lobe. Tests for constructional apraxia include having the patient fill in the numbers on a clock face, copy geometric figures, or build figures with blocks.

H. Integrative Motor Function

Apraxia is the inability to perform previously learned tasks, such as finger snapping or clapping the hands together, despite intact motor and sensory function. Unilateral apraxias are commonly caused by contralateral premotor frontal cortex lesions. Bilateral apraxias, such as gait apraxia, may be seen with bifrontal or diffuse cerebral lesions.

Gait & Station

It is useful to observe the patient standing and walking early in the neurologic examination, since these activities may reveal additional neurologic abnormalities associated with disturbed cognitive function.

Cranial Nerves

In patients with impaired cognitive function, abnormalities associated with cranial nerves may suggest the underlying cause.

A. Lesions of the Eyes and Ears

1. Papilledema suggests an intracranial mass, hypertensive encephalopathy, or other process that increases intracranial pressure.

2. In the confused patient, **pupillary constriction** suggests opiate ingestion; **dilated pupils** are characteristic of anticholinergic intoxication but may also be a manifestation of generalized sympathetic hyperactivity. **Small, irregular pupils** that react poorly to light—but better to accommodation—can be seen in neurosyphilis.

3. Sedative drugs and Wernicke's encephalopathy produce **nystagmus** or **ophthalmoplegia**. Selective impairment of vertical gaze (especially downward) occurs early in progressive supranuclear palsy.

B. Pseudobulbar Palsy

This syndrome is characterized by dysarthria, dysphagia, hyperactive jaw jerk and gag reflexes, and uncontrollable laughing or crying unrelated to emotional state (**pseudobulbar affect**). It results from bilateral interruption of the corticobulbar and corticospinal tracts. Dementing processes that produce this syndrome include progressive supranuclear palsy and multiinfarct dementia.

C. Multiple Cranial Neuropathies

These can accompany infectious or noninfectious meningitis or AIDS dementia complex.

Motor Findings

A. Acute Confusional State

In the acutely confused patient, a variety of motor abnormalities may suggest the cause.

1. Hemiparesis is most apt to be due to an intracranial structural lesion, although focal neurologic signs may be present in metabolic disorders such as hypoglycemia and nonketotic hyperglycemia.

2. Tremor is common in sedative drug or ethanol withdrawal and other states accompanied by autonomic hyperactivity.

3. Asterixis, a flapping tremor of the outstretched hands or feet, is seen in hepatic, renal, and pulmonary encephalopathy and in drug intoxication.

4. Myoclonus, which consists of rapid shocklike muscle contractions, can occur with uremia, cerebral hypoxia, or hyperosmolar nonketotic states.

5. Cerebellar signs such as broad-based ataxic gait and, often, dysmetria on heel-knee-shin maneuver accompany Wernicke's encephalopathy and sedative drug intoxication.

B. DEMENTIA

Motor signs are useful in the differential diagnosis of dementia.

1. Chorea—Huntington's disease, Wilson's disease.

2. Tremor, rigidity, or bradykinesia—Wilson's disease, acquired hepatocerebral degeneration.

3. Myoclonus—Creutzfeldt-Jakob disease, AIDS dementia complex.

4. Ataxia—Spinocerebellar degenerations, Wilson's disease, paraneoplastic syndromes, Creutzfeldt-Jakob disease, AIDS dementia complex.

5. Paraparesis—Vitamin B_{12} deficiency, hydrocephalus, AIDS dementia complex.

Abnormalities of Sensation & Tendon Reflexes

Dementias associated with prominent sensory abnormalities and loss of tendon reflexes include vitamin B_{12} deficiency, neurosyphilis, and AIDS dementia complex.

Primitive Reflexes

A number of reflexes that are present in infancy and subsequently disappear may be released by frontal lobe dysfunction in later life. It is presumed that such release results from loss of cortical inhibition of these primitive reflexes (frontal release signs), which include palmar and plantar grasps as well as palmomental, suck, snout, rooting, and glabellar reflexes. Although these responses are often seen in both acute confusional states and dementia, many can also occur in normal elderly adults. Their presence alone does not constitute evidence of cognitive dysfunction.

1. The **palmar grasp** reflex is elicited by stroking the skin of the patient's palm with the examiner's fingers. If the reflex is present, the patient's fingers close around those of the examiner. The force of the patient's grasp may increase when the examiner attempts to withdraw the fingers, and the patient may be unable to voluntarily release the grasp.

2. The **plantar grasp** reflex consists of flexion and adduction of the toes in response to stimulation of the sole of the foot.

3. The **palmomental reflex** is elicited by scratching along the length of the palm of the hand and results in contraction of ipsilateral chin (mentalis) and perioral (orbicularis oris) muscles.

4. The **suck reflex** consists of involuntary sucking movements following the stimulation of the lips.

5. The **snout reflex** is elicited by gently tapping the lips and results in their protrusion.

6. In the **rooting reflex,** stimulation of the lips causes them to deviate toward the stimulus.

7. The **glabellar reflex** is elicited by repetitive tapping on the forehead. Normal subjects blink only in response to the first several taps; persistent blinking is an abnormal response (**Myerson's sign**).

LABORATORY INVESTIGATIONS

Laboratory studies are critical in diagnosing disorders of cognitive function. Useful investigations are listed in Tables 1–6 and 1–7; those most likely to establish or support a diagnosis in acute confusional states are complete blood count, arterial blood gases and pH, serum sodium, serum glucose, serum urea nitrogen and creatinine, liver function tests, drug screens, blood cultures, stool test for occult blood, lumbar puncture, brain computed tomography (CT) scan or magnetic resonance imaging (MRI), and electroencephalogram (EEG).

Some of these studies can yield a specific diagnosis. Abnormal arterial blood gas or cerebrospinal fluid (CSF) profiles, for example, narrow the differential diagnosis to one or a few possibilities (Tables 1–8 and 1–9).

Reversible dementia may be diagnosed on the basis of laboratory studies (see Table 1–7). The most common reversible dementias are those due to intracranial masses, normal pressure hydrocephalus, thyroid dysfunction, and vitamin B_{12} deficiency.

■ II. ACUTE CONFUSIONAL STATES

Common causes of acute confusional states are listed in Table 1–10.

Table 1–6. Laboratory studies in acute confusional states.

Test	Most Useful in Diagnosis of	Test	Most Useful in Diagnosis of
Blood		**ECG**	Anticholinergic intoxication, vascular disorders
WBC	Meningitis, encephalitis, sepsis		
PT and PTT	Hepatic encephalopathy	**Cerebrospinal fluid**	
Arterial blood gas	Hepatic encephalopathy, pulmonary encephalopathy, uremia, sepsis	WBC, RBC	Meningitis, encephalitis, subarachnoid hemorrhage
Sodium	Hyponatremia	Gram's stain	Bacterial meningitis
Serum urea nitrogen and creatinine	Uremia	AFB stain	Tuberculous meningitis
		India ink stain	Cryptococcal meningitis
Glucose	Hyperglycemia, hypoglycemia	Cultures	Infectious meningitis
Osmolality	Alcohol intoxication, hyperglycemia	Cytology	Leptomeningeal metastases
Liver function tests, ammonia	Hepatic encephalopathy, Reye's syndrome	Glutamine	Hepatic encephalopathy
		VDRL	Syphilitic meningitis
Thyroid function tests	Hyperthyroidism, hypothyroidism	Cryptococcal antigen	Cryptococcal meningitis
Calcium	Hypercalcemia, hypocalcemia	Polymerase chain reaction	Bacterial meningitis, tuberculous meningitis, syphilitic meningitis, Lyme disease, viral meningitis and encephalitis, AIDS, leptomeningeal metastases
Drug screen	Drug intoxications		
Cultures	Meningitis, sepsis		
FTA or MHA-TP	Syphilitic meningitis		
HIV antibody titer	AIDS and related disorders	**CT brain scan or MRI**	Cerebral infarction, intracranial hemorrhage, head trauma, toxoplasmosis, herpes simplex encephalitis, subarachnoid hemorrhage
Urine, gastric aspirate			
Drug screen	Drug intoxication		
Stool		**EEG**	Complex partial seizures, herpes simplex encephalitis, nonconvulsive seizures
Guaiac	Hepatic encephalopathy		

DRUGS

Many drugs can cause acute confusional states, especially when taken in greater than customary doses, in combination with other drugs, by patients with altered drug metabolism from hepatic or renal failure, by the elderly, or in the setting of preexisting cognitive impairment. A partial list of drugs that can produce acute confusional states is provided in Table 1–11.

ETHANOL INTOXICATION

Ethanol intoxication produces a confusional state with nystagmus, dysarthria, and limb and gait ataxia. In nonalcoholics, signs correlate roughly with blood ethanol levels, but chronic alcoholics, who have developed tolerance to ethanol, may have very high levels without appearing intoxicated. Laboratory studies useful in con-

firming the diagnosis include blood alcohol levels and serum osmolality. In alcohol intoxication, serum osmolality determined by direct measurement exceeds the calculated osmolality ($2 \times$ serum sodium $+ \frac{1}{20}$ serum glucose $+ \frac{1}{3}$ serum urea nitrogen) by 22 mosm/L for every 100 mg/dL of ethanol present. Intoxicated patients are at high risk for head trauma. Alcohol ingestion may cause life-threatening hypoglycemia, and chronic alcoholism increases the risk of bacterial meningitis. Treatment is not required unless a withdrawal syndrome ensues, but alcoholic patients should receive thiamine to prevent Wernicke's encephalopathy (see below).

ETHANOL WITHDRAWAL

Three common withdrawal syndromes are recognized (Figure 1–3). Because of the associated risk of Wernicke's encephalopathy (discussed later), patients pre-

Table 1–7. Laboratory studies in dementia.

Test	Most Useful in Diagnosis of
Blood	
Hematocrit, mean corpuscular volume (MCV), peripheral blood smear, vitamin B_{12} level	Vitamin B_{12} deficiency
Thyroid function tests	Hypothyroidism
Liver function tests	Acquired hepatocerebral degeneration, Wilson's disease
Ceruloplasmin, copper	Wilson's disease
FTA or MHA-TP	Neurosyphilis
HIV antibody titer	AIDS dementia complex
Cerebrospinal fluid	
VDRL	Neurosyphilis
Cytology	Leptomeningeal metastases
CT scan or MRI	Brain tumor, chronic subdural hematoma, multiinfarct dementia, normal pressure hydrocephalus
EEG	Creutzfeldt-Jakob disease

Table 1–8. Arterial blood gases in acute confusional states.

Pattern	Differential Diagnosis
Metabolic acidosis (with increased anion gap)	Diabetic ketoacidosis, lactic acidosis (postictal, shock, sepsis), toxins (methanol, ethylene glycol, salicylates,[1] paraldehyde), uremia
Respiratory alkalosis	Hepatic encephalopathy, pulmonary insufficiency, salicylates,[1] sepsis
Respiratory acidosis	Pulmonary insufficiency, sedative drug overdose

[1] Sepsis and salicylates produce a combined acid-base disorder.

senting with these syndromes should be given thiamine, 100 mg/d, intravenously or intramuscularly, until a normal diet can be ensured.

1. Tremulousness & Hallucinations

This self-limited condition occurs within 2 days after cessation of drinking and is characterized by tremulousness, agitation, anorexia, nausea, insomnia, tachycardia, and hypertension. Confusion, if present, is mild. Illusions and hallucinations, usually visual, occur in about 25% of patients. Treatment with diazepam, 5–20 mg, or chlordiazepoxide, 25–50 mg, orally every 4 hours, will terminate the syndrome and prevent more serious consequences of withdrawal.

2. Seizures

Ethanol withdrawal seizures occur within 48 hours of abstinence, and within 7–24 hours in about two-thirds of cases. Roughly 40% of patients who experience seizures have a single seizure; more than 90% have between one and six seizures. In 85% of the cases, the interval between the first and last seizures is 6 hours or less. Anticonvulsants are usually not required, as seizures cease spontaneously in most cases. Unusual features such as focal seizures, prolonged duration of seizures (>6–12 hours), more than six seizures, status epilepticus, or a prolonged postictal state should prompt a search for other causes or complicating factors, such as head trauma or infection. The patient should be observed for 6–12 hours to make certain that atypical features are not present. Because patients with withdrawal seizures may develop delirium tremens, diazepam or chlordiazepoxide is sometimes given prophylactically.

3. Delirium Tremens

This most serious ethanol withdrawal syndrome typically begins 3–5 days after cessation of drinking and lasts for up to 72 hours. It is characterized by confusion, agitation, fever, sweating, tachycardia, hypertension, and hallucinations. Death may result from concomitant infection, pancreatitis, cardiovascular collapse, or trauma. Treatment consists of diazepam, 10–20 mg intravenously, repeated every 5 minutes as needed until the patient is calm, and correction of fluid and electrolyte abnormalities and hypoglycemia. The total requirement for diazepam may exceed 100 mg/h. Concomitant β-adrenergic receptor blockade with atenolol, 50–100 mg/d, has also been recommended.

SEDATIVE DRUG INTOXICATION

The classic signs of sedative drug overdose are confusional state or coma, respiratory depression, hypotension, hypothermia, reactive pupils, nystagmus or absence of ocular movements, ataxia, dysarthria, and hyporeflexia. The most commonly used sedative-hypnotic drugs are benzodiazepines and barbiturates.

Table 1–9. Cerebrospinal fluid profiles in acute confusional states.

	Appearance	Opening Pressure	Red Blood Cells	White Blood Cells	Glucose	Protein	Glutamine	Smears	Cultures
Normal	Clear, colorless	70–200 mm H$_2$O	0/μL	≤5 mononuclear/μL	≥45 mg/dL	≤45[1] mg/dL	<25 μg/dL	–	–
Bacterial meningitis	Cloudy	↑	Normal	↑↑ (PMN)[2]	↓↓	↑↑	Normal	Gram's stain +	+
Tuberculous meningitis	Normal or cloudy	↑	Normal	↑ (MN)[3,5]	↓	↑	Normal	AFB stain +	±
Fungal meningitis	Normal or cloudy	Normal or ↑	Normal	↑ (MN)	↓	↑	Normal	India ink prep + (Cryptococcus)	±
Viral meningitis/ encephalitis	Normal	Normal or ↑	Normal[4]	↑ (MN)[5]	Normal[6]	Normal or ↑	Normal	—	±
Parasitic meningitis/ encephalitis	Normal or cloudy	Normal or ↑	Normal	↑ (MN,E)[7]	Normal	Normal or ↑	Normal	Amebas may be seen on wet mount	±
Leptomeningeal metastases	Normal or cloudy	Normal or ↑	Normal	Normal or ↑ (MN)	↓↓	Normal or ↑	Normal	Cytology +	–
Subarachnoid hemorrhage	Pink-red (supernatant yellow)	↑	↑	Normal or ↑ (PMN)[8]	Normal or ↑[8]	↑	Normal	–	–
Hepatic encephalopathy	Normal	Normal	Normal	Normal	Normal	Normal	↑	–	–

[1] Lumbar cerebrospinal fluid.

[2] PMN, polymorphonuclear predominance.

[3] MN, mononuclear (lymphocytic or monocytic) predominance.

[4] Red blood cell count may be elevated in herpes simplex encephalitis.

[5] PMN predominance may be seen early in course.

[6] Glucose may be decreased in herpes or mumps infections.

[7] E, eosinophils often present.

[8] Pleocytosis and low glucose, sometimes seen several days after hemorrhage, reflect chemical meningitis caused by subarachnoid blood.

+, positive; –, negative; ±, can be positive or negative.

Glutethimide or very high doses of barbiturates may produce large, fixed pupils. Decerebrate and decorticate posturing can occur in coma that is caused by sedative drug overdose. The diagnosis can be confirmed by toxicologic analysis of blood, urine, or gastric aspirate, but blood levels of short-acting sedatives do not correlate with clinical severity.

Management is directed at supporting the patient's respiratory and circulatory function while the drug is being cleared. Complications include aspiration pneumonia and pulmonary edema caused by fluid overload. Barring the development of infections or cardiovascular complications, patients who arrive at the hospital with adequate cardiopulmonary function should survive without sequelae.

Table 1–10. Common causes of acute confusional states.

Metabolic Disorders	**Infectious and Noninfectious Meningitis/Encephalitis**
Drugs[1]	Bacterial meningitis
Ethanol intoxication	Tuberculous meningitis
Ethanol withdrawal	Syphilitic meningitis
Sedative drug intoxication	Viral meningoencephalitis
Sedative drug withdrawal	Herpes simplex virus encephalitis
Opioids	AIDS
Anticholinergics	Fungal meningitis
Phencyclidine	Parasitic infections
Endocrine disorders	Leptomeningeal metastases
Hypothyroidism	
Hyperthyroidism	**Vascular Disorders**
Hypoglycemia	Hypertensive encephalopathy
Hyperglycemia	Subarachnoid hemorrhage
Electrolyte disorders	Vertebrobasilar ischemia
Hyponatremia	Right (nondominant) hemisphere infarction
Hypocalcemia	Systemic lupus erythematosus
Hypercalcemia	Disseminated intravascular coagulation
Nutritional disorders	Thrombotic thrombocytopenic purpura
Wernicke's encephalopathy	
Vitamin B_{12} deficiency	**Head Trauma**
Organ system failure	Concussion
Hepatic encephalopathy	Intracranial hemorrhage
Reye's syndrome	
Uremia	**Seizures**
Dialysis disequilibrium	Postictal state
Pulmonary encephalopathy	Complex partial seizure
Organ transplantation	

[1] See also Table 1–11.

SEDATIVE DRUG WITHDRAWAL

Clinical Findings

Like ethanol, sedative drugs can produce confusional states or seizures when intake is stopped abruptly. The frequency and severity of withdrawal syndromes depend upon the duration of drug intake and the dose and half-life of the drug. They occur most often in patients taking large doses for at least several weeks. Intermediate- or short-acting agents are those most likely to produce withdrawal symptoms when discontinued.

Withdrawal syndromes commonly develop 1–3 days after cessation of short-acting agents but may not appear until a week or more after longer-acting drugs are discontinued. Symptoms are identical to those of ethanol withdrawal and are similarly self-limited. Myoclonus and seizures may appear after 3–8 days, however, and may require treatment. Seizures usually occur only when the average daily drug intake is several times the usual therapeutic dose. A syndrome indistinguishable from delirium tremens may also occur, and also tends to be restricted to patients taking several times the drug's daily sedative dose.

Sedative drug withdrawal syndrome can be confirmed by evaluating the patient about 1 hour after administering pentobarbital, 200 mg orally or intramuscularly. The absence of signs of sedative drug intoxication (sedation, nystagmus, dysarthria, or ataxia) establishes that the patient is tolerant to sedative drugs and makes sedative drug withdrawal a likely diagnosis, although other causes must be excluded. Sedative drug withdrawal is treated with a long-acting barbiturate such as phenobarbital, administered orally to maintain a calm state without signs of intoxication, and tapered over about 2 weeks.

OPIOIDS

Opioids can produce analgesia, mood changes, confusional states, coma, respiratory depression, pulmonary edema, nausea and vomiting, pupillary constriction, hypotension, urinary retention, and reduced gastroin-

Table 1–11. Therapeutic drugs associated with acute confusional states.

Acyclovir	Disulfiram
Amantadine	Ergot alkaloids
Aminocaproic acid	Ethanol
Amphetamines	Ganciclovir
Anticholinergics	Hallucinogens
Anticonvulsants	Isoniazid
Antidepressants	Ketamine
Antihistamines (H_1 and H_2)	Levodopa
Antipsychotics	Lidocaine
L-Asparaginase	Methylphenidate
Baclofen	Methylxanthines
Barbiturates	Nonsteroidal antiinflammatory
Benzodiazepines	drugs
β-Adrenergic	Opioids
receptor antagonists	Penicillin
Cephalosporins	Phenylpropanolamine
Chloroquine	Quinacrine
Clonidine	Quinidine
Cocaine	Quinine
Corticosteroids	Salicylates
Cycloserine	Selegiline
Cyclosporine	Thyroid hormones
Digitalis glycosides	

testinal motility. Their chronic use is associated with tolerance and physical dependence.

Examination may reveal needle tracks or the abovementioned signs, but the cardinal features of opioid overdose are pinpoint pupils—which usually constrict in bright light—and respiratory depression. These features can also result from pontine hemorrhage, but opioid

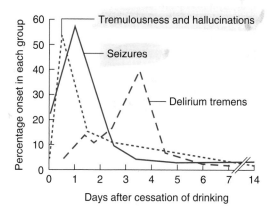

Figure 1–3. Ethanol withdrawal syndromes in relation to the time since cessation of drinking. (Data from Victor M, Adams RD: The effect of alcohol on the nervous system. Res Publ Assoc Res Nerv Ment Dis 1952;32:526–573.)

overdose can be distinguished by the patient's response to the opioid antagonist **naloxone.** After administration of naloxone, pupillary dilation and full recovery of consciousness occur promptly. When large doses of opioids or multiple drug ingestions are involved, however, slight dilation of the pupils may be the only observable effect.

Treatment involves intravenous administration of naloxone, 0.4–0.8 mg, and sometimes ventilatory support. Because naloxone's action may be as short as 1 hour—and many opioids are longer-acting—it should be readministered as the patient's condition dictates. With appropriate treatment, patients should recover uneventfully.

ANTICHOLINERGIC DRUGS

Muscarinic anticholinergic drugs are used to treat gastrointestinal disturbances, parkinsonism, motion sickness, and insomnia. Antipsychotic drugs, tricyclic antidepressants, and many antihistamines also exhibit prominent anticholinergic activity. Overdose with any of these agents can produce a confusional state with agitation, hallucinations, fixed and dilated pupils, blurred vision, dry skin and mucous membranes, flushing, fever, urinary retention, and tachycardia. In some cases, the diagnosis can be confirmed by toxicologic analysis of blood or urine. Symptoms usually resolve spontaneously, but treatment may be required, especially if life-threatening cardiac arrhythmias occur. In such cases, the cholinesterase inhibitor physostigmine can reverse the abnormality by interfering with the breakdown of acetylcholine. However, physostigmine may produce bradycardia and seizures, so it is rarely used.

PHENCYCLIDINE

Phencyclidine (PCP) can produce drowsiness, agitation, disorientation, amnesia, hallucinations, paranoia, and violent behavior. Neurologic examination may show large or small pupils, horizontal and vertical nystagmus, ataxia, hypertonicity, hyperreflexia, and myoclonus. There may be analgesia to a surprising degree. In severe cases, complications include hypertension, malignant hyperthermia, status epilepticus, coma, and death. Benzodiazepines may be useful for sedation and treating muscle spasms, and antihypertensives, anticonvulsants, and dantrolene (for malignant hyperthermia) may be required. Symptoms and signs usually resolve within 24 hours.

ENDOCRINE DISTURBANCES
HYPOTHYROIDISM

Profound hypothyroidism (**myxedema**) may produce a confusional state, coma, or dementia. Cognitive disturbances include flat affect, psychomotor retardation, agitation, and psychosis. The neurologic examination may show dysarthria, deafness, or ataxia, but the most characteristic abnormality is delayed relaxation of the tendon reflexes. Untreated, the condition can progress to seizures and coma.

Laboratory abnormalities include low thyroid hormone [triiodothyronine(T_3) and tetraiodothyronine (T_4)] levels and elevated thyroid-stimulating hormone (TSH) and serum cholesterol. Hypoglycemia and hyponatremia may occur, and arterial blood gases may reveal respiratory acidosis. CSF protein is typically elevated; CSF pressure is occasionally increased. Treatment is of the underlying thyroid disorder and, in severe myxedema madness or coma, rapid thyroid replacement with levothyroxine together with hydrocortisone for the possible coexistent adrenal insufficiency.

HYPERTHYROIDISM

Acute exacerbation of hyperthyroidism (**thyrotoxic crisis**) may cause a confusional state, coma, or death. In younger patients, agitation, hallucinations, and psychosis are common (**activated crisis**), whereas those over age 50 tend to be apathetic and depressed (**apathetic crisis**). Seizures may occur. Neurologic examination shows an exaggerated physiologic (action) tremor and hyperreflexia; ankle clonus and extensor plantar responses are rare. The diagnosis is confirmed by assaying thyroid hormones (T_3 and T_4) in the blood. Treatment includes correction of hyperthermia, fluid and electrolyte disorders, cardiac arrhythmias, and congestive heart failure, and administration of antithyroid drugs (propylthiouracil or methimazole), iodide, propranolol, and hydrocortisone. The underlying disorder that precipitated thyrotoxic crisis should also be sought.

HYPOGLYCEMIA

Prompt treatment of hypoglycemia is essential because hypoglycemic encephalopathy may progress rapidly from a reversible to an irreversible stage, and definitive therapy can be quickly and easily administered.

The most common cause is insulin overdose in diabetic patients, but oral hypoglycemic drugs, alcoholism, malnutrition, hepatic failure, insulinoma, and non-insulin-secreting fibromas, sarcomas, or fibrosarcomas may also be responsible. Neurologic symptoms usually develop over minutes to hours. Although no strict correlation between blood glucose levels and the severity of neurologic dysfunction can be demonstrated, prolonged hypoglycemia at levels of 30 mg/dL or lower invariably leads to irreversible brain damage.

Clinical Findings

Early signs of hypoglycemia include tachycardia, sweating, and pupillary dilation, which may be followed by a confusional state with somnolence or agitation. Neurologic dysfunction progresses in a rostral-caudal fashion (see Chapter 10), and may mimic a mass lesion causing transtentorial herniation. Coma ensues, with spasticity, extensor plantar responses, and decorticate or decerebrate posturing. Signs of brain stem dysfunction subsequently appear, including abnormal ocular movements and loss of pupillary reflexes. Respiratory depression, bradycardia, hypotonia, and hyporeflexia ultimately supervene, at which point irreversible brain damage is imminent.

Hypoglycemic coma is often associated with focal neurologic signs and focal or generalized seizures.

Treatment

The diagnosis is confirmed by measuring blood glucose levels, but treatment with glucose—50 mL of 50% dextrose intravenously—should be begun *immediately*, before the blood glucose level is known. Improvement in the level of consciousness is evident within minutes after glucose administration in patients with reversible hypoglycemic encephalopathy. The consequences of inadvertently worsening what later proves to be hyperglycemic encephalopathy are never as serious as those of a failure to treat hypoglycemia.

HYPERGLYCEMIA

Two hyperglycemic syndromes, **diabetic ketoacidosis** and **hyperosmolar nonketotic hyperglycemia,** can produce encephalopathy or coma. Either syndrome, distinguished by a variety of clinical and laboratory features (Table 1–12), may be the presenting manifestation of diabetes. Impaired cerebral metabolism, intravascular coagulation from hyperviscosity, and brain edema from rapid correction of hyperglycemia contribute to pathogenesis. Whereas the severity of hyperosmolarity correlates well with depression of consciousness, the degree of systemic acidosis does not.

Clinical Findings

Symptoms include blurred vision, dry skin, anorexia, polyuria, and polydipsia. Physical examination may show hypotension and other signs of dehydration, especially in hyperosmolar nonketotic hyperglycemia. Deep, rapid (Kussmaul) respiration characterizes diabetic ketoacidosis. Impairment of consciousness varies from mild confusion to coma. Focal neurologic signs and generalized or focal seizures are common in hyperosmolar nonketotic hyperglycemia. Laboratory findings are summarized in Table 1–12.

Treatment & Prognosis

Treatment of diabetic ketoacidosis includes insulin, fluid and electrolyte (especially potassium and phosphate)

Table 1–12. Features of hyperglycemic encephalopathies.

	Diabetic Ketoacidosis	Hyperosmolar Nonketotic State
Patient age	Young	Middle-aged to elderly
Type of diabetes	Juvenile-onset or insulin-dependent	Adult-onset
Blood glucose (mg/dL)	300–600	>800
Serum osmolality (mosm/L)	<350	>350
Ketosis	+	−
Metabolic acidosis	+	−
Coma	Uncommon	Common
Focal neurologic signs	−	+
Seizures	−	+

+, present; −, absent.

replacement, and antibiotics for concomitant infections. Blood glucose levels should be allowed to remain at 200–300 mg/dL for 24 hours to reduce the risk of brain edema. Deaths are usually related to sepsis, cardiovascular or cerebrovascular complications, or renal failure. In hyperosmolar nonketotic hyperglycemia, fluid replacement is most important; 0.5 N saline is administered except to patients with circulatory collapse, who should receive normal saline. Insulin is also required. Death is usually due to misdiagnosis or coexisting disease.

HYPOADRENALISM

Adrenocortical insufficiency produces fatigue, weakness, weight loss, anorexia, hyperpigmentation of the skin, hypotension, nausea and vomiting, abdominal pain, and diarrhea or constipation. Neurologic manifestations include confusional states, seizures, or coma. Treatment is administration of hydrocortisone and correction of hypovolemia, hypoglycemia, electrolyte disturbances, and precipitating illnesses.

HYPERADRENALISM

Hyperadrenalism (**Cushing's syndrome**) usually results from the administration of exogenous glucocorticoids.

Clinical features include truncal obesity, facial flushing, hirsutism, menstrual irregularities, hypertension, weakness, cutaneous striae, acne, and ecchymoses. Neuropsychiatric disturbances are common and include depression or euphoria, anxiety, irritability, memory impairment, psychosis, delusions, and hallucinations; fully developed acute confusional states are rare. The diagnosis is confirmed by elevated 24-hour urine-free cortisol level or a defective response to a low-dose dexamethasone suppression test. When a pituitary tumor is the cause, the usual treatment is transsphenoidal hypophysectomy.

ELECTROLYTE DISORDERS

HYPONATREMIA

Clinical Findings

Hyponatremia, particularly when acute, causes brain swelling due to hypoosmolality of extracellular fluid. Symptoms include headache, lethargy, confusion, weakness, muscle cramps, nausea, and vomiting. Neurologic signs include confusional state or coma, papilledema, tremor, asterixis, rigidity, extensor plantar responses, and focal or generalized seizures. Hyponatremia may also produce focal signs by unmasking preexisting structural brain lesions. Neurologic complications are usually associated with serum sodium levels less than 120 meq/L (Figure 1–4), but may be seen following a rapid fall to 130 meq/L—while chronic hyponatremia with levels as low as 110 meq/L may be asymptomatic.

Treatment

Treatment is most effective when the underlying cause of hyponatremia is corrected. Immediate management includes water restriction or, for severe symptoms, infusion of hypertonic saline with or without intravenous furosemide. Excessively rapid correction of hyponatremia may cause **central pontine myelinolysis,** a disorder of white matter that can produce a confusional state, paraparesis or quadriparesis, dysarthria, dysphagia, hyper- or hyporeflexia, and extensor plantar responses. Severe cases can result in the locked-in syndrome (see Chapter 10), coma, or death. MRI may show pontine and extrapontine white matter lesions. There is no treatment, so prevention is essential, and may best be achieved by restricting water intake and using small amounts of hypertonic saline to raise the serum sodium concentration to 125–130 mmol/L, at a rate not exceeding 8 mmol/L/d.

HYPERCALCEMIA

Symptoms include thirst, polyuria, constipation, nausea and vomiting, abdominal pain, anorexia, and flank pain

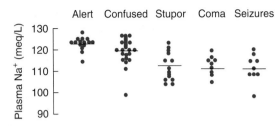

Figure 1–4. Relationship between plasma sodium concentration and neurologic manifestations of hyponatremia. (Reproduced, with permission, from Arieff AI, Llach F, Massry SG: Neurologic manifestations and morbidity of hyponatremia: correlation with brain water and electrolytes. Medicine 1976;55:121–129.)

from nephrolithiasis. Neurologic symptoms are always present with serum calcium levels higher than 17 mg/dL (8.5 meq/L) and include headache, weakness, and lethargy.

Physical examination may show dehydration, abdominal distention, focal neurologic signs, myopathic weakness, and a confusional state that can progress to coma. Seizures are rare. The myopathy spares bulbar muscles and tendon reflexes are usually normal. The diagnosis is confirmed by an elevated serum calcium level, and sometimes increased parathyroid hormone levels and a shortened QT interval on the ECG. Severe hypercalcemia is treated initially by vigorous intravenous hydration with 0.45% or 0.9% saline and usually requires central venous pressure monitoring. Patients with hypercalcemia should also be evaluated for occult cancer.

HYPOCALCEMIA

Symptoms include irritability, delirium, psychosis with hallucinations, depression, nausea, vomiting, abdominal pain, and paresthesias of the circumoral region and distal extremities. The most characteristic physical signs are those of overt or latent tetany. Neural hyperexcitability is exhibited by contraction of facial muscles in response to percussion of the facial (VII) nerve anterior to the ear (**Chvostek's sign**). **Carpopedal spasm** may occur spontaneously or following tourniquet-induced limb ischemia (**Trousseau's sign**). Cataracts and papilledema are sometimes present, and chorea has been reported. Seizures or laryngospasm can be life-threatening. Serum calcium levels are below 9 mg/dL (4.5 meq/L), but calcium is also decreased in hypoalbuminemia without affecting ionized calcium and hypocalcemia with normal ionized calcium is asymptomatic. The ECG may show a prolonged QT interval. Treatment is with intravenous calcium gluconate and seizures, if present, are treated with phenytoin or phenobarbital.

NUTRITIONAL DISORDERS
WERNICKE'S ENCEPHALOPATHY

Wernicke's encephalopathy is usually a complication of chronic alcoholism, but also occurs in other disorders associated with malnutrition. It is caused by deficiency of **thiamine** (vitamin B_1). Pathologic features include neuronal loss, demyelination, and gliosis in periventricular gray matter. Proliferation of small blood vessels and petechial hemorrhages may be seen. The areas most commonly involved are the medial thalamus, mammillary bodies, periaqueductal gray matter, cerebellar vermis, and oculomotor, abducens, and vestibular nuclei.

Clinical Findings

The classic syndrome comprises the triad of **ophthalmoplegia, ataxia,** and **confusional state.** The most common ocular abnormalities are nystagmus, abducens (VI) nerve palsy, and horizontal or combined horizontal-vertical gaze palsy. Ataxia affects gait primarily; ataxia of the arms is uncommon, as is dysarthria. The mental status examination reveals global confusion with a prominent disorder of immediate recall and recent memory. The confusional state progresses to coma in a small percentage of patients. Most patients have associated neuropathy with absent ankle jerks. Hypothermia and hypotension may occur due to hypothalamic involvement. Pupillary abnormalities, including mild anisocoria, or a sluggish reaction to light, are occasionally seen.

The peripheral blood smear may show macrocytic anemia and MRI may show atrophy of the mammillary bodies.

Treatment

Treatment requires prompt administration of thiamine. An initial dose of 100 mg is given intravenously, before or with dextrose, to avoid precipitating or exacerbating the disorder. Parenteral thiamine is continued for several days. The maintenance requirement for thiamine—about 1 mg/d—is usually available in the diet, although enteric absorption of thiamine is impaired in alcoholics.

Prognosis

Following treatment, ocular abnormalities usually begin to improve within 1 day and ataxia and confusion within a week. Ophthalmoplegia, vertical nystagmus, and acute confusion are entirely reversible, usually within 1 month. Horizontal nystagmus and ataxia, however, resolve completely in only about 40% of cases. The major long-term complication of Wernicke's encephalopathy is Korsakoff's syndrome.

VITAMIN B$_{12}$ DEFICIENCY

Vitamin B$_{12}$ (cyanocobalamin) deficiency produces peripheral neuropathy, subacute combined degeneration of the spinal cord, nutritional amblyopia (visual loss), and cognitive dysfunction that ranges from a mild confusional state to dementia or psychosis (megaloblastic madness). Neurologic abnormalities may precede the development of macrocytic anemia. The most frequent cause of vitamin B$_{12}$ deficiency is **pernicious anemia,** a defect in the production of intrinsic factor associated with gastric atrophy and achlorhydria, which is most common in those of northern European ancestry.

Clinical Findings

The presenting symptoms are usually due to anemia or orthostatic lightheadedness, but may also be neurologic. Distal paresthesias, gait ataxia, a bandlike sensation of tightness around the trunk or limbs, and Lhermitte's sign (an electric-shocklike sensation along the spine precipitated by neck flexion) may be present. Physical examination may show low-grade fever, glossitis, lemon-yellow discoloration of the skin, and cutaneous hyperpigmentation. Cerebral involvement produces confusion, depression, agitation, or psychosis with hallucinations. Spinal cord involvement is manifested by impaired vibratory and joint position sense, sensory gait ataxia and spastic paraparesis with extensor plantar responses. Associated peripheral nerve involvement may cause loss of tendon reflexes in the legs and urinary retention.

Hematologic abnormalities include macrocytic anemia, leukopenia with hypersegmented neutrophils, and thrombocytopenia with giant platelets. Because folate deficiency can produce identical changes, the diagnosis must be confirmed by the serum vitamin B$_{12}$ level. When this is low, **Schilling's test** determines whether defective intestinal absorption of vitamin B$_{12}$ (as in pernicious anemia) is the cause. In pernicious anemia, the urinary excretion of orally administered vitamin B$_{12}$ is abnormally low, and this abnormality can be corrected by coadministration of intrinsic factor.

Diagnosis may be difficult when cerebral symptoms occur without anemia or spinal cord disease, requiring that the serum vitamin B$_{12}$ level be determined routinely in patients with cognitive disorders, myelopathy, or peripheral neuropathy, whether or not anemia is present.

Treatment

Treatment of neurologic manifestations is by prompt intramuscular administration of cyanocobalamin, after blood is drawn to determine the serum vitamin B$_{12}$ level. Daily injections are continued for 1 week, and Schilling's test is performed to determine the cause of deficiency. If, as in pernicious anemia, deficiency is not correctable by dietary supplementation or treatment of intestinal malabsorption, intramuscular vitamin B$_{12}$ (typically 100 μg) are given at weekly intervals for several months and monthly thereafter. The reversibility of neurologic complications depends upon their duration. Abnormalities present for more than 1 year are less likely to resolve with treatment. Encephalopathy may begin to clear within 24 hours after the first vitamin B$_{12}$ dose, but full neurologic recovery, when it occurs, may take several months.

ORGAN SYSTEM FAILURE

HEPATIC ENCEPHALOPATHY

Hepatic encephalopathy occurs as a complication of cirrhosis, portosystemic shunting, chronic active hepatitis, or fulminant hepatic necrosis following viral hepatitis. Alcoholism is the most common underlying disorder. The syndrome may be chronic and progressive or acute in onset; in the latter case, gastrointestinal hemorrhage is a frequent precipitating cause.

Liver disease produces cerebral symptoms by impairing hepatocellular detoxifying mechanisms or by the portosystemic shunting of venous blood. As a result, ammonia and other toxins accumulate in the blood and diffuse into the brain. Increased activity of γ-aminobutyric acid (GABA)-containing neuronal pathways in the brain and elevated levels of endogenous benzodiazepines may be involved in the pathogenesis of cerebral symptoms.

Clinical Findings

Symptoms of encephalopathy may precede systemic symptoms such as nausea, anorexia, and weight loss. Recent gastrointestinal bleeding, consumption of high-protein foods, use of sedatives or diuretics, or systemic infection may provide a clue to the cause of clinical decompensation.

Physical examination may reveal systemic signs of liver disease. Cognitive disturbances include somnolence, agitation, and coma. Ocular reflexes are usually brisk. Nystagmus, tonic downward ocular deviation, and disconjugate eye movements may be seen. The most helpful neurologic sign of a metabolic disturbance, although not restricted to liver disease, is **asterixis**—a flapping tremor of the outstretched hands or feet that results from impaired postural control. Other motor abnormalities include tremor, myoclonus, paratonic rigidity, spasticity, decorticate or decerebrate posturing, and extensor plantar responses. Focal neurologic signs and focal or generalized seizures may occur.

Laboratory studies may show elevated serum bilirubin, transaminases, ammonia, prothrombin time (PT) and partial thromboplastin time (PTT), and respiratory alkalosis. The most specific CSF abnormality is elevated **glutamine** (Figure 1–5). The EEG may be diffusely slow with triphasic waves.

Treatment

Treatment includes restricting dietary protein, reversing electrolyte disturbances and hyperglycemia, discontinuing drugs that may have caused decompensation, providing antibiotics, and correcting coagulopathy with fresh-frozen plasma or vitamin K. Oral or rectal administration of lactulose, 20–30 g three or four times daily, decreases colonic pH and ammonia absorption. Neomycin, 1–3 g orally four times daily, may reduce ammonia-forming bacteria in the colon. Some success has also been reported with the benzodiazepine receptor antagonist flumazenil. Orthotopic liver transplantation is required in some cases. Prognosis in hepatic encephalopathy correlates best with the severity of hepatocellular rather than neurologic dysfunction.

REYE'S SYNDROME

Reye's syndrome is a rare disorder characterized by encephalopathy or coma with laboratory evidence of hepatic dysfunction. It usually occurs in children several days after a viral illness, especially varicella or influenza B. Administration of salicylates appears to be an additional risk factor. The incidence of Reye's syndrome has declined dramatically in recent years, at least partly as a result of the avoidance of aspirin in treating children with febrile illnesses.

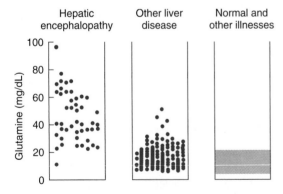

Figure 1–5. Range of CSF glutamine concentrations in hepatic encephalopathy. (Reproduced, with permission, from Plum F: The CSF in hepatic encephalopathy. Exp Biol Med 1971;4:34–41.)

UREMIA

Renal failure, particularly when acute in onset or rapidly progressive, may produce encephalopathy or coma with hyperventilation and prominent motor manifestations. These include tremor, asterixis, myoclonus, and tetany. Focal or generalized seizures and focal neurologic signs are common, and decorticate or decerebrate posturing may occur. Laboratory abnormalities include elevated serum urea nitrogen, creatinine and potassium, and metabolic acidosis, but their severity correlates poorly with symptoms. The EEG is diffusely slow and may show triphasic waves or paroxysmal spikes or sharp waves.

Acute management includes hydration, protein and salt restriction, and treatment of complications such as seizures. Long-term management requires reversing the cause (eg, urinary tract obstruction), dialysis, or kidney transplantation. Although dialysis reverses the encephalopathy, clinical improvement often lags behind normalization of serum urea nitrogen and creatinine. Dialysis itself can produce an encephalopathy, termed **dialysis disequilibrium syndrome,** that is thought to result from hypoosmolarity. This is most common with a patient's first hemodialysis and can be prevented by correcting uremia more gradually or using briefer periods of dialysis at reduced rates of blood flow.

PULMONARY ENCEPHALOPATHY

Patients with chronic lung disease or brainstem or neurologic disorders that affect respiratory function may develop encephalopathy related to hypoventilation. Symptoms include headache, confusion, and somnolence. Examination shows papilledema, asterixis or myoclonus, and confusional state or coma. Tendon reflexes are often decreased, but pyramidal signs may be present, and seizures occur occasionally. Arterial blood gases show respiratory acidosis. Treatment involves ventilatory support to decrease hypercapnia and to maintain adequate oxygenation.

ORGAN TRANSPLANTATION

Treatment of organ failure by transplantation can lead to acute confusional states as a consequence of surgical complications, immunosuppresive drug treatment, opportunistic infection, lymphoproliferative disorders, or transplant rejection. The problems encountered depend on the time in relation to transplantation and on the organ transplanted.

Surgical complications that may produce encephalopathy include hypotension, hypoxia, thromboembolism, and air embolism, and are most common with heart and liver transplants.

Immunosuppressive drugs used to prevent transplant rejection can cause acute confusional states by direct effects on the nervous system or as a consequence of immunological impairment. Cyclosporine and tacrolimus (FK-506) produce encephalopathy that may be associated with seizures, tremor, visual disturbances, weakness, sensory symptoms, or ataxia. MRI shows abnormalities in the subcortical white matter. Symptoms are often associated with excessively high drug levels in the blood and may improve with reduction of drug dosage. Corticosteroids can produce psychosis, which may respond to substituting dexamethasone, and corticosteroid withdrawal is sometimes associated with lethargy, headache, myalgia, and arthralgia. OKT3 causes encephalopathy, aseptic meningitis, and seizures. Gabapentin is often used to treat seizures in transplant recipients because of its relative lack of pharmacokinetic interaction with other drugs typically given to these patients.

Infections causing confusional states are most prominent following bone marrow transplantation, but are also common after transplantation of other organs. They are comparatively rare in the first month following transplantation and, when they occur, usually reflect preexisting infection in the recipient or in the donor organ, or a perioperative complication. Within this period, the most frequent organisms are gram-negative bacteria, herpes simplex virus, and fungi. Opportunistic infections are more common between 1 and 6 months posttransplant and include acute *Listeria* meningitis or encephalitis; chronic meningitis from *Cryptococcus* or *Mycobacterium tuberculosis;* and brain abscesses related to infection with *Aspergillus, Nocardia,* or *Toxoplasma.* Beyond 6 months, cytomegalovirus, *Toxoplasma, Cryptococcus, Listeria,* or *Nocardia* infection may be seen.

Posttransplant lymphoproliferative disorder is related to immunosuppression and may be associated with primary central nervous system lymphoma.

Transplant rejection may also produce encephalopathy, especially in recipients of kidney transplants.

MENINGITIS, ENCEPHALITIS, & SEPSIS

BACTERIAL MENINGITIS

Bacterial meningitis is a leading cause of acute confusional states and one in which early diagnosis greatly improves the outcome. Predisposing conditions include systemic (especially respiratory) or parameningeal infection, head trauma, anatomic meningeal defects, prior neurosurgery, cancer, alcoholism, and other immunodeficiency states. The etiologic organism varies with age and with the presence of predisposing conditions (Table 1–13).

Pathogenesis & Pathology

Bacteria typically gain access to the central nervous system by colonizing the mucous membranes of the nasopharynx, leading to local tissue invasion, bacteremia, and hematogenous seeding of the subarachnoid space. Bacteria can also spread to the meninges directly, through anatomic defects in the skull or from parameningeal sites such as the paranasal sinuses or middle ear. Polysaccharide bacterial capsules, lipopolysaccharides, and outer membrane proteins may contribute to the bacterial invasion and virulence. The low levels of antibody and complement present in the subarachnoid space are inadequate to contain the infection. The resulting inflammatory response is associated with the release of inflammatory cytokines, including interleukins 1 and 6 and tumor necrosis factor α, that promote blood-brain barrier permeability, vasogenic cerebral edema, changes in cerebral blood flow, and perhaps direct neuronal toxicity.

Pathologically, bacterial meningitis is characterized by leptomeningeal and perivascular infiltration with polymorphonuclear leukocytes and an inflammatory exudate. These changes tend to be most prominent over the cerebral convexities in *Streptococcus pneumoniae* and *Haemophilus* infection and over the base of the brain with *Neisseria meningitidis.* Brain edema, hydrocephalus, and cerebral infarction may occur, although actual bacterial invasion of the brain is rare.

Clinical Findings

A. Symptoms and Signs

At presentation, most patients have had symptoms of meningitis for 1 to 7 days. These include fever, confusion, vomiting, headache, and neck stiffness, but the full syndrome is often not present.

Physical examination may show fever and signs of systemic or parameningeal infection, such as skin abscess or otitis. A petechial rash is seen in 50–60% of patients with *N meningitidis* meningitis. Signs of meningeal irritation are seen in about 80% of cases, but are often absent in the very young and very old, or with profoundly impaired consciousness. These signs include neck stiffness on passive flexion, thigh flexion upon flexion of the neck (Brudzinski's sign), and resistance to passive extension of the knee with the hip flexed (Kernig's sign). The level of consciousness, when altered, ranges from mild confusion to coma. Focal neurologic signs, seizures, and cranial nerve palsies may occur.

B. Laboratory Findings

Peripheral blood may reveal polymorphonuclear leukocytosis from systemic infection or leukopenia due to immunosuppression. The causative organism can be cultured from the blood in 40–90% of meningitis cases.

Table 1–13. Etiologic agents and empirical antibiotic treatment in bacterial meningitis, based on age and predisposing condition.

Age or Condition	Etiologic Agents	Antibiotics of Choice
Less than 3 months	*S agalactiae* *E coli* *L monocytogenes*	Ampicillin, 100 mg/kg intravenously every 8 hours + cefotaxime, 50 mg/kg intravenously every 6 hours or ceftriaxone, 50–100 mg/kg intravenously every 12 hours
3 months to 8 years	*N meningitidis* *S pneumoniae* *H influenzae*	Cefotaxime, 50 mg/kg intravenously every 6 hours or ceftriaxone, 50–100 mg/kg intravenously every 12 hours + vancomycin, 15 mg/kg intravenously every 6 hours, to maximum of 4 g/d
18 to 50 years	*S pneumoniae* *N meningitidis*	Cefotaxime, 2 g intravenously every 6 hours or ceftriaxone, 2 g intravenously every 12 hours + vancomycin, 15 mg/kg intravenously every 6 hours, to maximum of 4 g/d
Older than 50 years	*S pneumoniae* *L monocytogenes* Gram-negative bacilli	Ampicillin, 2 g intravenously every 4 hours + cefotaxime, 2 g intravenously every 6 hours or ceftriaxone, 2 g intravenously every 12 hours
Impaired cellular immunity	*L monocytogenes* Gram-negative bacilli	Ampicillin, 100 mg/kg intravenously every 8 hours (neonate) or 2 g intravenously every 4 hours (adult) + ceftazidime, 50–100 mg/kg intravenously every 8 hours, to maximum of 2 g every 8 hours
Head trauma, neurosurgery, or CSF shunt	Staphylococci Gram-negative bacilli *S pneumoniae*	Vancomycin, 15 mg/kg intravenously every 6 hours, to maximum of 4 g/d + ceftazidime, 50–100 mg/kg intravenously every 8 hours, to maximum of 2 g every 8 hours

Adapted from Quagliarello VJ, Scheld WM: Treatment of bacterial meningitis. N Engl J Med 1997; 336:708–716.

X-rays of the chest, sinuses, or mastoid bones may indicate a primary site of infection. A brain CT or MRI scan may show contrast enhancement of the cerebral convexities, the base of the brain, or the ventricular ependyma. The EEG is usually diffusely slow, and focal abnormalities suggest the possibility of focal cerebritis, abscess formation, or scarring.

Although these studies may be helpful, the essential test in all cases of suspected meningitis is prompt lumbar puncture and CSF examination. CSF pressure is elevated in about 90% of cases, and the appearance of the fluid ranges from slightly turbid to grossly purulent. CSF white cell counts of 1000–10,000/mL are usually seen, consisting chiefly of polymorphonuclear leukocytes, although mononuclear cells may predominate in *Listeria monocytogenes* meningitis. Protein concentrations of

100–500 mg/dL are most common. The CSF glucose level is lower than 40 mg/dL in about 80% of cases and may be too low to measure. Gram-stained smears of CSF identify the causative organism in 70–80% of cases. CSF culture, which is positive in about 80% of cases, provides a definitive diagnosis and allows determination of antibiotic sensitivity. The polymerase chain reaction has also been used with CSF specimens to diagnose bacterial meningitis, including *H influenzae, N meningitidis,* and *L monocytogenes* meningitis.

Differential Diagnosis

Signs of meningeal irritation may also be seen with subarachnoid hemorrhage, but the distinction is easily made because lumbar puncture yields bloody CSF in that condition. Early viral meningitis can produce polymorphonuclear pleocytosis and symptoms identical to those of bacterial meningitis, but a repeat lumbar puncture after 6–12 hours should demonstrate a shift to lymphocytic predominance in viral meningitis, and the CSF glucose level is normal.

Prevention

Children should be routinely immunized against *H influenzae* by vaccination. A vaccine is also available for some strains of *N meningitidis* and is recommended for military recruits, college students, and travelers to areas of ongoing epidemics. The risk of contracting *H influenzae* or *N meningitidis* meningitis can be reduced in household and other close contacts of affected patients by the prophylactic administration of rifampin, 20 mg/kg/d orally, given as a single daily dose for 4 days (*H influenzae*) or as two divided doses for 2 days (*N meningitidis*).

Treatment

Unless the physical examination shows focal neurologic abnormalities or papilledema, lumbar puncture should be performed immediately; if the CSF is not clear and colorless, antibiotic treatment (see below) is started without delay. When focal signs or papilledema are present, blood and urine should be taken for culture, antibiotics begun, and a brain CT scan obtained. If the scan shows no focal lesion that would contraindicate lumbar puncture, the puncture is then performed.

The initial choice of antibiotics is empirical, based upon the patient's age and predisposing factors (see Table 1–13). Therapy is adjusted as indicated when the Gram's stain or culture and sensitivity results become available (Table 1–14). Lumbar puncture can be repeated to assess the response to therapy. CSF should be sterile after 24 hours, and a decrease in pleocytosis and in the proportion of polymorphonuclear leukocytes should occur within 3 days.

The use of corticosteroids as an adjunct to antibiotic treatment of bacterial meningitis is controversial, and is based primarily on their ability to reduce hearing loss and neurologic sequelae in children with *H influenzae* meningitis. Nonetheless, some authorities recommend dexamethasone, 0.15 mg/kg intravenously every 6 hours for the first 4 days of antibiotic therapy in children under 2 months of age, and in adults with a positive Gram's stain and increased intracranial pressure.

Prognosis

Complications of bacterial meningitis include headache, seizures, hydrocephalus, syndrome of inappropriate secretion of antidiuretic hormone (SIADH), residual neurologic deficits (including cognitive disturbances and cranial—especially VIII—nerve abnormalities), and death. A CT scan will confirm suspected hydrocephalus and fluid and electrolyte status should be carefully monitored to detect SIADH. *N meningitidis* infections may be complicated by adrenal hemorrhage related to meningococcemia, resulting in hypotension and often death (Waterhouse-Friderichsen syndrome).

Morbidity and mortality from bacterial meningitis are high. Fatalities occur in about 20% of affected adults, and more often with some pathogens (eg, *S pneumoniae,* gram-negative bacilli) than others (eg, *H influenzae, N meningitidis*). Factors that worsen prognosis include extremes of age, delay in diagnosis and treatment, complicating illness, stupor or coma, seizures, and focal neurologic signs.

TUBERCULOUS MENINGITIS

Tuberculous meningitis must be considered in patients who present with a confusional state, especially if there is a history of pulmonary tuberculosis, alcoholism, corticosteroid treatment, HIV infection, or other conditions associated with impaired immune responses. It should also be considered in patients from areas (eg, Asia, Africa) or groups (eg, the homeless and inner-city drug users) with a high incidence of tuberculosis.

Pathogenesis & Pathology

Tuberculous meningitis usually results from reactivation of latent infection with *Mycobacterium tuberculosis.* Primary infection, typically acquired by inhaling bacillus-containing droplets, may be associated with metastatic dissemination of blood-borne bacilli from the lungs to the meninges and the surface of the brain. Here the organisms remain in a dormant state in tubercles that can rupture into the subarachnoid space at a later time, resulting in tuberculous meningitis.

The main finding is a basal meningeal exudate containing primarily mononuclear cells. Tubercles may be seen on the meninges and surface of the brain. The ventricles may be enlarged as a result of hydrocephalus, and their surfaces may show ependymal exudate or granular ependymitis. Arteritis can result in cerebral infarction, and basal inflammation and fibrosis can compress cranial nerves.

Clinical Findings

A. SYMPTOMS AND SIGNS

Symptoms have usually been present for less than 4 weeks at the time of presentation and include fever, lethargy or confusion, and headache. Weight loss, vom-

Table 1–14. Treatment of bacterial meningitis of known cause.

Etiologic Agents	Antibiotics of Choice	Duration of Treatment (days)
Gram's stain		
Cocci		
Gram-positive	Vancomycin, 15 mg/kg intravenously every 6 hours, to maximum of 4 g/d; substitute rifampin (600 mg/d) for vancomycin in adults receiving dexamethasone + ⌈ cefotaxime, 50 mg/kg intravenously every 6 hours (neonates) or ceftriaxone, 50–100 mg/kg intravenously every 12 hours (children); 2 g intravenously every 12 hours (adults) ⌋	—
Gram-negative	Penicillin G, 300,000 units/kg/d intravenously, to maximum of 24 million units/d	—
Bacilli		
Gram-positive	⌈ Ampicillin, 100 mg/kg intravenously every 8 hours (children); 2 g intravenously every 4 hours (adults) or penicillin G, 300,000 units/kg/d intravenously, to maximum of 24 million units/d ⌋ + gentamicin, 1.5 mg/kg intravenous loading dose followed by 1–2 mg/kg intravenously every 8 hours	—
Gram-negative	⌈ Cefotaxime, 50 mg/kg intravenously every 6 hours (neonates) or ceftriaxone, 50–100 mg/kg intravenously every 12 hours (children); 2 g intravenously every 12 hours (adults) or ceftazidime, 50–100 mg/kg intravenously every 8 hours, to maximum of 2 g every 8 hours ⌋ + gentamicin, 1.5 mg/kg intravenous loading dose followed by 1–2 mg/kg intravenously every 8 hours	—
CSF culture		
S pneumoniae	Vancomycin, 15 mg/kg intravenously every 6 hours, to maximum of 4 g/d; subsititute rifampin (600 mg/d) for vancomycin in adults receiving dexamethasone + ⌈ cefotaxime, 50 mg/kg intravenously every 6 hours (neonates) or ceftriaxone, 50–100 mg/kg intravenously every 12 hours (children); 2 g intravenously every 12 hours (adults) ⌋	10–14
H influezae	Ceftriaxone, 50–100 mg/kg intravenously every 12 hours (children); 2 g intravenously every 12 hours (adults)	7
N meningitidis	Penicillin G, 300,000 units/kg/d intravenously, to maximum of 24 million units/d	7
L monocytogenes	Ampicillin, 100 mg/kg intravenously every 8 hours (children); 2 g intravenously every 4 hours (adults) + gentamicin, 1.5 mg/kg intravenous loading dose followed by 1–2 mg/kg intravenously every 8 hours	14–21
S agalactiae	Penicillin G, 300,000 units/kg/d intravenously, to maximum of 24 million units/d	14–21

continued

Table 1–14. Treatment of bacterial meningitis of known cause. *(continued)*

Etiologic Agents	Antibiotics of Choice	Duration of Treatment (days)
Enterobacteriaceae	Cefotaxime, 50 mg/kg intravenously every 6 hours (neonates) or ceftriaxone, 50–100 mg/kg intravenously every 12 hours (children); 2 g intravenously every 12 hours (adults) + gentamicin, 1.5 mg/kg intravenous loading dose followed by 1–2 mg/kg intravenously every 8 hours	21
Pseudomonas aeruginosa, acinetobacter	Ceftazidime, 50–100 mg/kg intravenously every 8 hours, to maximum of 2 g every 8 hours + gentamicin, 1.5 mg/kg intravenous loading dose followed by 1–2 mg/kg intravenously every 8 hours	21

Adapted from Quagliarello VJ, Scheld WM: Treatment of bacterial meningitis. N Engl J Med 1997;336:708–716.

iting, neck stiffness, visual impairment, diplopia, focal weakness, and seizures may also occur. A history of contact with known cases of tuberculosis is usually absent.

Fever, signs of meningeal irritation, and a confusional state are the most common findings on physical examination, but all may be absent. Papilledema, ocular palsies, and hemiparesis are sometimes seen. Complications include spinal subarachnoid block, hydrocephalus, brain edema, cranial nerve palsies, and stroke caused by vasculitis or compression of blood vessels at the base of the brain.

B. LABORATORY FINDINGS

Only one-half to two-thirds of patients show a positive skin test for tuberculosis or evidence of active or healed tubercular infection on chest x-ray. The diagnosis is established by CSF analysis. CSF pressure is usually increased, and the fluid is typically clear and colorless but may form a clot upon standing. Lymphocytic and mononuclear cell pleocytosis of 50–500 cells/mL is most often seen, but polymorphonuclear pleocytosis can occur early and may give an erroneous impression of bacterial meningitis. CSF protein is usually more than 100 mg/dL and may exceed 500 mg/dL, particularly in patients with spinal subarachnoid block. The glucose level is usually decreased and may be less than 20 mg/dL. Acid-fast smears of CSF should be performed in all cases of suspected tuberculous meningitis, but they are positive in only a minority of cases. Definitive diagnosis is most often made by culturing *M tuberculosis* from the CSF, a process that usually takes several weeks and requires large quantities of spinal fluid for maximum yield. However, the polymerase chain reaction has

also been used for diagnosis. Finally, the CT scan may show contrast enhancement of the basal cisterns and cortical meninges, or hydrocephalus.

Differential Diagnosis

Many other conditions can cause a subacute confusional state with mononuclear cell pleocytosis, including syphilitic, fungal, neoplastic, and partially treated bacterial meningitis. These can be diagnosed by appropriate smears, cultures, and serologic and cytologic examinations.

Treatment

Treatment should be started as early as possible; it should not be withheld while awaiting culture results. The decision to treat is based on the CSF findings described above; lymphocytic pleocytosis and decreased glucose are particularly suggestive, even if acid-fast smears are negative.

Four drugs are used for initial therapy, until culture and susceptibility test results are known. These are isoniazid, 300 mg; rifampin, 600 mg; pyrazinamide, 25 mg/kg; and ethambutol, 15 mg/kg, each given orally once daily. For susceptible strains, ethambutol can be discontinued, and triple therapy continued for 2 months, followed by 4–10 months of treatment with isoniazid and rifampin alone. Pyridoxine, 50 mg/d, can be used to decrease the likelihood of isoniazid-induced polyneuropathy. Complications of therapy include hepatic dysfunction (isoniazid, rifampin, and pyrazinamide), polyneuropathy (isoniazid), optic neuritis (ethambutol), seizures (isoniazid), and ototoxicity (streptomycin).

Corticosteroids (eg, prednisone, 60 mg/d orally in adults or 1–3 mg/kg/d orally in children, tapered gradually over 3–4 weeks) are indicated as adjunctive therapy in patients with spinal subarachnoid block. They may also be indicated in seriously ill patients with focal neurologic signs or with increased intracranial pressure from cerebral edema. The risk of using corticosteroids may be high, however, especially if tuberculous meningitis has been mistakenly diagnosed in a patient with fungal meningitis. Therefore, if fungal meningitis has not been excluded, antifungal therapy (see below) should be added along with corticosteroids.

Prognosis

Even with appropriate treatment, about one-third of patients with tuberculous meningitis succumb. Coma at the time of presentation is the most significant predictor of a poor prognosis.

SYPHILITIC MENINGITIS

Acute or subacute syphilitic meningitis usually occurs within 2 years after primary syphilitic infection. It is most common in young adults, affects men more often than women, and requires prompt treatment to prevent the irreversible manifestations of tertiary neurosyphilis.

In about one-fourth of patients with *Treponema pallidum* infection, treponemes gain access to the central nervous system, where they produce a meningitis that is usually asymptomatic (asymptomatic neurosyphilis). Asymptomatic invasion of the central nervous system is associated with CSF pleocytosis, elevated protein, and positive serologic tests for syphilis.

Clinical Findings

A. SYMPTOMS AND SIGNS

In a few patients, syphilitic meningitis is a clinically apparent acute or subacute disorder. At the time of presentation, symptoms such as headache, nausea, vomiting, stiff neck, mental disturbances, focal weakness, seizures, deafness, and visual impairment have usually been present for up to 2 months.

Physical examination may show signs of meningeal irritation, confusion or delirium, papilledema, hemiparesis, and aphasia. The cranial nerves most frequently affected are (in order) the facial (VII), acoustic (VIII), oculomotor (III), trigeminal (V), abducens (VI), and optic (II) nerves, but other nerves may be involved as well. Fever is typically absent.

B. LABORATORY FINDINGS

The diagnosis is established by CSF findings. Opening pressure is normal or slightly elevated. Pleocytosis is lymphocytic or mononuclear in character, with white cell counts usually in the range of 100–1000/mL. Protein may be mildly or moderately elevated (< 200 mg/dL) and glucose mildly decreased. CSF VDRL and serum FTA or MHA-TP tests are usually positive. Protein electrophoretograms of CSF may show discrete γ-globulin bands (oligoclonal bands) not visible in normal CSF.

Treatment

Acute syphilitic meningitis is usually a self-limited disorder with no or minimal sequelae. More advanced manifestations of neurosyphilis, including vascular and parenchymatous disease (eg, tabes dorsalis, general paresis, optic neuritis, myelitis), can be prevented by adequate treatment of the early syphilitic infection.

Syphilitic meningitis is treated with aqueous penicillin G, $2–4 \times 10^6$ units intravenously every 4 hours for 10 days. For penicillin-allergic patients, tetracycline or erythromycin, 500 mg orally every 6 hours for 20 days, can be substituted. The CSF should be examined every 6 months until all findings are normal. Another course of therapy must be given if the CSF cell count or protein remains elevated.

LYME DISEASE

Clinical Findings

Lyme disease is a tick-borne disorder that results from systemic infection with the spirochete *Borrelia burgdorferi*. Most cases occur during the summer months. Primary infection may be manifested by an expanding erythematous annular skin lesion (**erythema migrans**) that usually appears over the thigh, groin, or axilla. Less distinctive symptoms include fatigue, headache, fever, neck stiffness, joint or muscle pain, anorexia, sore throat, and nausea. Neurologic involvement may be delayed for up to 10 weeks and is characterized by meningitis or meningoencephalitis and disorders of the cranial or peripheral nerves or nerve roots. Cardiac abnormalities (conduction defects, myocarditis, pericarditis, cardiomegaly, or heart failure) can also occur at this stage. Lyme meningitis usually produces prominent headache that may be accompanied by signs of meningeal irritation, photophobia, pain when moving the eyes, nausea, and vomiting. When encephalitis is present, it is usually mild and characterized by insomnia, emotional lability, or impaired concentration and memory.

The CSF usually shows a lymphocytic pleocytosis with 100–200 cells/mL, slightly elevated protein, and normal glucose. Oligoclonal immunoglobulin G (IgG) bands may be detected. Definitive diagnosis is usually made by serologic testing for *B burgdorferi,* preferably by enzyme-linked immunosorbent assay (ELISA) followed by Western blot, but the polymerase chain reaction, which can amplify spirochetal DNA in synovial fluid, blood, or CSF, has also been used.

Treatment

Preventive measures include avoiding tick-infested areas and using insect repellents and protective clothing when avoidance is impossible. A Lyme disease vaccine is also available, but its use is controversial.

For patients with Lyme disease and Bell's palsy, treatment is with doxycycline (100 mg twice daily) or amoxicillin (500 mg three times daily), each given orally for 3–4 weeks. With meningitis or other central nervous system (CNS) involvement, intravenous treatment is indicated with ceftriaxone (2 g intravenously daily), penicillin G (20–24 million units intravenously daily in six divided doses), or cefotaxime (2 g intravenously every 8 hours), continued for 2–4 weeks.

Symptoms typically resolve within 10 days in treated cases. Untreated or inadequately treated infections may lead to recurrent oligoarthritis, and chronic neurologic disorders including memory, language, and other cognitive disturbances; focal weakness; and ataxia. In such cases, a CT scan or MRI may show hydrocephalus, lesions in white matter resembling those seen in multiple sclerosis, or abnormalities suggestive of cerebral infarction. Subtle chronic cognitive or behavioral symptoms should not be attributed to Lyme encephalitis in the absence of serologic evidence of *B burgdorferi* exposure, CSF abnormalities, or focal neurologic signs. The peripheral neurologic manifestations of Lyme disease are discussed in Chapter 6.

VIRAL MENINGITIS & ENCEPHALITIS

Viral infections of the meninges (**meningitis**) or brain parenchyma (**encephalitis**) often present as acute confusional states. Children and young adults are frequently affected. Viral meningitis is most often caused by enteric viruses (Table 1–15) and viral encephalitis by childhood exanthems, arthropod-borne agents, and herpes simplex type 1 (Table 1–16). Some forms of viral encephalitis tend to show a restricted geographic distribution. However, the speed and volume of international travel can permit these disorders to spread, as was observed recently for West Nile virus in the northeastern United States.

Pathology

Viral infections can affect the central nervous system in three ways—hematogenous dissemination of a systemic viral infection (eg, arthropod-borne viruses); neuronal spread of the virus by axonal transport (eg, herpes simplex, rabies); and autoimmune postinfectious demyelination (eg, varicella, influenza). Pathologic changes in viral meningitis consist of an inflammatory meningeal reaction mediated by lymphocytes. Encephalitis is characterized by perivascular cuffing, lymphocytic infiltration, and microglial proliferation mainly involving subcortical gray matter regions. Intranuclear or intracytoplasmic inclusions are often seen.

Clinical Findings

A. SYMPTOMS AND SIGNS

Clinical manifestations include fever, headache, neck stiffness, photophobia, pain with eye movement, and mild impairment of consciousness. Patients usually do not appear as ill as those with bacterial meningitis. Systemic viral infection may cause skin rash, pharyngitis, lymphadenopathy, pleuritis, carditis, jaundice, organomegaly, diarrhea, or orchitis, and these findings may suggest a particular etiologic agent. Because viral encephalitis involves the brain directly, marked alterations of consciousness, seizures, and focal neurologic signs can occur. When signs of meningeal irritation and brain dysfunction coexist, the condition is termed **meningoencephalitis.**

B. LABORATORY FINDINGS

CSF analysis is the most important laboratory test. CSF pressure is normal or increased, and a lymphocytic or monocytic pleocytosis is present, with cell counts usually less than 1000/mL. (Higher counts can be seen in lymphocytic choriomeningitis or herpes simplex encephalitis.) A polymorphonuclear pleocytosis can occur early in viral meningitis, while red blood cells may be seen with herpes simplex encephalitis. Protein is normal or slightly increased (usually 80–200 mg/dL). Glucose is usually normal, but may be decreased in mumps, herpes zoster, or herpes simplex encephalitis. Gram's stains and bacterial, fungal, and acid-fast bacillius (AFB) cultures are negative. Oligoclonal bands and CSF protein electrophoresis abnormalities may be present. An etiologic diagnosis can often be made by virus isolation, polymerase chain reaction, or acute- and convalescent-phase CSF antibody titers.

Blood counts may show a normal white cell count, leukopenia, or mild leukocytosis. Atypical lymphocytes in blood smears and a positive heterophil (Monospot) test suggest infectious mononucleosis. Serum amylase is frequently elevated in mumps; abnormal liver function tests are associated with both hepatitis viruses and infectious mononucleosis. The EEG is diffusely slow, especially if there is direct cerebral involvement.

Differential Diagnosis

The differential diagnosis of meningitis with mononuclear cell pleocytosis includes partially treated bacterial meningitis as well as syphilitic, tuberculous, fungal, par-

Table 1–15. Etiologic agents in viral meningitis.

Virus	Incidence	Seasonal Variation	Source	Susceptible Population	Systemic Involvement	Laboratory Findings
Echoviruses	30%	Summer, fall	Fecal-oral	Children, members of affected families	Maculopapular, vesicular, or petechial skin rash; gastroenteritis	—
Coxsackievirus A	10%	Summer, fall	Fecal-oral	Children, members of affected families	Maculopapular, vesicular, or petechial skin rash; herpangina; gastroenteritis	—
Coxsackievirus B	40%	Summer, fall	Fecal-oral	Children, members of affected families	Maculopapular, vesicular, or petechial skin rash; pleuritis, pericarditis, myocarditis, orchitis; gastroenteritis	—
Mumps virus	15%	Late winter, spring	Inhalation	Children, male more than female	Parotitis, orchitis, oophoritis, pancreatitis	Amylase ↑; CSF glucose may be ↓
Herpes simplex virus (type 2)	Uncommon	—	Genital infection	Neonates with affected mothers	Vesicular genital lesions	—
Adenovirus	Uncommon	—	Inhalation	Infants, children	Pharyngitis, pneumonitis	—
Lymphocytic choriomeningitis virus	Uncommon	Late fall, winter	Mouse	Laboratory workers	Pharyngitis, pneumonitis	Marked CSF pleocytosis (1000–10,000 WBC/μL)
Hepatitis viruses	Uncommon	—	Fecal-oral, venereal, transfusion	Intravenous drug users, male homosexuals, blood recipients	Jaundice, arthritis	Liver function abnormalities
Epstein–Barr virus (infectious mononucleosis)	Uncommon	—	Oral contact	Teenagers, young adults	Lymphadenopathy, pharyngitis, maculopapular skin rash, palatal petechiae, splenomegaly	Atypical lymphocytes, positive heterophil, liver function abnormalities

asitic, neoplastic, and other meningitides. Evidence of systemic viral infection and CSF wet mounts, stained smears, cultures, and cytologic examination can distinguish among these possibilities. When presumed early viral meningitis is associated with a polymorphonuclear pleocytosis of less than 1000 white blood cells/mL and normal CSF glucose, one of two strategies can be used. The patient can be treated for bacterial meningitis until the results of CSF cultures are known, or treatment can be withheld and lumbar puncture repeated in 6–12 hours. If the meningitis is viral in origin, the second sample should show a mononuclear cell pleocytosis.

Table 1-16. Etiologic agents in viral encephalitis.

Type of Encephalitis	Vector	Geographic Distribution	Comments
Childhood exanthems			
Measles, varicella, mumps, rubella	Human	Worldwide	Uncommon in USA because of vaccination.
Arthropod-borne (Arbo) viruses			
Alphaviruses			
Eastern equine	Mosquito	USA (Atlantic and Gulf coasts), Caribbean, South America	Children usually affected; mortality 50–75%; neurologic sequelae common
Western equine	Mosquito	Western and central USA, South America	Infants and adults >50 years usually affected; mortality 5–15%; neurologic sequelae uncommon except in infants
Venezuelan equine	Mosquito	Florida, southwestern USA, Central and South America	Adults usually affected; mortality 1%; neurologic sequelae rare
Flaviviruses			
Japanese B	Mosquito	China, Southeast Asia, India, Japan	Vaccine available
St. Louis	Mosquito	USA (rural west and midwest, New Jersey, Florida, Texas), Caribbean, Central and South America	Adults >50 years most often affected; mortality 2–20%; neurologic sequelae in about 20%
Murray Valley	Mosquito	Australia, New Guinea	
West Nile	Mosquito	Middle East, Africa, Europe, Central Asia, northeastern USA	
Rocio	Mosquito	Brazil	
Kyasanur Forest	Tick	India	
Powassan	Tick	New York, Ontario	
Russian spring-summer	Tick	Northern Europe, Siberia	
Louping-ill	Tick	United Kingdom	
Bunyaviruses			
California (including LaCrosse)	Mosquito	North America	Children usually affected; mortality <1%; neurologic sequelae uncommon
Rift Valley	Mosquito	Africa	
Orbiviruses			
Colorado tick fever	Tick	Western and Rocky Mountain states of USA	
Other			
Herpes simplex (type 1)	Human	Worldwide	Focal neurologic signs common; responds to treatment with acyclovir
Herpes simplex (type 2)	Human	Worldwide	Encephalitis usually affects neonates; causes meningitis in older children and adults
Rabies	Wild and domestic mammals	Worldwide	Invariably fatal unless vaccine and antiserum administered before symptoms occur following bite by affected animal

A disorder that may be clinically indistinguishable from viral encephalitis is the **immune-mediated encephalomyelitis** that may follow viral infections such as influenza, measles, or chickenpox. Progressive neurologic dysfunction typically begins a few days after the viral illness but can also occur either simultaneously or up to several weeks later. Neurologic abnormalities result from perivenous demyelination, which often severely affects the brainstem. The CSF shows a lymphocytic pleocytosis, usually with cell counts of 50–150/mL, and mild protein elevation.

Treatment

Except for herpes simplex encephalitis, which is discussed separately (see below), no specific therapy for viral meningitis and encephalitis is available. Corticosteroids are of no proven benefit except in immune-mediated postinfectious syndromes. Headache and fever can be treated with acetaminophen, but aspirin should be avoided, especially in children and young adults, because of its association with Reye's syndrome (see p. 20). Seizures usually respond to phenytoin or phenobarbital. Supportive measures in comatose patients include mechanical ventilation and intravenous or nasogastric feeding.

Prognosis

Symptoms of viral meningitis usually resolve spontaneously within 2 weeks regardless of the causative agent, although residual deficits may be seen. The outcome of viral encephalitis varies with the specific virus—for example, eastern equine and herpes simplex virus infections are associated with severe morbidity and high mortality rates. Mortality rates as high as 20% have also been reported in immune-mediated encephalomyelitis following measles infections.

HERPES SIMPLEX VIRUS (HSV) ENCEPHALITIS

HSV is the most common cause of sporadic fatal encephalitis in the United States. About two-thirds of cases involve patients over 40 years of age. Primary herpes infections most often present as stomatitis (HSV type 1) or a venereally transmitted genital eruption (HSV type 2). The virus migrates along nerve axons to sensory ganglia, where it persists in a latent form and may be subsequently reactivated. It is not clear whether HSV type 1 encephalitis, the most common type in adults, represents a primary infection or a reactivation of latent infection. Neonatal HSV encephalitis usually results from acquisition of type 2 virus during passage through the birth canal of a mother with active genital lesions. Central nervous system involvement by HSV type 2 in adults usually causes meningitis, rather than encephalitis.

Pathology

HSV type 1 encephalitis is an acute, necrotizing, asymmetric hemorrhagic process with lymphocytic and plasma cell reaction, and usually involves the medial temporal and inferior frontal lobes. Intranuclear inclusions may be seen in neurons and glia. Patients who recover may show cystic necrosis of the involved regions.

Clinical Findings

A. SYMPTOMS AND SIGNS

The clinical syndrome may include headache, stiff neck, vomiting, behavioral disorders, memory loss, anosmia, aphasia, hemiparesis, and focal or generalized seizures. Active herpes labialis is seen occasionally, but does not reliably implicate HSV as the cause of encephalitis. HSV encephalitis is usually rapidly progressive over several days and may result in coma or death. The most common sequelae in patients who survive are memory and behavior disturbances, reflecting the predilection of HSV for limbic structures.

B. LABORATORY FINDINGS

The CSF in HSV type 1 encephalitis most often shows increased pressure, lymphocytic or mixed lymphocytic and polymorphonuclear pleocytosis (50–100 white blood cells/mL), mild protein elevation, and normal glucose. Red blood cells, xanthochromia, and decreased glucose are seen in some cases. The virus generally cannot be isolated from the CSF, but viral DNA has been detected by the polymerase chain reaction in some cases. The EEG may show periodic slow-wave complexes arising from one or both temporal lobes, and CT scans and MRI may show abnormalities in one or both temporal lobes. These can extend to frontal or parietal regions and are sometimes enhanced with the infusion of contrast material (Figure 1–6). However, imaging studies may also be normal.

Differential Diagnosis

The symptoms and signs are not specific for herpes virus infection. The greatest diagnostic difficulty is distinguishing between HSV encephalitis and brain abscess, and the two disorders often cannot be differentiated on clinical grounds alone. Other CNS infections and vasculitis can also mimic HSV encephalitis. Definitive diagnosis can be made by biopsy of affected brain areas, with the choice of biopsy site guided by the EEG, CT, or MRI findings. However, because treatment is most effective when begun early and is comparatively safe, the most common approach is to treat patients with possible HSV

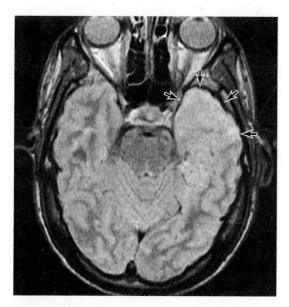

Figure 1–6. T2-weighted MRI in herpes simplex encephalitis. Note the lack of differentiation between gray and white matter, because of edema, in the left anterior temporal lobe **(arrows)** compared with the right. (Courtesy of A Gean.)

encephalitis as described below and to reserve biopsy for those who fail to improve.

Treatment

The most effective drug is **acyclovir**, given intravenously at a dosage of 10–15 mg/kg every 8 hours, with each dose given over 1 hour. Treatment is continued for 14–21 days. Complications include erythema at the infusion site, gastrointestinal disturbances, headache, skin rash, tremor, seizures, and encephalopathy or coma. Treatment is started as early as possible, since outcome is greatly influenced by the severity of dysfunction at the time treatment is initiated.

Prognosis

Patients under the age of 30 years and those who are only lethargic at the onset of treatment are more likely to survive than are older or comatose patients. The mortality rate is about 25% at 18 months in patients given acyclovir.

ACQUIRED IMMUNODEFICIENCY SYNDROME (AIDS)

AIDS is caused by infection with human immunodeficiency virus type 1 (HIV-1) and is characterized by opportunistic infections, malignant neoplasms (typically non-Hodgkin's lymphoma or Kaposi's sarcoma), and a variety of neurologic disturbances. Transmission occurs through sexual activity or by transfer of virus-contaminated blood or blood products. Individuals at particular risk of infection include those who engage in unprotected sexual intercourse, intravenous drug users who share needles, hemophiliacs who have received factor VIII transfusions, and their sexual partners.

Neurologic complications of AIDS include dementia (see below), myelopathy (see Chapter 5), neuropathy (see Chapter 6), myopathy (see Chapter 5), and stroke (see Chapter 9). In addition to the disorders that produce acute confusional states in persons without AIDS, patients with AIDS are at increased risk for direct HIV infection of the nervous system, other opportunistic infections, and certain tumors (Table 1–17). Treatment of AIDS is discussed in the section on AIDS dementia complex later in this chapter.

1. HIV-1 Meningitis

Patients infected with HIV-1 can develop a syndrome characterized by headache, fever, signs of meningeal irritation, cranial nerve (especially VII) palsies, other focal neurologic abnormalities, or seizures. This usually occurs at about the time of HIV-1 seroconversion. An acute confusional state is occasionally present. HIV-1 meningitis is associated with mononuclear pleocytosis of up to about 200 cells/mL. Symptoms usually resolve spontaneously within about 1 month. Other causes of pleocytosis associated with AIDS, including cryptococcal meningitis, herpes simplex encephalitis, and cerebral toxoplasmosis, must be excluded.

2. Cryptococcal Meningitis

Cryptococcal meningitis occurs in 5–10% of patients with AIDS. Clinical features include headache, confusion, stiff neck, fever, nausea and vomiting, seizures, and cranial nerve palsies. Because the CSF is otherwise normal in about 20% of patients with AIDS and cryptococcal meningitis, CSF cryptococcal antigen titers should always be obtained. Laboratory abnormalities and recommended treatment are discussed in the section on fungal meningitis below.

3. Herpes Simplex & Varicella-Zoster Encephalitis

Whereas HSV encephalitis in immunocompetent adults is almost always due to type 1 virus, either type 1 or type 2 HSV can produce the disorder in patients with AIDS. The focal neurologic signs and CSF abnormalities usually associated with HSV encephalitis may be absent in AIDS, and the disorder may follow a more indolent

Table 1–17. Causes of acute confusional states in patients with AIDS.

Meningitis
HIV-1 meningitis
Cryptococcal meningitis
Encephalitis
Herpes simplex encephalitis
Varicella-zoster encephalitis
Cytomegalovirus encephalitis
Intracerebral mass lesions
Cerebral toxoplasmosis
Primary central nervous system lymphoma
Metabolic encephalopathies
Pulmonary encephalopathy (related to *Pneumocystis carinii* - pneumonia)
Drug toxicity
Stroke
Seizures

course. Varicella-zoster virus, a herpesvirus that rarely causes encephalitis in immunocompetent individuals, may do so in patients with AIDS. Treatment is as described above (see p 31) for HSV encephalitis.

4. Cytomegalovirus Encephalitis

Cytomegalovirus, another herpesvirus, has been implicated as a cause of retinitis and polyradiculomyelitis (see Chapter 5) in patients with AIDS. Cytomegalovirus can also be identified in CSF and biopsy specimens from patients with AIDS who are neurologically asymptomatic, acutely confused, or demented. Death usually occurs within a few weeks, although therapeutic responses to antiviral treatment with ganciclovir and foscarnet have been reported.

5. Cerebral Toxoplasmosis

Cerebral toxoplasmosis produces intracerebral mass lesions in patients with AIDS, although its frequency appears to be declining as antitoxoplasma drugs such as trimethoprim-sulfamethoxazole are widely used for prophylaxis against *Pneumocystis carinii* pneumonia in patients with AIDS. A confusional state lasting days to weeks exists at the time of presentation in about 30% of patients. Other clinical features include fever, focal neurologic abnormalities such as cranial nerve palsies or hemiparesis, seizures, headache, and signs of meningeal irritation. Serologic tests for toxoplasmosis are unreliable in patients with AIDS. MRI is more sensitive than CT scanning and typically reveals one or more lesions, which often show a contrast enhancement of the rim and are commonly located in the basal ganglia.

Because toxoplasmosis is readily treatable, patients with AIDS and intracerebral mass lesions that are not obviously due to stroke should be treated for presumed toxoplasmosis, as described in the section on parasitic infections below. Up to 90% of patients respond favorably to therapy within the first few weeks and the majority survive longer than 6 months.

6. Primary Central Nervous System Lymphoma

Primary central nervous system lymphoma is the most common brain tumor associated with AIDS. Systemic non-Hodgkin's lymphoma also occurs with increased frequency, but usually produces lymphomatous meningitis (see below) rather than intracerebral masses. Clinical features of primary central nervous system lymphoma include confusional state, hemiparesis, aphasia, seizures, cranial nerve palsies, and headache; signs of meningeal irritation are uncommon. CSF commonly shows elevated protein and mild mononuclear pleocytosis, and glucose may be low; cytology is rarely positive. MRI is more sensitive than CT scanning and shows single or multiple contrast-enhanced lesions, which may not be distinguishble from those seen with toxoplasmosis. Patients with AIDS and one or more intracerebral mass lesions that fail to respond to treatment for toxoplasmosis within 3 weeks should undergo brain biopsy for diagnosis of lymphoma. Although corticosteroids and radiation therapy may prolong survival, most patients die within a few months.

7. Other Disorders

Pneumocystis carinii pneumonia in patients with AIDS may lead to hypoxia and a resulting confusional state. Patients with AIDS, especially those with central nervous system involvement, may be especially sensitive to drugs (eg, antidepressants) and metabolic disorders, and the antiretroviral drug zidovudine can produce a confusional state. Stroke can occur in patients with AIDS, especially when it is complicated by cryptococcal meningitis, and may produce an acute confusional state. Seizures are common in patients with AIDS, especially those with AIDS dementia complex, cerebral toxoplasmosis, or cryptococcal meningitis, and both complex partial seizures and the postictal state that follows generalized tonic-clonic seizures are associated with confusional states.

FUNGAL MENINGITIS

In a small fraction of patients with systemic fungal infections (mycoses), fungi invade the central nervous system to produce meningitis or focal intraparenchymal lesions (Table 1–18). Several fungi are opportunistic organisms that cause infection in patients with cancer, those receiving corticosteroids or other immunosuppressive drugs, and other debilitated hosts. Intravenous drug abuse is a potential route for infection with *Candida* and *Aspergillus*. Diabetic acidosis is strongly correlated with rhinocerebral mucormycosis. In contrast, meningeal infections with *Coccidioides, Blastomyces,* and *Actinomyces* usually occur in previously healthy individuals. *Cryptococcus* (the most common cause of fungal meningitis in the United States) and *Histoplasma* infection can occur in either healthy or immunosuppressed patients. Cryptococcal meningitis is the most common fungal infection of the nervous system in AIDS, but *Coccidioides* and *Histoplasma* infections can also occur in this setting. Geographic factors are also important in the epidemiology of certain mycoses (see Table 1–18).

Pathogenesis & Pathology

Fungi reach the central nervous system by hematogenous spread from the lungs, heart, gastrointestinal or genitourinary tract, or skin, or by direct extension from parameningeal sites such as the orbits or paranasal sinuses. Invasion of the meninges from a contiguous focus of infection is particularly common in mucormycosis but may also occur in aspergillosis and actinomycosis.

Pathologic findings in fungal infections of the nervous system include a primarily mononuclear meningeal exudative reaction, focal abscesses or granulomas in the brain or spinal epidural space, cerebral infarction related to vasculitis, and ventricular enlargement caused by communicating hydrocephalus.

Clinical Findings

Fungal meningitis is usually a subacute illness that clinically resembles tuberculous meningitis. A history of a predisposing condition such as carcinoma, hematologic malignancy, AIDS, diabetes, organ transplantation, treatment with corticosteroids or cytotoxic agents, prolonged antibiotic therapy, or intravenous drug use increases the suspicion of opportunistic infection. Patients should also be asked about recent travel through areas where certain fungi are endemic.

A. Symptoms and Signs

Common symptoms include headache and lethargy or confusion. Nausea, vomiting, visual loss, seizures, or focal weakness may be noted, while fever may be absent. In a diabetic patient with acidosis, complaints of facial or eye pain, nasal discharge, proptosis, or visual loss should urgently alert the physician to the likelihood of *Mucor* infection.

Careful examination of the skin, orbits, sinuses, and chest may reveal evidence of systemic fungal infection. Neurologic examination may show signs of meningeal irritation, a confusional state, papilledema, visual loss, ptosis, exophthalmos, ocular or other cranial nerve palsies, and focal neurologic abnormalities such as hemiparesis. Because some fungi (eg, *Cryptococcus*) can cause spinal cord compression, there may be evidence of spine tenderness, paraparesis, pyramidal signs in the legs, and loss of sensation over the legs and trunk.

B. Laboratory Findings

Blood cultures should be obtained. Serum glucose and arterial blood gas levels should be determined in diabetic patients. The urine should be examined for *Candida*. Chest x-ray may show hilar lymphadenopathy, patchy or miliary infiltrates, cavitation, or pleural effusion. The CT scan or MRI may demonstrate intracerebral mass lesions associated with *Cryptococcus* (Figure 1–7) or other organisms, a contiguous infectious source in the orbit or paranasal sinuses, or hydrocephalus.

CSF pressure may be normal or elevated, and the fluid is usually clear, but may be viscous in the presence of numerous cryptococci. Lymphocytic pleocytosis of up to 1000 cells/mL is common, but a normal cell count or polymorphonuclear pleocytosis can be seen in early fungal meningitis and normal cell counts are common in immunosuppressed patients. *Aspergillus* infection typically produces a polymorphonuclear pleocytosis. CSF protein, which may be normal initially, subsequently rises, usually to levels not exceeding 200 mg/dL. Higher levels (<1 g/dL) suggest possible subarachnoid block. Glucose is normal or decreased but rarely below 10 mg/dL. Microscopic examination of Gram-stained and acid-fast smears and India ink preparations may reveal the infecting organism (see Table 1–18). Fungal cultures of CSF and other body fluids and tissues should be obtained, but are often negative. In suspected mucormycosis, biopsy of the affected tissue (usually nasal mucosa) is essential. Useful CSF serologic studies include cryptococcal antigen and *Coccidioides* complement-fixing antibody. Cryptococcal antigen is more sensitive than India ink for detecting *Cryptococcus,* and should always be looked for in both CSF and serum when that organism is suspected, as in patients with AIDS.

Differential Diagnosis

Fungal meningitis may mimic brain abscess and other subacute or chronic meningitides, such as those due to tuberculosis or syphilis. CSF findings and contrast CT scans are useful in differential diagnosis.

Treatment & Prognosis

For most organisms causing fungal meningitis, treatment is begun with **amphotericin B deoxycholate,** 1

Table 1–18. Etiologic agents in fungal meningitis.

Name	Geographic Distribution	Opportunistic Infection	Systemic Involvement	Distinctive CSF Findings	Treatment
Cryptococcus neoformans	Nonspecific	Sometimes (including AIDS)	Lungs, skin, bones, joints	Viscous fluid, positive India ink prep, positive cryptococcal antigen	Amphotericin B + flucytosine (amphotericin B or amphotericin B + fluconazole for AIDS patients)
Coccidioides immitis	Southwestern USA	No	Lungs, skin, bones	Positive complement fixation	Amphotericin B (intravenous and intrathecal), fluconazole, or itraconazole
Candida species	Nonspecific	Yes	Mucous membranes, skin, esophagus, genitourinary tract, heart	Positive Gram's stain	Amphotericin B + flucytosine
Aspergillus species	Nonspecific	Yes	Lungs, skin	Polymorphonuclear pleocytosis	Amphotericin B
Mucor species	Nonspecific	Yes, diabetics	Orbits, paranasal sinuses		Amphotericin B + correction of hyperglycemia and acidosis
Histoplasma capsulatum	Eastern and midwestern USA	Sometimes	Lungs, skin, mucous membranes, heart, viscera		Amphotericin B
Blastomyces dermatitidis	Mississippi River Valley	No	Lungs, skin, bones, joints, viscera		Amphotericin B
Actinomyces israelii[1]	Nonspecific	No	Jaw, lungs, abdomen, orbits, sinuses, skin	Sulfur granules, positive Gram's stain, AFB smear	Penicillin G or tetracycline
Nocardia species[1]	Nonspecific	Yes	Lungs, skin	Positive Gram's stain, AFB smear	Sulfonamides

[1] *Actinomyces* and *Nocardia* are filamentous bacteria that are traditionally considered together with fungi.

mg intravenously as a test dose given over 20–30 minutes, followed the next day by 0.3 mg/kg intravenously in 5% dextrose, given over 2–3 hours. The dose is then increased daily in 5- to 10-mg increments until a maximal dose of 0.5–1.5 mg/kg/d is reached. Treatment is usually continued for 12 weeks.

Nephrotoxicity is common with amphotericin B and may force interruption of therapy for 2–5 days. Newer, lipid-based formulations (eg, amphotericin B lipid complex, amphotericin B cholesteryl sulfate, liposomal amphotericin B) are less nephrotoxic, and can be used in patients who develop such toxicity on amphotericin B deoxycholate.

In patients with *Coccidioides* meningitis or those not responding to intravenous therapy, intrathecal amphotericin B (usually administered via an Ommaya reservoir) is added. The drug is given as a 0.1-mg test dose diluted in 10 mL of CSF, with or without added corticosteroids, and increased to 0.25–0.5 mg every other day. Because administration of amphotericin into the CSF may produce side effects, may require instillation at multiple sites, and may be unsuccessful, another approach is to give fluconazole, 400–600 mg/d, or itraconazole, 200 mg twice daily with meals, by the oral route. In this case, treatment must be continued indefinitely.

In cryptococcal meningitis, **flucytosine,** 100 mg/kg/d orally, added to amphotericin B and given in

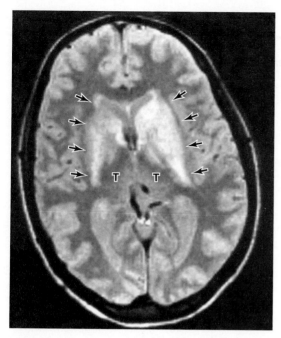

Figure 1–7. T2-weighted MRI in cryptococcal meningitis. Note the bilateral increase in signal in the basal ganglia (**arrows**) with relative sparing of the thalami (T). This is due to the presence of gelatinous fungal pseudocysts in the territory of the lenticulostriate arteries. (Courtesy of A Gean.)

four divided doses, reduces the duration of therapy from 12 to 6 weeks. The dose of flucytosine must be reduced in renal failure; the major side effect is bone marrow suppression, which is usually reversible. Because of this toxicity, flucytosine is usually omitted when treating cryptococcal meningitis in patients with AIDS. For patients with AIDS and cryptococcal meningitis who do not respond to amphotericin B alone, **fluconazole** can be added at an initial dose of 400 mg, followed by 200 mg/d, orally or intravenously, for at least 10–12 weeks after CSF cultures are negative. Long-term maintenance therapy with fluconazole, 100–200 mg/d orally, may also reduce the likelihood of recurrence following successful treatment of cryptococcal meningitis in patients with AIDS.

Rapid correction of hyperglycemia and acidosis must be combined with amphotericin B treatment and surgical debridement of necrotic tissue in diabetics with mucormycosis.

Mortality rates remain high in fungal meningitis. The complications of therapy are frequent, and neurologic residua are common.

PARASITIC INFECTIONS

Protozoal and helminthic infections are important causes of central nervous system disease, particularly in immunosuppressed patients (including those with AIDS), and in certain regions of the world (Table 1–19). Rickettsias, the parasitic bacteria that cause Rocky Mountain spotted fever, rarely affect the nervous system.

1. *Malaria*

Malaria is caused by the protozoan *Plasmodium falciparum* or another *Plasmodium* species that is transferred to humans by the female *Anopheles* mosquito. Clinical features include fever, chills, myalgia, nausea and vomiting, anemia, renal failure, hypoglycemia, and pulmonary edema. Although malaria is the most common parasitic infection of humans worldwide, cerebral involvement is rare. Plasmodia reach the central nervous system in infected red blood cells and cause occlusion of cerebral capillaries. Neurologic involvement becomes apparent weeks after infection. In addition to acute confusional states, cerebral malaria can produce seizures and, rarely, focal neurologic abnormalities. The diagnosis is made by finding plasmodia in red blood cells of peripheral blood smears. The CSF may show increased pressure, xanthochromia, mononuclear pleocytosis, or mildly elevated protein.

Prophylaxis

Malaria prophylaxis is recommended for travelers to areas where the disease is endemic and consists of chloroquine phosphate, 500 mg orally weekly, beginning 1–2 weeks before travel and continuing until 4 weeks after returning. If exposure to chloroquine-resistant strains is expected, treatment options include mefloquine (250 mg orally weekly for 4 weeks, beginning 1–2 weeks before travel and continuing until 4 weeks after returning), doxycycline (100 mg orally daily, beginning 1–2 days before travel and continuing until 4 weeks after returning), or atovaquone/proguanil (250/100 mg orally daily, beginning 1–2 days before travel and continuing until 1 week after returning).

Treatment

Chloroquine-sensitive cerebral malaria is treated with chloroquine, 10 mg base/kg by continuous intravenous infusion over 8 hours followed by 15 mg base/kg over 24 hours, or 3.5 mg base/kg by the intramuscular or subcutaneous route every 6 hours to a cumulative dose of ~25 mg base/kg. **Chloroquine-resistant** cerebral malaria is treated with quinidine, 10 mg base/kg by intravenous infusion over 1 hour followed by 0.02 mg base/kg/min,

Table 1–19. Parasitic infections of the central nervous system.

Parasite	Epidemiologic and Geographic Factors	Clinical Syndrome	Laboratory Findings	Treatment
Protozoa				
Plasmodium falciparum (malaria)	Africa, South America, Southeast Asia, Oceania	Acute confusional state, coma, seizures	Anemia, organisms within red blood cells on peripheral blood smear	Chloroquine (chloroquine sensitive) or quinidine or quinine sulfate (chloroquine resistant)
Toxoplasma gondii	Malignancy or immunosuppression (including AIDS)	Single or multiple focal mass lesions; meningoencephalitis; encephalopathy ± asterixis, myoclonus, or seizures	Positive CT/MRI brain scan; positive Sabin-Feldman dye test; positive IgM antibody; CSF: normal or lymphocytic pleocytosis, organism on wet mount	Pyrimethamine and sulfadiazine
Naegleria fowleri (primary amebic meningoencephalitis)	Freshwater swimming in southeastern USA	Acute fulminant meningoencephalitis with prominent headache and meningeal signs	CSF: polymorpho-nuclear pleocytosis, motile organisms on wet mount	Amophotericin B with or without rifampin and chloramphenicol or ketoconazole
Acanthamoeba or *Hartmanella* species (granulo-matous amebic encephalitis)	Chronic illness or immunosuppression	Subacute-chronic meningoencephalitis, often with seizures and focal neurologic signs	CSF: lymphocytic or polymorphonuclear pleocytosis, sluggish organisms on wet mount	None proven
Helminths				
Taenia solium (cysticercosis)	Latin America	Mass lesion or meningoencephalitis, often presenting with headache or seizures	CSF: lymphocytic pleocytosis, eosinophilia, positive complement fixation or hemagglutination; calcifications on soft tissue x-rays or brain CT scan	Albendazole or praziquantel, corticosteroids, surgical excision of solitary lesion, shunting for hydrocephalus
Angiostrongylus cantonensis (eosinophilic meningitis)	Hawaii, Asia	Acute-subacute meningitis with headache; stiff neck, vomiting, fever, and paresthesias in about half of patients; self-limited course of 1–2 weeks	Peripheral blood eosinophilia; CSF: eosinophilic and lymphocytic pleocytosis	Mebendazole, lev-amisole, albendazole, thiabendazole, or ivermectin
Rickettsia				
Rickettsia rickettsii (Rocky Mountain spotted fever)	Southeastern USA	Acute fever, headache, rash; confusion uncommon	Positive Weil-Felix reaction	Chloramphenicol or doxycycline

or with quinine dihydrochloride (not available in the United States), 20 mg/kg by intravenous infusion over 4 hours followed by 10 mg/kg infused over 2–8 hours every 8 hours. Each of these regimens is continued until oral therapy with chloroquine, amodiaquine, or sulfadoxine and pyrimethamine (for chloroquine-sensitive malaria) or with mefloquine, quinine, or quinidine (for chloroquine-resistant malaria) can be substituted.

Cerebral edema is not a consistent finding in cerebral malaria, and corticosteroids are *not* helpful and may be deleterious. The mortality rate in cerebral malaria is 20–50% and reaches 80% in cases complicated by coma and seizures.

2. Toxoplasmosis

Toxoplasmosis results from ingestion of *Toxoplasma gondii* cysts in raw meat or cat excrement and is usually asymptomatic. Symptomatic infection is associated with underlying malignancy (especially Hodgkin's disease), immunosuppressive therapy, or AIDS.

Clinical Findings

Systemic manifestations include skin rash, lymphadenopathy, myalgias, arthralgias, carditis, pneumonitis, and splenomegaly. Central nervous system involvement can take several forms (see Table 1–19).

The CSF may be normal, or it may show mild mononuclear cell pleocytosis or slight protein elevation. MRI is superior to CT scanning for demonstrating cerebral toxoplasmosis, and typically shows ring-enhancing lesions (Figure 1–8). The diagnosis is made by blood tests demonstrating a high (≥1:32,000) or rising Sabin-Feldman dye test titer or IgM antibodies to *Toxoplasma* by indirect immunofluorescence. Accurate diagnosis requires appropriate serologic studies in the immunosuppressed patient who develops neurologic symptoms.

Treatment

Treatment is with pyrimethamine, 25–100 mg/d orally and sulfadiazine, 1–1.5 g orally four times daily, and is continued for 3–4 weeks in immunocompetent patients and for at least several months in immunodeficient patients. Clindamycin, 600 mg orally four times a day, may be substituted for sulfonamides in patients who develop drug sensitivity rashes. Folinic acid (leucovorin), 10 mg orally daily, is added to prevent pyrimethamine-induced leukopenia and thrombocytopenia.

3. Primary Amebic Meningoencephalitis

The free-living ameba *Naegleria fowleri* causes primary amebic meningoencephalitis in previously healthy young patients exposed to polluted water. Amebas gain entry to the central nervous system through the cribriform plate, producing a diffuse meningoencephalitis that affects the base of the frontal lobes and posterior fossa. It is characterized by headache, fever, nausea and vomiting, signs of meningeal irritation, and disordered mental status. The CSF shows a polymorphonuclear pleocytosis with elevated protein and low glucose; highly motile, refractile trophozoites can be seen on wet mounts of centrifuged CSF. The disease is usually fatal within 1 week, although treatment with amphotericin B, 1 mg/kg/d intravenously, may be effective, as may a combination of amphotericin B, rifampin, and chloramphenicol or ketoconazole.

4. Granulomatous Amebic Encephalitis

Granulomatous amebic encephalitis results from infection with *Acanthamoeba/Hartmanella* species and commonly occurs with chronic illness or immunosuppression. The disorder typically lasts for from 1 week to 3 months and is characterized by subacute or chronic meningitis and granulomatous encephalitis. The cerebellum, brainstem, basal ganglia, and cerebral hemispheres are affected. An acute confusional state is the

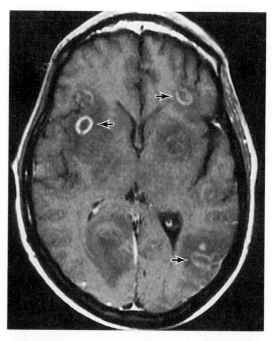

Figure 1–8. T1-weighted, gadolinium-enhanced MRI in cerebral toxoplasmosis complicating HIV infection. Note the multiple ring-enhanced lesions **(arrows)** with surrounding edema. (Courtesy of A Gean.)

most common clinical finding. Fever, headache, and meningeal signs each occur in only about half of patients. Seizures, hemiparesis cranial nerve palsies, cerebellar ataxia, and aphasia may occur. Pleocytosis may be primarily lymphocytic or polymorphonuclear; protein is elevated, and glucose is low or normal. Sluggishly motile trophozoites may be seen on wet mounts. Successful treatment has not been reported.

5. Cysticercosis

Cysticercosis is common in Mexico, Central and South America, western and southern Africa, India, China, and southeast Asia. The disease follows ingestion of larvae of the pork tapeworm (*Taenia solium*) and affects the brain in 60–90% of cases. Larvae undergo hematogenous dissemination, forming cysts in the brain, ventricles, and subarachnoid space. Neurologic manifestations of cysticercosis result from the mass effect of intraparenchymal cysts, obstruction of CSF flow by intraventricular cysts, or inflammation that causes basilar meningitis. They include seizures, headache, focal neurologic signs, hydrocephalus, myelopathy, and subacute meningitis. Peripheral blood eosinophilia, soft tissue calcifications, or parasites in the stool suggest the diagnosis. The CSF typically shows a lymphocytic pleocytosis (<100 cells/mL), with eosinophils usually present. Opening pressure is often increased but may be decreased with spinal subarachnoid block; if this is suspected, myelography should be performed. Protein is increased to 50–100 mg/dL, and glucose is 20–50 mg/dL in most cases. Complement fixation and hemagglutination studies can assist in the diagnosis. The CT scan or MRI may show contrast-enhanced mass lesions with surrounding edema, intracerebral calcifications, or ventricular enlargement (Figure 1–9).

The indications for treatment of cerebral cysticercosis are controversial. However, patients with symptomatic neurologic involvement (usually seizures) and either meningitis or one or more noncalcified intraparenchymal cysts should be treated. Intraventricular, subarachnoid, and racemose cysts respond poorly to treatment, and calcified cysts do not require treatment. Albendazole, 15 mg/kg/d in three doses taken with meals, and continued for 8 days, is the preferred therapy. Praziquantel, 50 mg/kg/d in three divided doses, can also be used, but blood levels are reduced by anticonvulsants and corticosteroids, which are often also required in these patients. Patients with seizures should also receive anticonvulsants. Corticosteroids are indicated for increased intracranial pressure or lesions near the cerebral aqueduct or intraventricular foramina; these may progress to cause obstructive hydrocephalus. Single accessible intraparenchymal lesions can be removed surgically, and shunting is required for intraventricular lesions causing hydrocephalus.

6. Angiostrongylus Cantonensis Meningitis

Angiostrongylus cantonensis is endemic to southeast Asia and to Hawaii and other Pacific islands. Infection is transmitted by ingestion of infected raw mollusks and produces meningitis with CSF eosinophilia (Table 1–20). Most patients complain of headache, and about half report stiff neck, vomiting, fever, and paresthesias. Most patients have a CSF leukocytosis of 150–1500/mL, mild elevation of protein, and normal glucose. The acute illness usually resolves spontaneously in 1–2 weeks, although paresthesias may persist longer.

Levamisole, albendazole, thiabendazole, mebendazole, and ivermectin have been used for treatment; mebendazole 100 mg twice daily orally for 5 days may be preferable. Analgesics, corticosteroids, and reduction of CSF pressure by repeated lumbar punctures may be of value.

7. Rocky Mountain Spotted Fever

Rocky Mountain spotted fever is caused by *Rickettsia rickettsii,* an intracellular parasite transmitted to humans by tick bites. *R rickettsii* damages endothelial cells, leading to vasculitis, microinfarcts, and petechial hemorrhage. Initial symptoms include fever, headache, and a characteristic rash that involves the palms and soles and spreads centrally. Neurologic involvement, which is

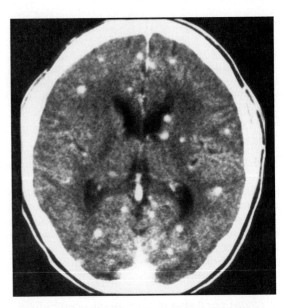

Figure 1–9. Contrast-enhanced CT scan in cerebral cysticercosis. Note the multiple bilateral, small, rounded areas of high density, which represent intraparenchymal cysts. (Courtesy of A Gean.)

Table 1–20. Causes of CSF eosinophilia.

Common causes
  Taenia solium (cysticercosis)
  Angiostrongylus cantonensis (eosinophilic meningitis)
Uncommon causes
  Other helminthic infections
  Coccidioides immitis meningitis
  Hematologic malignancies with meningeal infiltration
  Foreign matter (including myelography dye) in subarachnoid space
Possible causes (less well documented)
  Neurosyphilis
  Tuberculous meningitis
  Nonhematologic malignancies with meningeal infiltration
  Lymphocytic choriomeningitis
  Polyarteritis nodosa
  Allergic reactions

---

uncommon, produces a confusional state and, less often, coma or focal neurologic abnormalities. The CSF is normal or shows a mild mononuclear pleocytosis. Treatment is with chloramphenicol, 25–50 mg/kg/d orally or intravenously in four divided doses, or doxycycline, 200 mg/d orally or intravenously, and is continued for 7 days. Neurologic residua may occur.

LEPTOMENINGEAL METASTASES

Diffuse metastatic seeding of the leptomeninges may complicate systemic cancer (especially acute lymphocytic leukemia, non-Hodgkin's lymphoma, melanoma, acute myelogenous leukemia, carcinoma of the breast, Hodgkin's lymphoma, carcinoma of the lung, carcinoma of the gastrointestinal tract, and sarcoma), producing neurologic syndromes with prominent cognitive dysfunction. Primary brain tumors may be associated with meningeal gliomatosis, and medulloblastomas and pineal tumors have a particular propensity for meningeal dissemination.

Neoplastic meningitis usually occurs from 3 months to 5 years after the diagnosis of cancer, but may be the presenting manifestation or occur after many years of illness—sometimes in apparently cured patients. Its most frequent symptoms are headache and cognitive disorders, including lethargy, confusion, and memory impairment. Nausea, vomiting, seizures, and gait abnormalities are also common.

Clinical Findings

A. SYMPTOMS AND SIGNS

Abnormal neurologic signs are often more striking than the symptoms and usually suggest involvement at multiple levels of the neuraxis. The symptoms and signs most often seen when the patient presents with leptomeningeal metastases are listed in Table 1–21.

B. LABORATORY FINDINGS

The most useful diagnostic procedure is lumbar puncture, which may show increased opening pressure, pleocytosis and elevated protein, and markedly decreased or even immeasurably low glucose (see Table 1–21). Neoplastic meningitis is diagnosed by finding malignant cells in the CSF; large volumes of fluid and repeated lumbar punctures increase the yield of cytologic studies. Several biochemical markers for leptomeningeal metastases can be identified in CSF. These include carcinoembryonic antigen, human chorionic gonadotropin, and α-fetoprotein, which are specific for leptomeningeal metastases, as well as β_2-microglobulin, β-glucuronidase, and lactic dehydrogenase isozyme V, which can also be elevated in inflammatory disorders. Where clinically indicated, MRI or a metrizamide CT study of the spine, or myelography is performed to exclude the possibility of intraparenchymal metastasis or spinal cord compression by epidural metastasis.

Differential Diagnosis

Neoplastic meningitis can simulate infectious meningitis, metabolic encephalopathy, intraparenchymal or spinal epidural metastasis, remote effects of carcinoma, or chemotherapeutic drug toxicity and may coexist with any of these conditions.

Treatment & Prognosis

Untreated, leptomeningeal metastases are typically associated with death within about 2 months. Leptomeningeal leukemia and lymphoma can be successfully treated with radiation and chemotherapy, and some patients with breast cancer or small-cell lung cancer also respond to these approaches. However, even with treatment, most patients with leptomeningeal metastases from solid tumors live only a few months.

SEPSIS

Systemic sepsis can produce an encephalopathy that may be related to impaired cerebral blood flow, disruption of the blood-brain barrier, or cerebral edema. Gram-negative infections are the most common cause. Clinical findings include bacteremia and often liver or kidney failure. The EEG is often abnormal. Therapy involves supportive measures, such as assisted ventilation, and treatment of the underlying infection. Mortality is high, but can be prevented by prompt diagnosis and treatment.

Table 1–21. Presenting symptoms, signs, and CSF findings with leptomeningeal metastases.

Feature	Percentage of Patients
Symptoms	
Gait disturbance	46
Headache	38
Altered mentation	25
Weakness	22
Back pain	18
Nausea or vomiting	12
Radicular pain	12
Paresthesias	10
Signs	
Lower motor neuron weakness	78
Absent tendon reflex	60
Cognitive disturbance	50
Extensor plantar response	50
Dermatomal sensory deficit	50
Ophthalmoplegia	30
Facial weakness	25
Hearing loss	20
Neck meningeal signs	16
Seizures	14
Papilledema	12
Facial sensory deficit	12
Leg meningeal signs	12
CSF findings	
Protein increased[1]	81
Pleocytosis[2]	57
Positive cytology	54
Opening pressure elevated[3]	50
Glucose decreased[4]	31
Normal	3

[1] >50 mg/dL.
[2] >5 white blood cells/mm³.
[3] >160 mm CSF.
[4] <40 mg/dL.
Data from Posner JB: *Neurologic Complications of Cancer.* Davis, 1997.

VASCULAR DISORDERS

HYPERTENSIVE ENCEPHALOPATHY

A sudden increase in blood pressure, with or without preexisting chronic hypertension, may result in encephalopathy and headache, which develop over a period of several hours to days. Vomiting, visual disturbances, focal neurologic deficits, and focal or generalized seizures can also occur. Blood pressure in excess of 250/150 mm Hg is usually required to precipitate the syndrome in patients with chronic hypertension; previously normotensive patients may be affected at lower pressures. Coexisting renal failure appears to increase the risk of hypertensive encephalopathy.

Cerebrovascular spasm, impaired autoregulation of cerebral blood flow, and intravascular coagulation have all been proposed as the cause of neurological symptoms. These processes can lead to small infarcts and petechial hemorrhages that affect the brainstem most prominently and other subcortical gray and white matter regions to a lesser extent.

Clinical Findings

The physical findings most useful in confirming the diagnosis are those seen on ophthalmoscopy. Retinal arteriolar spasm is almost invariably present. Papilledema, retinal hemorrhages, and exudates are usually present. Lumbar puncture may show normal or elevated CSF pressure and protein. Low-density areas suggestive of edema in the posterior regions of hemispheric white matter are seen on CT scan and corresponding T2 hyperintense areas are seen on MRI (Figure 1–10); the changes are reversible with treatment. Blood studies are important to detect uremia.

Differential Diagnosis

Hypertensive encephalopathy is a diagnosis of exclusion. Stroke and subarachnoid hemorrhage also produce encephalopathy with acutely elevated blood pressure, and when focal neurologic abnormalities are present, stroke is by far the most likely diagnosis. Elevated blood pressure, headache, papilledema, and altered consciousness are also seen with intracranial hemorrhage; where this is a consideration, it can be excluded by CT scan or MRI.

Prevention

Hypertensive encephalopathy is best prevented by early treatment of uncomplicated hypertension and by prompt recognition of elevated blood pressure in settings—such as acute glomerulonephritis or eclampsia—in which it tends to occur in previously normotensive patients.

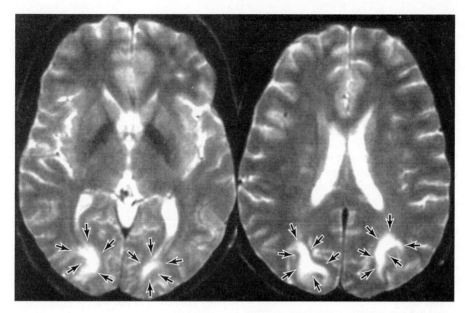

Figure 1–10. Axial T2-weighted images of the brain of a 39-year-old woman who developed hypertensive encephalopathy in the setting of chronic renal failure. Areas of abnormal high intensity **(arrows)** represent edema affecting posterior parietal and occipital regions, white matter more than gray. Similar imaging changes can sometimes be seen following generalized seizures and with certain drugs, particularly cyclosporine and chemotherapeutic agents. Imaging abnormalities typically resolve with treatment of the underlying condition. (Courtesy of HA Rowley.)

Treatment

The diagnosis of hypertensive encephalopathy is established when lowering the blood pressure results in rapid resolution of symptoms. This is accomplished with sodium nitroprusside, given by continuous intravenous infusion at an initial rate of 0.5 mg/kg/min, and increased to as much as 3–10 mg/kg/min as required. Alternative approaches include diazoxide, 50–100 mg by intravenous bolus every 5–10 minutes (to a maximum of 600 mg) or 10–30 mg/min by constant intravenous infusion, or labetalol, 20–80 mg by intravenous bolus every 5–10 minutes (to a maximum of 600 mg) or 0.5–2 mg/min by constant intravenous infusion. The patient must be carefully monitored and the infusion rate adjusted to maintain a therapeutic effect *without producing hypotension.* In the first hour of treatment, mean arterial blood pressure should be reduced by no more than 20–25% and diastolic pressure should not be allowed to fall below 100 mm Hg. Treatment should be terminated immediately if neurologic function worsens. Untreated hypertensive encephalopathy can result in stroke, coma, or death but prompt treatment usually produces full clinical recovery.

SUBARACHNOID HEMORRHAGE

Subarachnoid hemorrhage must receive early consideration in the differential diagnosis of an acute confusional state. This disorder is discussed in Chapter 2.

VERTEBROBASILAR ISCHEMIA

Transient ischemia or stroke in the distribution of the posterior cerebral circulation can produce an acute confusional state. Vertebrobasilar ischemia is discussed in Chapter 9.

RIGHT (NONDOMINANT) HEMISPHERIC INFARCTION

Agitated confusion of sudden onset can result from infarction (usually embolic) in the territory of the inferior division of the nondominant (usually right) middle cerebral artery. If the superior division is spared, there is no hemiparesis. Agitation may be so pronounced as to suggest an alcohol withdrawal syndrome, but autonomic hyperactivity is absent. The diagnosis is confirmed by CT brain scan or MRI. Rarely, isolated anterior cerebral artery infarcts or posterior cerebral artery infarcts cause acute confusion.

SYSTEMIC LUPUS ERYTHEMATOSUS

Systemic lupus erythematosus (SLE) is the most common autoimmune cause of encephalopathy. SLE is nine times more common in women than in men and usually has its onset between the ages of 10 and 40 years. Neurologic involvement is reported in 37–75% of patients. The clinical features that correlate best with nervous system involvement are active mucocutaneous or visceral vasculitis and thrombocytopenia, but clinically active systemic disease need not be present for neurologic symptoms to occur. Neuropathologic findings include fibrinoid degeneration of arterioles and capillaries, microinfarcts, and intracerebral hemorrhages. True vasculitis of cerebral blood vessels is rare.

Clinical Findings

A. SYMPTOMS AND SIGNS

The most common neurologic features are seizures and an altered mental status. Cognitive disturbances include acute confusional states, schizophreniform psychosis, depression, and mania. Seizures are usually generalized but may be focal. Less common neurologic manifestations include visual impairment from optic nerve involvement, ptosis, diplopia, hemiparesis, paraparesis, tremor, chorea, cerebellar ataxia, and polyneuropathy.

B. LABORATORY FINDINGS

Laboratory abnormalities in SLE include antinuclear antibodies, anemia, hypocomplementemia, antinative DNA antibodies, leukopenia, and autoantibodies against ribosomal P proteins. No laboratory finding is diagnostic of nervous system involvement, but CSF shows mild elevation of protein or a modest—usually mononuclear—pleocytosis in about one-third of cases. The EEG frequently shows diffuse slowing or focal abnormalities

Differential Diagnosis

Even in patients with known SLE, encephalopathy can be caused by a variety of factors other than cerebral lupus per se. Coagulopathy, infection, uremia, and emboli from endocarditis must be excluded. A common dilemma is the need to distinguish cerebral lupus from steroid-induced psychosis in patients receiving corticosteroid therapy for SLE. Cerebral lupus is by far the more frequent problem, particularly in patients receiving low or tapering doses of steroids.

Treatment

Cerebral lupus is treated with corticosteroids, beginning at 60 mg/d of prednisone or the equivalent. In patients already receiving steroids, the dose should be or increased by the equivalent of 5–10 mg/d of prednisone. After symptoms resolve, steroids should be tapered to a low maintenance dose. Seizures are treated with anticonvulsants.

Prognosis

Neurologic symptoms of SLE improve in more than 80% of patients treated with corticosteroids, but may also resolve without treatment. Cerebral involvement in SLE has not been shown to adversely affect the overall prognosis.

DISSEMINATED INTRAVASCULAR COAGULATION

Disseminated intravascular coagulation (DIC) results from pathologic activation of the coagulation and fibrinolytic systems, usually in the setting of a severe underlying systemic disease. The principal manifestation is hemorrhage. DIC tends to occur at the extremes of age, but patients of any age can be affected. Common findings in the brain include small multifocal infarctions and petechial hemorrhages involving both gray and white matter. Subdural hematoma, subarachnoid hemorrhage, and hemorrhagic infarction in the distribution of large vessels may also occur.

Clinical Findings

Neurologic manifestations are common and include confusional states, coma, focal signs, and seizures. They may precede the definitive hematologic abnormalities of hypofibrinogenemia, thrombocytopenia, fibrin degradation products, and prolonged prothrombin time. Microangiopathic hemolytic anemia may also occur.

Differential Diagnosis

Disorders that must be excluded include metabolic encephalopathy, meningoencephalitis, metastatic involvement of the brain or meninges, or stroke caused by nonbacterial thrombotic (marantic) endocarditis. Thrombotic thrombocytopenic purpura (TTP) is distinguished by its tendency to occur in previously healthy patients and its association with normal plasma fibrinogen and normal or only slightly elevated fibrin degradation products.

Treatment

Treatment is directed at the underlying disease. Transfusion of red blood cells, platelets, and coagulation factors from fresh-frozen plasma may be indicated. Transfused platelets are often rapidly destroyed, however, and transfused coagulation factors may be converted to anticoagulant fibrin degradation products and worsen the hemorrhagic tendency. Heparin has sometimes been advocated because of its ability to inhibit the coagulation cascade, but its utility is uncertain. Prognosis is related to the severity of the underlying disease.

THROMBOTIC THROMBOCYTOPENIC PURPURA

Thrombotic thrombocytopenic purpura (TTP) is a rare multisystem disorder defined by the pentad of thrombocytopenic purpura, microangiopathic hemolytic anemia, neurologic dysfunction, fever, and renal disease. In most cases, the cause is thought to be an IgG-mediated autoimmune reaction against a von Willebrand factor-cleaving protease, which allows unusually large multimers of von Willebrand factor to accumulate in the plasma, where they stimulate platelet aggregation. The result is platelet-fibrin thrombus formation with occlusion of small blood vessels, especially at arteriolar-capillary junctions. Pathologic findings in the brain include disseminated microinfarcts and, less frequently, petechial hemorrhages that are present mainly in gray matter. The antiplatelet drugs ticopidine and clopidogrel can precipitate TTP, but how this occurs is unclear.

Clinical Findings

A. Symptoms and Signs

Patients most often present with altered consciousness, headache, focal neurologic signs, or seizures or with cutaneous hemorrhages in the form of purpura, ecchymoses, or petechiae. Other symptoms include malaise, fatigue, generalized weakness, nausea, vomiting, diarrhea, fever, and abdominal pain. Bleeding from sites other than the skin may occur. Neurologic symptoms may be fleeting and recurrent. The physical examination is helpful in documenting fever, cutaneous hemorrhage, and neurologic dysfunction. TTP usually follows an acute, fulminant course but can be a chronic progressive or remitting and relapsing disorder lasting from months to years. What accounts for the defect in von Willebrand factor-cleaving protease activity in chronic cases is unknown.

B. Laboratory Findings

Hematologic studies show a Coombs-negative hemolytic anemia with hemoglobin levels usually less than 10 g/dL, normochromic red blood cell indices, fragmented and misshapen erythrocytes, and often nucleated red cells. Platelet counts are less than 20,000/mL in about half the cases and less than 60,000/mL in almost all cases; the white blood cell count is normal or elevated. Coagulation studies are normal or slightly abnormal in most patients: PT and PTT are normal in about 90% of cases and fibrinogen is normal in 80%. Fibrin degradation products are normal in about 50% of cases and slightly elevated in about 25%. Renal involvement may cause hematuria, proteinuria, or azotemia. Spinal fluid is usually normal, but protein may be elevated. Antemortem pathologic diagnosis may be made by gingival biopsy or splenectomy.

Differential Diagnosis

DIC is also associated with hemolytic anemia or thrombocytopenia. Idiopathic thrombocytopenic purpura (ITP) is not accompanied by microangiopathic hemolytic anemia or by evidence of multisystem disease. The hemolytic anemias of SLE, autoimmune hemolytic anemia (AIHA), and Evans syndrome (both ITP and AIHA) are Coombs-positive.

Treatment & Prognosis

Plasmapheresis is the mainstay of therapy and is sometimes combined with prednisone and antiplatelet agents (aspirin, 325 mg three times daily and dipyridamole, 75 mg three times daily). With treatment, >80% of patients recover, although relapses may occur.

HEAD TRAUMA

Blunt head trauma can produce a confusional state or coma. Acceleration or deceleration forces and physical deformation of the skull can cause shearing of white matter, contusion from contact between the inner surface of the skull and the polar regions of the cerebral hemispheres, torn blood vessels, vasomotor changes, brain edema, and increased intracranial pressure.

CONCUSSION

Concussion is characterized by transient loss of consciousness for seconds to minutes without demonstrable structural defects. Unconsciousness is associated with normal pupillary and ocular reflexes, flaccidity, and extensor plantar responses. The return of consciousness is followed by a confusional state that usually lasts from minutes to hours, and is characterized by prominent retrograde and anterograde amnesia (see below). Patients with simple concussion usually recover uneventfully, although headache, dizziness, or mild cognitive impairment may persist for weeks. When unconsciousness is prolonged, delayed in onset after a lucid interval, or associated with focal neurologic abnormalities, the possibility of posttraumatic intracranial hemorrhage should be considered.

INTRACRANIAL HEMORRHAGE

③ Traumatic intracranial hemorrhage can be epidural, subdural, or intracerebral. **Epidural hematoma** most often results from a lateral skull fracture that lacerates the middle meningeal artery or vein. Patients may or may not lose consciousness initially, but in either event a lucid interval lasting several hours to 1–2 days is followed by the rapid evolution—over hours—of headache, progressive obtundation, hemiparesis, and finally ipsilateral pupillary dilatation from uncal herniation. Death may follow if treatment is delayed.

Subdural hematoma after head injury can be acute, subacute, or chronic. In each case, headache and altered consciousness are the principal manifestations. Delay in diagnosis and treatment may lead to a fatal outcome. In contrast to epidural hematoma, the time between trauma and the onset of symptoms is typically longer, the hemorrhage tends to be located over the cerebral convexities, and associated skull fractures are uncommon. Subdural hematoma in the posterior fossa is uncommon.

Intracerebral contusion (bruising) or **hemorrhage** related to head injury is usually located at the frontal or temporal poles. Blood typically enters the CSF, resulting in signs of meningeal irritation and sometimes hydrocephalus. Focal neurologic signs are usually absent or subtle.

The diagnosis of posttraumatic intracranial hemorrhage is made by CT scan or MRI. Epidural hematoma tends to appear as a biconvex, lens-shaped, extraaxial mass that may cross the midline or the tentorium but not the cranial sutures. Subdural hematoma is typically crescent-shaped and may cross the cranial sutures but not the midline or tentorium. Midline structures may be displaced contralaterally.

Epidural and subdural hematomas are treated by surgical evacuation. The decision to use surgery to treat intracerebral hematoma depends upon the clinical course and location. Evacuation, decompression, or shunting for hydrocephalus may be indicated.

SEIZURES

POSTICTAL STATE

Generalized tonic-clonic (grand mal) seizures are typically followed by a transient confusional state (postictal state) that resolves within 1–2 hours. Disturbances of recent memory and of attention are prominent. When postictal confusion does not clear rapidly, an explanation for the **prolonged postictal state** must be sought. This occurs in three settings: status epilepticus, an underlying structural brain abnormality (eg, stroke, intracranial hemorrhage), and an underlying diffuse cerebral disorder (eg, dementia, meningitis or encephalitis, metabolic encephalopathy). Patients with an unexplained prolonged postictal state should be evaluated with blood chemistry studies, lumbar puncture, EEG, and CT scan or MRI.

COMPLEX PARTIAL SEIZURES

Complex partial (formerly called **temporal lobe** or **psychomotor**) seizures produce alterations in consciousness characterized by confusion alone, or by cognitive, affective, psychomotor, or psychosensory symptoms. Complex partial seizures rarely cause diagnostic problems in the patient presenting with an acute confusional state, because spells are typically brief and stereotypical, psychomotor manifestations are often obvious to the observer, and patients themselves may describe classic cognitive, affective, or psychosensory symptoms (see Chapter 8).

Complex partial seizures produce a confusional state that may be characterized by a withdrawn or unresponsive state or by agitated behavior. Automatisms such as staring, repetitive chewing, swallowing, lip-smacking, or picking at clothing are characteristic. Complex partial status epilepticus, which is rare, lasts for hours to days. The diagnosis is made or confirmed by EEG.

PSYCHIATRIC DISORDERS

Symptoms similar to those associated with acute confusional states—incoherence, agitation, distractibility, hypervigilance, delusions, and hallucinations—can also be seen in a variety of psychiatric disorders. These include psychotic disorders (schizophrenia, schizophreniform disorder, schizoaffective disorder, delusional disorder, brief psychotic disorder), mood (depressive and bipolar) disorders, anxiety disorders (posttraumatic stress disorder), and factitious disorders. Such diagnoses may be mistakenly assigned to patients with acute confusional states; conversely, patients with psychiatric disturbances may be thought—incorrectly—to have organic disease.

Unlike acute confusional states, psychiatric disorders are rarely acute in onset but typically develop over a period of at least several weeks. The history may reveal previous psychiatric disease or hospitalization or a precipitating psychological stress. Physical examination may show abnormalities related to autonomic overactivity, including tachycardia, tachypnea, and hyperreflexia but no definitive signs of neurologic dysfunction. Routine laboratory studies are normal in the psychiatric disorders listed above, but are useful for excluding organic disorders.

Although the mental status examination in acute confusional states is often characterized by disorientation and fluctuating consciousness, patients with psychiatric disorders tend to maintain a consistent degree of cognitive impairment and to be oriented to person, place, and time. Disorientation as to person, especially in the face of preserved orientation in other spheres, is virtually diagnostic of psychiatric disease. Patients with psychiatric disorders exhibit a normal level of consciousness, usually appearing awake and alert, and memory is intact. Disturbances in the content and form of thought (eg, persecutory delusions, delusions of reference, loosening of associations), perceptual abnormalities (eg, auditory hallucinations), and flat or inappropriate affect are common, however.

Psychiatric consultation should be sought regarding diagnosis and management.

■ III. DEMENTIA

Dementia is an acquired, generalized, and usually progressive impairment of cognitive function that affects the content, but not the level, of consciousness. Although its incidence increases with advancing age (it has been estimated to affect 5–20% of individuals over age 65), dementia is not an invariable accompaniment of aging. It reflects instead a disorder that affects the cerebral cortex, its subcortical connections, or both.

Minor changes in neurologic function, including alterations in memory and other cognitive spheres, can occur with normal aging (Table 1–22). Enlargement of ventricles and cerebral cortical sulci seen on CT or MRI scans (Figure 1–11) is also common with normal aging. These findings should not by themselves be considered indicative of dementia.

APPROACH TO DIAGNOSIS

The first step in evaluating a patient with a disorder of cognitive function is to classify the disorder as either a disturbance of the level of consciousness (wakefulness or arousal), such as an acute confusional state or coma, or a disturbance of the content of consciousness, in which wakefulness is preserved. The latter category includes both global cognitive disorders (dementia) and more circumscribed deficits, such as aphasia and amnestic syndromes. This distinction is important because the initial classification of the disorder determines the subsequent diagnostic approach. The most common problem in this area is distinguishing dementia from an acute confusional state, such as that produced by drug intoxication. The clinical features presented in Table 1–1 may be useful in making this distinction. Another common problem is differentiating between dementia and so-called pseu-

dodementia, such as that produced by depression (see below).

In the clinical evaluation of patients with suspected dementia, it is important to try to find the cause, even though only about 10% of dementias are reversible. The possibility of reversing or arresting the disorder through appropriate treatment and dramatically improving the quality and duration of life justifies a thorough diagnostic investigation. A diagnosis is important in other cases for purposes of providing a prognosis and genetic counseling, or alerting family members and medical personnel to the risk of a transmissible disease. As better treatments are developed for dementing disorders that are unresponsive or poorly responsive to current therapy, the importance of arriving at an etiologic diagnosis of dementia will continue to increase.

History

Because dementia implies deterioration in cognitive ability, it is important to establish that the patient's level of functioning has declined. Data that can help to establish the cause of dementia include the time course of deterioration; associated symptoms such as headache, gait disturbance, or incontinence; family history of a similar condition; concurrent medical illnesses; and the use of alcohol and prescribed or unprescribed drugs.

General Physical Examination

The general physical examination can contribute to the etiologic diagnosis when it reveals signs of a systemic disease responsible for the dementia. Particularly helpful signs are listed in Table 1–3.

Mental Status Examination

The mental status examination helps to determine whether it is the level or the content of consciousness that is impaired and whether the cognitive dysfunction is global or circumscribed. A disorder of the level of consciousness is suggested by sleepiness, inattention, impairment of immediate recall, or disorientation as to place or time. Abnormalities in these areas are unusual in dementia until the disorder is far advanced.

To determine the scope of the cognitive dysfunction (global or circumscribed), various spheres of cognition are tested in turn. These include memory, language, parietal lobe functions (pictorial construction, right-left discrimination, localization of objects in space), and frontal lobe or diffuse cerebral cortical functions (judgment, abstraction, thought content, the ability to perform previously learned acts). Multiple areas of cognitive function are impaired in dementia. The Minimental Status Examination (see Table 1–5) provides a useful bedside screening test when dementia is suspected.

Table 1–22. Neurologic changes in normal aging.

Cognitive
  Memory loss (benign senescent forgetfulness)
Neuroophthalmologic
  Small, sluggishly reactive pupils
  Impaired upgaze
  Impaired convergence
Motor
  Muscular atrophy (intrinsic hand and foot muscles)
  Increased muscle tone
  Flexion (stooped) posture
  Gait disorders (small-stepped or broad-based gait)
Sensory
  Impaired vision
  Impaired hearing
  Impaired taste
  Impaired olfaction
  Decreased vibration sense
Reflexes
  Primitive reflexes
  Absent abdominal reflexes
  Absent ankle jerks

Neurologic Examination

Certain disorders that produce dementia also affect vision, coordination, or motor or sensory function. Detecting such associated neurologic abnormalities can help to establish an etiologic diagnosis. Neurologic signs suggesting causes of dementia are listed in Table 1–3.

Laboratory Investigations

Laboratory studies that can help to identify the cause of dementia are listed in Table 1–7.

DIFFERENTIAL DIAGNOSIS

Common Causes of Dementia

Although a wide variety of diseases can produce dementia (Table 1–23), it is generally agreed that Alzheimer's disease is the most common cause. Dementia with Lewy bodies, which has been recognized as a distinct entity rather than simply concurrent Alzheimer's disease and Parkinson's disease, may be second in frequency. Vascular dementia, sometimes referred

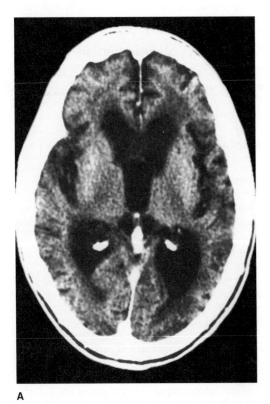
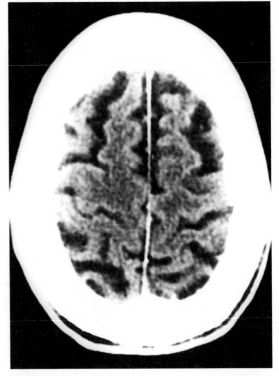

A **B**

Figure 1–11. CT scan in cerebrocortical atrophy, showing ventricular dilation **(A)** and prominent cortical sulci **(B)**.

Table 1–23. Causes of dementia.

Disorder	Distinctive Features
Cerebral disorders	
Without extrapyramidal features	
Alzheimer's disease	Prominent memory loss, language impairment, visuospatial disturbance, depression, anxiety, delusions
Pick's disease	Apathy, disinhibition, anosognosia, logorrhea, echolalia, palilalia
Creutzfeldt-Jakob disease	Myoclonus, ataxia, periodic EEG complexes
Normal-pressure hydrocephalus	Incontinence, gait disorder
With extrapyramidal features	
Dementia with Lewy bodies (includes diffuse Lewy body-disease and Lewy-body variant of Alzheimer's disease)	Fluctuating cognitive function, visual hallucinations, parkinsonism
Corticobasal ganglionic degeneration	Parkinsonism, apraxia (including orofacial apraxia that can mimic aphasia), cortical sensory loss, alien-hand syndrome
Huntington's disease	Chorea, psychosis
Progressive supranuclear palsy	Supranuclear ophthalmoplegia, pseudobulbar palsy, axial dystonia in extension
Systemic disorders	
Cancer	
Brain tumor	Headache, focal neurologic signs, papilledema
Meningeal neoplasia	Focal weakness or sensory deficit, areflexia, pyramidal signs, headache
Infection	
AIDS	Opportunistic infections, memory loss, psychomotor retardation, ataxia, pyramidal signs, white matter lesions on MRI brain scan
Neurosyphilis	Reactive CSF VDRL, psychosis, Argyll-Robertson pupils, facial tremor, strokes, tabes dorsalis
Progressive multifocal leukoencephalopathy	Visual disturbances, white matter lesions on MRI brain scan
Metabolic disorders	
Alcoholism	Prominent memory loss, nystagmus, gait ataxia
Hypothyroidism	Myxedema, hair loss, skin changes, hypothermia, headache, hearing loss, tinnitus, vertigo, ataxia, delayed relaxation of tendon reflexes
Vitamin B_{12} deficiency	Macrocytic anemia, low serum vitamin B_{12} level, psychosis, sensory disturbance, spastic paraparesis
Organ failure	
Dialysis dementia	Dysarthria, myoclonus, seizures
Non-Wilsonian hepatocerebral degeneration	Cirrhosis, esophageal varices, fluctuating mental status, dysarthria, pyramidal and extrapyramidal signs, ataxia
Wilson's disease	Cirrhosis, dysarthria, pyramidal and extrapyramidal signs, ataxia, Kayser-Fleischer pigmented corneal rings, decreased serum ceruloplasmin
Trauma	Headache, variable pyramidal and extrapyramidal signs
Vascular disorders	
Chronic subdural hematoma	Headache, hemiparesis, extraaxial collection on CT or MRI brain scan
Vascular dementia	Hypertension, diabetes, stepwise progression of deficits, hemiparesis, aphasia, infarcts on CT or MRI brain scan
Pseudodementia	
Depression	Depressed mood, anhedonia, anorexia, weight loss, insomnia or hypersomnia, suicidality

to as multiinfarct dementia, is the next most common. Other causes of dementia, including reversible dementias, are comparatively rare.

Treatable Causes of Dementia

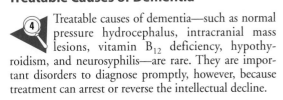 Treatable causes of dementia—such as normal pressure hydrocephalus, intracranial mass lesions, vitamin B_{12} deficiency, hypothyroidism, and neurosyphilis—are rare. They are important disorders to diagnose promptly, however, because treatment can arrest or reverse the intellectual decline.

Other Important Causes of Dementia

Diagnosing dementia caused by Huntington's disease allows patients with this disorder (and their families) to benefit from genetic counseling. If Creutzfeldt-Jakob disease or AIDS dementia complex is diagnosed, precautions can be instituted against transmission; the course of AIDS dementia complex may also be modified by antiviral treatment. Progressive multifocal leukoencephalopathy may indicate underlying immunosuppression from HIV infection, lymphoma, leukemia, or another disorder.

Controversial Causes of Dementia

Some disorders to which dementia is often attributed may not directly cause the disorder. For example, the existence of a primary alcoholic dementia is questionable, since dementia in alcoholic patients may be the result of related problems such as head trauma or nutritional deficiency.

Pseudodementias

About 15% of patients referred for evaluation of possible dementia instead have other disorders (pseudodementias), such as depression. Drug intoxication, commonly cited as a cause of dementia in the elderly, actually produces an acute confusional state, rather than dementia.

CEREBRAL DISORDERS WITHOUT EXTRAPYRAMIDAL FEATURES

ALZHEIMER'S DISEASE

Alzheimer's disease is the most common cause of dementia. Its incidence rises from less than 1% per year to more than 7% per year, and its prevalence from 3% to almost 50%, between the ages of 65 and 85 years. This translates into a prevalence of 10–20 million cases worldwide. Men and women are affected with equal frequency, when adjusted for age.

Alzheimer's disease is a progressive, degenerative disorder of uncertain cause, although abnormal metabolism and deposition of β-**amyloid** protein appears to be closely linked to pathogenesis (see below).

The disease is defined by characteristic histopathologic features, especially neurofibrillary tangles and neuritic (senile) plaques. **Neuritic plaques** are extracellular deposits that contain the proteins β-amyloid, presenilin 1, presenilin 2, α_1-antichymotrypsin, apolipoprotein E, α_2-macroglobulin, and ubiquitin. **Neurofibrillary tangles** are intracellular deposits containing hyperphosphorylated tau (a microtubule-associated protein) and ubiquitin.

Pathogenesis

A. GENETICS

Alzheimer's disease is usually sporadic, but a genetic basis can be identified in about 5% of cases (Table 1–24).

Patients with **trisomy 21** (**Down's syndrome**) have a high incidence of Alzheimer's disease beginning in the fourth decade.

Familial Alzheimer's disease with autosomal dominant inheritance is genetically heterogeneous. In some families there are mutations in the gene for **amyloid precursor protein (APP)** on chromosome 21. In other kindreds, familial Alzheimer's disease has an especially early onset and more virulent course and is linked to mutations in the gene for **presenilin 1,** a transmembrane protein, on chromosome 14. Mutations in another transmembrane protein, **presenilin 2,** have been associated with familial Alzheimer's disease in a German kindred. Some cases of familial Alzheimer's disease are not caused by these defects, and mutations at other sites are presumed responsible.

Genetic factors may also modify susceptibility to Alzheimer's disease without being directly causal. In late-onset familial (and to a lesser extent sporadic) Alzheimer's disease, the risk of being affected and the age at onset are related to the number of **apolipoprotein E ε-4** (*APOE4*) alleles on chromosome 19. How the *APOE4* allele (or the absence of other *APOE* alleles) confers disease susceptibility is unclear. It has been speculated that apolipoprotein E produced by astrocytes may be taken up into neurons and interact abnormally with microtubule-associated proteins, like tau, to produce paired helical filaments in neurofibrillary tangles. Other proteins that may be involved in pathogenesis include α_2-macroglobulin and its receptor, low density lipoprotein-related protein-1.

B. β-AMYLOID

β-Amyloid is the principal constituent of neuritic plaques and is also deposited in cerebral and meningeal blood vessels in Alzheimer's disease. β-Amyloid is a 40- to 42-amino-acid peptide produced by proteolytic cleavage of the transmembrane protein, APP (Figure 1–12). Normal processing of APP involves its cleavage by an enzyme called α-**secretase** to form the 40-amino-acid fragment β-amyloid 1–40, which is secreted and cleared from the brain. In Alzheimer's disease, APP is cleaved abnormally. The first cleavage is in the extracellular region of APP by an enzyme called β-**secretase,** which has been identified as the transmembrane protease **BACE** (β-site APP cleaving enyme). Then γ-**secretase** acts within the transmembrane region to generate the abnormal β-amyloid 1–42, which is secreted and accumulates in extracellular plaques. Presenilins 1 and 2 appear to be involved in this latter cleavage step.

β-Amyloid, especially in its aggregated form, can be toxic to neurons under some circumstances. It has therefore been suggested that the abnormal accumulation of β-amyloid in Alzheimer's disease is responsible for the death of selectively vulnerable neurons. However, others have cited the lack of a clear correlation between the extent of amyloid deposition in the brain and the severity of dementia as evidence against the amyloid hypothesis.

C. CHOLINERGIC DEFICIENCY

Cholinergic neurons are lost and the acetylcholine-synthesizing enzyme **choline acetyltransferase** is markedly depleted in the cerebral cortex and hippocampus of patients with Alzheimer's disease. Degeneration of the nucleus basalis of Meynert (the principal origin of cortical cholinergic innervation) and of the cholinergic septal-hippocampal tract may underlie this abnormality. The cholinergic deficiency in Alzheimer's disease has led to the therapeutic use of acetylcholinesterase inhibitors, which enhance cholinergic neurotransmission by inhibiting acetylcholine breakdown (see below).

Clinical Findings

A. EARLY MANIFESTATIONS

Impairment of recent memory is typically the first sign of Alzheimer's disease—often noticed only by family members. As the memory disorder progresses, the patient becomes disoriented to time and then to place. Aphasia, anomia, and acalculia may develop, forcing the patient to leave work or give up the management of family finances. The depression apparent in the earlier stages of the disorder may give way to an agitated, restless state. Apraxias and visuospatial disorientation ensue, causing the patient to become lost easily. Primitive reflexes are commonly found. A frontal lobe gait disorder may become apparent, with short, slow, shuffling steps, flexed posture, wide base, and difficulty in initiating walking.

B. LATE MANIFESTATIONS

In the late stages, previously preserved social graces are lost, and psychiatric symptoms, including psychosis with paranoia, hallucinations, or delusions, may be prominent. Seizures occur in some cases. Examination at this stage may show extrapyramidal rigidity and bradykinesia. Rare and usually late features of the disease include myoclonus, incontinence, spasticity, extensor plantar responses, and hemiparesis. Mutism, incontinence, and a bedridden state are terminal manifestations, and death typically occurs from 5 to 10 years after the onset of symptoms.

Table 1–24. Genes implicated in Alzheimer's disease.

Gene	Gene Locus	Protein	Genotype	Phenotype
APP	21q21.3–q22.05	Amyloid β A4 precursor protein	Various missense mutations	Familial Alzheimer's disease (autosomal dominant)
PS1	14q24.3	Presenilin 1 (PS1)	Various missense mutations	Familial Alzheimer's disease (autosomal dominant) with early onset (age 35–55)
PS2	1q31–q42	Presenilin 2 (PS2)	Various missense mutations	Familial Alzheimer's disease (autosomal dominant) in Volga Germans
APOE	19q13.2	Apolipoprotein E	APOE4 polymorphism	Increased susceptibility to Alzheimer's disease
Multiple	21	Unknown	Trisomy 21 or chromosome 21-to-14 or 21-to-21 translocation	Down's syndrome (early-onset Alzheimer's disease)

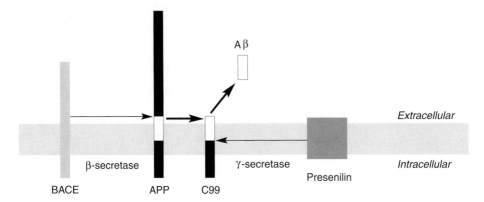

Figure 1–12. Molecular mechanisms of disease: Proteolytic processing of APP to form β-amyloid. (Adapted from Vassar R, Citron M. Aβ-generating enzymes: recent advances in β- and γ-secretase research. Neuron 2000;27:419–422.)

Investigative Studies

Laboratory investigations do not assist in the diagnosis—except to exclude other disorders. The CT scan or MRI often shows cortical atrophy and enlarged ventricles, but such changes may also be seen in elderly nondemented patients. Cognitive testing may be useful in some cases in helping to distingish between Alzheimer's disease and other causes of dementia.

Differential Diagnosis

Early Alzheimer's disease may resemble depression or pure memory disorders such as the Korsakoff amnestic syndrome (see below). More advanced Alzheimer's disease must be distinguished from Lewy body dementia, multiinfarct dementia, Creutzfeldt-Jakob disease, and other dementing disorders (see below).

Treatment

No currently available treatment has been shown unequivocally to reverse existing deficits or to arrest disease progression. Because cholinergic neuronal pathways degenerate and choline acetyltransferase is depleted in the brains of patients with Alzheimer's disease, cholinergic replacement therapy has been used in an effort at symptomatic treatment of cognitive dysfunction (Table 1–25). The acetylcholinesterase inhibitors tacrine, donepezil, rivastigmine, galantamine, physostigmine, metrifonate, and eptastigmine have all been shown to produce small (~5%) improvements in tests of cognitive function. Among these drugs, tacrine, donepezil, rivastigmine, and galantamine are available in the United States. Side effects include nausea, vomiting, diarrhea, and dizziness; tacrine also elevates serum transaminase levels. The better side-effect profile of donepezil and its once-daily dosage schedule have made it the agent of choice. Several drugs have also been tested for their ability to delay the progression of Alzheimer's disease, including α-tocopherol, selegiline, idebenone, propentofylline, *Gingko biloba,* and acetyl-L-carnitine. Of these, only α-tocopherol and selegiline have shown evidence of slight benefit. Antipsychotic drugs, antidepressants, and anxiolytics may be useful in controlling behavioral disturbances associated with Alzheimer's disease.

Prognosis

Early in the course of the disease, patients can usually remain at home and continue social, recreational, and limited professional activities. Early diagnosis can allow patients time to plan orderly retirement from work, to arrange for management of their finances, and to discuss with physicians and family members the management of future medical problems. Patients in advanced stages of the disease may require care in a nursing facility and the use of psychoactive medications. These patients must be protected and prevented from injuring themselves and their families by injudicious actions or decisions. Death from inanition or infection generally occurs 5–10 years after the first symptoms.

FRONTOTEMPORAL DEMENTIA

The frontotemporal dementias, including Pick's disease, can sometimes be distinguished from Alzheimer's disease during life by their generally earlier onset, more prominent behavioral than cognitive dysfunction at presentation, and preferential atrophy of the frontal and anterior

Table 1–25. Drugs used in the treatment of Alzheimer's disease.

Indication	Drug Class	Drug	Dose	Toxicity
Cognitive dysfunction	Acetylcholinesterase inhibitor	Tacrine (Cognex)	10 mg orally four times per day; may be increased to 20 mg orally four times per day after 6 weeks	Abdominal cramps, nausea, vomiting, diarrhea, hepatocellular toxicity (liver enzymes should be monitored twice monthly for 4 months)
		Donepezil (Aricept)	5 mg orally at bedtime; may be increased to 10 mg orally at bedtime after 4–6 weeks	Nausea, diarrhea, vomiting, insomnia, fatigue, muscle cramps, anorexia
		Rivastigmine (Exelon)	1.5–6 mg orally twice per day	Nausea, vomiting, diarrhea, anorexia
		Galantamine (Reminyl)	4–12 mg orally twice per day	Nausea, vomiting, dizziness, diarrhea, anorexia, weight loss
Behavioral disturbance	Antipsychotic	Haloperidol (Haldol)	0.5–2 mg orally at bedtime, or every 4–6 hours	Parkinsonism, akathisia, tardive dyskinesia, increased cognitive dysfunction
		Loxapine (Loxitane)	50–250 mg orally daily	Parkinsonism, akathisia, tardive dyskinesia, increased cognitive dysfunction
		Risperidone (Risperdal)	2–4 mg orally daily	Parkinsonism, akathisia, tardive dyskinesia, increased cognitive dysfunction
		Thioridazine (Mellaril)	25–300 mg orally daily	Parkinsonism, akathisia, tardive dyskinesia, increased cognitive dysfunction
		Thiothixene (Navane)	2–20 mg orally daily	Parkinsonism, akathisia, tardive dyskinesia, increased cognitive dysfunction
	Antidepressant	Citalopram (Celexa)	20–40 mg orally daily	Insomnia, anorexia, ejaculatory failure, nausea, diarrhea
		Fluoxetine (Prozac)	5–20 mg orally with breakfast	Insomnia, anorexia, ejaculatory failure, nausea, diarrhea
		Paroxetine (Paxil)	5–20 mg orally with breakfast, or in two divided daily doses	Insomnia, anorexia, ejaculatory failure, nausea, diarrhea
	Anxiolytic	Carbamazepine (Tegretol)	400–1200 mg orally in two (extended-release form) or four divided doses	Ataxia

Adapted from Mayeux R, Sano M: Treatment of Alzheimer's disease. N Engl J Med 1999;341:1670–1679.

temporal lobes on CT scan or MRI of the brain. However, definitive diagnosis is usually not possible during life, and relies instead on histopathological features. These include the distinctively circumscribed pattern of lobar atrophy, the presence of Pick cells and Pick inclusion bodies, the absence of amyloid plaque and neurofibrillary tangles characteristic of Alzheimer's disease, and inclusions in neurons and glia that contain the microtubule-associated protein, tau. This latter feature accounts for the classification of frontotemporal dementia as a **tauopathy.** Familial occurrence of frontotemporal dementia has been documented and mapped to chomosome 17 (17q21). There is no treatment.

CREUTZFELDT-JAKOB DISEASE

Creutzfeldt-Jakob disease is an invariably fatal transmissible disorder of the central nervous system characterized by rapidly progressive dementia and variable focal involvement of the cerebral cortex, basal ganglia, cerebellum, brainstem, and spinal cord. The annual incidence is about 1:1,000,000 population. The naturally acquired disease occurs in patients 16–82 years of age, with a peak incidence between 60 and 64 years and an equal sex incidence. More than one member of a family is affected in 5–10% of cases. Conjugal cases are rare.

Although transmission from humans to animals has been demonstrated experimentally, documented human-to-human transmission (by corneal transplantation, cortical electrode implantation, or administration of human growth hormone) is rare. The infectious agent is present in the brain, spinal cord, eyes, lungs, lymph nodes, kidneys, spleen, liver, and CSF, but not other body fluids.

Pathogenesis

A proteinaceous infectious particle (**prion**) is the etiologic agent. Familial cases, which are uncommon, have been associated with mutations in a form of the prion protein (cellular isoform, or PrP^c) that is expressed by normal neurons but whose function is unknown. In sporadic cases, an abnormal prion protein (scrapie isoform, or PrP^{Sc}), which differs from PrP^c in its secondary (folding) structure, has been proposed as the infectious agent. In both circumstances, the result is accumulation of abnormal PrP^{Sc} prions in brain tissue. To explain the ability of PrP^{Sc} prions to replicate in the brain (despite the fact that they contain no detectable nucleic acids), it has been suggested that infectious PrP^{Sc} prions induce a conformational change in normally expressed PrP^c prions that converts them to the PrP^{Sc} form.

Prions have also been implicated in diseases of animals and in three other rare human disorders (Table 1–26)—**kuru,** a dementing disease of Fore-speaking tribes of New Guinea (apparently spread by cannibalism); **Gerstmann-Straussler syndrome,** a familial disorder characterized by dementia and ataxia; and **fatal familial insomnia,** which produces disturbances of sleep and of autonomic, motor, and endocrine function.

Clinical Findings

The clinical picture may be that of a diffuse central nervous system disorder or of a more localized dysfunction (Table 1–27). Dementia is present in virtually all cases and may begin as a mild global cognitive impairment or a focal cortical disorder such as aphasia, apraxia, or agnosia. Progression to akinetic mutism or coma typically ensues over a period of months. Psychiatric symptoms including anxiety, euphoria, depression, labile affect, delusions, hallucinations, and changes in personality or behavior may be prominent.

Aside from cognitive abnormalities, the most frequent clinical manifestations are myoclonus (often induced by a startle), extrapyramidal signs (rigidity, bradykinesia, tremor, dystonia, chorea, or athetosis), cerebellar signs, and extrapyramidal signs. Visual field defects, cranial nerve palsies, and seizures occur less often.

A distinct variant of Creutzfeldt-Jakob disease is thought to result from the transmission of **bovine spongiform encephalopathy ("mad cow disease")** to humans. This variant is characterized by earlier onset (mean age, about 30 years), a more prolonged course (greater than 1 year), invariable cerebellar involvement, prominent early psychiatric abnormalities, and diffuse amyloid plaques.

Investigative Studies

The EEG may show periodic sharp waves or spikes (Figure 1–13), which are absent in the variant form described above. CSF protein may be elevated (<100 mg/dL) and levels of 14–3–3, a normal brain protein that is also elevated in herpes simplex virus encephalitis, are increased. MRI scans may show hyperintense signals in the basal ganglia on T_2-weighted images. Definitive diagnosis is by immunodetection of PrP^{Sc} in brain tissue obtained at biopsy or, in familial cases, by detection of mutant forms of PrP^c in DNA from lymphocytes.

Differential Diagnosis

A variety of other disorders must be distinguished from Creutzfeld-Jakob disease. Alzheimer's disease is often a consideration, especially in patients with a less fulminant course and a paucity of cerebellar and extrapyramidal signs. Where subcortical involvement is prominent, Parkinson's disease, cerebellar degeneration, or progressive supranuclear palsy may be suspected. Striking focal signs raise the possibility of an intracerebral mass lesion. Acute metabolic disorders that produce altered mentation and myoclonus (eg, sedative drug withdrawal) can mimic Creutzfeldt-Jakob disease.

Prognosis

No treatment is currently available. The disease is usually relentlessly progressive and, although transient improvement may occur, is invariably fatal. In most sporadic cases, death occurs within 1 year after the onset of symptoms: the mean duration of illness in these patients is 7 months. Depending on the specific mutation present, familial forms of the disease may have similar short or much longer courses.

NORMAL-PRESSURE HYDROCEPHALUS

Normal-pressure hydrocephalus, a potentially reversible cause of dementia, is characterized by the clinical triad of dementia, gait apraxia, and incontinence. It may be idiopathic or secondary to conditions that interfere with cerebrospinal fluid absorption, such as meningitis or subarachnoid hemorrhage. The dementia is often mild and insidious in onset, and is typically preceded by gait

Table 1–26. Prion diseases.[1]

Human diseases
  Creutzfeldt-Jakob disease (sporadic)
  Creutzfeldt-Jakob disease (familial)
  Creutzfeldt-Jakob disease (new variant)
  Fatal familial insomnia
  Gerstmann-Straussler-Scheinker disease
  Kuru
Animal diseases
  Bovine spongiform encephalopathy
  Feline spongiform encephalopathy
  Scrapie (sheep and goats)
  Transmissible mink encephalopathy
  Wasting disease of deer and elk
  Transmissible spongiform encephalopathy of captive wild
    ruminants

[1]Adapted from Johnson RT, Gibbs CJ: Creutzfeldt-Jakob disease and related transmissible spongiform encephalopathies. N Engl J Med 1998;339:1994–2004.

Table 1–27. Clinical features of sporadic Creutzfeldt-Jakob disease.[1]

Feature	Percentage
Cognitive	
Memory loss	100
Behavioral abnormalities	57
Other	73
Motor	
Myoclonus	78
Cerebellar ataxia	71
Pyramidal signs	62
Extrapyramidal signs	56
Lower motor neuron signs	12
Visual disturbances	42
Periodic EEG complexes	60

[1] Data from Brown P et al: Human spongiform encephalopathy: the National Institutes of Health series of 300 cases of experimentally transmitted disease. Ann Neurol 1994;35:513.

disorder and incontinence. It is characterized initially by mental slowness and apathy and later by global cognitive dysfunction. Deterioration of memory is common, but aphasia and agnosia are rare.

Pathophysiology

Normal-pressure hydrocephalus is sometimes called **communicating** (because the lateral, third, and fourth ventricles remain in communication) or **nonobstruc-** tive hydrocephalus (because the flow of CSF between the ventricles is not obstructed). It is presumed to be due to impaired CSF absorption from arachnoid granulations in the subarachnoid space over the convexity of the hemispheres (Figure 1–14), eg, from meningeal fibrosis and adhesions following meningitis or subarachnoid hemorrhage. In contrast, **noncommunicating** or **obstructive hydrocephalus** is caused by a blockade of CSF circulation *within* the ventricular system (eg, by an intraventricular cyst or tumor) and is associated with increased CSF pressure and often with headache and papilledema.

Clinical Findings

Normal-pressure hydrocephalus usually develops over a period of weeks to months; a gait disorder is often the initial manifestation. This typically takes the form of **gait apraxia,** characterized by unsteadiness on standing and difficulty in initiating walking even though there is no weakness or ataxia. The patient can perform the leg movements associated with walking, bicycling, or kicking a ball and can trace figures with the feet while lying or sitting but is unable to do so when the legs are bearing weight. The patient typically appears to be glued to the floor, and walking, once under way, is slow and shuffling. Pyramidal signs, including spasticity, hyperreflexia, and extensor plantar responses, are sometimes present. Motor perseveration (the inappropriate repetition of motor activity) and grasp reflexes in the hands and feet may occur. Urinary incontinence is a later development, and patients may be unaware of it; fecal incontinence is uncommon.

Investigative Studies

Lumbar puncture reveals normal or low opening pressure. The CT scan or MRI typically shows enlarged lateral ventricles without increased prominence of cortical sulci (Figure 1–15). Radionuclide cisternography classically shows isotope accumulation in the ventricles, delayed clearance, and failure of ascent over the cerebral convexities. This pattern is not necessarily present in patients who respond to shunting, however. Transient improvement in gait, cognitive testing, or sphincteric function following the removal of 30–50 mL of CSF by lumbar puncture is probably the best predictor of a favorable clinical response to shunting (see below).

Differential Diagnosis

A variety of conditions that produce dementia must be considered in the differential diagnosis. Alzheimer's disease tends to follow a longer course, often with prominent focal cortical dysfunction and enlarged cortical sulci shown in a CT scan or MRI. Parkinsonism may be

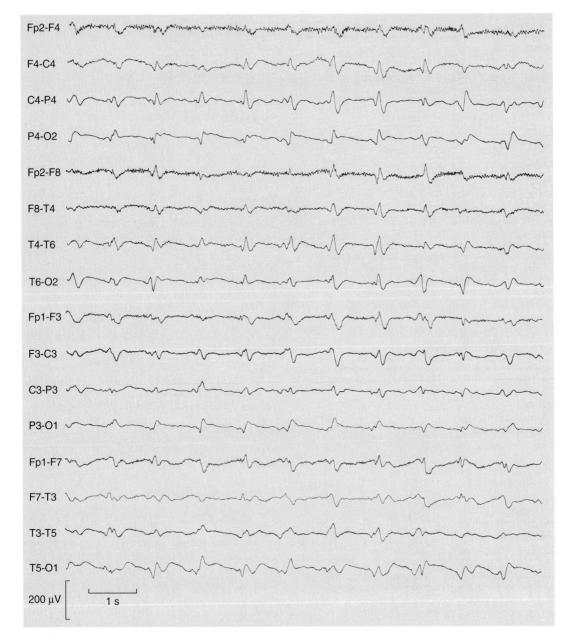

Figure 1–13. Electroencephalogram of a patient with Creutzfeldt-Jakob disease, showing triphasic waves with sharpened outlines; these occur repetitively about once every second.

simulated by the gait disorder but can be distinguished by extrapyramidal rigidity, tremor, and response to antiparkinsonian medications. Vascular dementia should be suspected if the disorder follows a stepwise course, or pseudobulbar palsy, focal sensorimotor signs, or a history of stroke is encountered.

Treatment

Some patients, especially those with hydrocephalus from meningitis or subarachnoid hemorrhage, recover or improve following ventriculoatrial, ventriculoperitoneal, or lumboperitoneal shunting. In idiopathic nor-

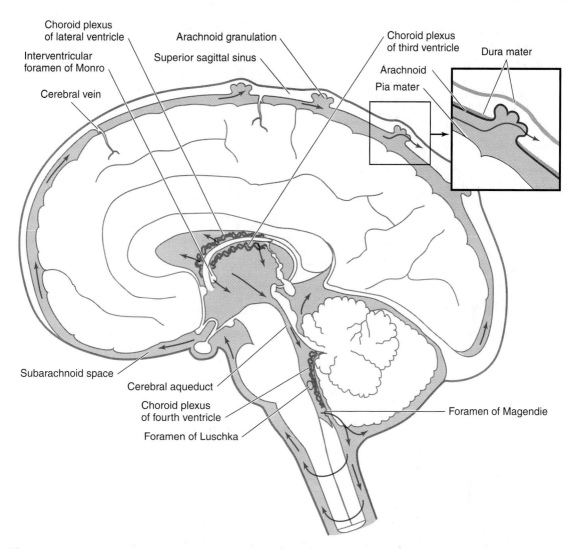

Figure 1–14. Circulation of cerebrospinal fluid (CSF). CSF is produced by the choroid plexus, which consists of specialized secretory tissue located within the cerebral ventricles. It flows from the lateral and third ventricles through the cerebral aqueduct and fourth ventricle and exits the ventricular system through two laterally situated foramina of Luschka and a single, medially located foramen of Magendie. CSF then enters and circulates through the subarachnoid space surrounding the brain and spinal cord. It is ultimately absorbed through arachnoid granulations into the venous circulation.

mal-pressure hydrocephalus, about one-half of patients have sustained improvement and about one-third have a good or excellent response (ie, return to work) after shunting. As noted above, a favorable response to the removal of CSF by lumbar puncture may be the best predictor of successful surgery. Complications of shunting occur in about one-third of patients and include shunt infection, subdural hematoma, and shunt malfunction that necessitates replacement.

CEREBRAL DISORDERS WITH EXTRAPYRAMIDAL FEATURES

DEMENTIA WITH LEWY BODIES

Dementia with Lewy bodies is probably the second most common cause of dementia, as up to one-fourth of elderly demented patients who come to autopsy have round, eosinophilic, intracytoplasmic neuronal inclu-

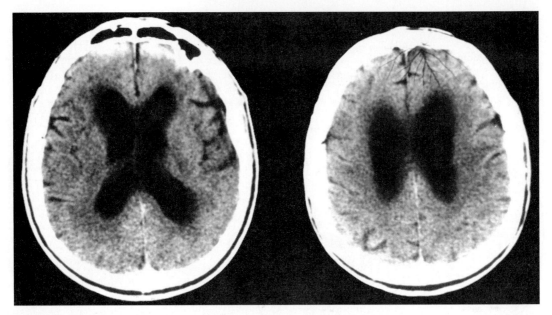

Figure 1–15. CT scan at two levels in normal-pressure hydrocephalus, showing enlarged lateral ventricles without enlargement of the cortical sulci.

sions (**Lewy bodies**) in the cerebral cortex and brainstem. These contain α-synuclein, a protein that is also found in Lewy bodies in Parkinson's disease, and tau, which is present in Alzheimer's disease and frontotemporal dementia (see above). Dementia with Lewy bodies is found in patients with (Lewy-body variant of Alzheimer's disease) and without (diffuse Lewy-body disease) histopathological features of Alzheimer's disease, and is probably a heterogeneous disorder. In contrast to Alzheimer's disease, it is characterized clinically by cognitive decline without prominent early memory impairment. Other distinctive features include fluctuating cognitive ability, well-formed visual hallucinations, and signs of parkinsonism, especially rigidity and bradykinesia. These patients may respond well to anticholinesterase drugs such as tacrine or donepezil (Table 1–25), but are especially sensitive to extrapyramidal side effects of antipsychotic drugs, which should therefore be avoided or used with caution.

CORTICOBASAL GANGLIONIC DEGENERATION

This dementing disorder is also associated with parkinsonism, especially rigidity, bradykinesia, postural instability, and action (but rarely resting) tremor, as well as with a variety of asymmetric cortical motor and sensory defects. These include apraxias affecting the eye movements, speech, and limbs, the latter of which may pro-

duce the alien-hand sign, in which the limb moves seemingly of its own accord.

HUNTINGTON'S DISEASE

Huntington's disease is an autosomal dominant heredodegenerative condition characterized by a movement disorder, psychiatric symptoms, and dementia. The cause is an expanded CAG trinucleotide repeat coding for a polyglutamine tract in the huntingtin gene on chromosome 4 (4p16.3).

Dementia, which usually becomes apparent after chorea and psychiatric symptoms have been present for a few years, precedes chorea in about one-fourth of cases. A memory disturbance affecting all aspects of memory is an early and prominent feature; aphasia, apraxia, agnosia, and global cognitive dysfunction tend to occur later. Huntington's disease is discussed further in Chapter 7.

PROGRESSIVE SUPRANUCLEAR PALSY

Progressive supranuclear palsy is an idiopathic degenerative disorder that primarily affects subcortical gray matter regions of the brain. The classic clinical features are supranuclear ophthalmoplegia, pseudobulbar palsy, axial dystonia with or without extrapyramidal rigidity of the limbs, and dementia. The disorder of movement is a conspicuous feature of this syndrome, which is discussed further in Chapter 7.

SYSTEMIC DISORDERS

CANCER

1. Brain Tumor

Brain tumors produce dementia and related syndromes by a combination of local and diffuse effects, including edema, compression of adjacent brain structures, increased intracranial pressure, and impairment of cerebral blood flow. The tumors most likely to produce generalized cerebral syndromes are gliomas arising in the frontal or temporal lobes or the corpus callosum. Although such lesions tend to infiltrate subcortical white matter extensively, they initially give rise to few focal neurologic signs.

The dementia associated with brain tumor is characterized by prominent mental slowness, apathy, impaired concentration, and subtle alterations in personality. Depending on the areas of involvement, memory disorder, aphasia, or agnosia may be seen early. Brain tumors ultimately produce headache, seizures, or focal sensorimotor disturbances. Brain tumor is covered in detail in Chapter 2.

2. Meningeal Neoplasia

Meningeal neoplasia, discussed above (see p. 39) as a cause of confusional states, may also produce dementia that is commonly associated with headache as well as symptoms and signs of dysfunction at multiple sites in the nervous system. The diagnosis is established by cytologic studies of the CSF.

INFECTION

1. AIDs

AIDS dementia complex is the most common neurologic complication of AIDS. Although especially common in severely immunosuppressed patients late in the course of the disease, it can also be an early or presenting manifestation.

Pathogenesis

AIDS dementia complex results from invasion of the brain by a retrovirus, **human immunodeficiency virus type 1** (**HIV-1**). The virus appears to reach the central nervous system early in the course of systemic HIV-1 infection; monocytes, macrophages, and microglia are the principal cell types affected. Neurologic involvement at this stage may be asymptomatic, or it can produce transient symptomatic HIV-1 meningitis (see above). The infection then seems to be contained until progressive immunosuppression impairs the normal host defense mechanisms, leading to increased HIV-1 production in the brain and, perhaps, the emergence of neurotropic strains. Productive viral infection within the brain seems to be associated with multinucleated cells.

HIV-1 does not appear to replicate within neurons, astrocytes, or oligodendrocytes *in vivo*, and the loss of these cell types is not prominent in brains of patients with AIDS dementia complex. It has therefore been suggested that neuronal function is impaired by an indirect neurotoxic mechanism. This might involve cytokines released from HIV-infected monocytes or macrophages, viral products such as the HIV-1 envelope protein gp120, or molecules that mimic the effects of excitotoxic amino acids.

Pathology

The earliest histopathologic sign is pallor of subcortical and periventricular cerebral white matter associated with reactive astrocytosis but few inflammatory changes. More advanced cases are associated with parenchymal and perivascular infiltration by macrophages, microglia, lymphocytes, and multinucleated cells; the last are thought to result from the virus-induced fusion of macrophages. These changes affect the white matter, basal ganglia, thalamus, and pons and are accompanied by reactive astrocytosis. Spongy vacuolation of white matter occurs infrequently. Neuronal loss has been reported. The spinal cord may also be affected by a vacuolar myelopathy (see Chapter 5) resembling that caused by vitamin B_{12} deficiency.

Clinical Findings

The onset is usually insidious and is associated with cognitive and behavioral symptoms, such as forgetfulness, apathy, social withdrawal, and motor symptoms, including impaired balance, leg weakness, and deterioration of handwriting (Table 1–28). Examination at this early stage may also show cerebellar ataxia, pyramidal signs such as hyperreflexia and extensor plantar responses, weakness in one or both legs, postural tremor, and dysarthria. As the disease progresses, hypertonia, fecal and urinary incontinence, primitive reflexes, myoclonus, seizures, quadriparesis, and organic psychosis with delusions and visual hallucinations can occur.

Investigative Studies

Antibodies to HIV are detectable in the blood. The CSF is usually abnormal and may show a mild to moderate elevation of protein (<200 mg/dL), a modest, usually mononuclear pleocytosis (<50 cells/μL), and oligoclonal bands. CT scans and MRI usually demonstrate cerebrocortical atrophy with ventricular dilation and may also show diffuse involvement of subcortical white matter (Figure 1–16).

Table 1–28. Clinical features of AIDS dementia complex.[1]

Feature	Percentage of Patients	
	Early Stage	Late Stage
Symptoms		
Memory loss	80	74
Behavioral changes (eg, social withdrawal)	30	11
Depression	30	16
Motor symptoms (eg, imbalance, weakness, deteriorated handwriting)	20	21
Apathy	15	58
Confusion	15	42
Hallucinations	5	11
Signs		
Cognitive		
Psychomotor retardation	61	84
Dementia	39	100
Psychosis	5	16
Mutism	0	40
Motor		
Ataxia	34	71
Hypertonia	22	44
Tremor	16	45
Paraparesis or quadriparesis	13	33
Monoparesis or hemiparesis	5	2
Myoclonus	0	20
Other		
Hyperreflexia	36	78
Primitive reflexes	22	38
Seizures	7	20
Incontinence	0	47
Investigative studies[2]		
CSF		
Mononuclear pleocytosis	19	
Increased protein	66	
Decreased glucose	1	
Oligoclonal IgG bands	25	
Imaging		
Cerebral cortical atrophy (CT)	79	
Cerebral cortical atrophy (MRI)	55	
White matter lesions (CT)	11	
White matter lesions (MRI)	35	

[1] Adapted from Navia BA et al: The AIDS dementia complex. 1. Clinical features. 2. Neuropathology. Ann Neurol 1986; 19:517–524 and 525–535, and McArthur JC: Neurologic manifestations of AIDS. Medicine 1987;66:407–437.

[2] All stages.

Treatment

Combination pharmacotherapy of HIV infection can prolong life by inhibiting replication of HIV and improving immue function. The available drugs fall into three classes: nucleoside reverse transcriptase inhibitors (abacavir, didanosine, lamivudine, stavudine, zalcitabine, zidovudine), nonnucleoside reverse transcriptase inhibitors (delavirdine, efavirenz, nevirapine), and protease inhibitors (amprenavir, indinavir, nelfinavir, ritonavir, saquinavir). Most drug combinations used clinically include two nucleosides together with either a nonnucleoside or a protease inhibitor.

Side effects vary, but certain class-specific patterns have been noted. Nucleosides can cause fatal lactic acidosis with hepatic steatosis, nonnucleosides are associated with skin rash (including Stevens-Johnson syndrome with nevirapine), and protease inhibitors may produce gastrointestinal disturbances and increased blood levels of aminotransferases. Neurologic side effects of drugs used to treat HIV include myopathy (zidovudine), neuropathy (stavudine, didanosine, zalcitabine), paresthesias (ritonavir, amprenavir), and nightmares and hallucinations (efavirenz).

Prognosis

The course may be steadily progressive, or it can be acutely exacerbated by concurrent pulmonary infection. Patients usually die 1–9 months after the onset of dementia from aspiration or opportunistic infection.

2. Neurosyphilis

Neurosyphilis was a common cause of dementia before the widespread use of penicillin permitted effective treatment of early syphilis. Dementia from neurosyphilis is now rare, but the resurgence of syphilis in recent years suggests that it may become more common.

Clinical Findings

A. Early Syphilis

Syphilis is caused by *Treponema pallidum* transmitted by sexual contact, which results in infection in about one-third of encounters with infected individuals. Primary syphilis is characterized by local skin lesions (chancres) that usually appear within 1 month of exposure. There are no neurologic symptoms. Hematogenous spread of *T pallidum* produces symptoms and signs of secondary syphilis within 1–6 months. These include fever, skin rash, alopecia, anogenital skin lesions, and ulceration of mucous membranes; neurologic symptoms are still uncommon at this stage. **Meningeal syphilis,** the earliest form of symptomatic neurosyphilis, is most often

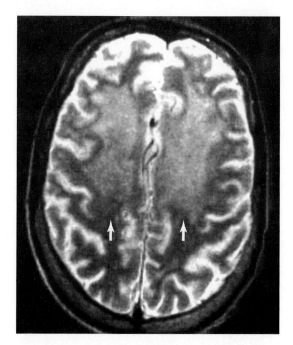

Figure 1–16. T2-weighted MRI in AIDS dementia complex, showing extensive, bilaterally symmetrical increases in signal intensity **(arrows)** in white matter (centrum semiovale) of the frontal lobes.

seen 2–12 months after primary infection. Clinical features include headache, stiff neck, nausea and vomiting, and cranial nerve (especially II, VII, or VIII) involvement.

B. Meningovascular Syphilis

This delayed manifestation of neurosyphilis occurs 4–7 years into the course of the disease and usually presents with transient ischemic attacks or stroke (see Chapter 9).

C. Late (Parenchymatous) Neurosyphilis

This produces the syndromes of general paresis and tabes dorsalis, which can occur separately or together (taboparesis); either one can occur in combination with optic atrophy.

1. **General paresis**—A chronic meningoencephalitis caused by active spirochetal infection, this was the usual cause of dementia and psychiatric disorders related to neurosyphilis in the prepenicillin era. Onset is with gradual memory loss or altered affect, personality, or behavior. This is followed by global intellectual deterioration with grandiosity, depression, psychosis, and focal weakness. Terminal features include incontinence, seizures, or strokes. Neurologic examination may show

tremor of the face and tongue, paucity of facial expression, dysarthria, and pyramidal signs.

2. **Taboparesis**—In taboparesis—the coexistence of tabes dorsalis (see Chapter 6) with general paresis—signs and symptoms include Argyll Robertson pupils (see Chapter 4), lancinating pains, areflexia, posterior column sensory deficits with sensory ataxia and Romberg's sign, incontinence, impotence, Charcot (hypertrophic) joints, and genu recurvatum (hyperextended knees). Optic atrophy may also be present.

Investigative Studies

Treponemal serologic blood tests (FTA-ABS or MHA-TP) are reactive in almost all patients with active neurosyphilis, but nontreponemal blood tests (VDRL or RPR) can be negative; therefore, a treponemal blood test should be obtained in all suspected cases. If this is nonreactive, neurosyphilis is effectively excluded; if it is reactive, lumbar puncture should be performed to confirm the diagnosis of neurosyphilis and provide a baseline CSF profile against which to gauge the efficacy of subsequent treatment. The CSF in active neurosyphilis shows a lymphocytic pleocytosis and reactive nontreponemal CSF serology in almost all cases. The exceptions are acute syphilitic meningitis and meningovascular syphilis, in which pleocytosis may precede seroconversion so that nontreponemal CSF tests are falsely negative early on, and end-stage tabes dorsalis, in which the CSF can be normal. Other CSF abnormalities include protein elevation, increased γ-globulin, and the presence of oligoclonal bands.

Treatment

Neurosyphilis is treated with a 10-day course of aqueous penicillin G, $2–4 \times 10^6$ units intravenously every 4 hours. Tetracycline or erythromycin can be used for patients allergic to penicillin. Fever and leukocytosis may occur shortly after therapy is started (**Herxheimer's reaction**) but are transient. Failure of the CSF to return to normal within 6 months requires retreatment. Neither failure of treatment nor relapse is convincingly more common in HIV-1-infected patients.

Prognosis

After penicillin (or other antibiotic) treatment for general paresis, the clinical condition may improve or stabilize; in some cases it continues to deteriorate. Patients with persistent CSF abnormalities or symptomatic progression despite therapy should be retreated. Patients with reactive CSF serological tests but no pleocytosis are unlikely to respond to penicillin therapy but are usually treated nevertheless.

3. Progressive Multifocal Leukoencephalopathy

Progressive multifocal leukoencephalopathy results from infection with a papovavirus called **JC virus**. Antibodies are present in most adults, but symptomatic infection is rare. It is most common in patients with AIDS, lymphoma or leukemia, carcinoma, sarcoidosis, tuberculosis, or pharmacologic immunosuppression following organ transplantation, and rare in those with normal immune function. The virus infects oligodendrocytes, leading to diffuse and patchy demyelination that primarily affects white matter of the cerebral hemispheres but also involves the brainstem and cerebellum.

The course is subacute and progressive, leading to death in 3–6 months. Fever and systemic symptoms are absent. Dementia and focal cortical dysfunction are prominent. Signs of the latter include hemiparesis, visual deficits, aphasia, dysarthria, and sensory impairment. Ataxia and headache are uncommon and seizures do not occur.

The CSF is usually normal but may show a mild increase in pressure, white cell count, or protein. The CT scan or MRI shows multifocal white matter abnormalities (Figure 1–17). When the diagnosis is in doubt, it can be established by brain biopsy.

The disorder is almost uniformly fatal, and treatment with such antiviral agents as cytosine arabinoside, adenine arabinoside, or amantadine has generally been unsuccessful.

METABOLIC DISORDERS

1. Alcoholism

Certain complications of alcoholism can cause dementia. These include acquired hepatocerebral degeneration from alcoholic liver disease, chronic subdural hematoma from head trauma, and nutritional deficiency states.

Pellagra, caused by deficiency of nicotinic acid (niacin), affects neurons in the cerebral cortex, basal ganglia, brainstem, cerebellum, and anterior horns of the spinal cord. Systemic involvement is manifested by diarrhea, glossitis, anemia, and erythematous skin lesions. Neurologic involvement may produce dementia; psychosis; confusional states; pyramidal, extrapyramidal, and cerebellar signs; polyneuropathy; and optic neuropathy. Treatment is with nicotinamide, but the neurologic deficits may persist despite treatment.

Marchiafava Bignami syndrome is characterized by necrosis of the corpus callosum and subcortical white matter and occurs most often in malnourished alcoholics. The course can be acute, subacute, or chronic. Clinical features include dementia, spasticity, dysarthria, gait disorder, and coma. The diagnosis can sometimes be made by CT scan or MRI. No specific treatment is available, but cessation of drinking and improvement of nutrition are advised. The outcome is variable: patients may die, survive with dementia, or recover.

Alcoholic dementia due to direct toxic effects of ethanol on the brain has been proposed to occur, but no distinctive abnormalities have been identified in the brains of demented alcoholics. Dementia in alcoholics is more likely to result from one or more of the metabolic and traumatic disorders mentioned above.

2. Hypothyroidism

Hypothyroidism (myxedema), which is discussed above as a cause of acute confusional states, can also produce a reversible dementia or chronic organic psychosis. The dementia is a global disorder characterized by mental slowness, memory loss, and irritability. Focal cortical deficits do not occur. Psychiatric manifestations are typically prominent and include depression, paranoia, visual and auditory hallucinations, mania, and suicidal behavior.

Patients with myxedema may complain of headache, hearing loss, tinnitus, vertigo, weakness, or paresthesia. Examination may show deafness, dysarthria, or cerebellar ataxia. The most suggestive finding is delayed relaxation of the tendon reflexes. Diagnosis and treatment are discussed above (see p. 16). Cognitive dysfunction is usually reversible with treatment.

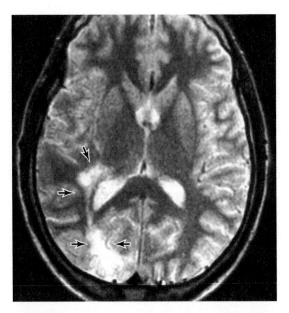

Figure 1–17. T2-weighted MRI in progressive multifocal leukoencephalopathy, showing abnormally high signal intensity **(arrows)** in white matter of the right parietal and occipital lobes. (Courtesy of A Gean.)

3. *Vitamin B₁₂ Deficiency*

Vitamin B_{12} deficiency is a rare cause of reversible dementia and organic psychosis. Like the acute confusional state associated with vitamin B_{12} deficiency (see above), dementia can occur with or without hematologic and other neurologic manifestations. The dementia consists of global cognitive dysfunction with mental slowness, impaired concentration, and memory disturbance; aphasia and other focal cortical disorders do not occur. Psychiatric manifestations are often prominent and include depression, mania, and paranoid psychosis with visual and auditory hallucinations. Laboratory findings and treatment are discussed above (see p. 19).

ORGAN FAILURE

1. *Dialysis Dementia*

This rare disorder typically occurs in patients receiving chronic hemodialysis. Clinical features include dysarthria, myoclonus, and seizures. These are initially intermittent, but later become permanent, and dementia supervenes. The EEG shows paroxysmal high-voltage slowing with intermixed spikes and slow waves; these abnormalities can be reversed by diazepam. Aluminum in the dialysate is a major etiologic suspect, and removing trace metals from the dialysate has decreased the syndrome's incidence. Mean survival is 6 months.

2. *Non-Wilsonian Hepatocerebral Degeneration*

Acquired (non-Wilsonian) hepatocerebral degeneration is an uncommon complication of chronic hepatic cirrhosis with spontaneous or surgical portosystemic shunting. Symptoms may be related to failure of the liver to detoxify ammonia. Neurologic symptoms precede hepatic symptoms in about one-sixth of patients.

Clinical Findings

Systemic manifestations of chronic liver disease are usually present. The neurologic syndrome is fluctuating but progressive over 1–9 years, and may be punctuated by episodes of acute hepatic encephalopathy (see p. 19). Dementia, dysarthria, and cerebellar, extrapyramidal, and pyramidal signs are the most common features. Dementia is marked by mental slowness, apathy, impaired attention and concentration, and memory disturbance. Cerebellar signs include gait and limb ataxia and dysarthria; nystagmus is rare. Extrapyramidal involvement may produce rigidity, resting tremor, dystonia, chorea, or athetosis. Asterixis, myoclonus, hyperreflexia, and extensor plantar responses are common; paraparesis is rare.

Laboratory studies show abnormal hepatic blood chemistries and elevated blood ammonia, but the degree of abnormality bears no direct relationship to the severity of neurologic symptoms. The CSF is normal, except for increased glutamine and occasional mild elevation of protein.

Differential Diagnosis

Wilson's disease can be distinguished by its earlier onset, Kayser-Fleischer rings and abnormal copper metabolism. Alcoholic cerebellar degeneration primarily affects gait and is not accompanied by extrapyramidal or pyramidal signs.

Treatment & Prognosis

Patients may benefit from a low-protein diet, lactulose, neomycin, liver transplantation, or portosystemic shunting, and improvement following levodopa or bromocriptine therapy has been described. Death results from progressive liver failure or variceal bleeding.

3. *Wilson's Disease*

Wilson's disease (hepatolenticular degeneration) is a rare but treatable autosomal recessive hereditary disorder of copper metabolism that produces dementia and extrapyramidal symptoms. The disease results from mutations in the ATP7B gene on chromosome 13 (13q14.3–q21.1), which codes for the β polypeptide of a copper-transporting ATPase. Wilson's disease is discussed further in Chapter 7.

TRAUMA

Severe open or closed head injury, particularly when followed by prolonged unconsciousness, may cause impaired memory and concentration, personality changes, headache, focal neurologic disorders, or seizures. Cognitive impairment is nonprogressive, and the cause is usually obvious. Delayed, progressive posttraumatic dementia in boxers (**dementia pugilistica**) is characterized by cheerful or labile affect, mental slowness, memory deficit, and irritability. Associated neurologic abnormalities include tremor, rigidity, bradykinesia, dysarthria, cerebellar ataxia, pyramidal signs, and seizures. Neuroradiologic investigations may show cortical atrophy and cavum septi pellucidi.

VASCULAR DISORDERS

1. *Chronic Subdural Hematoma*

Chronic subdural hematoma usually affects patients aged 50–70 years, often after minor head trauma. Other risk factors include alcoholism, cerebral atrophy, epilepsy, the use of anticoagulation, ventricular shunts, and long-term hemodialysis. The onset of symptoms may be delayed for months after trauma. Hematomas are bilateral in about one-sixth of cases.

Clinical Findings

Headache is the initial symptom in most patients. Confusion, dementia, hemiparesis, and vomiting may ensue. The most frequent signs are cognitive disturbance, hemiparesis, papilledema, and extensor plantar responses. Aphasia, visual field defects, and seizures are uncommon, but can occur.

The hematoma can usually be seen on CT scan or MRI (Figure 1–18) as an extraaxial crescent-shaped area of decreased density, with ipsilateral obliteration of cortical sulci and often ventricular compression. The scan should be carefully reviewed for evidence of bilateral subdural collections. Isodense collections may become more apparent after contrast infusion. In a few cases, demonstration of the hematoma may require cerebral arteriography, which should always be undertaken bilaterally.

Treatment

Unless contraindicated by medical problems or spontaneous improvement, symptomatic hematomas should be surgically evacuated.

2. Vascular Dementia

Vascular dementia is thought to be the third most common cause of dementia, after Alzheimer's disease and dementia with Lewy bodies. Most patients with this diagnosis have either multiple large cortical infarcts from occlusion of major cerebral arteries or several smaller infarcts (**lacunar state**; see Chapter 9) affecting subcortical white matter, basal ganglia, or thalamus.

The relationship between cerebral vascular disease and dementia is poorly characterized. For example, the number of strokes, their locations, and the total infarct volume required for strokes to produce dementia are uncertain, making it often difficult to determine if strokes are the cause of dementia in a given patient. Whether dementia can result from cerebrovascular disease without frank infarction, as is commonly presumed to exist when periventricular white matter lesions are detected by neuroimaging, is also controversial. Thus, the absence of neuroradiologic signs of cerebrovascular disease argues strongly against a vascular basis for dementia, but the presence of vascular lesions does not prove that they are causal. This is especially true when another cause of dementia, such as Alzheimer's disease, coexists with cerebrovascular disease.

Clinical Findings

As classically described, patients with multiinfarct dementia have a history of hypertension, a stepwise progression of deficits, a more or less abrupt onset of dementia, and focal neurologic symptoms or signs. Because extensive pathologic changes may already exist at presentation, it is assumed that patients can remain functionally well compensated until a new and perhaps otherwise innocuous infarct tips the balance.

The neurologic examination commonly shows pseudobulbar palsy with dysarthria, dysphagia, and pathologic emotionality (**pseudobulbar affect**), focal motor and sensory deficits, ataxia, gait apraxia, hyperreflexia, and extensor plantar responses.

Investigative Studies

The MRI (Figure 1–19) may show multiple small subcortical lucencies. Extensive areas of low density in subcortical white matter are seen in **Binswanger's disease** (**subcortical arteriosclerotic encephalopathy**), which may be a related condition. MRI is more sensitive than CT for detecting these abnormalities.

Additional laboratory studies should be performed to exclude cardiac emboli, polycythemia, thrombocytosis, cerebral vasculitis, and meningovascular syphilis as causes of multiple infarctions, particularly in younger patients or those without a history of hypertension.

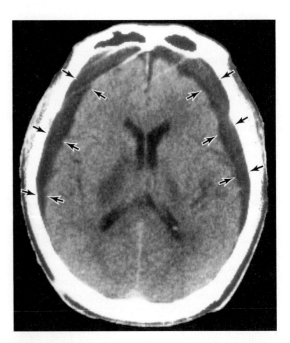

Figure 1–18. CT scan in chronic subdural hematoma, showing bilateral low-density collections between the inner table of the skull and the cerebral hemispheres (**arrows**).

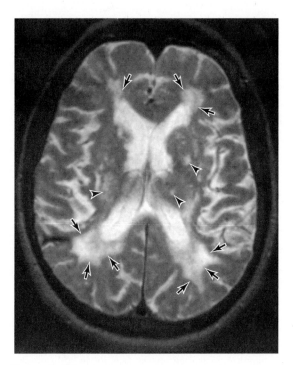

Figure 1–19. T2-weighted MRI in multiinfarct dementia, showing foci of abnormal high signal intensity adjacent to the lateral ventricles **(arrows)** and within the basal ganglia **(arrowheads)**.

Treatment

Hypertension, when present, should be treated to reduce the incidence of subsequent infarction and to prevent other end-organ diseases. Antiplatelet agents (discussed in Chapter 9) may help to reduce the risk of future strokes.

PSEUDODEMENTIA

Depression is the disorder most commonly mistaken for dementia. Because depression is common and usually treatable, distinguishing between the two conditions is important. Both dementia and depression can be characterized by mental slowness, apathy, self-neglect, withdrawal, irritability, difficulty with memory and concentration, and changes in behavior and personality. In addition, depression can be a feature of dementing illnesses, and the two frequently coexist. Clinical features that help in the differentiation are listed in Table 1–29. When depression is being considered, psychiatric consultation should be obtained. If depression is identified as a significant problem and is not correctable by treatment of an underlying disease or by a change in medication, it should be treated directly. Modes of treatment include psychotherapy, tricyclic and related antidepressants, selective serotonin reuptake inhibitors, monoamine oxidase inhibitors, and electroconvulsive therapy.

■ IV. AMNESTIC SYNDROMES

A disorder of memory (**amnestic syndrome**) may occur as one feature of an acute confusional state or dementia, or as an isolated abnormality (Table 1–30). The latter condition is discussed in this section.

Memory

Memory is a complex function that can be viewed for clinical purposes as comprising phases of **registration**, **storage**, and **retrieval**. Autopsy and imaging studies of the brains of patients with memory disorders suggest that the hippocampus and related structures, such as the dorsomedial nucleus of the thalamus, are important in

Table 1–29. Dementia and the pseudodementia of depression: distinguishing features.

Dementia	Depression
Insidious onset	Abrupt onset
Progressive deterioration	Plateau of dysfunction
No history of depression	History of depression may exist
Patient typically unaware of extent of deficits and does not complain of memory loss	Patient aware of and may exaggerate deficits and frequently complains of memory loss
Somatic complaints uncommon	Somatic complaints or hypochondriasis common
Variable affect	Depressed affect
Few vegetative symptoms	Prominent vegetative symptoms
Impairment often worse at night	Impairment usually not worse at night
Neurologic examination and laboratory studies may be abnormal	Neurologic examination and laboratory studies normal

Table 1–30. Causes of amnestic syndromes.

Acute
    Accompanying acute confusional states
    Head trauma
    Hypoxia or ischemia
    Bilateral posterior cerebral artery occlusion
    Transient global amnesia
    Alcoholic blackouts
    Wemicke's encephalopathy
    Dissociative (psychogenic) amnesia
Chronic
    Accompanying dementias
    Alcoholic Korsakoff amnestic syndrome
    Postencephalitic amnesia
    Brain tumor
    Paraneoplastic limbic encephalitits

---

memory processing. Bilateral damage to these regions results in impairment of **short-term memory,** which is manifested clinically by the inability to form new memories. **Long-term memory,** which involves retrieval of previously learned information, is relatively preserved, perhaps because well-established memories are stored diffusely in the cerebral cortex. Some patients with amnestic syndromes may attempt to fill in gaps in memory with false recollections (**confabulation**), which can take the form of elaborate contrivances or of genuine memories misplaced in time. The longest-standing and most deeply ingrained memories, however, such as one's own name, are almost always spared in organic memory

disturbances. In contrast, such personal memories may be prominently or exclusively impaired in **dissociative (psychogenic) amnesia.**

The cellular basis of memory is poorly understood, but repetitive neuronal firing produces lasting pre- and postsynaptic changes that facilitate neurotransmission at hippocampal synapses (**long-term potentiation**). These changes appear to involve the release of glutamate, which stimulates the entry of calcium into postsynaptic neurons, and the production of retrograde signals that act on presynaptic nerve terminals to increase transmitter release upon subsequent firing.

ACUTE AMNESIA

HEAD TRAUMA

Head injuries resulting in loss of consciousness are invariably associated with an amnestic syndrome. Patients seen shortly after such an injury exhibit a confusional state in which they are unable to incorporate new memories (**anterograde, or posttraumatic amnesia;** see Figure 1–20), although they may behave in an apparently normal automatic fashion. In addition, **retrograde amnesia** is present, covering a variable period prior to the trauma. Features characteristic of **transient global amnesia** (see below) may be seen.

As full consciousness returns, the ability to form new memories is restored. Events occurring in the confusional interval tend to be permanently lost to memory, however. Exceptions are islands of memory, for a lucid interval

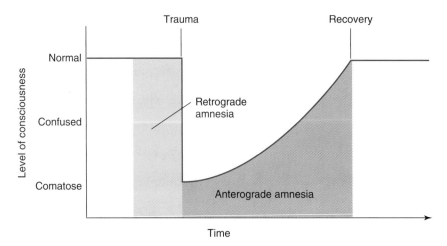

Figure 1–20. Retrograde and anterograde amnesia in posttraumatic memory disorders. Head trauma may produce transient coma, followed by a confusional state during which the patient is unable to form new memories. With recovery, this ability is restored, but there is persistent amnesia for the period of coma and confusion (**anterograde amnesia**) and for a variable period preceding the trauma (**retrograde amnesia**); the latter deficit may improve with time.

between trauma and unconsciousness, or for periods of lesser impairment in the course of a fluctuating posttraumatic confusional state. The period of retrograde amnesia begins to shrink, with the most remote memories the first to return. The severity of the injury tends to correlate with the duration of confusion and with the extent of permanent retrograde and posttraumatic amnesia.

HYPOXIA OR ISCHEMIA

Because of the selective vulnerability of pyramidal neurons in the Sommer sector (h1 sector of Scholz) of the hippocampus, conditions resulting in cerebral hypoxia or ischemia, such as cardiac arrest or carbon monoxide poisoning, can produce amnestic syndromes. Amnesia tends to occur in patients in whom coma has lasted at least 12 hours. There is severe impairment of the ability to incorporate new memories, with relative preservation of registration and remote memory; patients typically appear to have an isolated disorder of short-term memory. A period of retrograde amnesia preceding the insult may occur. Patients exhibit a lack of concern about their impairment and sometimes confabulate. Amnesia following cardiac arrest may be the sole manifestation of neurologic dysfunction, or it may coexist with other cerebral watershed syndromes, such as bibrachial paresis, cortical blindness, or visual agnosia (see Chapter 9). Recovery often occurs within several days, although deficits may persist.

Amnestic syndromes from **carbon monoxide poisoning** are frequently associated with affective disturbances. Other associated abnormalities include focal cortical and extrapyramidal dysfunction. Acute carbon monoxide poisoning is suggested by cherry-red coloration of the skin and mucous membranes, elevated carboxyhemoglobin levels, or cardiac arrhythmia. The CT brain scan may show lucencies in the basal ganglia and dentate nuclei.

BILATERAL POSTERIOR CEREBRAL ARTERY OCCLUSION

The posterior cerebral artery supplies the medial temporal lobe, thalamus, posterior internal capsule, and occipital cortex (Figure 1–21). Ischemia or infarction in this territory, typically when bilateral, may produce a transient or permanent amnestic syndrome. Emboli in the vertebrobasilar system (see Chapter 9) are frequent causes of such disorders.

The amnestic syndrome is usually associated with unilateral or bilateral hemianopia and sometimes with visual agnosia, alexia without agraphia, anomia, sensory disturbances, or signs of upper midbrain dysfunction (especially impaired pupillary light reflex). Recent memory tends to be selectively impaired, with relative preservation of remote memory and registration.

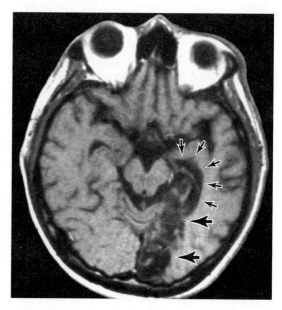

Figure 1–21. T1-weighted MRI in a patient with an old left posterior cerebral artery occlusion, showing tissue loss in the medial temporal **(small arrows)** and occipital **(large arrows)** lobes and associated dilation of the temporal and occipital horns of the lateral ventricle. (Courtesy of A Gean.)

The CT scan shows lucencies—which may or may not be enhanced by use of contrast material—in any combination of the above-mentioned regions. Evaluation and treatment are described in Chapter 9.

TRANSIENT GLOBAL AMNESIA

Transient global amnesia is a syndrome of acute memory loss that tends to occur in middle-aged or elderly patients with risk factors for atherosclerotic disease, especially a prior ischemic event in the posterior cerebral circulation. The disorder is recurrent in fewer than 10% of patients.

A primary disorder of short-term memory that can last for minutes or days, it typically lasts for hours. Patients appear agitated and perplexed and may repeatedly inquire about their whereabouts, the time, and the nature of what they are experiencing. Knowledge of personal identity is preserved, as are remote memories and registration. New memories cannot be formed, however, which accounts for the patient's repetitive questions. Retrograde amnesia for a variable period preceding the episode may be present, but this period shrinks as the episode resolves.

The patient's obvious concern about the condition distinguishes transient global amnesia from most other organically based amnestic syndromes and may give rise to the suspicion that amnesia is psychogenic. A CT scan or MRI may demonstrate focal thalamic or temporal lobe abnormalities. Diffusion-weighted MRI has shown signal abnormalities in the temporal lobe during spells of transient global amnesia. These are compatible with cellular edema and may be related to spreading depression—a wave of cellular depolarization accompanied by cellular swelling in the brain.

ALCOHOLIC BLACKOUTS

Short-term consumption of large amounts of ethanol by alcoholic or nonalcoholic individuals may lead to "blackouts"—transient amnestic episodes that are not due to global confusion, seizures, head trauma, or the Wernicke-Korsakoff syndrome. These spells are characterized by an inability to form new memories, without impairment of long-term memory or immediate recall. Although the cause is unknown, alcoholic blackouts may result from ethanol-induced depression of synaptic (especially serotonin- or glutamate-mediated) neurotransmission. The disorder is self-limited and no specific treatment is required, but reduction of the ethanol intake should be counseled, and thiamine should be given to treat possible Wernicke's encephalopathy (see p. 18).

WERNICKE'S ENCEPHALOPATHY

Wernicke's encephalopathy is caused by thiamine deficiency and classically produces an acute confusional state, ataxia, and ophthalmoplegia. Amnesia may be the major or sole cognitive disturbance, however, especially after thiamine treatment is begun and other cognitive abnormalities improve. Because patients with Wernicke's encephalopathy usually present with global confusion rather than isolated amnesia, the disorder is discussed more fully above (see p. 18).

DISSOCIATIVE (PSYCHOGENIC) AMNESIA

Amnesia may be a manifestation of a dissociative disorder or of malingering. In such patients a prior psychiatric history, additional psychiatric symptoms, or a precipitating emotional stress can often be identified. Dissociative amnesia is characterized by an isolated or a disproportionate loss of traumatic or stressful personal memories. Dissociative amnesia is usually localized in time to the immediate aftermath of a traumatic experience or selective for some but not other events during such a period. Less frequent patterns include systematized amnesia restricted to certain categories of information, continuous amnesia for events from some time in the past up to and including the present, and generalized amnesia. In some cases, patients may be unable to remember even their own name—an exceedingly rare finding in organic amnesia. Despite such disorientation

to person, orientation to place and time may be preserved. In addition, recent memories may be less affected than remote memories—the reverse of the pattern customarily seen in amnesia caused by organic disease. Examination under hypnosis or after administration of amobarbital sodium may be helpful in establishing that amnesia is of psychogenic origin.

CHRONIC AMNESIA

ALCOHOLIC KORSAKOFF AMNESTIC SYNDROME

The Korsakoff amnestic syndrome, which occurs in chronic alcoholism and other malnourished states, is thought to be caused by thiamine deficiency. It is usually preceded by one or more episodes of Wernicke's encephalopathy (see p. 18), but such a history may be lacking. The memory disorder may be related to bilateral degeneration of the dorsomedial thalamic nuclei.

An amnestic syndrome of variable severity follows recovery from Wernicke's encephalopathy in about three-fourths of cases and is often associated with polyneuropathy and other residua such as nystagmus or gait ataxia. The essential defect is an inability to form new memories, resulting in significant impairment of short-term memory. Long-term memory is also frequently affected, although to a lesser extent. Registration is intact. Patients are typically apathetic and lack insight into their disorder. They may attempt to reassure the physician that no impairment exists and try to explain away their obvious inability to remember. Confabulation is often, but not invariably, a feature.

Korsakoff's syndrome can be prevented or its severity decreased by prompt administration of thiamine to patients with Wernicke's encephalopathy. Patients with established Korsakoff's syndrome should also receive thiamine to prevent the progression of deficits, although existing deficits are unlikely to be reversed.

POSTENCEPHALITIC AMNESIA

Patients who recover from acute viral encephalitis—particularly that caused by **herpes simplex virus** (see p. 30)—may be left with a permanent and static amnestic syndrome. The syndrome is similar to that produced by chronic alcoholism in that an inability to form new memories is its outstanding feature. Remote memories are affected to a lesser extent than are recent ones, and registration is intact. Confabulation may occur. Often there is total amnesia for the period of the acute encephalitis.

Patients may also exhibit other symptoms of limbic system disease. These include docility, indifference, flatness of mood and affect, inappropriate jocularity and sexual allusions, hyperphagia, impotence, repetitive stereotyped motor activity, and the absence of goal-oriented activity. Complex partial seizures, with or without secondary generalization, may occur.

BRAIN TUMOR

Brain tumor is a rare cause of amnestic syndrome. Tumors that can present in this manner include those that are located in the third ventricle or that compress its floor or walls from without. The amnestic syndrome closely resembles Korsakoff's syndrome. In addition, patients with deep midline tumors often exhibit marked lethargy, headache, endocrine disturbances, visual field deficits, or papilledema.

The diagnosis of brain tumor is made by CT scan or MRI. Treatment consists of surgery or irradiation or both, depending upon the type of tumor and its location.

PARANEOPLASTIC LIMBIC ENCEPHALITIS

An inflammatory and degenerative disorder of gray matter regions of the central nervous system can occur as a remote effect of systemic cancer. When limbic structures are primarily affected, the clinical picture is that of an amnestic syndrome. The disorder is thought to be autoimmune in origin since, as in other paraneoplastic neurologic syndromes, antineuronal autoantibodies can be detected (see p. 120).

Paraneoplastic limbic encephalitis is most often associated with small cell cancer of the lung, and symptoms typically precede diagnosis of the underlying cancer. Histopathologic findings include neuronal loss, reactive gliosis, microglial proliferation, and perivascular lymphocytic cuffing. Gray matter of the hippocampus, cingulum, piriform cortex, inferior frontal lobes, insula, and amygdala is characteristically affected. Symptoms develop over several weeks. The disorder is characterized by profound impairment of recent memory, corresponding to the inability to learn new material. Remote memory is less impaired, and registration is unaffected; confabulation occurs in some cases. Affective symptoms, either anxiety or depression, are common early features. Hallucinations and complex partial or generalized seizures may occur. In many instances, the amnestic syndrome progresses to a global dementia. Depending upon the extent to which gray matter regions outside the limbic system are involved, cerebellar, pyramidal, bulbar, and peripheral nerve disturbances may coexist with the amnestic disorder.

The CSF may also show a modest mononuclear pleocytosis and mildly elevated protein. Diffuse slowing or bitemporal slow waves and spikes are sometimes seen on EEG. An MRI may reveal abnormal signal intensity in the medial temporal lobes. About 60% of patients have antineuronal antibodies in serum or CSF. Anti-Hu antibodies are most common and are usually associated with small-cell lung cancer and anti-Ta antibodies are seen in patients with testicular cancer; in both groups, prognosis is poor. Patients with neither anti-Hu nor anti-Ta antibodies have a better outcome and often improve after treatment of the underlying tumor.

The paraneoplastic amnestic syndrome can be static, it can progress, or it can remit. Excluding other, especially treatable disorders is of primary importance. Korsakoff's syndrome caused by thiamine deficiency should especially be considered, because patients with cancer are susceptible to nutritional deficiency and thiamine administration may prevent these symptoms from worsening.

REFERENCES

ACUTE CONFUSIONAL STATES (GENERAL)

Plum F, Posner JB: *The Diagnosis of Stupor and Coma,* 3rd ed. Vol 19 of: *Contemporary Neurology Series.* Davis, 1980.

Drugs

Khantzian EJ, McKenna GJ: Acute toxic and withdrawal reactions associated with drug use and abuse. Ann Intern Med 1979; 90:361–372.

Meador KJ: Cognitive side effects of medications. Neurol Clin 1998;16:141–155.

Endocrine Disturbances

Chen HC, Marsharani U: Hashimoto's encephalopathy. South Med J 2000;93:504–506.

Malouf R, Brust JC: Hypoglycemia: causes, neurologic manifestations, and outcome. Ann Neurol 1985;17:421–430.

Oelkers W: Adrenal insufficiency. N Engl J Med 1996; 335:1206–1212.

Electrolyte Disorders

Adrogué HJ, Madias NE. Hyponatremia. N Engl J Med 2000; 342:1581–1589.

Bilezikian JP: Management of acute hypercalcemia. N Engl J Med 1992;326:1196–1203.

Nutritional Disorders

Charness ME, Simon RP, Greenberg DA: Ethanol and the nervous system. N Engl J Med 1989;321:442–454.

Toh BH et al: Pernicious anemia. N Engl J Med 1997;337: 1441–1448.

Organ System Failure

Burn DJ, Bates D: Neurology and the kidney. J Neurol Neurosurg Psychiat 1998;65:810–821.

Patchell RA: Neurological complications of organ transplantation. Ann Neurol 1994;36:688–703.

Riordan SM, Williams R: Treatment of hepatic encephalopathy. N Engl J Med 1997;337:473–479.

Meningitis & Encephalitis

Berenguer J et al: Tuberculous meningitis in patients infected with the human immunodeficiency virus. N Engl J Med 1993; 326:668–672.

Gottfredsson M, Perfect JR: Fungal meningitis. Semin Neurol 2000;20:307–322.

Hook EW, Marra CM: Acquired syphilis in adults. N Engl J Med 1992;326:1060–1069.

Iseman MD: Treatment of multidrug-resistant tuberculosis. N Engl J Med 1993;329:784–791.

Liu LX, Weller PF: Drug therapy: antiparasitic drugs. N Engl J Med 1996;334:1178–1184.

Luft BJ et al: Toxoplasmic encephalitis in patients with the acquired immunodeficiency syndrome. N Engl J Med 1993; 329:995–1000.

Marra CM: Encephalitis in the 21st century. Semin Neurol 2000; 20:323–327.

McJunkin JE et al: La Crosse encephalitis in children. N Engl J Med 2001;344:801–807.

Newton CR, Hien TT, White N: Cerebral malaria. J Neurol Neurosurg Psychiat 2000;69:433–441.

Papadopoulos MC et al: Pathophysiology of septic encephalopathy: a review. Crit Care Med 2000;28:3019–3024.

Posner JB: *Neurologic complications of cancer.* Davis, 1995.

Quagliarello VJ, Scheld WM: Treatment of bacterial meningitis. N Engl J Med 1997;336:708–716.

Rosenstein NE et al: Meningococcal disease. N Engl J Med 2001; 344:1378–1388.

Simon RP: Neurosyphilis. Neurology 1994;44:2228–2230.

Simpson DM, Tagliati M: Neurologic manifestations of HIV infection. Ann Intern Med 1994;121:769–785.

Steere AC: Lyme disease. N Engl J Med 2001;345:115–125.

Whitley RJ: Viral encephalitis. N Engl J Med 1990;323: 242–250.

Vascular Disorders

Levi M, ten Cate, H: Disseminated intravascular coagulation. N Engl J Med 1999;341:586-592.

Mills JA: Systemic lupus erythematosus. N Engl J Med 1994; 330: 1871–1879.

Raife TJ, Montgomery RR: von Willebrand factor and thrombotic thrombocytopenic purpura. Curr Opin Hematol 2000; 7: 278–283.

Schievink WI: Intracranial aneurysms. N Engl J Med 1997; 336: 28–40.

Vaughan CJ, Delanty N: Hypertensive mergencies. Lancet 2000; 356:411–417.

Head Trauma

White RJ, Likavec MJ: The diagnosis and initial management of head injury. N Engl J Med 1992;327:1507–1511.

Psychiatric Disorders

Hillard JR: Emergency treatment of acute psychosis. J Clin Psychiatry 1998;59(Suppl 1):57–60.

Richards CF, Gurr DE: Psychosis. Emerg Med Clin North Am 2000;18:253–262.

DEMENTIA (GENERAL)

Geldmacher DS, Whitehouse PJ: Evaluation of dementia. N Engl J Med 1996;335:330–336.

Martin JB. Molecular basis of the neurodegenerative disorders. N Engl J Med 1999;340:1970–1980.

Alzheimer's Disease

Martin JB. Molecular basis of the neurodegenerative disorders. N Engl J Med 1999;340:1970–1980.

Mayeux R, Sano M. Treatment of Alzheimer's disease. N Engl J Med 1999;341:1670–1679.

Vassar R, Citron M: Aβ-generating enzymes: recent advances in β- and γ-secretase research. Neuron 2000;27:419–422.

Other Cerebral Disorders

Johnson RT, Gibbs CJ Jr: Creutzfeldt-Jakob disease and related transmissible spongiform encephalopathies. N Engl J Med 1998;339:1994–2004.

McKeith IG et al: Consensus guidelines for the clinical and pathologic diagnosis of dementia with Lewy bodies (DLB): report of the consortium on DLB international workshop. Neurology 1996;47:1113–1124.

Mendez MF et al: Frontotemporal dementia versus Alzheimer's disease: differential cognitive features. Neurology 1996;47:1189–1194.

Poser S et al: How to improve the clinical diagnosis of Creutzfeldt-Jakob disease. Brain 1999;122:2345–2351.

Prusiner SB: Neurodegenerative diseases and prions. N Engl J Med 2001;344:1516–1526.

Riley DE et al: Cortical-basal ganglionic degeneration. Neurology 1990;40:1203–1212.

Vanneste JA: Diagnosis and management of normal-pressure hydrocephalus. J Neurol 2000;247:5–14.

Will RG et al: Diagnosis of new variant Creutzfeldt-Jakob disease. Ann Neurol 2000;47:575–582.

Systemic Disorders

Berger JR, Major EO: Progressive multifocal leukoencephalopathy. Semin Neurol 1999;19:193–200.

Hook EW, Marra CM: Acquired syphilis in adults. N Engl J Med 1992;326:1060–1069.

Iantosca MR, Simon RH: Chronic subdural hematoma in adult and elderly patients. Neurosurg Clin N Am 2000; 11:447–454.

Roman GC: Vascular dementia today. Rev Neurol (Paris) 1999; 155(Suppl 4):S64–S72.

Simon RP: Neurosyphilis. Neurology 1994;44:2228–2230.

Simpson DM, Tagliati M: Neurologic manifestations of HIV infection Ann Intern Med 1994;121:769–785.

Victor M: Alcoholic dementia. Can J Neurol Sci 1994;21:88–99.

Toh BH et al: Pernicious anemia. N Engl J Med 1997; 337: 1441–1448.

Pseudodementia

Raskind MA: The clinical interface of depression and dementia. J Clin Psychiatry 1998;59(Suppl 10):9–12.

AMNESTIC SYNDROMES

Cabeza R, Nyberg L: Neural bases of learning and memory: functional neuroimaging evidence. Curr Opin Neurol 2000; 13:415–421.

Caronna JJ: Diagnosis, prognosis, and treatment of hypoxic coma. Adv Neurol 1979;26:1–15.

Charness ME, Simon RP, Greenberg DA: Ethanol and the nervous system. N Engl J Med 1989;321:442–454.

Gultekin SH et al: Paraneoplastic limbic encephalitis: neurological symptoms, immunological findings and tumour association in 50 patients. Brain 2000;123:1481–1494.

Jordan BD: Chronic traumatic brain injury associated with boxing. Semin Neurol 2000;20:179–185.

Martin SJ, Grimwood PD, Morris RG: Synaptic plasticity and memory: an evaluation of the hypothesis. Annu Rev Neurosci 2000;23:649–711.

Pantoni L, Lamassa M, Inzitari D: Transient global amnesia: a review emphasizing pathogenic aspects. Acta Neurol Scand 2000;102:275–283.

Headache & Facial Pain

CONTENTS

KEY CONCEPTS

 Headache results from disorders that affect pain-sensitive structures of the head and neck, such as meninges, blood vessels, and muscle.

 Headaches that are new in onset or different from previous headaches are those most likely to be caused by a serious illness, whereas headaches of long standing usually have a benign cause.

 Signs of meningeal irritation—such as neck stiffness on passive flexion in the anteroposterior direction or hip and knee flexion in response to passive neck flexion—must be sought in patients with acute headache; detecting these signs is critical in the rapid diagnosis of meningitis, and directs the diagnostic evaluation toward urgent lumbar puncture and away from imaging procedures.

 Subarachnoid hemorrhage from a ruptured intracranial aneurysm can often be diagnosed by the presence of subarachnoid blood on a noncontrast CT scan; however, in the absence of this finding, a lumbar puncture showing no blood in the cerebrospinal fluid is required to exclude the diagnosis.

 High blood pressure alone does not cause chronic headache.

 For maximum effect, drugs for migraine should be taken immediately at the onset of symptoms.

Headache occurs in all age groups and is the seventh leading reason for medical office visits; the causes are myriad (Table 2–1). Although most often a benign condition (especially when chronic and recurrent), headache of new onset may be the earliest or the principal manifestation of serious systemic or intracranial disease and therefore requires thorough and systematic evaluation.

An etiologic diagnosis of headache is based on understanding the pathophysiology of head pain; obtaining a history, with characterization of the pain as acute, subacute, or chronic; performing a careful physical examination; and formulating a differential diagnosis.

APPROACH TO DIAGNOSIS

PATHOPHYSIOLOGY OF HEADACHE & FACIAL PAIN

Pain-Sensitive Structures

 Headache is caused by traction, displacement, inflammation, vascular spasm, or distention of

Table 2–1. Causes of headache and facial pain.

Acute onset
  Common causes
    Subarachnoid hemorrhage
      Other cerebrovascular diseases
      Meningitis or encephalitis
      Ocular disorders (glaucoma, acute iritis)
  Less common causes
    Seizures
      Lumbar puncture
      Hypertensive encephalopathy
      Coitus
  Subacute onset
    Giant cell (temporal) arteritis
    Intracranial mass (tumor, subdural hematoma, abscess)
    Pseudotumor cerebri (benign intracranial hypertension)
    Trigeminal neuralgia (tic douloureux)
    Glossopharyngeal neuralgia
    Posttherpetic neuralgia
    Hypertension (including pheochromocytoma and the
      use of monoamine oxidase inhibitors plus tyramine)
    Atypical facial pain
  Chronic
    Migraine
    Cluster headache
    Tension headache
    Cervical spine disease
    Sinusitis
    Dental disease

the pain-sensitive structures in the head or neck. Isolated involvement of the bony skull, most of the dura, or most regions of brain parenchyma does not produce pain.

A. PAIN-SENSITIVE STRUCTURES WITHIN THE CRANIAL VAULT

These include the venous sinuses (eg, sagittal sinus); the anterior and middle meningeal arteries; the dura at the base of the skull; the trigeminal (V), glossopharyngeal (IX), and vagus (X) nerves; the proximal portions of the internal carotid artery and its branches near the Circle of Willis; the brainstem periaqueductal gray matter; and the sensory nuclei of the thalamus.

B. EXTRACRANIAL PAIN-SENSITIVE STRUCTURES

These include the periosteum of the skull; the skin; the subcutaneous tissues, muscles, and arteries; the neck muscles; the second and third cervical nerves; the eyes, ears, teeth, sinuses, and oropharynx; and the mucous membranes of the nasal cavity.

Radiation or Projection of Pain

The trigeminal (V) nerve carries sensation from intracranial structures in the anterior and middle fossae of the skull, above the cerebellar tentorium. Discrete intracranial lesions in these locations produce pain that radiates in the trigeminal nerve distribution (Figure 2–1).

The glossopharyngeal (IX) and vagus (X) nerves supply part of the posterior fossa; pain originating in this area may also be referred to the ear or throat (eg, glossopharyngeal neuralgia).

The upper cervical nerves transmit stimuli arising from infratentorial and cervical structures; therefore, pain from posterior fossa lesions projects to the second and third cervical dermatomes (Figure 2–1).

HISTORY

Classification & Approach to the Differential Diagnosis

A. ACUTE HEADACHES AND FACIAL PAIN

Headaches that are new in onset and clearly different from any the patient has experienced previously are commonly a symptom of serious illness and therefore demand prompt evaluation. The sudden onset of "the worst headache I've ever had in my life" (classic subarachnoid hemorrhage), diffuse headache with neck stiffness and fever (meningitis), and head pain centered about one eye (acute glaucoma) are striking examples. Acute headaches may also accompany more benign processes such as viral syndromes or other febrile illnesses.

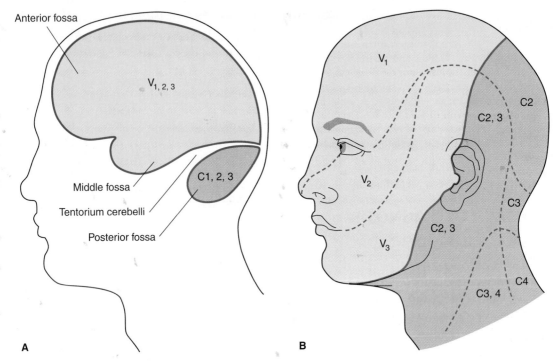

Figure 2–1. Innervation of pain-sensitive intracranial compartments **A** and corresponding extracranial sites of pain radiation **B**. The trigeminal (V) nerve, especially its ophthalmic (V_1) division, innervates the anterior and middle cranial fossae; lesions in these areas can produce frontal headache. The upper cervical nerve roots (especially C2) innervate the posterior fossa; lesions here can cause occipital headache.

B. SUBACUTE HEADACHES AND FACIAL PAIN

Subacute headaches occur over a period of weeks to months. Such headaches may also signify serious medical disorders, especially when the pain is progressive or when it develops in elderly patients. Inquiries should be made about recent head trauma (subdural hematoma or postconcussive syndrome); a history of malaise, fever, or neck stiffness (subacute meningitis); other neurologic abnormalities or weight loss (primary or metastatic brain tumor); symptoms of vasculitis, especially giant cell arteritis; and medical conditions (eg, optic neuritis in multiple sclerosis; cutaneous herpes zoster) or medications predisposing to any of the disorders listed in Table 2–1.

C. CHRONIC HEADACHES AND FACIAL PAIN

Headaches that have occurred for years (eg, migraine or tension headaches) usually have a benign cause, although each acute attack may be profoundly disabling. When treating these patients, it is important to determine whether the present headache is similar to those suffered previously or is new—and thus represents a different process.

Precipitating Factors

Precipitating factors can provide a guide to the cause of headache. Such factors include recent eye or dental surgery; acute exacerbation of chronic sinusitis or hay fever; systemic viral infection; tension, emotional stress, or fatigue; menses; hunger; ice cream; foods containing nitrite (hot dogs, salami, ham, and most sausage), phenylethylamine (chocolate), or tyramine (cheddar cheese); and bright lights. Precipitation of headache by alcohol is especially typical of cluster headache. Chewing and eating commonly trigger glossopharyngeal neuralgia, tic douloureux, and the jaw claudication of giant cell arteritis; these activities also trigger pain in patients with temporomandibular joint dysfunction. The use of oral contraceptive agents or other drugs such as nitrates may precipitate or exacerbate migraine and even lead to stroke. Intense headache can occur in response to coughing in patients with structural lesions in the posterior fossa; in other instances no specific cause for cough headache can be identified.

Prodromal Symptoms

Prodromal symptoms or auras, such as scintillating scotomas or other visual changes, often occur with migraine;

they may also occur in patients with a seizure disorder who present with postictal headaches.

Characteristics of Pain

Headache or facial pain is most often described as throbbing; a dull, steady ache; or a jabbing, lancinating pain. **Pulsating, throbbing** pain is frequently ascribed to migraine, but it is equally common in patients with tension headache. A steady sensation of **tightness** or **pressure** is also commonly seen with tension headache. The pain produced by intracranial mass lesions is typically **dull** and **steady**. **Sharp**, **lancinating** pain suggests a neuritic cause such as trigeminal neuralgia. **Ice pick-like** pain may be described by patients with migraine, cluster headache, or giant cell arteritis.

Headache of virtually any description can occur in patients with migraine or brain tumors, however, so the character of the pain alone does not provide a reliable etiologic guide.

Location of Pain

Unilateral headache is an invariable feature of cluster headache and occurs in the majority of migraine attacks; most patients with tension headache report bilateral pain.

Ocular or **retroocular** pain suggests a primary ophthalmologic disorder such as acute iritis or glaucoma, optic (II) nerve disease (eg, optic neuritis), or retroorbital inflammation (eg, Tolosa-Hunt syndrome). It is also common in migraine or cluster headache.

Paranasal pain localized to one or several of the sinuses, often associated with tenderness in the overlying periosteum and skin, occurs with acute infection or outlet obstruction of these structures.

Headache from intracranial mass lesions may be **focal** ("it hurts right here"), but even in such cases it is replaced by bioccipital and bifrontal pain when the intracranial pressure becomes elevated.

Bandlike or **occipital** discomfort is commonly associated with tension headaches. Occipital localization can also occur with meningeal irritation from infection or hemorrhage and with disorders of the joints, muscles, or ligaments of the upper cervical spine.

Pain within the **first division of the trigeminal nerve** (Figure 2–1B), characteristically described as burning in quality, is a common feature of postherpetic neuralgia.

Lancinating pain localized to the **second** or **third division of the trigeminal nerve** (Figure 2–1B) suggests tic douloureux.

The **pharynx** and **external auditory meatus** are the most frequent sites of pain caused by glossopharyngeal neuralgia.

Associated Symptoms

Manifestations of underlying systemic disease can aid in the etiologic diagnosis of headache and should always be sought.

Recent weight loss may accompany cancer, giant cell arteritis, or depression.

Fever or **chills** may indicate systemic infection or meningitis.

Dyspnea or other symptoms of heart disease raise the possibility of subacute infective endocarditis and resultant brain abscess.

Visual disturbances suggest an ocular disorder (eg, glaucoma), migraine, or an intracranial process involving the optic nerve or tract or the central visual pathways.

Nausea and **vomiting** are common in migraine and posttraumatic headache syndromes and can be seen in the course of mass lesions. Some patients with migraine also report that diarrhea accompanies the attacks.

Photophobia may be prominent in migraine and acute meningitis or subarachnoid hemorrhage.

Myalgias often accompany tension headaches, viral syndromes, and giant cell arteritis.

Ipsilateral rhinorrhea and **lacrimation** during attacks typify cluster headache.

Transient loss of consciousness may be a concomitant of both migraine and glossopharyngeal neuralgia.

Other Features of Headache

A. TEMPORAL PATTERN OF HEADACHE

Headaches from mass lesions are commonly maximal on awakening, as are sinus headaches. Headaches from mass lesions, however, increase in severity over time. Cluster headaches frequently awaken patients from sleep; they often recur at the same time each day or night. Tension headaches can develop whenever stressful situations occur and are often maximal at the end of a workday. Migraine headaches are episodic and may be worse during menses (Figure 2–2).

B. CONDITIONS RELIEVING HEADACHE

Migraine headaches are frequently relieved by darkness, sleep, vomiting, or pressing on the ipsilateral temporal artery, and their frequency is often diminished during pregnancy. Postlumbar-puncture headaches are typically relieved by recumbency, whereas headaches caused by intracranial mass lesions may be less severe with the patient standing.

C. CONDITIONS EXACERBATING HEADACHE

Discomfort exacerbated by rapid changes in head position or by events that transiently raise intracranial pressure, such as coughing and sneezing, is often associated with an intracranial mass but can occur in migraine.

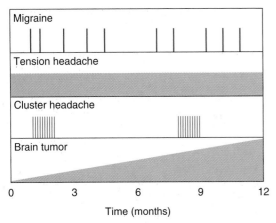

Figure 2–2. Temporal patterns of headache. Migraine headache is episodic and may occur at varying intervals. Tension headache may be present every day. Cluster headache occurs in bouts separated by symptom-free periods. Headache caused by brain tumor often increases in severity with time.

Anger, excitement, or irritation can precipitate or worsen both migraine and tension headaches. Stooping, bending forward, sneezing, or blowing the nose characteristically worsens the pain of sinusitis. Postural headache (maximal when upright, nearly absent when lying down) occurs with low cerebrospinal fluid (CSF) pressure caused by lumbar puncture, head injury, or spontaneous spinal fluid leak.

Fluctuations in intensity and duration of the headache with no obvious cause, especially when associated with similar fluctuations in mental status, are seen with subdural hematoma.

D. History of Headache

The characteristics of the present headache should be compared with those of previous occurrences, since headache with features different from those previously experienced calls for careful investigation.

PHYSICAL EXAMINATION

A general physical examination is mandatory, since headache is a nonspecific accompaniment of many systemic disorders. If possible, the patient should be observed during an episode of headache or facial pain.

Vital Signs

A. Temperature

Although fever suggests a viral syndrome, meningitis, encephalitis, or brain abscess, headache from these causes can occur without fever. Moreover, headache can accompany any systemic infectious illness.

B. Pulse

Tachycardia can occur in a tense, anxious patient with a tension headache or accompany any severe pain. Paroxysmal headache associated with tachycardia and perspiration is characteristic of pheochromocytoma.

C. Blood Pressure

Hypertension per se rarely causes headache unless the blood pressure elevation is acute, as with pheochromocytoma, or very high, as with early hypertensive encephalopathy. Chronic hypertension, however, is the major risk factor for stroke, which can be associated with acute headache. Subarachnoid hemorrhage is commonly followed by marked acute blood pressure elevation.

D. Respiration

Hypercapnia from respiratory insufficiency from any cause can elevate intracranial pressure and produce headache.

General Physical Examination

A. Weight Loss

Weight loss or cachexia in a patient with headache suggests the presence of cancer or chronic infection. Polymyalgia rheumatica-giant cell arteritis syndromes can also be accompanied by weight loss.

B. Skin

Focal cellulitis of the face or overlying the skull indicates local infection, which may be the source of intracranial abscess or venous sinus thrombosis. Cutaneous abnormalities elsewhere may suggest vasculitis (including that from meningococcemia), endocarditis, or cancer. The neurofibromas or café-au-lait spots of von Recklinghausen's disease (neurofibromatosis) may be associated with benign or malignant intracranial tumors that can produce headache. Cutaneous angiomas sometimes accompany arteriovenous malformations (AVMs) of the central nervous system and may be associated with chronic headache—or acute headache if they bleed. Herpes zoster that affects the face and head most often involves the eye and the skin around the periorbital tissue, causing facial pain.

C. Scalp, Face, and Head

Scalp tenderness is characteristic of migraine headache, subdural hematoma, giant cell arteritis, and postherpetic neuralgia. Nodularity, erythema, or tenderness over the temporal artery suggests giant cell arteritis. Localized tenderness of the superficial temporal artery also accompanies acute migraine. Recent head trauma or a mass lesion can cause a localized area of tenderness.

Paget's disease, myeloma, or metastatic cancer of the skull may produce head pain that is boring in quality and associated with skull tenderness. In Paget's disease, arteriovenous shunting within bone may make the scalp feel warm.

Disorders of the eyes, ears, or teeth may cause headache. Tooth percussion may reveal periodontal abscess. Sinus tenderness may indicate sinusitis. A bruit over the orbit or skull suggests an intracranial AVM, a carotid artery-cavernous sinus fistula, an aneurysm, or a meningioma. Lacerations of the tongue raise the possibility of postictal headache. Ipsilateral conjunctival injection, lacrimation, Horner's syndrome, and rhinorrhea occur with cluster headache. Temporomandibular joint disease is accompanied by local tenderness and crepitus.

D. NECK

Cervical muscle spasms occur with tension and migraine headaches, cervical spine injuries, cervical arthritis, or meningitis. Carotid bruits may be associated with cerebrovascular disease.

Meningeal signs must be carefully sought, especially if the headache is of recent onset. Meningeal irritation causes nuchal rigidity mainly in the anteroposterior direction, whereas cervical spine disorders restrict movement in all directions. Discomfort or hip and knee flexion during neck flexion (Brudzinski's sign) readily indicates meningeal irritation (Figure 2–3).

Meningeal signs may be absent or difficult to demonstrate in the early stages of subacute (eg, tuberculous) meningitis, in the first few hours after subarachnoid hemorrhage, and in comatose patients.

E. HEART AND LUNG

Brain abscess may be associated with congenital heart disease, which is evidenced by murmurs or cyanosis. Lung abscess may also be a source of brain abscess.

NEUROLOGIC EXAMINATION

Mental Status Examination

During the mental status examination, patients with acute headache may demonstrate confusion, as is commonly seen with subarachnoid hemorrhage and meningitis. Dementia may be the major feature of intracranial tumor, particularly one in the frontal lobe.

Cranial Nerve Examination

Cranial nerve abnormalities may suggest and localize an intracranial tumor or other mass lesion. Papilledema, the hallmark of increased intracranial pressure, may be seen in space-occupying intracranial lesions, carotid artery-cavernous sinus fistula, pseudotumor cerebri, or hypertensive encephalopathy. Superficial retinal (sub-hyaloid) hemorrhages are characteristic of subarachnoid hemorrhage in adults. Ischemic retinopathy may be found in patients with vasculitis.

Progressive oculomotor nerve palsy, especially when it causes pupillary dilatation, may be the presenting sign of an expanding posterior-communicating-artery aneurysm, or it may reflect increasing intracranial pressure and incipient herniation. Decreased pupillary reactivity occurs in optic neuritis. Extraocular muscle palsies occur in Tolosa-Hunt syndrome. Proptosis suggests an orbital mass lesion or carotid artery-cavernous sinus fistula.

Decreased sensation over the area of pain—most commonly the first division of the trigeminal nerve—is found in postherpetic neuralgia. Trigger areas eliciting pain in and about the face and pharynx suggest trigeminal and glossopharyngeal neuralgia, respectively.

Motor Examination

Asymmetric motor function or gait ataxia in a patient with a history of subacute headache demands complete evaluation to exclude intracranial mass lesions.

Sensory Examination

Focal or segmental sensory impairment or diminished corneal sensation (corneal reflex) is strong evidence against a benign cause of pain.

HEADACHES OF ACUTE ONSET

Sudden onset of new headache may be a symptom of serious intracranial or systemic disease; it must be investigated promptly and thoroughly.

SUBARACHNOID HEMORRHAGE

Spontaneous (nontraumatic) subarachnoid hemorrhage (bleeding into the subarachnoid space) is usually the result of a ruptured cerebral arterial aneurysm or an AVM. Rupture of a berry aneurysm accounts for about 75% of cases, with an annual incidence of 6 per 100,000. Rupture occurs most often during the fifth and sixth decades, with an approximately equal sex distribution. Hypertension has not been conclusively demonstrated to predispose to the formation of aneurysms, but acute elevation of blood pressure (eg, at orgasm) may be responsible for their rupture. Intracranial AVMs, a less frequent cause of subarachnoid hemorrhage (10%), occur twice as often in men and usually bleed in the second to fourth decades, although a significant incidence extends into the 60s. Blood in the sub-

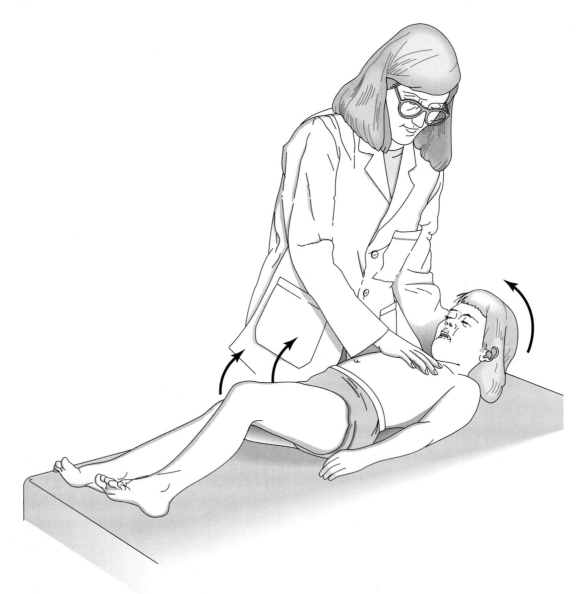

Figure 2–3. Brudzinski's sign. With the patient supine and the examiner's hand on the patient's chest, passive neck flexion **(arrow at right)** results in flexion at the hips **(arrows at left)**, which is often asymmetric. The sign is present with meningeal irritation from disorders such as infectious meningitis or subarachnoid hemorrhage.

arachnoid space can also result from intracerebral hemorrhage, embolic stroke, and trauma.

Pathology

Cerebral artery aneurysms are most commonly congenital "berry" aneurysms, which result from developmental weakness of the vessel wall, especially at sites of branching. These aneurysmal dilatations arise from intracranial arteries about the circle of Willis at the base of the brain (Figure 2–4) and are multiple in about 20% of cases. Other congenital abnormalities, including polycystic kidney disease and coarctation of the aorta, may be associated with berry aneurysms. Occasionally, systemic infections such as infective endocarditis disseminate to a cerebral artery and cause aneurysm formation; such "mycotic" aneurysms account for 2–3% of aneurysmal ruptures. Mycotic aneurysms are usually more distal (along the course of cerebral arteries) than are berry aneurysms.

AVMs consist of abnormal vascular communications that permit arterial blood to enter the venous system without passing through a capillary bed. They are most common in the middle cerebral artery distribution.

Pathophysiology

Rupture of an intracranial artery elevates intracranial pressure and distorts pain-sensitive structures, producing headache. Intracranial pressure may reach systemic perfusion pressure and acutely decrease cerebral blood flow; together with the concussive effect of the rupture, this is thought to cause the loss of consciousness that occurs at the onset in about 50% of patients. Rapid elevation of intracranial pressure can also produce subhyaloid retinal hemorrhages (Figure 2–5).

Because aneurysmal hemorrhage is usually confined to the subarachnoid space, it does not produce a focal cerebral lesion. Prominent focal findings on neurologic examination are accordingly uncommon except with

middle cerebral artery aneurysms. Ruptured AVMs, however, produce focal abnormalities that correspond to their parenchymal location.

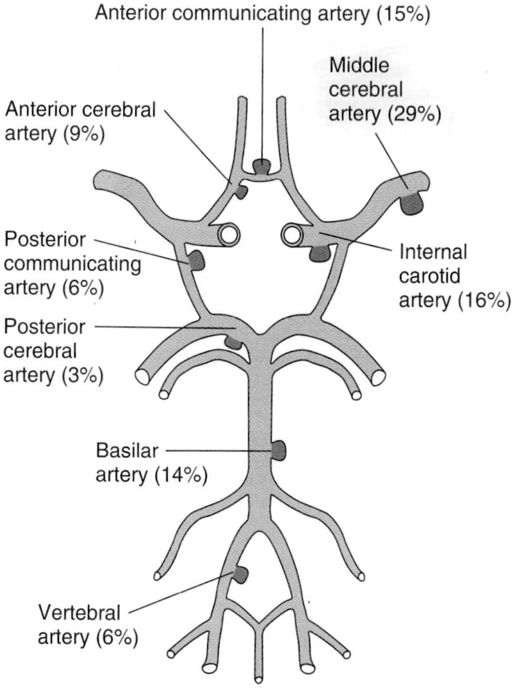

Clinical Findings

A. SYMPTOMS AND SIGNS

The classic (but not invariable) presentation of subarachnoid hemorrhage is the sudden onset of an unusually severe generalized headache ("the worst headache I ever had in my life"). The absence of headache essentially precludes the diagnosis. Loss of consciousness is frequent, as are vomiting and neck stiffness. Symptoms may begin at any time of day and during either rest or exertion.

The most significant feature of the headache is that it is *new*. Milder but otherwise similar headaches may have occurred in the weeks prior to the acute event. These earlier headaches are probably the result of small prodromal hemorrhages (sentinel, or warning, hemorrhages) or aneurysmal stretch.

The headache is not always severe, however, especially if the subarachnoid hemorrhage is from a ruptured AVM rather than an aneurysm. Although the duration of the hemorrhage is brief, the intensity of the headache may remain unchanged for several days and may subside only slowly over the next 2 weeks. A recrudescent headache usually signifies recurrent bleeding.

Anterior communicating artery (15%)

Middle cerebral artery (29%)

Anterior cerebral artery (9%)

Posterior communicating artery (6%)

Internal carotid artery (16%)

Posterior cerebral artery (3%)

Basilar artery (14%)

Vertebral artery (6%)

Figure 2–4. Frequency and distribution of intracranial aneurysms.

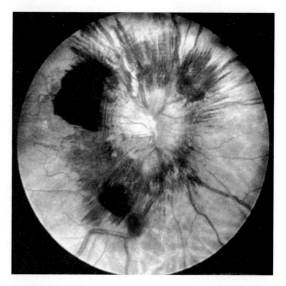

Figure 2–5. Peripapillary intraretinal (streak-like) and preretinal or subhyaloid (globular) hemorrhages associated with a sudden increase in intracranial pressure caused by aneurysmal rupture. (Courtesy of WF Hoyt.)

Blood pressure frequently rises precipitously as a result of the hemorrhage. Meningeal irritation may induce temperature elevations to as high as 39°C (102.2°F) during the first 2 weeks. There is frequently confusion, stupor, or coma. Nuchal rigidity and other evidence of meningeal irritation (see Figure 2–3) are common, but these signs may not occur for several hours after the onset of the headache. Preretinal globular subhyaloid hemorrhages (found in 20% of cases) are most suggestive of the diagnosis (see Figure 2–5). Because bleeding occurs mainly in the subarachnoid space in patients with aneurysmal rupture, prominent focal signs are uncommon on neurologic examination. When present, they may bear no relationship to the site of the aneurysm. An exception is oculomotor nerve palsy occurring ipsilateral to a posterior communicating artery aneurysm. Bilateral extensor plantar responses and VI nerve palsies are frequent in such cases. Ruptured AVMs may produce focal signs, such as hemiparesis, aphasia, or a defect of the visual fields, that help to localize the intracranial lesion.

B. LABORATORY FINDINGS

Patients presenting with subarachnoid hemorrhage are generally investigated first by computed tomography (CT) scan (Figure 2–6), which will usually confirm that hemorrhage has occurred and may help to identify a focal source. CT brain scanning will detect subarachnoid blood in more than 90% of patients with aneurysmal rupture. The test is highly sensitive on the day bleeding occurs; it is most sensitive in patients with altered consciousness. Intracerebral or intraventricular blood, associated hydrocephalus, and infarction can also be identified. Aneurysms may not be evident on the CT scan, but most AVMs can be seen with contrast. Magnetic resonance imaging (MRI) is especially useful in detecting small AVMs localized to the brainstem (an area poorly seen on CT scan). If the CT scan fails to confirm the clinical diagnosis of subarachnoid hemorrhage, lumbar puncture is performed.

The CSF examination usually reveals markedly elevated pressure, often above the maximum recordable value (600 mm H_2O) using the standard CSF manometer; the fluid is grossly bloody and contains from 100,000 to more than 1 million red cells/mm³. As a result of the breakdown of hemoglobin from red cells, the supernatant of the centrifuged CSF becomes yellow (xanthochromic) within several hours (certainly by 12 hours) following the hemorrhage (see Chapter 11). White cells are initially present in the spinal fluid in the same proportion to red cells as in the peripheral blood.

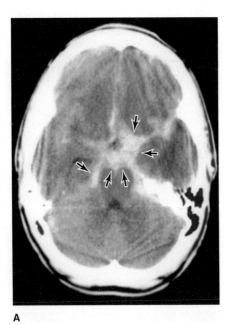

A

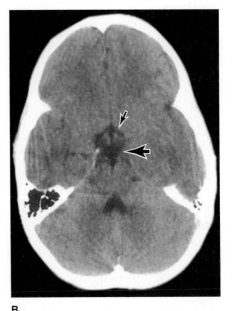

B

Figure 2–6. **A:** Nonenhanced brain CT scan from a patient with an acute aneurysmal subarachnoid hemorrhage. Areas of high density **(arrows)** represent blood in the subarachnoid space at the base of the brain (most aneurysms occur in this region about the Circle of Willis, see Figure 2–4). **B:** A normal unenhanced brain CT scan of the same region. Interpeduncular cistern, arrow; suprasellar cistern, small arrow. (Courtesy of C Jungreis.)

The chemical meningitis caused by blood in the subarachnoid space, however, may produce a pleocytosis of several thousand white blood cells during the first 48 hours and a reduction in CSF glucose between the fourth and eighth days after the hemorrhage. In the absence of pleocytosis, CSF glucose following subarachnoid hemorrhage is normal. The peripheral blood white count is often modestly elevated but rarely exceeds 15,000 cells/mm^3. The electrocardiogram (ECG) may reveal a host of abnormalities: peaked or deeply inverted T waves, short PR interval, or tall U waves.

Once the diagnosis is confirmed, four-vessel cerebral arteriography is undertaken. Cerebral angiography of both the carotid and vertebral arteries should be performed to visualize the entire cerebral vascular anatomy, since multiple aneurysms occur in 20% of patients and AVMs are frequently supplied from multiple vessels. Angiography can be performed at the earliest time convenient for radiology department personnel; emergency studies in the middle of the night are rarely indicated. Angiography is a prerequisite to the rational planning of surgical treatment and is therefore not necessary for patients who are not surgical candidates, eg, those who are deeply comatose.

Differential Diagnosis

The history of a sudden severe headache with confusion or obtundation, nuchal rigidity, a nonfocal neurologic examination, and bloody spinal fluid is highly specific for subarachnoid hemorrhage.

Hypertensive intracerebral hemorrhage is also manifested by obtundation and hemorrhagic spinal fluid, but there are prominent focal findings. Bacterial meningitis is excluded by the CSF examination. Ruptured mycotic aneurysm is suggested by other signs of endocarditis. Traumatic spinal puncture can be excluded as the cause of bloody CSF by examination of the centrifuged CSF specimen. Because blood that results from traumatic lumbar puncture has not yet undergone enzymatic breakdown to bilirubin, centrifugation of the spinal fluid specimen reveals a colorless supernatant.

Complications & Sequelae

A. RECURRENCE OF HEMORRHAGE

Recurrence of aneurysmal hemorrhage (20% over 10–14 days) is the major acute complication and roughly doubles the mortality rate. Recurrence of hemorrhage from AVM is less common in the acute period.

B. INTRAPARENCHYMAL EXTENSION OF HEMORRHAGE

Although it is common for hemorrhages from an AVM to involve the cerebral parenchyma, this is far less common with aneurysm. Nevertheless, rupture of an aneurysm of the anterior cerebral or middle cerebral artery may direct a jet of blood into brain parenchyma, producing hemiparesis, aphasia, and sometimes transtentorial herniation.

C. ARTERIAL VASOSPASM

Delayed arterial narrowing, termed vasospasm, occurs in vessels surrounded by subarachnoid blood and can lead to parenchymal ischemia in more than one-third of cases. Clinical ischemia typically does not appear before Day 4 after the hemorrhage, peaks at Day 10–14, and then spontaneously resolves. The diagnosis can be confirmed by transcranial Doppler or cerebral angiography. The severity of spasm is related to the amount of subarachnoid blood, and therefore is less common where less blood is usually seen, such as in traumatic subarachnoid hemorrhage or AVM.

D. ACUTE OR SUBACUTE HYDROCEPHALUS

Acute or subacute hydrocephalus may develop during the first day—or after several weeks—as a result of impaired CSF absorption in the subarachnoid space. Progressive somnolence, nonfocal findings, and impaired upgaze should suggest the diagnosis.

E. SEIZURES

Seizures occur in fewer than 10% of cases and only following damage to the cerebral cortex. Decorticate or decerebrate posturing is common, however, and may be mistaken for seizures.

F. OTHER COMPLICATIONS

Although inappropriate secretion of antidiuretic hormone and resultant diabetes insipidus can occur, they are uncommon.

Treatment

A. MEDICAL TREATMENT

Medical treatment is traditionally directed toward preventing elevation of arterial or intracranial pressure that might rerupture the aneurysm or AVM. Typical measures include absolute bed rest with the head of the bed elevated 15–20 degrees, mild sedation, and analgesics for headache. Drugs impairing platelet function (eg, aspirin) should be avoided. Because patients who are hypertensive on admission have an increased mortality risk, reducing the blood pressure (to approximately 160/100 mm Hg) is prudent. Bed rest and mild sedation are often adequate in this regard. Hypotension should be prevented, however, to ensure adequate cerebral perfusion. Intravenous fluids should be administered with care, since overhydration can exacerbate cerebral swelling. Intravenous fluids should be isoosmotic to minimize free water exacerbating brain edema. Normal saline can be given in amounts to ensure normovolemia. Hyponatremia is frequently seen, and usually represents, at least in part, cerebral salt wasting; it should be managed with sodium replacement such as NaCl orally or 3% normal saline intravenously rather than fluid restriction. Prophylactic use of the calcium channel antagonist drug **nimodipine**, 60 mg orally (or by nasogastric tube) every 4 hours for 21 days, may reduce the ischemic sequelae of cerebral vasospasm in patients with a ruptured aneurysm. Vasospasm is treated by induced hypertension with phenylephrine or dopamine; this intervention is more safely performed after definitive surgical treatment of the aneurysm. Although seizures are uncommon after aneurysmal rupture, the hypertension accompanying a seizure increases the risk of rerupture; a prophylactic anticonvulsant (eg, phenytoin, 300 mg/d) is therefore recommended routinely.

B. SURGICAL TREATMENT

1. Aneurysm—Definitive surgical therapy of a **ruptured aneurysm** consists of clipping the neck of the aneurysm or the endovascular placement of a coil to induce clotting. The neurologic examination is used to grade the patient's clinical state relative to surgical candidacy (Table 2–2). In patients who are fully alert (grades I and II) or only mildly confused (grade III), surgery has been shown to improve the clinical outcome. In contrast, stuporous (grade IV) or comatose (grade V) patients do not appear to benefit from the procedures. Although there is some controversy about the optimal timing of surgery, current evidence supports early intervention, within about 2 days following the hemorrhage. This approach reduces the period at risk for rebleeding and permits aggressive treatment of vasospasm with volume expansion and pharmacologic elevation of blood pressure.

Treatment of **unruptured aneurysm** is individualized. Surgery is favored by young age, previous rupture, family history of aneurysmal rupture, observed aneurysm growth, and low operative risk. Decreased life expectancy and asymptomatic small aneurysms favor conservative management.

2. AVMs—Surgically accessible AVMs may be removed by en bloc resection or obliterated by ligation of feeding vessels or embolization via local intraarterial catheter. Because the risk of an early second hemorrhage is much less with AVMs than with aneurysms, surgical treatment can be undertaken electively at a convenient time after the bleeding episode.

Prognosis

The mortality rate from aneurysmal subarachnoid hemorrhage is high. About 20% of patients die before reaching a hospital, 25% die subsequently from the initial hemorrhage or its complications, and 20% die from rebleeding if the aneurysm is not surgically corrected. Most deaths occur in the first few days after the hemorrhage. The probability of survival following aneurysmal rupture is related to the patient's state of consciousness and the elapsed time since the hemorrhage. On Day 1, the prognosis for survival for symptom-free and somnolent patients is, respectively, 60% and 30%; such patients still alive at 1 month have survival probabilities of 90% and 60%, respectively. Of survivors, half have permanent brain injury. Recovery from subarachnoid hemorrhage resulting from rupture of intracerebral AVMs occurs in nearly 90% of patients, and although recurrent hemorrhage remains a danger, conservative management compares favorably with surgical therapy.

OTHER CEREBROVASCULAR DISORDERS

Headache may be associated with—or may rarely be the presenting symptom of—**thrombotic** or **embolic stroke**. Compression of pain-sensitive structures is the mechanism of headache in **intracranial hemorrhage**, whereas pain-sensitive receptors in large cerebral arteries

Table 2–2. Clinical grading of patients with aneurysmal subarachnoid hemorrhage.

Grade	Level of Consciousness	Associated Clinical Features	Surgical Candidate
I	Normal	None or mild headache and stiff neck	Yes
II	Normal	Moderate headache and stiff neck; minimal neurologic deficit (eg, cranial nerve palsy) in some cases	Yes
III	Confusional state	Focal neurologic deficits in some cases	Yes
IV	Stupor	Focal neurologic deficits in some cases	No
V	Coma	Decerebrate posturing in some cases	No

are responsible for headache in thrombotic and embolic stroke. Lacunar strokes, which affect small arterial branches deep in the brain, are not as frequently associated with headache.

Headaches associated with ischemic stroke are typically mild to moderate in intensity, ipsilateral to the involved hemisphere, and nonthrobbing in character. Their location is determined by the pain projection sites of the involved arteries: posterior fossa strokes usually present with occipital headache, whereas carotid lesions usually produce frontal (trigeminal distribution) pain. **Transient ischemic attacks** may be associated with headache in as many as 50% of cases; in perhaps one-third of these, headaches precede the other symptoms.

Headache accompanying **retinal artery embolism** or posterior cerebral artery spasm or occlusion may be erroneously diagnosed as migraine because of the associated visual impairment.

Headache also occurs following **carotid endarterectomy** and may be associated with focal sensory or motor signs of contralateral hemispheric ischemia. This syndrome occurs in the presence of a patent carotid artery on the second or third postoperative day and typically produces intense throbbing anterior headache that is often associated with nausea.

Headache disorders associated with ischemic or hemorrhagic cerebral infarction require direct treatment of the cerebral lesion combined with the use of analgesics for symptomatic relief.

MENINGITIS OR ENCEPHALITIS

Headache is a prominent feature of inflammation of the brain (encephalitis) or its meningeal coverings (meningitis) caused by bacterial, viral, or other infections; granulomatous processes; neoplasms; or chemical irritants. The pain is caused by inflammation of intracranial pain-sensitive structures, including blood vessels at the base of the brain. The headache syndrome produced is commonly throbbing in character, bilateral, and occipital or nuchal in location. The headache is increased by sitting upright, moving the head, compressing the jugular vein, or performing other maneuvers (eg, sneezing, coughing) that transiently increase intracranial pressure. Photophobia may be prominent. The headache rarely presents suddenly but more commonly develops over hours to days, especially with subacute infections (eg, tuberculous meningitis).

Neck stiffness and other signs of meningeal irritation (see Figure 2–3) must be sought with care, since they may not be obvious either early in the course of the illness or when the brain parenchyma, rather than meninges, is the predominant site of involvement. Lethargy or confusion may also be a prominent feature.

The diagnosis is suggested by a CSF examination that shows an increased white blood cell count. Bacterial, syphilitic, tuberculous, viral, fungal, and parasitic infections may be distinguished by CSF VDRL, Gram's stain, acid-fast stain, India ink preparation and cryptococcal antibody assays, and cultures (see Table 1–9). Treatment of meningitis or encephalitis caused by these different organisms is discussed in Chapter 1.

OTHER CAUSES OF ACUTE HEADACHE

1. Seizures

Postictal headache that follows generalized tonic-clonic seizures is frequently accompanied by resolving lethargy, diffuse muscle soreness, or tongue laceration. Although this headache requires no specific treatment, it is important to differentiate it from subarachnoid hemorrhage and meningitis. If doubt exists, lumbar puncture should be undertaken.

2. Lumbar Puncture

Postlumbar-puncture headache is diagnosed by a history of lumbar puncture—and by the characteristic marked increase in pain in the upright position and relief with recumbency. The pain is typically occipital, comes on 24–48 hours after the procedure (although it may be later), and lasts 1–2 days, but may be prolonged. Headache is caused by persistent spinal subarachnoid leak with resultant traction on pain-sensitive structures at the base of the brain. The risk of this complication can be reduced by using a small-gauge needle (22 gauge or smaller) for the puncture and removing only as much fluid as needed for the studies to be performed. Lying flat afterward, for any length of time, does not lessen the incidence. Low-pressure headache syndromes are usually self-limited. When this is not the case, they may respond to the administration of caffeine sodium benzoate, 500 mg intravenously, which can be repeated after 45 minutes if headache persists or recurs upon standing. In persistent cases, the subarachnoid rent can be sealed by injection of autologous blood into the epidural space at the site of the puncture; this requires an experienced anesthesiologist. Headache similar in character to that caused by lumbar puncture occasionally occurs spontaneously. T1-weighted, gadolinium-enhanced MRI may show smooth enhancement of the pachymeninges and a "sagging brain"(Figure 2–7); the enhancement may be confused with disorders producing leptomeningeal inflammation. Low CSF pressure can also produce this MRI picture in the absence of headache.

3. Hypertensive Encephalopathy

Headache may be due to a sudden elevation in blood pressure caused by pheochromocytoma, sexual inter-

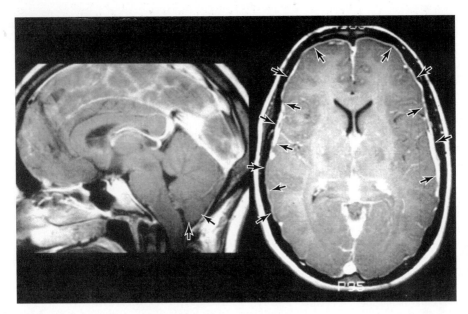

Figure 2–7. Spontaneous intracranial hypotension in a 27-year-old woman presenting with severe postural headaches. Sagittal and axial T1-weighted images obtained after gadolinium injections show features of "sagging brain": downward displacement of the cerebellar tonsils into the foramen magnum (**arrows, left image**), effacement of the brainstem cisterns (left image; compare with normal sagittal MRI Figure 11–3), and diffuse dural enhancement (**arrows, right image**). MRI abnormalities and symptoms reversed following an epidural blood patch. (Courtesy of HA Rowley.)

course, the combination of monoamine oxidase inhibitors and tyramine-containing foods such as cheddar cheese, or—the most important cause—malignant hypertension. Blood pressures of 250/150 mm Hg or higher—characteristic of malignant hypertension—produce cerebral edema and displace pain-sensitive structures. The pain is described as severe and throbbing. Other signs of diffuse or focal central nervous system dysfunction are present, such as lethargy, hemiparesis, or focal seizures; on CT or MRI images, posterior white matter changes may be seen (see Figure 1–10). Treatment is with antihypertensive drugs (see Chapter 1), but care must be taken to avoid hypotension, which can result in cerebral ischemia and stroke.

4. Coitus

Headache during sexual intercourse has been described as the presenting sign of subarachnoid hemorrhage; however, headache in this setting is more often of a benign nature. Men are more often affected than women. The pain may be either a dull, bilateral pain occurring during sexual excitement or a severe, sudden headache occurring at the time of orgasm, presumably caused by a marked increase in systemic blood pressure.

Persistent headache following orgasm—worse in the upright posture—has also been described. In the latter case, the symptoms are reminiscent of postlumbar-puncture headache and patients have low opening pressures at lumbar puncture. Each of these headaches—except for those associated with aneurysmal rupture—is benign and subsides over minutes to days.

Patients reporting severe headache in association with orgasm should be evaluated for possible subarachnoid hemorrhage as described on p 75. If no hemorrhage is found, prophylactic treatment with indomethacin, 50 mg orally prior to intercourse, may be effective.

5. Ocular Disorders

Pain about the eye may occur in migraine and cluster headache and is also the presenting feature of iritis and glaucoma. **Acute iritis** produces extreme eye pain that is associated with photophobia. The diagnosis is confirmed by slit lamp examination; acute management involves pharmacologic dilatation of the pupil. **Angle-closure glaucoma** produces pain within the globe that radiates to the forehead. When it occurs after middle age, such a pain syndrome should prompt diagnostic tonometry. Acute treatment is with glycerol, 1 mL/kg orally, followed by pilocarpine, 2%, two drops every 15 minutes.

HEADACHES OF SUBACUTE ONSET

GIANT CELL ARTERITIS

This disorder, also known as temporal arteritis, is characterized by a subacute granulomatous inflammation (consisting of lymphocytes, neutrophils, and giant cells) that affects the external carotid arterial system, particularly the superficial temporal artery, and the vertebral artery. Inflammation of the pain-sensitive arterial wall produces the headache. Thrombosis may occur in the most severely affected arteries.

This syndrome, which affects women twice as frequently as men, is uncommon before age 50 and is frequently associated with nonspecific signs and symptoms, such as malaise, myalgia, weight loss, arthralgia, and fever (the polymyalgia rheumatica complex). The headache can be unilateral or bilateral, fairly severe, and boring in quality. It is characteristically localized to the scalp, especially over the temporal arteries. Scalp tenderness may be especially apparent when lying with the head on a pillow or brushing the hair. Pain or stiffness in the jaw during chewing (jaw claudication) is highly suggestive of giant cell arteritis and is due to arterial ischemia in the muscles of mastication. Involvement of the ophthalmic artery leads to permanent blindness in 50% of untreated patients; in half of these, blindness will become bilateral. The visual loss is most often sudden in onset. Although episodes of transient prodromal blindness have been reported, blindness is unusual as an initial symptom; however, it often occurs within the first month.

The diagnosis is made by biopsy of affected temporal arteries, which are characteristically thickened and non-pulsatile as well as dilated and tender. The temporal arteries may be affected in a patchy manner, and serial sections may be necessary to demonstrate histologic vasculitis. The erythrocyte sedimentation rate (ESR) is almost invariably elevated. The mean Westergren ESR is about 100 mm/h in giant cell arteritis (range, 29–144 mm/h) and in polymyalgia rheumatica (range, 58–160 mm/h). The normal upper limit of the Westergren ESR in elderly patients is reported to be only as high as 40 mm/h.

Consideration of this diagnosis demands prompt inpatient evaluation if vision is to be preserved. Therapy for giant cell arteritis is prednisone, 40–60 mg/d orally, with decreasing dosage usually after about 3 months, depending upon the clinical response. The sedimentation rate returns rapidly toward normal with prednisone therapy and must be maintained within normal limits as the drug dose is tapered. Therapy should not be withheld pending biopsy diagnosis and should be continued despite negative biopsy findings if the diagnosis can be made with confidence on clinical grounds. Therapy generally has to be continued for 1–2 years. Although dramatic improvement in headache occurs within 2–3 days after institution of therapy, the blindness is usually irreversible.

INTRACRANIAL MASS

The new onset of headache in middle or later life should always raise concern about a mass lesion. A mass lesion, such as a brain tumor (Table 2–3), subdural hematoma, or abscess, may or may not produce headache depending upon whether it compresses or distorts pain-sensitive intracranial structures. Only 30% of patients with intracranial tumor present with headache as the first symptom, although 80% have such a complaint at the time of diagnosis. Subdural hematoma frequently presents with conspicuous headache, since its large size increases the likelihood of impinging upon pain-sensitive areas. Headaches associated with brain tumors are

Table 2–3. Symptoms of brain tumors.[1]

Symptom	Percent with Symptom		
	Low-Grade Glioma	*Malignant Glioma*	*Meningioma (Benign)*
Headache	40	50	36
Seizure	65–95	15–25	40
Hemiparesis	5–15	30–50	22
Altered mental status	10	40–60	21

[1] Modified from DeAngelis LM: Brain tumors. N Engl J Med 2001;344:114.

most often nonspecific in character, mild to moderate in severity, dull and steady in nature, and intermittent. The pain is characteristically bifrontal, worse ipsilaterally, and aggravated by a change in position or by maneuvers that increase intracranial pressure, such as coughing, sneezing, and straining at stool. The headache is classically maximal on awakening in the morning and is associated with nausea and vomiting.

An uncommon type of headache that suggests brain tumor is characterized by a sudden onset of severe pain reaching maximal intensity within seconds, persisting for minutes to hours, and subsiding rapidly. Altered consciousness or "drop attacks" may be associated. Although classically associated with third ventricular colloid cysts, these paroxysmal headaches can be associated with tumors at many different intracranial sites.

Suspicion of an intracranial mass lesion demands prompt evaluation, preferably with CT scan or MRI; brain tumor is excluded by a normal contrast-enhanced brain MRI scan. Lumbar puncture should not be used as a diagnostic screening test, since the results are nonspecific and the procedure may aggravate the symptoms of the intracerebral mass, sometimes with a fatal outcome.

PSEUDOTUMOR CEREBRI

Pseudotumor cerebri (benign intracranial hypertension) is characterized by a diffuse increase in intracranial pressure causing headache, papilledema, and diminished visual acuity. Diplopia may also occur as a result of abducens nerve palsy. Although pseudotumor can accompany many disorders (Table 2–4), most cases are idiopathic. In the idiopathic variety, women are affected much more commonly than men, with a peak incidence in the third decade. Diffuse headache is almost always a presenting symptom, and diplopia and blurred vision occur in 60% of cases. Although visual acuity is normal

Table 2–4. Disorders associated with pseudotumor cerebri.

Intracranial venous drainage obstruction (eg, venous sinus thrombosis, head trauma, polycythemia, thrombocytosis)
Endocrine dysfunction (eg, obesity, especially with marked menstrual irregularities; pregnancy; menarche; oral contraceptive therapy; withdrawal from steroid therapy; Cushing's disease; Addison's disease; hypoparathyroidism)
Vitamin and drug therapy (eg, hypervitaminosis A in children and adolescents; tetracycline in infants)
Other (eg, chronic hypercapnia, congestive heart failure, chronic meningitis, hypertensive encephalopathy)
Idiopathic

in 50% of patients at presentation, moderate to severe papilledema is seen in almost 90%. Visual loss from increased intracranial pressure can occur even in the idiopathic form; episodes of clouded vision precede the loss.

The course of the idiopathic disorder is generally self-limited over several months, with no sequelae if intracranial pressure is maintained at a relatively normal level to prevent secondary optic atrophy. Differentiating idiopathic pseudotumor cerebri from intracerebral mass lesions and from the disorders listed in Table 2–4 is critical; evaluation must include MRI or CT brain scanning. These studies typically show small (slitlike) ventricles in pseudotumor cerebri. Elevation of intracranial pressure can be documented by lumbar puncture. If a specific cause is identified, it must be treated appropriately.

Treatment with acetazolamide, 250 mg orally three times daily, with or without a diuretic (eg, furosemide), may be adequate to control mild intracranial hypertension. In other instances, prednisone, 60–80 mg/d orally, may be necessary. In refractory cases, repeated lumbar punctures or lumboperitoneal shunting procedures protect vision and decrease headache. Transorbital optic nerve sheath fenestration is also used to protect the optic nerve from the pressure injury that is thought to cause blindness.

TRIGEMINAL NEURALGIA

Trigeminal neuralgia (tic douloureux) is a facial-pain syndrome of unknown cause that develops in middle to late life. In many instances, the trigeminal nerve roots are close to some vascular structure, and microvascular compression of the nerve is believed to cause the disorder. Pain is confined mainly to the area supplied by the second and third divisions of the trigeminal nerve (Figure 2–8). Involvement of the first division or bilateral disease occurs in less than 5% of cases. Characteristically, lightninglike momentary jabs of excruciating pain occur and spontaneously abate. Occurrence during sleep is rare. Pain-free intervals may last for minutes to weeks, but long-term spontaneous remission is rare. Sensory stimulation of trigger zones about the cheek, nose, or mouth by touch, cold, wind, talking, or chewing can precipitate the pain. Physical examination discloses no abnormalities. Rarely, similar pain may occur in multiple sclerosis or brainstem tumors, and these possibilities should thus be considered in young patients and in all patients who show neurologic abnormalities on examination.

In idiopathic cases, CT scan and MRI fail to show any abnormality, and arteriography is similarly normal. Any vascular structure compressing the nerve roots is generally too small to be seen by these means.

Remission of symptoms with carbamazepine, 400–1200 mg/d orally in three divided doses, occurs within

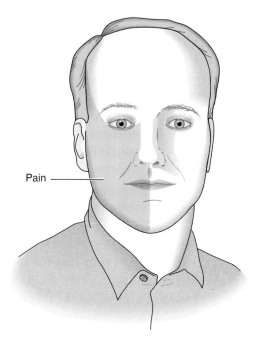

Pain

Figure 2–8. Distribution of symptoms in trigeminal neuralgia.

24 hours in such a high percentage of cases that some believe it to be diagnostic. Rarely, blood dyscrasia occurs as an adverse reaction to carbamazepine. Intravenous administration of phenytoin, 250 mg, will abort an acute attack, and phenytoin, 200–400 mg/d orally, may be effective in combination with carbamazepine if a second drug is necessary. Lamotrigine 400 mg/d or baclofen 10 mg three times daily–20 mg four times daily has been used in refractory cases. Posterior fossa microvascular decompressive surgery has been used in drug-resistant cases.

GLOSSOPHARYNGEAL NEURALGIA

Patients with glossopharyngeal neuralgia, an uncommon pain syndrome, present with either a paroxysmal pain that is identical in quality to that of trigeminal neuralgia, or a continuous burning or aching discomfort. The pain is localized to the oropharynx, the tonsillar pillars, the base of the tongue, or the auditory meatus. The trigger areas are usually around the tonsillar pillars, so that symptoms are initiated by swallowing or by talking. Paroxysms of pain can occur many times daily and may be accompanied by syncopal episodes caused by transient bradyarrhythmias. Men are affected more often than women, and symptoms begin at a somewhat younger age than in trigeminal neuralgia. The diagnosis

is established by the history and by reproducing pain through stimulation of the trigger zones (usually about the tonsillar regions). Examination reveals no abnormal neurologic signs. Application of local anesthetics to the trigger area may block the pain response. Carbamazepine or phenytoin therapy (as described above for trigeminal neuralgia) usually produces dramatic relief; microvascular decompression has been used.

POSTHERPETIC NEURALGIA

Herpes zoster—a vesicular skin eruption in dermatomal distribution, accompanied and followed by local pain and tenderness—is due to reactivation of varicella-zoster virus in patients with a history of varicella infection. It does not occur before age 50 and becomes increasingly common with advancing age (70% in those over 70 years), in immunocompromised patients, and in patients with certain malignant diseases (eg, leukemia, lymphoma). Postherpetic neuralgia is characterized by constant, severe, stabbing or burning, dysesthetic pain that may persist for months or years in a minority of patients, especially older ones. It occurs in the same dermatomal distribution as a previous bout of herpes zoster, conforming to the distribution of the involved nerve root, where residual scars may be present. When the head is involved, the first division of the trigeminal nerve is most commonly affected, so that pain is usually localized to the forehead on one side (Figure 2–9). Careful testing of the painful area reveals decreased cutaneous sensitivity to pinprick. The other major complication of trigeminal herpes is decreased corneal sensation with impaired blink reflex, which can lead to corneal abrasion, scarring, and ultimate loss of vision.

The intensity and duration of the cutaneous eruption and the acute pain of herpes zoster are reduced by 7 to 10 days of treatment with acyclovir (800 mg 5 times daily), famciclovir, or valacyclovir, but this treatment has not been shown to lessen the likelihood of postherpetic neuralgia. Corticosteroids (60 mg/d prednisone, orally for 2 weeks, with rapid tapering) taken during the acute herpetic eruption also reduce the incidence of acute herpetic pain, but have an uncertain effect on postherpetic pain. Once the postherpetic pain syndrome is established, the most useful treatment has been with tricyclic antidepressants such as amitriptyline, 25–150 mg/d orally, which are thought to act directly on central nervous system pain-integration pathways (rather than via an antidepressant effect). Tricyclic antidepressant drugs may be more effective when combined with a phenothiazine, as in the commercially available preparation Triavil. Carbamazepine, phenytoin, and gabapentin in anticonvulsant doses have also been used. Postherpetic neuralgia subsides within 6–12 months in many patients but in 50% of those over 70 years the pain per-

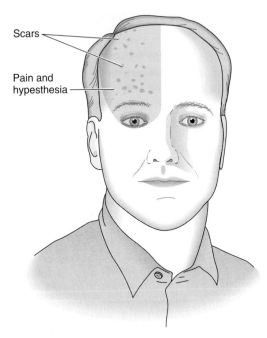

Scars

Pain and
hypesthesia

Figure 2–9. Distribution of symptoms and signs in postherpetic neuralgia.

sists. Lidocaine-prilocaine 2.5% cream, or lidocaine gel 5%, is effective topical therapy. Topical application of capsaicin cream (eg, Zostrix 0.025%), which depletes pain-mediating peptides from peripheral sensory neurons, can also be helpful but is poorly tolerated. In otherwise intractable cases, weekly intrathecal administration of methylprednisolone may reduce pain.

HYPERTENSION

⑤ Chronic hypertension is often invoked as a cause of headache, but evidence to support such a connection is sparse. In contrast, headache is a well-established complication of paroxysmal hypertension such as seen in patients with pheochromocytoma or those ingesting tyramine-rich foods while being treated with monoamine oxidase inhibitors. In pheochromocytoma, headache attacks are brief. They last less than 15 minutes in one-half of patients and are characteristically associated with perspiration and tachycardia. The headache is usually bilateral and may be precipitated by urination if the bladder is involved.

ATYPICAL FACIAL PAIN

Constant, boring, mainly unilateral lower facial pain for which no cause can be found is referred to as atypical facial pain. Unlike trigeminal neuralgia, it is not con-

fined to the trigeminal nerve distribution and is not paroxysmal. This idiopathic disorder must be distinguished from similar pain syndromes related to nasopharyngeal carcinoma, intracranial extension of squamous cell carcinoma of the face, or infection at the site of a tooth extraction. Treatment is with amitriptyline, 20–250 mg/d orally, alone or in combination with phenelzine, 30–75 mg/d orally. Dilantin can be an effective alternative, especially if a tricyclic is inappropriate.

CHRONIC HEADACHES

MIGRAINE

Migraine is manifested by headache that is usually unilateral and frequently pulsatile in quality; it is often associated with nausea, vomiting, photophobia, phonophobia, and lassitude. Visual or other neurologic auras occur in about 10% of patients. Two-thirds to three-fourths of cases of migraine occur in women; the onset is early in life—approximately 25% beginning during the first decade, 55% by 20 years of age, and more than 90% before age 40. A family history of migraine is present in most cases.

Genetics of Migraine

The aggregation of migraine within families has long been recognized, although consistent mendelian patterns of inheritance have not been found among the collective group of familial migraineurs. Presumably this reflects a variety of inheritance patterns, variable penetrance, and possibly multiple genes interacting with environmental factors in the multigenic/multifactorial pattern characteristic of complex diseases. Concordance rates in monozygotic twins of only 28–52 attest to the genetic component, but also predict a significant environmental contribution.

A rare subtype of migraine with aura, familial hemiplegic migraine, has a straightforward autosomal dominant, highly penetrant inheritance pattern indicative of a strong genetic component. Three genetic loci for familial hemiplegic migraine have been identified: one on chromosome 19p13 (associated with missense mutations in a brain-expressed, voltage-gated P/Q calcium channel gene) and two neighboring loci on chromosome 1q.

Pathogenesis

Intracranial vasoconstriction and extracranial vasodilatation have long been held to be the respective causes of the aura and headache phases of migraine. This theory received support from the efficacy of vasoconstrictive ergot alkaloids (eg, ergotamine) in aborting the acute migraine attack and vasodilators such as amyl nitrite in abolishing the migraine aura. More recent studies of regional cerebral blood flow during migraine attacks have demonstrated a reduction in regional flow, which begins in the occipital region, during the aura phase. The "spreading depression" in cerebral blood flow, however, proceeds according to cytoarchitectural patterns in the cerebral cortex and does not reflect the distribution of major vascular territories (Figure 2–10). In addition, the areas of decreased blood flow do not correspond to the cortical areas responsible for the particular aura, and regional cerebral blood flow may remain depressed after focal neurologic symptoms have resolved and headache has begun (Figure 2–11). Later in the headache phase, blood flow increases to parts of the cortex (cingulate, auditory, and visual association areas) and the contralateral brainstem (serotonergic dorsal raphe nucleus and adrenergic nucleus ceruleus); treatment with effective agents (sumatriptan, ergotamine) attenuates the cortical but not brainstem changes. These data imply that cerebral blood flow changes and headache generation in migraine may be secondary to a primary disturbance in neuronal function in the brainstem. Brainstem stimulation in the periaqueductal gray and dorsal raphe nucleus produces migraine-like headache in humans.

Serotonergic neurons ramify extensively throughout the brain, and many effective antimigraine drugs act as

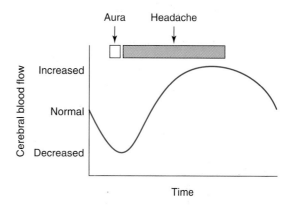

Figure 2–11. Time course of changes in cerebral blood flow in migraine with aura. (Adapted from Olesen J et al: Timing and topography of cerebral blood flow, aura, and headache during migraine attacks. Ann Neurol 1990;28:791–798.)

antagonists or partial agonists at central serotonin receptors. Serotonin in platelets decreases and urinary serotonin increases during the acute phase of a migraine attack. Depletion of serotonin by reserpine may precipitate migraine. The headache and other manifestations of migraine may thus reflect a disorder of central serotonergic neurotransmission. A link between neuronal initiation and trigeminovascular-mediated pain may be calcitonin gene-related peptide (CGRP), a potent vasodilator present in increased concentrations in venous blood during migraine and cluster headache, and at decreased levels after the administration of serotonin receptor agonists such as sumatriptan.

Clinical Findings

A. Migraine with Aura (Classic Migraine)

Classic migraine headache is preceded by transient neurologic symptoms—the aura. The most common auras are visual alterations, particularly hemianopic field defects and scotomas and scintillations that enlarge and spread peripherally (Figure 2–12). A throbbing unilateral headache ensues (Figure 2–13) with or following these prodromal features. The frequency of headache varies, but more than 50% of patients experience no more than one attack per week. The duration of episodes is greater than 2 hours and less than 1 day in most patients. Remissions are common during the second and third trimesters of pregnancy and after menopause. Especially in the elderly, prodromal symptoms may occur without headache (migraine equivalents). Although hemicranial pain is a hallmark of classic migraine, headaches can also be bilateral. Bilateral

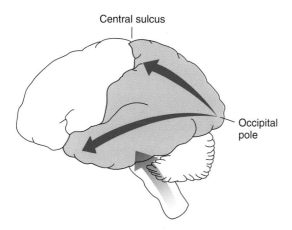

Figure 2–10. Direction of spread **(arrows)** and maximal extent (colored region) of depressed cerebral blood flow (CBF) in migraine with and without aura. These processes may be initiated by contralateral brainstem structures as increases in brainstem CBF during migraine persist after headache treatment with sumatriptan.

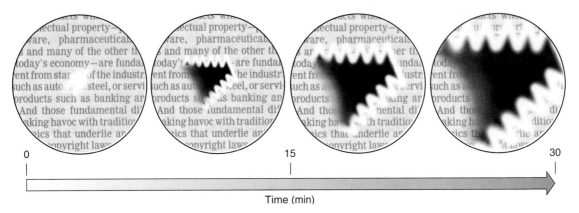

Time (min)

Figure 2–12. Successive maps of scintillating scotoma to show the evolution of fortification figures and associated scotoma in a patient with classic migraine. As the fortification moves laterally, a region of transient blindness remains.

headache, therefore, does not exclude the diagnosis of migraine, nor does an occipital location—a characteristic commonly attributed to tension headaches. During the headache, prominent associated symptoms include

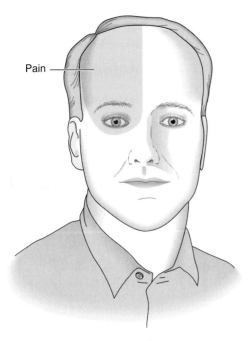

Pain

Figure 2–13. Distribution of pain in migraine. Hemicranial pain (the pattern shown) is most common, but the pain can also be holocephalic, bifrontal, or unilateral frontal in distribution or, less commonly, localized to the occiput or the vertex of the skull.

nausea, vomiting, photophobia, phonophobia, irritability, osmophobia, and lassitude. Uncommonly, migraines are associated with frank neurologic deficits that accompany, or persist beyond resolution of the pain phase. These may include hemiparesis, hemisensory loss, speech dysfunction, or visual disturbance. Vasomotor and autonomic symptoms are frequent; lightheadedness, vertigo, ataxia, or altered consciousness may represent vertebrobasilar ischemia. All these phenomena may be distinguished from stroke both by their gradual onset ("migrainous march") and spontaneous resolution. Stroke may very exceptionally occur as a consquence of migraine alone.

B. MIGRAINE WITHOUT AURA (COMMON MIGRAINE)

The common migraine headache lacks the classic aura, is usually bilateral and periorbital, and is seen more frequently in clinical practice. The pain may be described as throbbing. As the pain persists, associated cervical muscle contraction can compound the symptoms. Scalp tenderness is often present during the episode. Vomiting may occasionally terminate the headache.

A useful bedside test for both common and classic migraine is reducing headache severity by compressing the ipsilateral carotid or superficial temporal artery.

Precipitating Factors

Migraine attacks can be precipitated by certain foods (tyramine-containing cheeses; meat, such as hot dogs or bacon, with nitrite preservatives; chocolate containing phenylethylamine but not chocolate alone) and by food additives such as monosodium glutamate, a commonly used flavor enhancer. Fasting, emotion, menses, drugs (especially oral contraceptive agents and vasodilators such as nitroglycerin), and bright lights may also trigger attacks.

Treatment

Acute migraine attacks may respond to simple analgesics (eg, aspirin, acetaminophen, naprosyn). If not, they usually respond to ergot preparations or to the 5-hydroxytryptamine (5-HT) agonist sumatriptan. These drugs (Table 2–5A) must be taken immediately at the onset of symptoms to be maximally effective. Rapidly absorbed forms (eg, suppository, aerosol) are superior to oral or sublingual preparations. In severe cases, subcutaneous, nasal, intramuscular, or intravenous administration is used. Unfortunately, nausea, which is a prominent feature of migraine, is also a common side effect of the drugs, so that concomitant administration of an antiemetic (eg, metoclopramide, 10 mg subcutaneously or intravenously) may be necessary. Ergot alkaloids and 5-HT agonists are potent vasoconstrictors and are contraindicated in patients with significant hypertension or cardiac disease. Established migraine headaches may respond to dihydroergotamine, sumatriptan, or narcotic analgesics (eg, meperidine, 100 mg intramuscularly).

Several drugs are effective in the prophylactic treatment of migraine (Table 2–5B). Prophylactic treatment is indicated for patients who have frequent attacks—especially more than one per week—and those for whom the ergot alkaloids used for acute treatment are poorly tolerated or contraindicated. Three structurally unrelated agents—propranolol, amitriptyline, and valproic acid—are the mainstays of therapy. Each is effective in a substantial fraction of patients, and patients refractory to one agent may respond to another. The initial choice of medication is usually influenced by consideration of clinical side effects that may be especially troublesome for a particular patient. Propranolol, imipramine, and amitriptyline may be sedating, especially at the onset of treatment. The β-adrenergic-receptor-blocking properties of propranolol often preclude its use in patients with congestive heart failure, asthma, or insulin-dependent diabetes. It may also be associated with depression, hypotension, exercise intolerance, and impotence. The anticholinergic actions of amitriptyline may complicate glaucoma and prostatism. Valproic acid should be introduced gradually as nausea can be a problem; it is also particularly contraindicated in pregnancy.

Calcium channel antagonists such as verapamil or nicardepine are also efficacious in the prophylactic treatment of migraine. Drugs available in other countries or approved in the United States only for other indications include nimodipine and flunarizine; however, both common and classic migraine respond to these drugs. As discussed above, potential side effects should be taken into account in the choice of therapy. Verapamil, which has pronounced effects on cardiac and gastrointestinal calcium channels, may exacerbate atrioventricular, nodal heart block and congestive heart failure and frequently causes constipation. Nimodipine, which is more selective for vascular smooth muscle, is associated with a higher incidence of headache, lightheadedness, hypotension, and peripheral edema. It should not be used in conjuction with β-blockers. Nifedipine is ineffective.

Surprisingly, selective serotonin reuptake inhibitors have not been shown to be efficacious.

Migraine during pregnancy should be treated only with opiates, eg, meperidine 100–150 mg orally, as all other pharmacologic agents raise concerns regarding teratogenicity or complications of pregnancy.

ANALGESIC WITHDRAWAL HEADACHE

A common, frequently unsuspected, cause of intractable headache is overuse of analgesics. The patient, in futile attempts at relief, takes increasing amounts of medications (both prescription and over-the-counter drugs). When the high blood levels drop, even slightly, the headache rebounds; the result is daily, virtually constant, atypical headache, which may be superimposed on an underlying migraine pattern. Caffeine-containing analgesics are particularly responsible. The patient should be abruptly withdrawn from all such medications and caffeine. After a few weeks of drug withdrawal symptoms the underlying, usually less severe, headache pattern will reveal itself and can be more appropriately treated. Headaches during withdrawal can be managed with oral sumatriptan or parenteral dihydroergotamine.

CLUSTER HEADACHE

Cluster headache is a common headache syndrome seen much more frequently in men than in women. Cluster headaches characteristically begin at a later age than does migraine, with a mean age at onset of 25 years. There is rarely a family history of such headaches. The syndrome presents as clusters of brief, very severe, unilateral, constant nonthrobbing headaches that last from a few minutes to less than 2 hours. Unlike migraine headaches, cluster headaches are always unilateral, and usually recur on the same side in any given patient. The headaches commonly occur at night, awakening the patient from sleep, and recur daily, often at nearly the same time of day, for a cluster period of weeks to months. Between clusters, the patient may be free from headaches for months or years. Functional MRI imaging during attacks has shown activation of the ipsilateral hypothalamic gray.

The headache may begin as a burning sensation over the lateral aspect of the nose or as a pressure behind the

Table 2–5. Drug treatment of migraine headache.

Drug	Route[1]	Strength	Recommended Dose	Comments
A. Acute Treatment				
Simple analgesics				
Aspirin	PO	325 mg	650–1300 mg	May cause gastric pain
Naproxen sodium	PO	250, 375, 500 mg	375–750 mg	or bleeding and rebound
Ibuprofen	PO	300, 400, 600, 800 mg	400–800 mg	headache if used
Acetaminophen	PO	325 mg	650–1300 mg	frequently
Ergot preparations				
Ergotamine/caffeine (*Cafergot, Wigraine*)	PO	1/100 mg	2–6 tablets; max. 10 per week	May cause nausea and vomiting;
	PR	2/100 mg	2–6 tablets; max. 10 per week 1/4–2 suppositories; max. 5 per week	contraindicated by pregnancy or coronary or peripheral vascular disease
Dihydroergotamine	IM, SC, IV	1 mg/mL	1–2 mg IM or SC; 0.75–1.25 mg IV	Use dihydroergotamine with metoclopramide (see below)
	NS	4 mg/1 mL (2 mg/treatment)	1 spray to each nostril repeated in 15 minutes	
Narcotic analgesics				
Codeine/aspirin	PO	15, 30, 60/325 mg	30–120 mg codeine	
Codeine/acetaminophen	PO	7.5, 15, 30, 60/300 mg	30–120 mg codeine	
Meperidine	PO, IM	50, 100 mg	50–200 mg	
Butorphanol	NS	10 mg/mL (1 mg/spray)	1 spray every 3–4 hours as needed	
5-HT agonists				
Sumatriptan	NS	5, 20 mg/spray	40 mg/24 hours	10% incidence nausea, vomiting
	PO	25, 50, 100 mg	200 mg/24 hours	Contraindicated by
	SC	6 mg	12 mg	pregnancy or coronary
Rizatriptan	PO	5, 10 mg	30 mg/24 hours	or peripheral vascular
Zolmitriptan	PO	2.5, 5 mg	10 mg/24 hours	disease, and with
Naratriptan	PO	1, 2.5 mg	5 mg/24 hours	monoamine oxidase
Almotriptan	PO	6.25, 12.5 mg	12.5 mg/24 hours	inhibitors
Other agents				
Isometheptene/ dichloralphenazone/ acetaminophen (*Midrin*)	PO	65/100/325 mg	2–5 capsules	
Caffeine/butalbital/ aspirin (*Fiorinal*)	PO	40/50/325 mg	1–2 tablets or capsules	
Prochlorperazine	PR, IM, IV	2.5/10/10 mg	2.5–10 mg	Can cause hypotension and drug-induced dystonia
B. Prophylactic Treatment				
Antiinflammatory agents				
Aspirin	PO	325 mg	650 mg bid	May cause gastric pain or
Naproxen sodium	PO	275, 550 mg	500–825 mg bid	bleeding

continued

Table 2–5. Drug treatment of migraine headache. *(continued)*

Drug	Route[1]	Strength	Recommended Dose	Comments
Tricyclic antidepressants				
Amitriptyline[2]	PO	10, 25, 50, 75, 100, 150 mg	10–175 mg hs	May cause dry mouth, urinary retention, and sedation; contraindicated in glaucoma or prostatism
			10–175 mg hs	
Nortriptyline	PO	10, 25, 50, 75 mg	10–150 mg hs	
Protriptyline	PO	5, 10 mg	5–40 mg qhs	
Doxepin	PO	10, 25, 30, 75, 100, 150 mg	10–150 mg hs	
β-Receptor antagonists				
Propranolol	PO	10, 20, 40, 60, 80, 90 mg	20–160 mg bid	Listed in descending order of efficacy; symptomatic bradycardia may occur at high doses; contraindicated in asthma and congestive heart failure; not to be used with calcium blockers
	PO (long acting)	60, 80, 120, 160 mg	60–320 mg qd	
Nadolol	PO	40, 80, 120, 160 mg	40–240 mg qd	
Atenolol	PO	50, 100 mg	50–200 mg bid	
Timolol	PO	10, 20 mg	10–30 mg bid	
Metoprolol	PO	50, 100 mg	50–200 mg qd	
Ergot alkaloids				
Methysergide	PO	2 mg	2–8 mg qd	Occurrence of retroperitoneal fibrosis with urethral obstruction and mediastinal fibrosis, although uncommon, should be monitored with creatinine, ultrasonography, or intravenous urograms, and chest x-rays every 6 months; a drug holiday every 6 months is prudent
Cyproheptadine	PO	4 mg	4–8 mg tid	Drowsiness common early in treatment
Anticonvulsants				
Phenytoin	PO	100 mg	200–400 mg qd	
Valproic acid	PO	250 mg	250–1000 mg bid	
Topiramate	PO	15, 25, 100, 200 mg	50–100 mg qd	
Gabapentin	PO	100, 300, 400, 600, 800 mg	900–2400 mg qd	
Calcium channel antagonists				
Verapamil	PO	40, 80, 120 mg	80–160 mg tid	Contraindicated by severe left ventricular dysfunction, hypotension, sick sinus syndrome without artificial pacemaker, or second- or third-degree AV nodal block; constipation is most common side effect; not for use with β-blockers
	PO (long acting)	240 mg	240 mg qd–bid	
Nicardipine	PO	20 mg	20–40 mg tid	
Flunarizine	PO	5, 10 mg	5–15 mg/d	

continued

Table 2–5. Drug treatment of migraine headache. *(continued)*

Drug	Route[1]	Strength	Recommended Dose	Comments
Other agents				
Ergotamine/ phenobarbital/ belladonna (*Bellergal-S*)	PO	0.6/40/0.2 mg	1 tablet bid	May cause nausea and vomiting; contraindicated by pregnancy or coronary or peripheral vascular disease
Phenelzine	PO	15 mg	15–90 mg qd	
Prochlorperazine	PO, IM, IV	2.5–10 mg		
Hydroxyzine	IM	25–100 mg		
Metoclopramide	PO, IV, SC	10 mg		Adjunct to treatment; improves enteric drug absorption and reduces nausea; dystonia and akathisia may occur and respond to IV benadryl

[1] PO, oral; SL, sublingual; PR, rectal; IM, intramuscular; IV, intravenous; SC, subcutaneous; NS, nasal spray; bid, twice daily; hs, at bedtime; qd, every day.

[2] Other tricyclic agents such as imipramine and desipramine may also be used, are available in similar strengths, and are prescribed in similar doses.

eye (Figure 2–14). Ipsilateral conjunctival injection, lacrimation, nasal stuffiness, and Horner's syndrome are commonly associated with the attack (Figure 2–15). Episodes are often precipitated by the use of alcohol or vasodilating drugs, especially during a cluster siege.

At the onset of a headache cluster, treatment involves measures both to abort the acute attack and to prevent subsequent ones. Acute relief of pain within minutes may be achieved by sumatriptan (Table 2–5A), 100% oxygen (8–10 L/min for 10–15 minutes), or dihydroergotamine (Table 2–5A).

Several drugs used in the treatment of migraine (see Table 2–5), including 5-HT agonists, ergotamine, dihydroergotamine, methysergide, and calcium channel antagonists (verapamil, sustained-release), are also useful for preventing recurrent symptoms during an active bout of cluster headache. Ergotamine rectal suppositories or subcutaneous dihydroergotamine at bedtime may be especially helpful for nocturnal headaches. In addition, dramatic improvement is typically seen with administration of prednisone, 40–80 mg/d orally for 1 week, discontinued by tapering the dose over the following week. Pain may resolve within hours, and most patients who respond do so within 2 days. Alternatively, lithium carbonate or lithium citrate syrup, 300 mg orally three times daily, is highly effective in many cases. Serum lithium levels should be measured at weekly

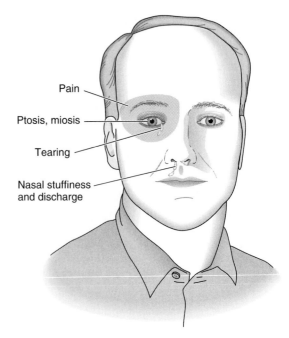

Figure 2–14. Distribution of symptoms and signs in cluster headache.

Pain

Ptosis, miosis

Tearing

Nasal stuffiness and discharge

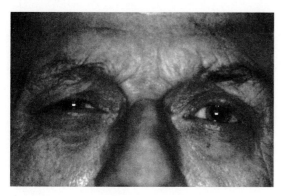

Figure 2–15. Right ptosis during acute cluster headache.

intervals for the first several weeks and should be maintained below 1.2 meq/L to reduce the likelihood of adverse effects (nausea, diarrhea, polyuria, renal failure, hypothyroidism, tremor, dysarthria, ataxia, myoclonus, and seizures). Chronic rather than episodic cluster headaches may respond dramatically to indomethacin, 25 mg three times daily. A bilateral variant, hypnic headache, lacking the autonomic components, occurs in the elderly. It is reponsive to lithium.

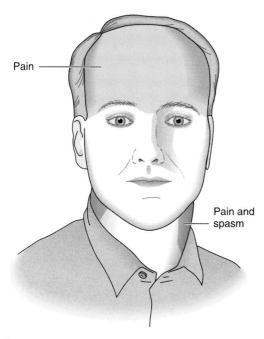

Pain

Pain and spasm

Figure 2–16. Distribution of symptoms and signs in tension headache.

TENSION-TYPE HEADACHE

Tension headache is the term used to describe chronic headaches of inapparent cause that lack features characteristic of migraine or cluster headache. The underlying pathophysiologic mechanism is unknown, and tension is unlikely to be primarily responsible. Contraction of neck and scalp muscles, which has also been proposed as the cause, is probably a secondary phenomenon. In its classic form (Figure 2–16), tension headache is a chronic disorder that begins after age 20. It is characterized by frequent (often daily) attacks of nonthrobbing, bilateral occipital head pain that is not associated with nausea, vomiting, or prodromal visual disturbance. The pain is sometimes likened to a tight band around the head. Women are more commonly affected than men. Although tension headache and migraine have been traditionally considered distinct disorders, many patients have headaches that exhibit features of both. Thus, some patients who are classified as having tension headaches experience throbbing headaches, unilateral head pain, or vomiting with attacks. In consequence, it may be more accurate to view tension headache and migraine as representing opposite poles of a single clinical spectrum.

Drugs used in the treatment of tension headache include many of the same agents used for migraine (see Table 2–5). Acute attacks may respond to aspirin, other nonsteroidal antiinflammatory drugs, acetaminophen, ergotamine, or dihydroergotamine. For prophylactic treatment, amitriptyline, imipramine, or selective serotonin reuptake inhibitors (eg, sertraline or fluoxetine) are often effective, and propranolol is useful in some cases. Although many patients respond to benzodiazepines such as diazepam, 5–30 mg/d orally, or chlordiazepoxide, 10–75 mg/d orally, these drugs should be used sparingly because of their addictive potential. Psychotherapy, physical therapy, and relaxation techniques can provide additional benefit in selected cases.

ICE PICK PAIN

Very brief, sharp, severe pains located in the scalp outside of the trigeminal distribution are named by their defining characteristic as "ice pick pains." They may be single or repetitive or occur in clusters, either at a single point or scattered over the scalp. The pains are electric-like jabs maximal in intensity in less than a second and then resolving rapidly; they are severe enough to cause involuntary flinching. They are more common in migraine and cluster patients, but occur in some headache-free individuals as well. Patients frequently seek medical attention because of the intensity of the pain. If the bouts of pain are repetitive, treatment may be indicated; the syndrome responds to indomethacin (25 mg three times daily).

CERVICAL SPINE DISEASE

Injury or degenerative disease processes involving the upper neck can produce pain in the occiput or referred to the orbital regions. The most important source of discomfort is irritation of the second cervical nerve root. In the lower cervical spine, disk disease or abnormalities of the articular processes refer pain to the ipsilateral arm or shoulder, not to the head. Cervical muscle spasm may occur, however.

Acute pain of cervical origin is treated with immobilization of the neck (eg, using a soft collar) and analgesics or antiinflammatory drugs.

SINUSITIS

Acute sinusitis can produce pain and tenderness localized to the affected frontal or maxillary sinus areas. Inflammation in the ethmoidal or sphenoidal sinuses produces a deep midline pain behind the nose. Sinusitis pain is increased by bending forward and by coughing or sneezing. Tenderness and accentuation of pain on percussion over the frontal or maxillary area are present on examination.

Sinusitis is treated with vasoconstrictor nose drops (eg, phenylephrine, 0.25%, instilled every 2–3 hours), antihistamines, and antibiotics. In refractory cases, sinus drainage may be necessary.

Patients who complain of chronic sinus headache rarely have recurrent inflammation of the sinuses; they are much more likely to have migraine or tension headaches.

DENTAL DISEASE

Temporomandibular joint dysfunction is a poorly defined syndrome that is characterized by preauricular facial pain, limitation of jaw movement, tenderness of the muscles of mastication, and "clicking" of the jaw with movement. Symptoms are often associated with malocclusion, bruxism, or clenching of the teeth, and may result from spasm of the masticatory muscles. Some patients benefit from local application of heat, jaw exercises, nocturnal use of a bite guard, or nonsteroidal antiinflammatory drugs.

Infected tooth extraction sites can also give rise to pain, which is characteristically constant, unilateral, and aching or burning in character. Although radiologic studies may be normal, injection of a local anesthetic at the extraction site relieves the symptoms. Treatment is with jaw bone curettage and antibiotics.

REFERENCES

Aurora SK, Welch KM: Migraine: imaging the aura. Curr Opin Neurol 2000;13:273–276.

Brew BJ, Miller J: Human immunodeficiency virus-related headache. Neurology 1993;43:1098–1100.

Broadley SA, Fuller GN: Lumbar puncture needn't be a headache. BMJ 1997;315:1324–1325.

Caselli RJ, Hunder GG: Giant cell (temporal) arteritis. Neurol Clin 1997;15:893–902.

DeAngelis LM: Brain tumors. N Engl J Med 2001;344:114–123.

Ferrari MD: Migraine. Lancet 1998;351:1043–1051.

Flippen C, Welch KM: Imaging the brain of migraine sufferers. Curr Opin Neurol 1997;10:226–230.

Forsyth PA, Posner JB: Headaches in patients with brain tumors: a study of 111 patients. Neurology 1993;43:1678–1683.

Friedman DI: Pseudotumor cerebri. Neurosurg Clin N Am 1999;10:609–621.

Gawel MJ, Worthington I, Maggisano A: A systematic review of the use of triptans in acute migraine. Can J Neurol Sci 2001:28:30–41.

Hunder GG: Giant cell arteritis and polymyalgia rheumatica. Med Clin North Am 1997;81:195–219.

Katusic S et al: Incidence and clinical features of trigeminal neuralgia, Rochester, Minnesota, 1945–1984. Ann Neurol 1990;27:89–95.

Kelly AM: Migraine: pharmacotherapy in the emergency department. West J Med 2000;173:189–193.

Kost RG, Straus SE: Postherpetic neuralgia—pathogenesis, treatment, and prevention. N Engl J Med 1996;335:32–42.

Kotani N et al: Intrathecal methylprednisolone for intractable postherpetic neuralgia. N Engl J Med 2000;343:1514–1519.

Lance JW, Goadsby PJ: *Mechanism and Management of Headache,* 6th ed. Butterworth-Heinemann, 1998.

May A, Goadsby PJ: The trigeminovascular system in humans: pathophysiologic implications for primary headache syndromes of the neural influences on the cerebral circulation. J Cereb Blood Flow Metab 1999;19:115–127.

Pascual J, Berciano J: Experience in the diagnosis of headaches that start in elderly people. J Neurol Neurosurg Psychiatry 1994;57:1255–1257.

Raskin NH: Headaches associated with organic diseases of the nervous system. Med Clin North Am 1978;62:459–466.

Raskin NH: Chemical headaches. Annu Rev Med 1981;32:63–71.

Raskin NH: *Headache,* 2nd ed. Churchill Livingstone, 1988.

Rushton JG, Stevens JC, Miller RH: Glossopharyngeal (vagoglossopharyngeal) neuralgia: a study of 217 cases. Arch Neurol 1981;38:201–205.

Schwartz BS et al: Epidemiology of tension-type headache. JAMA 1998;279:381–383.

Silberstein SD: Tension-type and chronic daily headache. Neurology 1993;32:1644–1649.

Solomon S, Cappa KG: The headache of temporal arteritis. J Am Geriatr Soc 1987;35:163–165.

Tomsak RL: Ophthalmologic aspects of headache. Med Clin North Am 1991;75:693–706.

Weiller C et al: Brainstem activation in spontaneous human migraine attacks. Nat Med 1995;1:658–660.

Welch KMA: Drug therapy of migraine. N Engl J Med 1993;329:1476–1483.

Woods RP, Iacoboni M, Mazziotta JC: Bilateral spreading cerebral hypoperfusion during spontaneous migraine headache. N Engl J Med 1994;331:1689–1692.

Disorders of Equilibrium

3

CONTENTS

KEY CONCEPTS

 Disorders of equilibrium can be produced by disorders that affect vestibular pathways, the cerebellum, or sensory pathways in the spinal cord or peripheral nerves.

 Disorders of equilibrium present with one or both of two cardinal symptoms: vertigo—an illusion of bodily or environmental movement, or ataxia—incoordination of limbs or gait.

 Cerebellar hemorrhage and infarction produce disorders of equilibrium that require urgent diagnosis, because surgical evacuation of the hematoma or infarct can prevent death from brainstem compression.

APPROACH TO DIAGNOSIS

Equilibrium is the ability to maintain orientation of the body and its parts in relation to external space. It depends on continuous visual, labyrinthine, and somatosensory (proprioceptive) input and its integration in the brainstem and cerebellum.

 Disorders of equilibrium result from diseases that affect central or peripheral vestibular pathways, the cerebellum, or sensory pathways involved in proprioception.

 Such disorders usually present with one of two clinical problems: **vertigo** or **ataxia.**

1. Vertigo

Vertigo is the illusion of movement of the body or the environment. It may be associated with other symptoms, such as **impulsion** (a sensation that the body is being hurled or pulled in space), **oscillopsia** (a visual illusion of moving back and forth), nausea, vomiting, or gait ataxia.

Distinction Between Vertigo & Other Symptoms

Vertigo must be distinguished from nonvertiginous dizziness, which includes sensations of light-headedness, faintness, or giddiness not associated with an illusion of movement. In contrast to vertigo, these sensations are produced by conditions that impair the brain's supply of blood, oxygen, or glucose—eg, excessive vagal stimulation, orthostatic hypotension, cardiac arrhythmias, myocardial ischemia, hypoxia, or hypoglycemia—and may culminate in loss of consciousness (**syncope;** see Chapter 8).

Differential Diagnosis

A. ANATOMIC ORIGIN

The first step in the differential diagnosis of vertigo is to localize the pathologic process in the peripheral or central vestibular pathways (Figure 3–1).

Peripheral vestibular lesions affect the labyrinth of the inner ear or the vestibular division of the acoustic (VIII) nerve. **Central** lesions affect the brainstem vestibular nuclei or their connections. Rarely, vertigo is of cortical origin, occurring as a symptom associated with complex partial seizures.

B. SYMPTOMS

Certain characteristics of vertigo, including the presence of any associated abnormalities, can help differentiate between peripheral and central causes (Table 3–1).

1. Peripheral vertigo tends to be intermittent, lasts

for briefer periods, and produces more distress than vertigo of central origin. **Nystagmus** (rhythmic oscillation of the eyeballs) is always associated with peripheral vertigo; it is usually unidirectional and never vertical (see below). Peripheral lesions commonly produce additional symptoms of inner ear or acoustic nerve dysfunction, ie, hearing loss and tinnitus.

2. Central vertigo may occur with or without nystagmus; if nystagmus is present, it can be vertical, unidirectional, or multidirectional and may differ in character in the two eyes. (Vertical nystagmus is oscillation in a vertical plane; that produced by upgaze or downgaze is not necessarily in the vertical plane.) Central lesions may produce intrinsic brainstem or cerebellar signs, such as motor or sensory deficits, hyperreflexia, extensor plantar responses, dysarthria, or limb ataxia.

2. Ataxia

Ataxia is incoordination or clumsiness of movement that is not the result of muscular weakness. It is caused by vestibular, cerebellar, or sensory (proprioceptive) disorders. Ataxia can affect eye movement, speech (producing dysarthria), individual limbs, the trunk, stance, or gait (Table 3–2).

Vestibular Ataxia

Vestibular ataxia can be produced by the same central and peripheral lesions that cause vertigo. Nystagmus is frequently present and is typically unilateral and most pronounced on gaze away from the side of vestibular involvement. Dysarthria does not occur.

Vestibular ataxia is gravity dependent: Incoordination of limb movements cannot be demonstrated when the patient is examined lying down but becomes apparent when the patient attempts to stand or walk.

Cerebellar Ataxia

Cerebellar ataxia is produced by lesions of the cerebellum or its afferent or efferent connections in the cerebellar peduncles, red nucleus, pons, or spinal cord (Figure 3–2). Because of the crossed connection between the frontal cerebral cortex and the cerebellum, unilateral frontal disease can also occasionally mimic a disorder of the contralateral cerebellar hemisphere. The clinical manifestations of cerebellar ataxia consist of irregularities in the rate, rhythm, amplitude, and force of voluntary movements.

A. HYPOTONIA

Cerebellar ataxia is commonly associated with hypotonia, which results in defective posture maintenance. Limbs are easily displaced by a relatively small force and, when shaken by the examiner, exhibit an increased

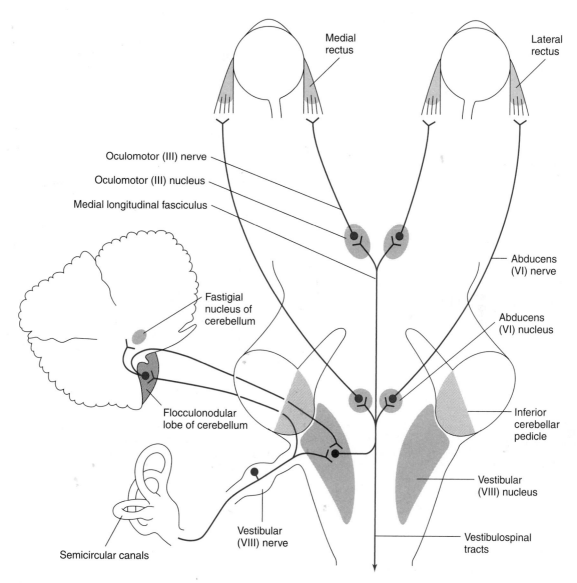

Figure 3–1. Peripheral and central vestibular pathways. The vestibular nerve terminates in the vestibular nucleus of the brainstem and in midline cerebellar structures that also project to the vestibular nucleus. From here, bilateral pathways in the medial longitudinal fasciculus ascend to the abducens and oculomotor nuclei and descend to the spinal cord.

range of excursion. The range of arm swing during walking may be similarly increased. Tendon reflexes take on a pendular quality, so that several oscillations of the limb may occur after the reflex is elicited, although neither the force nor the rate of the reflex is increased. When muscles are contracted against resistance that is then removed, the antagonist muscle fails to check the movement and compensatory muscular relaxation does

not ensue promptly. This results in rebound movement of the limb.

B. INCOORDINATION

In addition to hypotonia, cerebellar ataxia is associated with incoordination of voluntary movements. Simple movements are delayed in onset, and their rates of acceleration and deceleration are decreased. The rate,

Table 3–1. Characteristics of central and peripheral vertigo.

	Peripheral	Central
Vertigo	Often intermittent; severe	Often constant; usually less severe
Nystagmus	Always present; unidirectional, never vertical	May be absent; uni- or bidirectional, may be vertical
Associated findings		
Hearing loss or tinnitus	Often present	Rarely present
Intrinsic brain stem signs	Absent	Typically present

rhythm, amplitude, and force of movements fluctuate, producing a jerky appearance. Because these irregularities are most pronounced during initiation and termination of movement, their most obvious clinical manifestations include **terminal dysmetria,** or "overshoot," when the limb is directed at a target, and terminal **intention tremor** as the limb approaches the target. More complex movements tend to become decomposed into a succession of individual movements rather than a single smooth motor act (**asynergia**). Movements that involve rapid changes in direction or greater physiologic complexity, such as walking, are most severely affected.

C. ASSOCIATED OCULAR ABNORMALITIES

Because of the cerebellum's prominent role in the control of eye movements, ocular abnormalities are a frequent consequence of cerebellar disease. These include nystagmus and related ocular oscillations, gaze pareses, and defective saccadic and pursuit movements.

D. ANATOMIC BASIS OF DISTRIBUTION OF CLINICAL SIGNS

Various anatomic regions of the cerebellum (Figure 3–3) are functionally distinct, corresponding to the somatotopic organization of their motor, sensory, visual, and auditory connections (Figure 3–4).

1. Midline lesions—The middle zone of the cerebellum—the vermis and flocculonodular lobe and their associated subcortical (fastigial) nuclei—is involved in the control of axial functions, including eye movements, head and trunk posture, stance, and gait. Midline cerebellar disease therefore results in a clinical syndrome characterized by nystagmus and other disorders of ocular motility, oscillation of the head and trunk (**titubation**), instability of stance, and gait ataxia (Table 3–3). Selective involvement of the superior cerebellar vermis, as commonly occurs in alcoholic cerebellar degeneration, produces exclusively or primarily ataxia of gait, as would be predicted from the somatotopic map of the cerebellum (see Figure 3–4).

2. Hemispheric lesions—The lateral zones of the cerebellum (cerebellar hemispheres) help to coordinate movements and maintain tone in the ipsilateral limbs. The hemispheres also have a role in regulating ipsilateral gaze. Disorders affecting one cerebellar hemisphere

Table 3–2. Characteristics of vestibular, cerebellar, and sensory ataxia.

	Vestibular	Cerebellar	Sensory
Vertigo	Present	May be present	Absent
Nystagmus	Present	Often present	Absent
Dysarthria	Absent	May be present	Absent
Limb ataxia	Absent	Usually present (one limb, unilateral, legs only, or all limbs)	Present (typically legs only)
Stance	May be able to stand with feet together; typically worse with eyes closed	Unable to stand with feet together and eyes either open or closed	Often able to stand with feet together and eyes open but not with eyes closed (Romberg's sign)
Vibratory and position sense	Normal	Normal	Impaired
Ankle reflexes	Normal	Normal	Depressed or absent

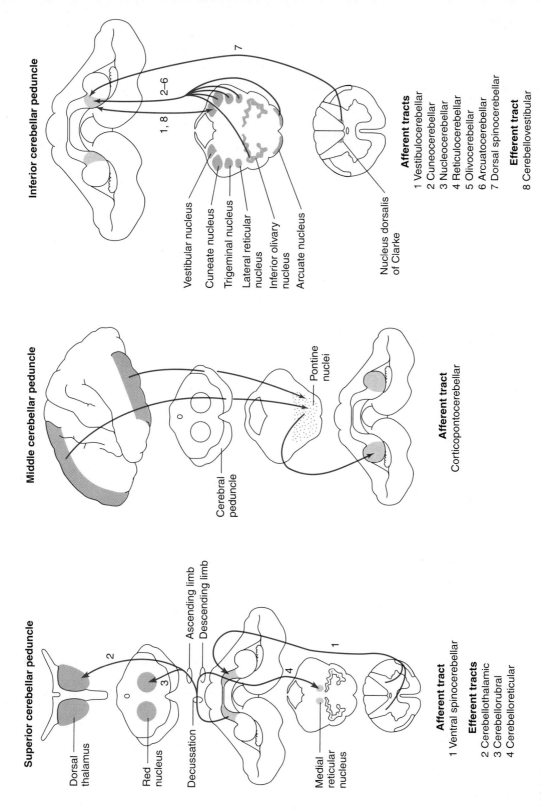

Superior cerebellar peduncle

Dorsal thalamus

Red nucleus

Ascending limb

Descending limb

Decussation

Medial reticular nucleus

Afferent tract
1 Ventral spinocerebellar

Efferent tracts
2 Cerebellothalamic
3 Cerebellorubral
4 Cerebelloreticular

Middle cerebellar peduncle

Cerebral peduncle

Pontine nuclei

Afferent tract
Corticopontocerebellar

Inferior cerebellar peduncle

Vestibular nucleus

Cuneate nucleus

Trigeminal nucleus

Lateral reticular nucleus

Inferior olivary nucleus

Arcuate nucleus

Nucleus dorsalis of Clarke

Afferent tracts
1 Vestibulocerebellar
2 Cuneocerebellar
3 Nucleocerebellar
4 Reticulocerebellar
5 Olivocerebellar
6 Arcuatocerebellar
7 Dorsal spinocerebellar

Efferent tract
8 Cerebellovestibular

Figure 3–2. Cerebellar connections in the superior, middle, and inferior cerebellar peduncles. The peduncles are indicated by gray shading and the areas to and from which they project by blue shading.

A

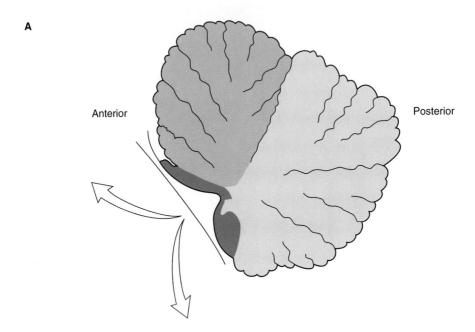

Anterior

Posterior

B

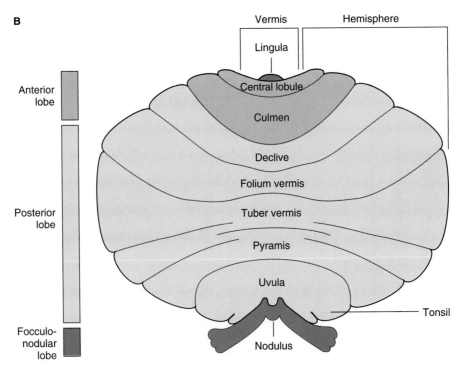

Vermis

Hemisphere

Lingula

Anterior lobe

Central lobule

Culmen

Declive

Folium vermis

Posterior lobe

Tuber vermis

Pyramis

Uvula

Tonsil

Focculo-nodular lobe

Nodulus

Figure 3–3. Anatomic divisions of the cerebellum in midsagittal view (**A**); unfolded (**arrows**) and viewed from behind (**B**).

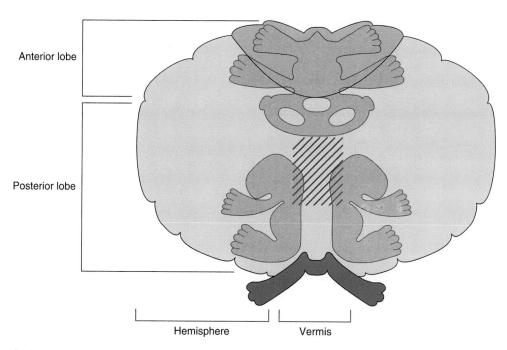

Figure 3–4. Functional organization of the cerebellum. The view is similar to that in Figure 3–3B but is of a monkey rather than a human cerebellum. The three cerebellar homunculi represent areas to which proprioceptive and tactile stimuli project, and the stripes represent areas to which auditory and visual stimuli project.

Table 3–3. Clinical patterns of cerebellar ataxia.

Pattern of Involvement	Signs	Causes
Midline	Nystagmus, head and trunk titubation, gait ataxia	Tumor, multiple sclerosis
Superior vermis	Gait ataxia	Wernicke's encephalopathy, alcoholic cerebellar degeneration, tumor, multiple sclerosis
Cerebellar hemisphere	Nystagmus, ipsilateral gaze paresis, dysarthria (especially left hemisphere lesion), ipsilateral hypotonia, ipsilateral limb ataxia, gait ataxia, falling to side of lesion	Infarction, hemorrhage, tumor, multiple sclerosis
Pancerebellar	Nystagmus, bilateral gaze paresis, dysarthria, bilateral hypotonia, bilateral limb ataxia, gait ataxia	Drug intoxications, hypothyroidism, hereditary cerebellar degeneration, paraneoplastic cerebellar degeneration, Wilson's disease, infections and parainfectious encephalomyelitis, Creutzfeldt-Jakob disease, multiple sclerosis

cause ipsilateral hemiataxia and hypotonia of the limbs as well as nystagmus and transient ipsilateral gaze paresis (an inability to look voluntarily toward the affected side). Cerebellar dysarthria may also occur with paramedian lesions in the left cerebellar hemisphere.

3. Diffuse disease—Many cerebellar disorders—typically toxic, metabolic, and degenerative conditions—affect the cerebellum diffusely. The clinical picture in such states combines the features of midline and bilateral hemisphere disease.

Sensory Ataxia

Sensory ataxia results from disorders that affect the proprioceptive pathways in peripheral sensory nerves, sensory roots, posterior columns of the spinal cord, or medial lemnisci. Thalamic and parietal lobe lesions are rare causes of contralateral sensory hemiataxia. Sensations of joint position and movement (**kinesthesis**) originate in pacinian corpuscles and unencapsulated nerve endings in joint capsules, ligaments, muscle, and periosteum. Such sensations are transmitted via heavily myelinated A fibers of primary afferent neurons, which enter the dorsal horn of the spinal cord and ascend uncrossed in the posterior columns (Figure 3–5). Proprioceptive information from the legs is conveyed in the medially located fasciculus gracilis, and information from the arms is conveyed in the more laterally situated fasciculus cuneatus. These tracts synapse on second-order sensory neurons in the nucleus gracilis and nucleus cuneatus in the lower medulla. The second-order neurons decussate as internal arcuate fibers and ascend in the contralateral medial lemniscus. They terminate in the ventral posterior nucleus of the thalamus, from which third-order sensory neurons project to the parietal cortex.

Sensory ataxia from polyneuropathy or posterior column lesions typically affects the gait and legs in symmetric fashion; the arms are involved to a lesser extent or spared entirely. Examination reveals impaired sensations of joint position and movement in the affected limbs, and vibratory sense is also commonly disturbed. Vertigo nystagmus, and dysarthria are characteristically absent.

HISTORY

Symptoms & Signs

A. VERTIGO

True vertigo must be distinguished from a light-headed or presyncopal sensation. Vertigo is typically described as spinning, rotating, or moving, but when the description is vague, the patient should be asked specifically if the symptom is associated with a sense of movement. The circumstances under which symptoms occur may

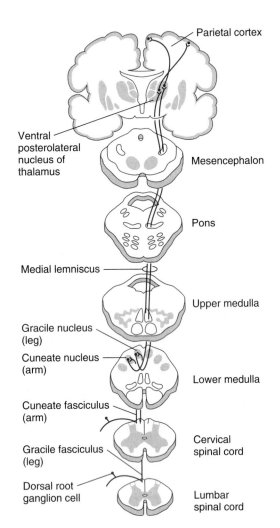

Figure 3–5. Pathway mediating proprioceptive sensation.

also be diagnostically helpful. Vertigo is often brought on by changes in head position. The occurrence of symptoms upon arising after prolonged recumbency is a common feature of orthostatic hypotension, and nonvertiginous dizziness related to pancerebral hypoperfusion may be immediately relieved by sitting or lying down. Such hypoperfusion states can lead to loss of consciousness, which is rarely associated with true vertigo. If the problem is identified as vertigo, associated symptoms may help to localize the site of involvement. Complaints of hearing loss or tinnitus strongly suggest a disorder of the peripheral vestibular apparatus (labyrinth or acoustic nerve). Dysarthria, dysphagia, diplopia, or focal weakness or sensory loss affecting the face or limbs indicates the likelihood of a central (brainstem) lesion.

B. Ataxia

Ataxia associated with vertigo suggests a vestibular disorder, whereas numbness or tingling in the legs is common in patients with sensory ataxia. Because proprioceptive deficits may, to some extent, be compensated for by other sensory cues, patients with sensory ataxia may report that their balance is improved by watching their feet when they walk or by using a cane or the arm of a companion for support. They thus find that they are much more unsteady in the dark and may experience particular difficulty in descending stairs.

Onset & Time Course

Establishing the time course of the disorder may suggest its cause. **Sudden** onset of disequilibrium occurs with infarcts and hemorrhages in the brainstem or cerebellum (eg, lateral medullary syndrome, cerebellar hemorrhage or infarction). **Episodic** disequilibrium of acute onset suggests transient ischemic attacks in the basilar artery distribution, benign positional vertigo, or Ménière's disease. Disequilibrium from transient ischemic attacks is usually accompanied by cranial nerve deficits, neurologic signs in the limbs, or both. Ménière's disease is usually associated with progressive hearing loss and tinnitus as well as vertigo.

Chronic, progressive disequilibrium evolving over weeks to months is most suggestive of a toxic or nutritional disorder (eg, vitamin B_{12} or vitamin E deficiency, nitrous oxide exposure). Evolution over months to years is characteristic of an inherited spinocerebellar degeneration.

Medical History

The medical history should be scrutinized for evidence of diseases that affect the sensory pathways (vitamin B_{12} deficiency, syphilis) or cerebellum (hypothyroidism, paraneoplastic syndromes, tumors), and drugs that produce disequilibrium by impairing vestibular or cerebellar function (ethanol, sedative drugs, phenytoin, aminoglycoside antibiotics, quinine, salicylates).

Family History

A hereditary degenerative disorder may be the cause of chronic, progressive cerebellar ataxia. Such disorders include spinocerebellar degenerations, Friedreich's ataxia, ataxia-telangiectasia, and Wilson's disease.

GENERAL PHYSICAL EXAMINATION

Various features of the general physical examination may provide clues to the underlying disorder. **Orthostatic hypotension** is associated with certain sensory disorders that produce ataxia—eg, tabes dorsalis, polyneu-

ropathies—and with some cases of spinocerebellar degeneration. The **skin** may show oculocutaneous telangiectasia (ataxia-telangiectasia), or it may be dry, with brittle hair (hypothyroidism) or have a lemon-yellow coloration (vitamin B_{12} deficiency). **Pigmented corneal (Kayser-Fleischer) rings** are seen in Wilson's disease (see Chapter 7).

Skeletal abnormalities may be present. Kyphoscoliosis is typical in Friedreich's ataxia; hypertrophic or hyperextensible joints are common in tabes dorsalis; and pes cavus is a feature of certain hereditary neuropathies. Abnormalities at the craniocervical junctions may be associated with Arnold-Chiari malformations or other congenital anomalies that involve the posterior fossa.

NEUROLOGIC EXAMINATION

Mental Status Examination

An **acute confusional state** with ataxia characterizes ethanol or sedative drug intoxication and Wernicke's encephalopathy.

Dementia with cerebellar ataxia is seen in Wilson's disease, Creutzfeldt-Jakob disease, hypothyroidism, paraneoplastic syndromes, and some spinocerebellar degenerations. Dementia with sensory ataxia suggests syphilitic taboparesis or vitamin B_{12} deficiency.

Korsakoff's amnestic syndrome and cerebellar ataxia are associated with chronic alcoholism.

Stance & Gait

Observation of stance and gait is helpful in distinguishing between cerebellar, vestibular, and sensory ataxias. In any ataxic patient, the stance and gait are wide-based and unsteady, often associated with reeling or lurching movements.

A. Stance

The ataxic patient asked to stand with the feet together may show great reluctance or an inability to do so. With persistent urging, the patient may gradually move the feet closer together but will leave some space between them. Patients with sensory ataxia and some with vestibular ataxia are, nevertheless, ultimately able to stand with the feet together, compensating for the loss of one source of sensory input (proprioceptive or labyrinthine) with another (visual). This compensation is demonstrated when the patient closes the eyes, eliminating visual cues. With sensory or vestibular disorders, unsteadiness increases and may result in falling (**Romberg's sign**). With a vestibular lesion, the tendency is to fall toward the side of the lesion. Patients with cerebellar ataxia are unable to compensate for their deficit by using visual input and are unstable on their feet whether the eyes are open or closed.

B. GAIT

1. The gait seen in **cerebellar ataxia** is wide-based, often with a staggering quality that might suggest drunkenness. Oscillation of the head or trunk (**titubation**) may be present. If a unilateral cerebellar hemisphere lesion is responsible, there is a tendency to deviate toward the side of the lesion when the patient attempts to walk in a straight line or circle or marches in place with eyes closed. **Tandem** (heel-to-toe) **gait,** which requires walking with an exaggerated narrow base, is always impaired.

2. In **sensory ataxia** the gait is also wide-based and tandem gait is poor. In addition, walking is typically characterized by lifting the feet high off the ground and slapping them down heavily (**steppage gait**) because of impaired proprioception. Stability may be dramatically improved by letting the patient use a cane or lightly rest a hand on the examiner's arm for support. If the patient is made to walk in the dark or with eyes closed, gait is much more impaired.

3. Gait ataxia may also be a manifestation of **conversion disorder** (conversion disorder with motor symptom or deficit) or **malingering.** Determining this can be particularly difficult, since isolated gait ataxia without ataxia of individual limbs can also be produced by diseases that affect the superior cerebellar vermis. The most helpful observation in identifying factitious gait ataxia is that such patients often exhibit wildly reeling or lurching movements from which they are able to recover without falling. In fact, recovery of balance from such awkward positions requires excellent equilibratory function.

Oculomotor (III), Trochlear (IV), Abducens (VI), & Acoustic (VIII) Nerves

Abnormalities of ocular and vestibular nerve function are typically present with vestibular disease and often present with lesions of the cerebellum. (Examination of cranial nerves III, IV, and VI is discussed in more detail in Chapter 5.)

A. OCULAR ALIGNMENT

The eyes are examined in the primary position of gaze (looking directly forward) to detect malalignment in the horizontal or vertical plane.

B. NYSTAGMUS AND VOLUNTARY EYE MOVEMENTS

The patient is asked to turn the eyes in each of the cardinal directions of gaze (left, up and left, down and left, right, up and right, down and right; see Chapter 5) to determine whether gaze paresis (impaired ability to move the two eyes coordinately in any of the cardinal directions of gaze) or gaze-evoked nystagmus is present. Nystagmus—an abnormal involuntary oscillation of the eyes—is characterized in terms of the positions of gaze in which it occurs, its amplitude, and the direction of its fast phase. **Pendular nystagmus** has the same velocity in both directions of eye movement; **jerk nystagmus** is characterized by both fast (vestibular-induced) and slow (cortical) phases. The direction of jerk nystagmus is defined by the direction of the fast component. Fast voluntary eye movements (**saccades**) are elicited by having the patient rapidly shift gaze from one target to another placed in a different part of the visual field. Slow voluntary eye movements (**pursuits**) are assessed by having the patient track a slowly moving target such as the examiner's finger.

1. Peripheral vestibular disorders produce unidirectional horizontal jerk nystagmus that is maximal on gaze away from the involved side. **Central** vestibular disorders can cause unidirectional or bidirectional horizontal nystagmus, vertical nystagmus, or gaze paresis. **Cerebellar** lesions are associated with a wide range of ocular abnormalities, including gaze pareses, defective saccades or pursuits, nystagmus in any or all directions, and ocular dysmetria (overshoot of visual targets during saccadic eye movements).

2. Pendular nystagmus is usually the result of visual impairment that begins in infancy.

C. HEARING

Preliminary examination of the acoustic (VIII) nerve should include otoscopic inspection of the auditory canals and tympanic membranes, assessment of auditory acuity in each ear, and Weber and Rinne tests performed with a 256-Hz tuning fork.

1. In the **Weber test,** unilateral sensorineural hearing loss (from lesions of the cochlea or cochlear nerve) causes the patient to perceive the sound produced by a vibrating tuning fork placed at the vertex of the skull as coming from the normal ear. With a conductive (external or middle ear) disorder, sound is localized to the abnormal ear.

2. The **Rinne test** may also distinguish between sensorineural and conductive defects in the affected ear. Air conduction (tested by holding the vibrating tuning fork next to the external auditory canal) normally produces a louder sound than does bone conduction (tested by placing the base of the tuning fork over the mastoid bone). This pattern also occurs with acoustic nerve lesions but is reversed in the case of conductive hearing loss (Table 3–4).

D. POSITIONAL TESTS

When patients indicate that vertigo occurs with a change in position, the Nylen-Bárány or Dix-Hallpike maneuver (Figure 3–6) is used to try to reproduce the precipitating circumstance. The head, turned to the right, is rapidly lowered 30 degrees below horizontal

Table 3–4. Assessment of hearing loss.

	Weber Test	Rinne Test
Normal	Sound perceived as coming from midline	Air conduction > bone conduction
Sensorineural hearing loss	Sound perceived as coming from normal ear	Air conduction > bone conduction
Conductive hearing loss	Sound perceived as coming from affected ear	Bone conduction > air conduction on affected side

while the gaze is maintained to the right. This process is repeated with the head and eyes turned first to the left and then straight ahead. The eyes are observed for nystagmus, and the patient is asked to note the onset, severity, and cessation of vertigo.

Positional nystagmus and **vertigo** are usually associated with peripheral vestibular lesions and are most often a feature of **benign positional vertigo.** This is typically characterized by severe distress, a latency of several seconds between assumption of the position and the onset of vertigo and nystagmus, a tendency for the response to remit spontaneously (fatigue) as the position is maintained, and attenuation of the response (habituation) as the offending position is repeatedly assumed (Table 3–5). Positional vertigo can also occur with central vestibular disease.

E. Caloric Testing

Disorders of the vestibuloocular pathways can be detected by caloric testing. The patient is placed supine with the head elevated 30 degrees to bring the superficially situated lateral semicircular canal into the upright position. Each ear canal is irrigated in turn with cold (33°C) or warm (44°C) water for 40 seconds, with at least 5 minutes between tests. Warm water tends to produce less discomfort than cold. ***Caution:*** Caloric testing should be preceded by careful otoscopic examination, and should not be undertaken if the tympanic membrane is perforated.

1. In the normal awake patient, cold-water caloric stimulation produces nystagmus with the slow phase toward and the fast phase away from the irrigated ear. Warm water irrigation produces the opposite response.

2. In patients with unilateral labyrinthine, vestibular nerve, or vestibular nuclear dysfunction, irrigation of the affected side fails to cause nystagmus or elicits nystagmus that is later in onset or briefer in duration than on the normal side.

Other Cranial Nerves

Papilledema associated with disequilibrium suggests an intracranial mass lesion, usually in the posterior fossa, that is causing increased intracranial pressure. Optic

neuropathy may be present in multiple sclerosis, neurosyphilis, or vitamin B_{12} deficiency. A depressed corneal reflex or facial palsy ipsilateral to the lesion (and the ataxia) can accompany cerebellopontine angle tumor. Weakness of the tongue or palate, hoarseness, or dysphagia results from lower brainstem disease.

Motor System

Examination of motor function in the patient with a disorder of equilibrium should determine the pattern and severity of ataxia and disclose any associated pyramidal, extrapyramidal, or peripheral nerve involvement that might suggest a cause. The clinical features that help distinguish cerebellar disease from diseases involving these other motor systems are summarized in Table 3–6.

A. Ataxia and Disorders of Muscle Tone

Muscle tone is assessed as discussed in Chapter 6. Truncal stability is assessed with the patient in the sitting position, and the limbs are examined individually.

1. Movement of the patient's arm is observed as his or her finger tracks back and forth between his or her own nose or chin and the examiner's finger. With mild cerebellar ataxia, an intention tremor characteristically appears near the beginning and end of each such movement, and the patient may overshoot the target.

2. When the patient is asked to raise the arms rapidly to a given height—or when the arms, extended and outstretched in front of the patient, are displaced by a sudden force—there may be overshoot (rebound). Impaired ability to check the force of muscular contractions can also be demonstrated by having the patient forcefully flex the arm at the elbow against resistance —and then suddenly removing the resistance. If the limb is ataxic, continued contraction without resistance may cause the hand to strike the patient at the shoulder or in the face.

3. Ataxia of the legs is demonstrated by the supine patient's inability to run the heel of the foot smoothly up and down the opposite shin.

4. Ataxia of any limb is reflected by irregularity in the rate, rhythm, amplitude, and force of rapid successive tapping movements.

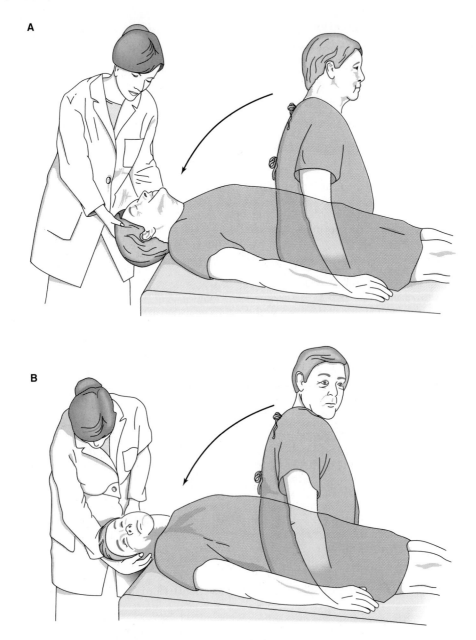

Figure 3–6. Test for positional vertigo and nystagmus. The patient is seated on a table with the head and eyes directed forward (**A**), and is then quickly lowered to a supine position with the head over the table edge, 45 degrees below horizontal. The patient's eyes are then observed for nystagmus, and the patient is asked to report any vertigo. The test is repeated with the patient's head and eyes turned 45 degrees to the right (**B**), and again with the head and eyes turned 45 degrees to the left (not shown).

5. Hypotonia is characteristic of cerebellar disorders; with unilateral cerebellar hemispheric lesions, the ipsilateral limbs are hypotonic.

6. Extrapyramidal hypertonia (rigidity) occurs with cerebellar ataxia in Wilson's disease, acquired hepatocerebral degeneration, Creutzfeldt-Jakob disease,

Table 3–5. Characteristics of positional nystagmus.

Feature	Peripheral Lesion	Central Lesion
Vertigo	Severe	Mild
Latency	2–40 seconds	No
Fatigability	Yes	No
Habituation	Yes	No

and certain types of olivopontocerebellar degeneration.

7. Ataxia with spasticity may be seen in multiple sclerosis, posterior fossa tumors or congenital anomalies, vertebrobasilar ischemia or infarction, olivopontocerebellar degeneration, Friedreich's and other hereditary ataxias, neurosyphilis, Creutzfeldt-Jakob disease, and vitamin B_{12} deficiency.

B. WEAKNESS

The pattern of any weakness should be determined. **Distal neuropathic weakness** can be caused by disorders that produce sensory ataxia, such as polyneuropathies and Friedreich's ataxia. **Paraparesis** may be superimposed on ataxia in vitamin B_{12} deficiency, multiple sclerosis, foramen magnum lesions, or spinal cord tumors. **Ataxic quadriparesis, hemiataxia** with **contralateral hemiparesis,** or **ataxic hemiparesis** suggests a brainstem lesion.

C. ABNORMAL INVOLUNTARY MOVEMENTS

Asterixis may occur in hepatic encephalopathy, acquired hepatocerebral degeneration, or other metabolic encephalopathies. **Myoclonus** occurs in the same conditions as asterixis and is a prominent manifestation of Creutzfeldt-Jakob disease. **Chorea** may be associated with cerebellar signs in Wilson's disease, acquired hepatocerebral degeneration, or ataxia-telangiectasia.

Sensory System

A. JOINT POSITION SENSE

In patients with sensory ataxia, joint position sense is always impaired in the legs and may be defective in the arms as well. Testing is accomplished by asking the patient to detect passive movement of the joints, beginning distally and moving proximally, to establish the upper level of deficit in each limb. Abnormalities of position sense can also be demonstrated by positioning one limb and having the patient, with eyes closed, place the opposite limb in the same position.

Table 3–6. Clinical features distinguishing cerebellar from other motor systems disorders.

	Cerebellar	Upper Motor Neuron[1]	Lower Motor Neuron[1]	Extrapyramidal[2]
Strength	Normal	Decreased	Decreased	Normal
Tone	Decreased	Increased (spastic)[3]	Normal	Increased (rigid)[3] or decreased
Tendon reflexes	Normal	Increased[3]	Decreased[3]	Normal
Plantar responses	Flexor	Extensor[3]	Flexor	Flexor
Atrophy	Absent	Absent	Present[3] or absent	Absent
Fasciculations	Absent	Absent	Present[3] or absent	Absent
Tremor	Intention tremor[3] or absent	Absent	Absent	Resting tremor[3] or absent
Chorea or athetosis	Absent	Absent	Absent	Present[3] or absent
Akinesia	Absent	Absent	Absent	Present[3] or absent
Ataxia	Present[3]	Absent	Absent	Absent

[1] Also see Chapter 5.

[2] Also see Chapter 7.

[3] Most helpful diagnostic features.

B. VIBRATORY SENSE

Perception of vibratory sensation is frequently impaired in patients with sensory ataxia. The patient is asked to detect the vibration of a 128-Hz tuning fork placed over a bony prominence. Again, successively more proximal sites are tested to determine the upper level of the deficit in each limb or over the trunk. The patient's threshold for appreciating the vibration is compared with the examiner's own ability to detect it in the hand that holds the tuning fork.

Reflexes

Tendon reflexes are typically hypoactive, with a pendular quality, in cerebellar disorders; unilateral cerebellar lesions produce ipsilateral hyporeflexia. Hyporeflexia of the legs is a prominent manifestation of Friedreich's ataxia, tabes dorsalis, and polyneuropathies that cause sensory ataxia. Hyperactive reflexes and extensor plantar responses may accompany ataxia caused by multiple sclerosis, vitamin B_{12} deficiency, focal brainstem lesions, and certain olivopontocerebellar or spinocerebellar degenerations.

INVESTIGATIVE STUDIES

Blood Studies

Blood studies may disclose the hematologic abnormalities associated with vitamin B_{12} deficiency, the decreased levels of thyroid hormones in hypothyroidism, the elevated hepatic enzymes and low ceruloplasmin and copper concentrations in Wilson's disease, immunoglobulin deficiency and elevated α-fetoprotein in ataxia-telangiectasia, antibodies to Purkinje cell antigens in paraneoplastic cerebellar degeneration, or genetic abnormalities associated with hereditary spinocerebellar degenerations.

Cerebrospinal Fluid Studies

The cerebrospinal fluid (CSF) shows elevated protein with cerebellopontine angle tumors (eg, acoustic neuroma), brainstem or spinal cord tumors, hypothyroidism, and some polyneuropathies. Increased protein with pleocytosis is commonly found with infectious or parainfectious encephalitis, paraneoplastic cerebellar degeneration, and neurosyphilis. Although elevated pressure and bloody CSF characterize cerebellar hemorrhage, lumbar puncture is contraindicated if cerebellar hemorrhage is suspected. CSF VDRL is reactive in tabes dorsalis, and oligoclonal immunoglobulin G (IgG) bands may be present in multiple sclerosis or other inflammatory disorders.

Imaging

The **computed tomography (CT) scan** is useful for demonstrating posterior fossa tumors or malformations,

cerebellar infarction or hemorrhage, and cerebellar atrophy associated with degenerative disorders. **Magnetic resonance imaging (MRI)** provides better visualization of posterior fossa lesions, including cerebellopontine angle tumors, and is superior to CT scanning for detecting the lesions of multiple sclerosis.

Evoked Potential Testing

Evoked potential testing, especially of optic pathways (visual evoked potentials), may be helpful in evaluating patients with suspected multiple sclerosis. Brainstem auditory evoked potentials may be abnormal in patients with cerebellopontine angle tumors even though CT scans show no abnormality.

Chest X-Ray & Echocardiography

The chest x-ray or echocardiogram may provide evidence of cardiomyopathy associated with Friedreich's ataxia. The chest x-ray may also show a lung tumor in paraneoplastic cerebellar degeneration.

Special Studies

In vestibular disorders, three additional special investigations may be of help.

A. AUDIOMETRY

This is useful when vestibular disorders are associated with auditory impairment; such testing can distinguish conductive, labyrinthine, acoustic nerve, and brainstem disease.

Tests of pure tone hearing are abnormal when sounds are transmitted through air with conductive hearing loss and when transmitted through either air or bone with labyrinthine or acoustic nerve disorders.

Speech discrimination is markedly impaired with acoustic nerve lesions, and is impaired less with disorders of the labyrinth. Speech discrimination is normal in conductive or brainstem involvement.

B. ELECTRONYSTAGMOGRAPHY (ENG)

This test can be used to detect and characterize nystagmus, including that elicited by caloric stimulation.

C. AUDITORY EVOKED RESPONSE

This test can localize vestibular disease to the peripheral vestibular pathways.

PERIPHERAL VESTIBULAR DISORDERS

A list of peripheral vestibular disorders and features helpful in the differential diagnosis is presented in Table 3–7.

BENIGN POSITIONAL VERTIGO

Positional vertigo occurs upon assuming a particular head position. It is usually associated with peripheral vestibular lesions but may also be due to central (brainstem or cerebellar) disease.

Benign positional vertigo is the most common cause of vertigo of peripheral origin, accounting for about 30% of cases. The most frequently identified cause is head trauma, but in most instances, no cause can be determined. The pathophysiologic basis of benign positional vertigo is thought to be **canalolithiasis**—stimulation of the semicircular canal by debris floating in the endolymph.

Table 3–7. Differential diagnosis of peripheral vestibular disorders.

| | Hearing Loss | | Other Cranial Nerve Palsies |
	Conductive	Sensorineural	
Benign positional vertigo	–	–	–
Ménière's disease	–	+	
Acute peripheral vestibulopathy	–	–	–
Otosclerosis	+	+	–
Head trauma	±	±	±
Cerebellopontine angle tumor	–	+	±
Toxic vestibulopathy			
Alcohol	–	–	–
Aminoglycosides	–	+	–
Salicylates	–	+	–
Quinine	–	+	–
Acoustic (VIII) neuropathy			
Basilar meningitis	–	+	±
Hypothyroidism	–	+	–
Diabetes	–	+	±
Paget's disease of the skull (osteitis deformans)	–	+	±

The syndrome is characterized by brief (seconds to minutes) episodes of severe vertigo that may be accompanied by nausea and vomiting. Symptoms may occur with any change in head position but are usually most severe in the lateral decubitus position with the affected ear down. Episodic vertigo typically continues for several weeks and then resolves spontaneously; in some cases it is recurrent. Hearing loss is not a feature.

Peripheral and central causes of positional vertigo can usually be distinguished on physical examination by means of the Nylen-Bárány or Dix-Hallpike maneuver (discussed earlier; see Figure 3–6). Positional nystagmus always accompanies vertigo in the benign disorder and is typically unidirectional, rotatory, and delayed in onset by several seconds after assumption of the precipitating head position. If the position is maintained, nystagmus and vertigo resolve within seconds to minutes. If the maneuver is repeated successively, the response is attenuated. In contrast, positional vertigo of central origin tends to be less severe, and positional nystagmus may be absent. There is no latency, fatigue, or habituation in central positional vertigo.

The mainstay of treatment in most cases of benign positional vertigo of peripheral origin (canalolithiasis) is the use of **repositioning maneuvers** that employ the force of gravity to move endolymphatic debris out of the semicircular canal and into the vestibule, where it can be reabsorbed. In one such maneuver (Figure 3–7), the head is turned 45 degrees in the direction of the affected ear (determined clinically, as described above), and the patient reclines to a supine position, with the head (still turned 45 degrees) hanging down over the end of the examining table. The head, still hanging down, is then turned 90 degrees in the opposite direction, to 45 degrees toward the opposite ear. Next, the patient rolls to a lateral decubitus position with the affected ear up, and the head still turned 45 degrees toward the unaffected ear and hanging down. Finally, the patient turns to a prone position and sits up. Vestibulosuppressant drugs (Table 3–8) may also be useful in the acute period, and vestibular rehabilitation, which promotes compensation for vestibular dysfunction through the recruitment of other sensory modalities, may be helpful as well.

MÉNIÈRE'S DISEASE

Ménière's disease is characterized by repeated episodes of vertigo lasting from minutes to days, accompanied by tinnitus and progressive sensorineural hearing loss. Most cases are sporadic, but familial occurrence has also been decribed, and may show anticipation, or earlier onset in successive generations. Some cases appear to be related to mutations in the **cochlin** gene on chromosome 14q12–q13. Onset is between the ages of 20 and

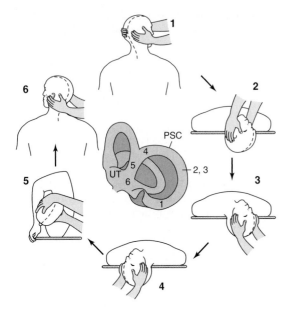

Figure 3–7. Repositioning treatment for benign positional vertigo resulting from canalolithiasis. In the example shown, repositioning maneuvers are used to move endolymphatic debris out of the posterior semicircular canal (PSC) of the right ear and into the utricle (UT), the larger of two membranous sacs in the vestibule of the labyrinth, where this debris can be reabsorbed. The numbers (1–6) refer to both the position of the patient and the corresponding location of debris within the labyrinth. The patient is seated and the head is turned 45 degrees to the right (1). The head is lowered rapidly to below the horizontal (2); the examiner shifts position (3); and the head is rotated rapidly 90 degrees in the opposite direction, so it now points 45 degrees to the left, where it remains for 30 seconds (4). The patient then rolls onto the left side without turning the head in relation to the body and maintains this position for another 30 seconds (5) before sitting up (6). This maneuver may need to be repeated until nystagmus is abolished. The patient must then avoid the supine position for at least 2 days. (Courtesy of Baloh, RW. Reproduced with permission from Samuels MA et al: *Office Practice of Neurology.* Churchill Livingstone, 1995.)

50 years in about three-fourths of cases, and men are affected more often than women. The cause is thought to be an increase in the volume of labyrinthine endolymph (**endolymphatic hydrops**), but the pathogenetic mechanism is unknown.

At the time of the first acute attack, patients may already have noted the insidious onset of tinnitus, hearing loss, and a sensation of fullness in the ear. Acute attacks are characterized by vertigo, nausea, and vomiting and recur at intervals ranging from weeks to years. Hearing deteriorates in a stepwise fashion, with bilateral involvement reported in 10–70% of patients. As hearing loss increases, vertigo tends to become less severe.

Physical examination during an acute episode shows spontaneous horizontal or rotatory nystagmus (or both) that may change direction. Although spontaneous nystagmus is characteristically absent between attacks, caloric testing usually reveals impaired vestibular function. The hearing deficit is not always sufficiently advanced to be detectable at the bedside. Audiometry shows low-frequency pure-tone hearing loss, however, that fluctuates in severity as well as impaired speech discrimination and increased sensitivity to loud sounds.

As has been noted, episodes of vertigo tend to resolve as hearing loss progresses. Treatment is with diuretics, such as hydrochlorothiazide and triamterene. The drugs listed in Table 3–8 may also be helpful during acute attacks. In persistent, disabling, drug-resistant cases, surgical procedures such as endolymphatic shunting, labyrinthectomy, or vestibular nerve section are helpful.

ACUTE PERIPHERAL VESTIBULOPATHY

This term is used to describe a spontaneous attack of vertigo of inapparent cause that resolves spontaneously and is not accompanied by hearing loss or evidence of central nervous system dysfunction. It includes disorders diagnosed as **acute labyrinthitis** or **vestibular neuronitis,** which are based on unverifiable inferences about the site of disease and the pathogenetic mechanism. A recent antecedent febrile illness can sometimes be identified, however.

The disorder is characterized by vertigo, nausea, and vomiting of acute onset, typically lasting up to 2 weeks. Symptoms may recur, and some degree of vestibular dysfunction may be permanent.

During an attack, the patient—who appears ill—typically lies on one side with the affected ear upward and is reluctant to move his or her head. Nystagmus with the fast phase away from the affected ear is always present. The vestibular response to caloric testing is defective in one or both ears with about equal frequency. Auditory acuity is normal.

Acute peripheral vestibulopathy must be distinguished from central disorders that produce acute vertigo, such as stroke in the posterior cerebral circulation. Central disease is suggested by vertical nystagmus, altered consciousness, motor or sensory deficit, or dysarthria. Treatment is with a 10- to 14-day course of prednisone, 20 mg orally twice daily, the drugs listed in Table 3–8, or both.

Table 3–8. Drugs used in the treatment of vertigo.[1]

Drug	Dosage[2]
Antihistamines	
Meclizine	25 mg PO q4–6h
Promethazine	25–50 mg PO, IM, or PR q4–6h
Dimenhydrinate	50 mg PO or IM q4–6h or 100 mg PR q8h
Anticholinergics	
Scopolamine	0.5 mg transdermally q3d
Benzodiazepines	
Diazepam	5–10 mg PO or IM q4–6h
Sympathomimetics	
Amphetamine	5–10 mg PO q4–6h
Ephedrine	25 mg PO q4–6h

[1] Adapted from Baloh RW, Honrubia V: *Clinical Neurophysiology of the Vestibular System,* 2nd ed. Vol 32 of *Contemporary Neurology Series.* Davis, 1990.

[2] PO, orally; IM, intramuscularly; PR, rectally.

OTOSCLEROSIS

Otosclerosis is caused by immobility of the stapes, the ear ossicle that transmits vibration of the tympanic membrane to the inner ear. Its most distinctive feature is conductive hearing loss, but sensorineural hearing loss and vertigo are also common; tinnitus is infrequent. Auditory symptoms usually begin before 30 years of age, and familial occurrence is common.

Vestibular dysfunction is most often characterized by recurrent episodic vertigo—with or without positional vertigo—and a sense of positional imbalance. More continuous symptoms may also occur, and the frequency and severity of attacks may increase with time.

Vestibular abnormalities on examination include spontaneous or positional nystagmus of the peripheral type and attenuated caloric responses, which are usually unilateral.

Hearing loss is always demonstrable by audiometry. It is usually of mixed conductive-sensorineural character, and is bilateral in about two-thirds of patients. In patients with episodic vertigo, progressive hearing loss, and tinnitus, otosclerosis must be distinguished from Ménière's disease. Otosclerosis (rather than Ménière's disease) is suggested by a positive family history, a tendency toward onset at an earlier age, the presence of conductive hearing loss, or bilateral symmetric auditory impairment. Imaging studies may also be diagnostically useful.

Treatment with a combination of sodium fluoride, calcium gluconate, and vitamin D may be effective. If not, surgical stapedectomy should be considered.

HEAD TRAUMA

Head trauma is the most common identifiable cause of benign positional vertigo. Injury to the labyrinth is usually responsible for posttraumatic vertigo; however, fractures of the petrosal bone may lacerate the acoustic nerve, producing vertigo and hearing loss. Hemotympanum or CSF otorrhea suggests such a fracture.

CEREBELLOPONTINE ANGLE TUMOR

The cerebellopontine angle is a triangular region in the posterior fossa bordered by the cerebellum, the lateral pons, and the petrous ridge (Figure 3–8). By far the most common tumor in this area is the histologically benign **acoustic neuroma** (also termed **neurilemoma, neurinoma,** or **schwannoma**), which typically arises from the neurilemmal sheath of the vestibular portion of the acoustic nerve in the internal auditory canal. Less common tumors at this site include **meningiomas** and primary **cholesteatomas** (epidermoid cysts). Symptoms are produced by compression or displacement of the cranial nerves, brainstem, and cerebellum and by obstruction of CSF flow. Because of their anatomic relationship to the acoustic nerve (see Figure 3–8), the trigeminal (V) and facial (VII) nerves are often affected.

Acoustic neuromas occur most often as isolated lesions in patients 30–60 years old, but they may also be a manifestation of neurofibromatosis. **Neurofibromatosis 1 (von Recklinghausen's disease)** is a common autosomal dominant disorder related to mutations in the **neurofibromin** gene on chromosome 17q11.2. In addition to unilateral acoustic neuromas, neurofibromatosis 1 is associated with café-au-lait spots on the skin, cutaneous neurofibromas, axillary or inguinal freckles, optic gliomas, iris hamartomas, and dysplastic bony lesions. **Neurofibromatosis 2** is a rare autosomal dominant disorder caused by mutations in the **neurofibromin 2** gene on chromosome 22q11.1–13.1. Its hallmark is bilateral acoustic neuromas, which may be accompanied by other tumors of the central or peripheral nervous system, including neurofibromas, meningiomas, gliomas, and schwannomas.

Clinical Findings

A. SYMPTOMS AND SIGNS

Hearing loss of insidious onset is usually the initial symptom. Less often, patients present with headache, vertigo, gait ataxia, facial pain, tinnitus, a sensation of fullness in the ear, or facial weakness. Although vertigo ultimately develops in 20–30% of patients, a nonspe-

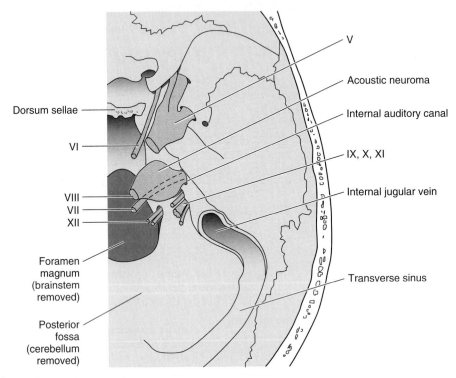

Dorsum sellae

VI

VIII
VII
XII

Foramen
magnum
(brainstem
removed)

Posterior
fossa
(cerebellum
removed)

V

Acoustic neuroma

Internal auditory canal

IX, X, XI

Internal jugular vein

Transverse sinus

Figure 3–8. Cerebellopontine angle tumor, viewed from above, with the brain removed to permit the cranial nerves and base of the skull to be seen. The tumor, a neuroma arising from the acoustic (VIII) nerve, may compress adjacent structures, including the trigeminal (V) and facial (VII) nerves, the brainstem, and the cerebellum.

cific feeling of unsteadiness is encountered more commonly. In contrast to Ménière's disease, there is a greater tendency for mild vestibular symptoms to persist between attacks. Symptoms may be stable or progress very slowly for months or years.

Unilateral hearing loss of the sensorineural type is the most common finding on physical examination. Other frequently noted abnormalities are ipsilateral facial palsy, depression or loss of the corneal reflex, and sensory loss over the face. Ataxia, spontaneous nystagmus, other lower cranial nerve palsies, and signs of increased intracranial pressure are less common. Unilateral vestibular dysfunction can usually be demonstrated with caloric testing.

B. Laboratory Findings

Audiometry shows a sensorineural pattern of deficit with high-frequency pure-tone hearing loss, poor speech discrimination, and marked tone decay. CSF protein is elevated in about 70% of patients, usually in the range of 50–200 mg/dL. The most useful diagnostic radiologic study is MRI of the cerebellopontine angle. Acoustic neuromas sometimes cause abnormalities of

the brainstem auditory evoked potentials at a time when radiologic studies show no abnormalities.

Differential Diagnosis

Acoustic neuroma must be distinguished from other cerebellopontine angle tumors, the most common being meningioma and cholesteatoma. Meningioma should be considered in patients whose initial symptoms indicate more than isolated acoustic nerve disease. Cholesteatoma is suggested by conductive hearing loss, early facial weakness, or facial twitching, with normal CSF protein. Metastatic carcinoma may also present as a lesion in the cerebellopontine angle.

Treatment

Treatment is complete surgical excision. In untreated cases, severe complications may result from brainstem compression or hydrocephalus.

TOXIC VESTIBULOPATHIES

Several drugs can produce vertigo by their effects on the peripheral vestibular system.

1. Alcohol

Alcohol causes an acute syndrome of positional vertigo because of its differential distribution between the cupula and endolymph of the inner ear. Alcohol initially diffuses into the cupula, reducing its density relative to the endolymph. This difference in density makes the peripheral vestibular apparatus unusually sensitive to gravity and thus to position. With time, alcohol also diffuses into the endolymph, and the densities of cupula and endolymph equalize, eliminating the gravitational sensitivity. As the blood alcohol level declines, alcohol leaves the cupula before it leaves the endolymph. This produces a second phase of gravitational sensitivity that persists until the alcohol diffuses out of the endolymph also.

Alcohol-induced positional vertigo typically occurs within 2 hours after ingesting ethanol in amounts sufficient to produce blood levels in excess of 40 mg/dL. It is characterized clinically by vertigo and nystagmus in the lateral recumbent position and is accentuated when the eyes are closed. The syndrome lasts up to about 12 hours and consists of two symptomatic phases separated by an asymptomatic interval of 1–2 hours. Other signs of alcohol intoxication, such as spontaneous nystagmus, dysarthria, and gait ataxia, are caused primarily by cerebellar dysfunction.

2. Aminoglycosides

Aminoglycoside antibiotics are widely recognized ototoxins that can produce both vestibular and auditory symptoms. Streptomycin, gentamicin, and tobramycin are the agents most likely to cause vestibular toxicity, and amikacin, kanamycin, and tobramycin are associated with hearing loss. Aminoglycosides concentrate in the perilymph and endolymph and exert their ototoxic effects by destroying sensory hair cells. The risk of toxicity is related to drug dosage, plasma concentration, duration of therapy, conditions—such as renal failure—that impair drug clearance, preexisting vestibular or cochlear dysfunction, and concomitant administration of other ototoxic agents.

Symptoms of vertigo, nausea, vomiting, and gait ataxia may begin acutely; physical findings include spontaneous nystagmus and the presence of Romberg's sign. The acute phase typically lasts for 1 to 2 weeks and is followed by a period of gradual improvement. Prolonged or repeated aminoglycoside therapy may be associated with a chronic syndrome of progressive vestibular dysfunction.

3. Salicylates

Salicylates, when used chronically and in high doses, can cause vertigo, tinnitus, and sensorineural hearing loss—all usually reversible when the drug is discontinued. Symptoms result from cochlear and vestibular end-organ damage. Chronic salicylism is characterized by headache, tinnitus, hearing loss, vertigo, nausea, vomiting, thirst, hyperventilation, and sometimes a confusional state. Severe intoxication may be associated with fever, skin rash, hemorrhage, dehydration, seizures, psychosis, or coma. The characteristic laboratory findings are a high plasma salicylate level (about or above 0.35 mg/mL) and combined metabolic acidosis and respiratory alkalosis.

Measures for treating salicylate intoxication include gastric lavage, administration of activated charcoal, forced diuresis, peritoneal dialysis or hemodialysis, and hemoperfusion.

4. Quinine & Quinidine

Both quinine and quinidine can produce the syndrome of **cinchonism,** which resembles salicylate intoxication in many respects. The principal manifestations are tinnitus, impaired hearing, vertigo, visual deficits (including disorders of color vision), nausea, vomiting, abdominal pain, hot flushed skin, and sweating. Fever, encephalopathy, coma, and death can occur in severe cases. Symptoms result from either overdosage or idiosyncratic reactions (usually mild) to a single small dose of quinine.

5. Cis-Platinum

This antineoplastic drug causes ototoxicity in about 50% of patients. Tinnitus, hearing loss, and vestibular dysfunction are most likely to occur with cumulative doses of 3–4 mg/kg; they may be reversible if the drug is discontinued.

ACOUSTIC NEUROPATHY

Involvement of the acoustic nerve by systemic disease is an uncommon cause of vertigo. **Basilar meningitis** from bacterial, syphilitic, or tuberculous infection or sarcoidosis can lead to compression of the acoustic and other cranial nerves, but hearing loss is a more common consequence than vertigo. Metabolic disorders associated with acoustic neuropathy include **hypothyroidism, diabetes,** and **Paget's disease.**

CEREBELLAR & CENTRAL VESTIBULAR DISORDERS

Many disorders can produce acute or chronic cerebellar dysfunction (Table 3–9). Several of these conditions may also be associated with central vestibular disorders,

Table 3–9. Differential diagnosis of cerebellar ataxia.

Acute
Drug intoxications: ethanol, sedative-hypnotics, anticonvulsants, hallucinogens
Wernicke's encephalopathy[1]
Vertebrobasilar ischemia or infarction[1]
Cerebellar hemorrhage
Inflammatory disorders

Chronic
Multiple sclerosis[1,2]
Alcoholic cerebellar degeneration
Phenytoin-induced cerebellar degeneration
Hypothyroidism
Paraneoplastic cerebellar degeneration
Hereditary spinocerebellar ataxias (SCA1–7)
Friedreich's ataxia[2]
Ataxia-telangiectasia
Wilson's disease
Acquired hepatolenticular degeneration
Creutzfeldt-Jakob disease
Posterior fossa tumor[1]
Posterior fossa malformations

---

[1] May also be associated with central vestibular dysfunction.
[2] May also produce sensory ataxia.

particularly Wernicke's encephalopathy, vertebrobasilar ischemia or infarction, multiple sclerosis, and posterior fossa tumors.

ACUTE DISORDERS

1. Drug Intoxication

Pancerebellar dysfunction manifested by nystagmus, dysarthria, and limb and gait ataxia is a prominent feature of many drug intoxication syndromes. Agents that produce such syndromes include ethanol, sedative-hypnotics (eg, barbiturates, benzodiazepines, meprobamate, ethchlorvynol, methaqualone), anticonvulsants (such as phenytoin), and hallucinogens (especially phencyclidine). The severity of symptoms is dose related; while therapeutic doses of sedatives or anticonvulsants commonly produce nystagmus, other cerebellar signs imply toxicity.

Drug-induced cerebellar ataxia is often associated with a confusional state, although cognitive function tends to be spared in phenytoin intoxication. The confusional state produced by ethanol and sedative drugs is characterized by somnolence, whereas hallucinogens are more often associated with agitated delirium. In most cases, only general supportive care is necessary. The distinctive features of intoxication with each of these groups of drugs are discussed in detail in Chapter 1.

2. Wernicke's Encephalopathy

Wernicke's encephalopathy (see also Chapter 1) is an acute disorder comprising the clinical triad of ataxia, ophthalmoplegia, and confusion. It is caused by thiamine (vitamin B_1) deficiency and is most common in chronic alcoholics, although it may occur as a consequence of malnutrition from any cause. The major sites of pathologic involvement are the medial thalamic nuclei, mammillary bodies, periaqueductal and periventricular brainstem nuclei (especially those of the oculomotor, abducens, and acoustic nerves), and superior cerebellar vermis. Cerebellar and vestibular involvement both contribute to the ataxia.

Ataxia affects gait primarily or exclusively; the legs themselves are ataxic in only about one-fifth of patients, and the arms in one-tenth. Dysarthria is rare. Other classic findings include an amnestic syndrome or global confusional state, horizontal or combined horizontal-vertical nystagmus, bilateral lateral rectus palsies, and absent ankle jerks. Caloric testing reveals bilateral or unilateral vestibular dysfunction. Conjugate gaze palsies, pupillary abnormalities, and hypothermia can also occur.

The diagnosis is established by the response to administration of thiamine, which is usually given initially in a dose of 100 mg intravenously. Ocular palsies tend to be the earliest deficits to improve and typically begin to do so within hours. Ataxia, nystagmus, and acute confusion start to resolve within a few days. Recovery from ocular palsies is invariably complete, but horizontal nystagmus may persist.

Ataxia is fully reversible in only about 40% of patients; where gait returns fully to normal, recovery typically takes several weeks to months.

3. Vertebrobasilar Ischemia & Infarction

Transient ischemic attacks and strokes in the vertebrobasilar system are often associated with ataxia or vertigo.

Internal Auditory Artery Occlusion

Vertigo of central vestibular origin with unilateral hearing loss results from occlusion of the internal auditory artery (Figure 3–9), which supplies the acoustic nerve. This vessel may originate from the basilar or anterior inferior cerebellar artery. Vertigo is accompanied by nystagmus, with the fast phase directed away from the involved side. Hearing loss is unilateral and sensorineural.

Lateral Medullary Infarction

Lateral medullary infarction produces **Wallenberg's syndrome** (Figure 3–10) and is most often caused by proximal vertebral artery occlusion. Clinical manifestations vary, depending on the extent of infarction. They typically consist of vertigo, nausea, vomiting, dysphagia, hoarseness, and nystagmus in addition to ipsilateral Horner's syndrome, limb ataxia, impairment of all sensory modalities over the face, and loss of light touch and position sense in the limbs. There is also impairment of pinprick and temperature appreciation in the contralateral limbs. Vertigo results from involvement of the vestibular nuclei and hemiataxia from involvement of the inferior cerebellar peduncle.

Cerebellar Infarction

The cerebellum is supplied by three arteries: the superior cerebellar, anterior inferior cerebellar, and posterior inferior cerebellar. The territory supplied by each of these vessels is highly variable, both from one individual to another and between the two sides of the cerebellum in a given patient. The superior, middle, and inferior cerebellar peduncles are typically supplied by the superior, anterior inferior, and posterior inferior cerebellar arteries, respectively.

Cerebellar infarction results from occlusion of a cerebellar artery (Figure 3–11); the clinical syndromes produced can be distinguished only by the associated brainstem findings. In each case, cerebellar signs include ipsilateral limb ataxia and hypotonia. Other symptoms and signs such as headache, nausea, vomiting, vertigo, nystagmus, dysarthria, ocular or gaze palsies, facial weakness or sensory loss, and contralateral hemiparesis or hemisensory deficit may be present. Brainstem infarction or compression by cerebellar edema can result in coma and death.

The diagnosis of cerebellar infarction is made by CT scan or MRI, which allows differentiation between infarction and hemorrhage; it should be obtained promptly. When brainstem compression occurs, surgical decompression and resection of infarcted tissue can be lifesaving.

Paramedian Midbrain Infarction

Paramedian midbrain infarction caused by occlusion of the paramedian penetrating branches of the basilar artery affects the third nerve root fibers and red nucleus (Figure 3–12). The resulting clinical picture (**Benedikt's syndrome**) consists of ipsilateral medial rectus palsy with a fixed dilated pupil and contralateral limb ataxia (typically affecting only the arm). Cerebellar signs result from involvement of the red nucleus, which receives a crossed projection from the cerebellum in the ascending limb of the superior cerebellar peduncle.

4. Cerebellar Hemorrhage

Most cerebellar hemorrhages are due to hypertensive vascular disease; less common causes include anticoagulation, arteriovenous malformation, blood dyscrasia, tumor, and trauma. Hypertensive cerebellar hemorrhages are usually located in the deep white matter of the cerebellum and commonly extend into the fourth ventricle.

The classic clinical picture of hypertensive cerebellar hemorrhage consists of the sudden onset of headache, which may be accompanied by nausea, vomiting, and vertigo, followed by gait ataxia and impaired consciousness, usually evolving over a period of hours. At the time of presentation, patients can be fully alert, confused, or comatose. In alert patients, nausea and vomiting are often prominent. The blood pressure is typically elevated, and nuchal rigidity may be present. The pupils are often small and sluggishly reactive. Ipsilateral gaze palsy (with gaze preference away from the side of hemorrhage) and ipsilateral peripheral facial palsy are common. The gaze preference cannot be overcome by caloric stimulation. Nystagmus and ipsilateral depression of the corneal reflex may occur. The patient, if alert, exhibits ataxia of stance and gait; limb ataxia is less common. In the late stage of brainstem compression, the legs are spastic and extensor plantar responses are present.

The CSF is frequently bloody, but lumbar puncture should be avoided if cerebellar hemorrhage is suspected, because it may lead to a herniation syndrome.

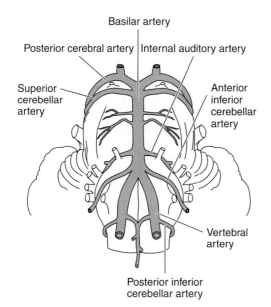

Basilar artery

Posterior cerebral artery | Internal auditory artery

Superior cerebellar artery

Anterior inferior cerebellar artery

Vertebral artery

Posterior inferior cerebellar artery

Figure 3–9. Principal arteries of the posterior fossa.

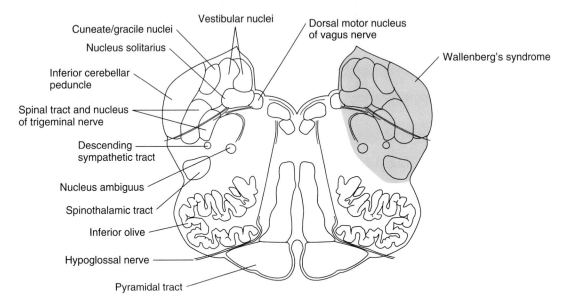

Cuneate/gracile nuclei
Vestibular nuclei
Dorsal motor nucleus of vagus nerve
Nucleus solitarius
Wallenberg's syndrome
Inferior cerebellar peduncle
Spinal tract and nucleus of trigeminal nerve
Descending sympathetic tract
Nucleus ambiguus
Spinothalamic tract
Inferior olive
Hypoglossal nerve
Pyramidal tract

Figure 3–10. Lateral medullary infarction (Wallenberg's syndrome) showing the area of infarction (shaded) and anatomic structures affected.

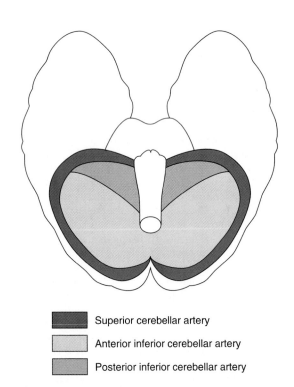

Superior cerebellar artery

Anterior inferior cerebellar artery

Posterior inferior cerebellar artery

Figure 3–11. Arterial supply of the cerebellum, viewed from below.

 The diagnostic procedure of choice is a CT scan. Treatment consists of surgical evacuation of the hematoma, a procedure that can be lifesaving.

5. Inflammatory Disorders

Acute inflammatory disorders of the cerebellum mediated by infection or immune mechanisms are important and often reversible causes of ataxia. Cerebellar ataxia caused by **viral infection** is one of the principal manifestations of St. Louis encephalitis. AIDS dementia complex and meningoencephalitis associated with varicella, mumps, poliomyelitis, infectious mononucleosis, and lymphocytic choriomeningitis can also produce cerebellar symptoms. **Bacterial infection** is a less common cause of cerebellar ataxia; 10–20% of brain abscesses are located in the cerebellum, however, and ataxia may be a feature of *Haemophilus influenzae* meningitis in children. A cerebellar syndrome has been described in legionnaires' disease, usually without clinical evidence of meningitis.

Several conditions that may occur following an acute febrile illness or vaccination produce cerebellar ataxia that is assumed to be of autoimmune origin.

Acute Cerebellar Ataxia of Childhood

Acute cerebellar ataxia of childhood is a syndrome characterized by severe gait ataxia that usually resolves com-

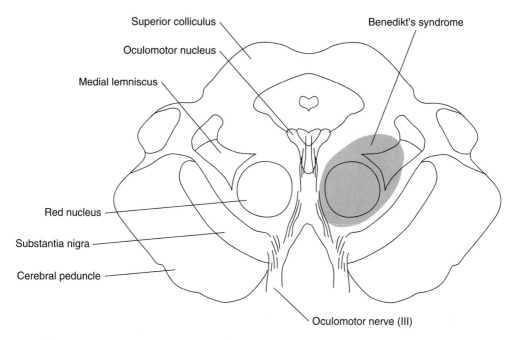

Figure 3–12. Paramedian midbrain infarction (Benedikt's syndrome). The area of infarction is indicated by shading.

pletely within months. It generally follows an acute viral infection or inoculation. A full discussion of cerebellar ataxia in childhood is beyond the scope of this chapter.

Acute Disseminated Encephalomyelitis

This immune-mediated disorder may cause demyelination and inflammatory changes in the cerebellar white matter, producing ataxia that is often associated with impaired consciousness, seizures, focal neurological signs, or myelopathy.

Fisher Variant of Guillain-Barré Syndrome

Cerebellar ataxia, external ophthalmoplegia, and areflexia constitute this variant of Guillain-Barré syndrome. Symptoms develop over a few days. Ataxia primarily affects the gait and trunk, with lesser involvement of the individual limbs; dysarthria is uncommon. CSF protein may be elevated. Respiratory insufficiency occurs rarely, and the usual course is of gradual and often complete recovery over weeks to months. The ataxia is similar to that of cerebellar disease, but it is not yet known whether it arises centrally or peripherally.

CHRONIC DISORDERS

1. Multiple Sclerosis

Multiple sclerosis can produce disorders of equilibrium of cerebellar, vestibular, or sensory origin. Cerebellar signs are associated with demyelinated areas (plaques) in the white matter of the cerebellum, cerebellar peduncles, or brainstem. As is the case with other manifestations of multiple sclerosis, these signs may remit and relapse.

Involvement of vestibular pathways in the brainstem produces vertigo, which may be acute in onset and sometimes positional. Vertigo, which is rarely the first symptom of multiple sclerosis, is not uncommon during the course of the disease.

Gait ataxia from cerebellar involvement is a presenting complaint in 10–15% of patients. Cerebellar signs are present in about one-third of patients on initial examination; they ultimately develop in twice that number.

Nystagmus is one of the most common physical findings; it can occur with or without other evidence of cerebellar dysfunction. Dysarthria also occurs frequently. When gait ataxia occurs, it is most often cerebellar rather than sensory in origin. Ataxia of the limbs is common; it is usually bilateral and tends to affect either both legs or all four limbs.

Evidence that a cerebellar disorder is due to multiple sclerosis may be found in a history of remitting and relapsing neurologic dysfunction that affects multiple sites in the central nervous system; from such associated abnormalities as optic neuritis, internuclear ophthalmoplegia, or pyramidal signs; or from laboratory investigations. CSF analysis may reveal oligoclonal bands, elevated IgG, increased protein, or a mild lymphocytic pleocytosis. Visual, auditory, or somatosensory evoked response recording can document subclinical sites of involvement. The CT scan or MRI may show areas of demyelination. It must be emphasized, however, that no laboratory finding is itself diagnostic of multiple sclerosis, and the history and neurologic examination must be primarily relied upon in arriving at such a diagnosis.

Multiple sclerosis is discussed in more detail in Chapter 5.

2. Alcoholic Cerebellar Degeneration

A characteristic cerebellar syndrome may develop in chronic alcoholics, probably as a result of nutritional deficiency. Affected patients typically have a history of daily or binge drinking lasting 10 or more years with associated dietary inadequacy. Most have experienced other medical complications of alcoholism: liver disease, delirium tremens, Wernicke's encephalopathy, or polyneuropathy. Alcoholic cerebellar degeneration is most common in men and usually has its onset between the ages of 40 and 60 years.

Degenerative changes in the cerebellum are largely restricted to the superior vermis (Figure 3–13); because this is also the site of cerebellar involvement in Wernicke's encephalopathy, both disorders may be part of the same clinical spectrum.

Alcoholic cerebellar degeneration is usually insidious in onset; it is gradually progressive, eventually reaching a stable level of deficit. Progression over weeks to months is more common than is deterioration over years; in occasional cases, ataxia appears abruptly or is mild and stable from the onset.

Gait ataxia is a universal feature and is almost always the problem that initially commands medical attention. The legs are also ataxic on heel-knee-shin testing in about 80% of patients. Commonly associated findings are distal sensory deficits in the feet and absent ankle reflexes—from polyneuropathy—and signs of malnutrition such as loss of subcutaneous tissue, generalized muscle atrophy, or glossitis. Less frequent manifestations include ataxia of the arms, nystagmus, dysarthria, hypotonia, and truncal instability.

CT scan or MRI may show cerebellar atrophy (Figure 3–14), but this is a nonspecific finding that can be encountered in any degenerative disorder that affects the cerebellum.

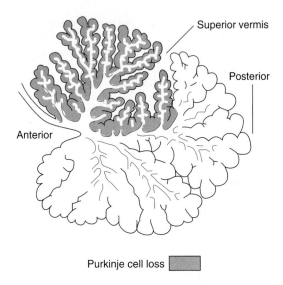

Figure 3–13. Distribution of disease in alcoholic cerebellar degeneration. Midsagittal view of the cerebellum showing loss of Purkinje cells, confined largely to the superior vermis.

Chronic cerebellar ataxia that begins in adulthood and primarily affects gait can also occur in hypothyroidism, paraneoplastic syndromes, idiopathic cerebellar degenerations, and anomalies at the craniocervical junction such as Arnold-Chiari malformation. The possibility of hypothyroidism or systemic cancer, which may be treatable, should be investigated with thyroid function tests, chest x-ray, and, in women, breast and pelvic examinations.

No specific treatment is available for alcoholic cerebellar degeneration. Nonetheless, all patients with this diagnosis should receive thiamine because of the apparent role of thiamine deficiency in the pathogenesis of Wernicke's encephalopathy, a closely related syndrome. Abstinence from alcohol, combined with adequate nutrition, leads to stabilization in most cases.

3. Phenytoin-Induced Cerebellar Degeneration

Chronic therapy with phenytoin, often with drug levels in the toxic range, may cause cerebellar degeneration that affects the cerebellar hemispheres and inferior and posterior vermis most severely, while the superior vermis is relatively spared. Clinical features include nystagmus, dysarthria, and ataxia affecting the limbs, trunk, and gait. Polyneuropathy may be present. Symptoms are typically irreversible, but tend to stabilize when the drug is discontinued.

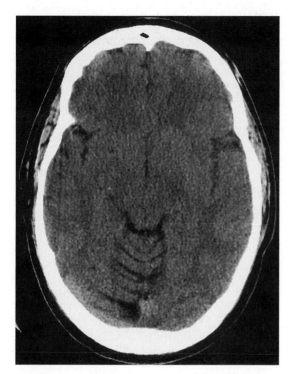

Figure 3–14. CT scan in alcoholic cerebellar degeneration, showing marked atrophy of the cerebellar vermis with relative sparing of the cerebellar hemispheres. (Courtesy of A Gean.)

4. Hypothyroidism

Among the neurologic disorders associated with hypothyroidism is a subacute or chronically progressive cerebellar syndrome. This condition may complicate hypothyroidism (of various causes) and is most common in middle-aged or elderly women. Symptoms evolve over a period of months to years. Systemic symptoms of myxedema usually precede the appearance of the cerebellar disorder, but patients occasionally present first with ataxia.

Gait ataxia is the most prominent finding and is present in all patients; ataxia of the limbs, which is also common, may be asymmetric. Dysarthria and nystagmus occur less frequently. Patients may exhibit other neurologic disorders related to hypothyroidism, including sensorineural hearing loss, carpal tunnel syndrome, neuropathy, or myopathy.

Laboratory studies show decreased blood levels of thyroid hormones, elevated thyroid-stimulating hormone (TSH), and often increased CSF protein.

Replacement therapy with levothyroxine, 25–50 μg, increased gradually to 100–200 μg/d orally, usually produces definite but incomplete improvement.

5. Paraneoplastic Cerebellar Degeneration

Cerebellar degeneration can also occur as a remote effect of systemic cancer. Lung cancer (especially small-cell), ovarian cancer, Hodgkin's disease, and breast cancer are the most commonly associated neoplasms.

Paraneoplastic degeneration affects the cerebellar vermis and hemispheres diffusely. The pathogenetic mechanism in many cases appears to involve antibodies to tumor cell antigens that cross-react with cerebellar Purkinje cells. Cerebellar symptoms may appear before or after the diagnosis of systemic cancer and typically develop over months. Although the disorder usually progresses steadily, it may stabilize; remission has been described with treatment of the underlying neoplasm.

Gait and limb ataxia are characteristically prominent, and dysarthria occurs in most cases. The limbs may be affected asymmetrically. Nystagmus is rare. Paraneoplastic involvement of other regions of the nervous system may produce associated dysphagia, dementia, memory disturbance, pyramidal signs, or neuropathy. Anti-Purkinje cell antibodies, such as anti-Yo (ovarian and breast cancer), or antinuclear antibodies, such as anti-Hu (small-cell lung cancer) and anti-Ri (breast cancer), can sometimes be detected in the blood (Table 3–10). The CSF may show a mild lymphocytic pleocytosis or elevated protein.

The diagnosis of paraneoplastic cerebellar degeneration is most difficult when the neurologic symptoms precede the discovery of underlying cancer. The frequent occurrence of dysarthria and dysphagia helps to distinguish this condition from the cerebellar syndromes produced by chronic alcoholism or hypothyroidism. Ataxia of the arms also suggests that alcohol is an unlikely cause. Wernicke's encephalopathy should always be considered because of the susceptibility of patients with cancer to malnutrition.

6. Autosomal Dominant Spinocerebellar Ataxias

The hereditary spinocerebellar degenerations (Table 3–11) are a group of inherited disorders characterized by slowly progressive cerebellar ataxia that affects gait early and severely and may eventually confine the patient to bed. These disorders show considerable clinical variability, even within a given family. Most autosomal dominant forms, termed **spinocerebellar ataxias** or **SCAs,** begin in adulthood and show **anticipation,** in which the age at onset decreases, the disease severity increases, or both, in successive generations.

Autosomal dominant spinocerebellar ataxia is genetically heterogeneous. The best characterized gene defects are expanded CAG trinucleotide repeats coding for

Table 3–10. Antineuronal autoantibodies in paraneoplastic syndromes.

	Antigen					
Syndrome	*Hu*	*Yo*	*Ri*	*Ma*	*Ta*	α_{1A}[1]
Cerebellar degeneration	+	+	+	+	+	
Limbic encephalitis	+		+	+		
Sensory neuronopathy	+					
Opsoclonus/myoclonus	+	+	+			
Lambert-Eaton syndrome						+

[1] P/Q-type voltage-gated calcium channel, α_{1A}-subunit.

polyglutamine tracts in proteins without known function (**ataxins**), and in the α_{1A}-subunit of the P/Q-type calcium channel, which is found on nerve terminals. Other types of mutations include expanded CTG trinucleotide (SCA8) and ATTCT pentanucleotide (SCA10) repeats. In many cases, the size of these expansions correlates with disease severity and inversely with age at onset.

The gain-of-function mutations seen in SCAs appear to alter the properties of the mutated protein, which cannot be processed normally. The abnormally processed fragments are conjugated with **ubiquitin,** a protein involved in nonlysosomal degradation of defective proteins, with which they are transported to the nucleus in a complex called a **proteasome.** The precise relationship of this accumulation to the neurotoxicity that results from these mutations is uncertain, but intranuclear protein aggregates may interfere with nuclear function.

Atrophy of the cerebellum and sometimes also of the brainstem may be apparent on CT or MRI scans (Figure 3–15). However, definitive diagnosis is by demonstrating one of the known SCA gene defects on genetic testing. There is no specific treatment for the spinocerebellar ataxias, but occupational and physical therapy and devices to assist ambulation may be helpful, and genetic counseling may be indicated.

7. Friedreich's Ataxia

Among the idiopathic degenerative disorders that produce cerebellar ataxia, Friedreich's ataxia merits separate consideration because it is the most common, and because of its unique clinical and pathologic features. Unlike most of the late-onset autosomal dominant spinocerebellar ataxias discussed above, Friedreich's ataxia begins in childhood. It is transmitted by autosomal recessive inheritance and is due to an expanded GAA trinucleotide repeat in a noncoding region of the **frataxin** gene on chromosome 9 (see Table 3–10). The recessive inheritance of Friedreich's ataxia suggests a loss-of-function mutation. Most affected patients are homozygous for the trinucleotide repeat expansion in the Friedreich's ataxia gene, but some are heterozygous, with the repeat affecting one allele and a point mutation on the other allele.

The pathologic findings are localized, for the most part, to the spinal cord. These include degeneration of the spinocerebellar tracts, posterior columns, and dorsal roots as well as depletion of the neurons in Clarke's column that are the cells of origin of the dorsal spinocerebellar tracts. Large myelinated axons of peripheral nerves and cell bodies of primary sensory neurons in dorsal root ganglia are also involved.

Clinical Findings

Detailed clinical evaluation of relatively large numbers of patients has allowed certain diagnostic criteria to be established (Table 3–11). Clinical manifestations almost always appear after age 4 years and before the end of puberty, with more expanded repeats correlating with earlier onset.

The initial symptom is progressive gait ataxia, followed by ataxia of all limbs within 2 years. During the same early period, knee and ankle tendon reflexes are lost and cerebellar dysarthria appears; reflexes in the arms and in some cases at the knees may be preserved. Joint position and vibration sense are impaired in the legs, typically adding a sensory component to the gait ataxia. Abnormalities of light touch, pain, and temperature sensation occur less frequently. Weakness of the legs—and less often the arms—is a later development and may be of the upper or lower motor neuron variety (or both).

Extensor plantar responses usually appear during the first 5 years of symptomatic disease. Pes cavus (high-

Table 3–11. Genetic and clinical features of hereditary spinocerebellar ataxias.

Disease	Gene	Protein	Gene Defect	Syndrome
Autosomal recessive				
FA[1]	FRDA1	Frataxin	GAA_n[2]	[3]
Autosomal dominant				
SCA1[4]	SCA1	Ataxin-1	CAG_n	ADCA I[5]
SCA 2	SCA2	Ataxin-2	CAG_n	ADCA I
SCA 3/MJD[6]	SCA3	Ataxin-3	CAG_n	ADCA I
SCA 4	SCA4	Unknown	Unknown	ADCA I
SCA 5	SCA5	Unknown	Unknown	ADCA III
SCA 6	CACNL1A4	Ca channel[7]	CAG_n	ADCA III
SCA 7	SCA7	Ataxin-7	CAG_n	ADCA II
SCA 8	SCA8	Unknown	CTG_n	ADCA I
SCA 10	SCA10	Ataxin-10	$ATTCT_n$	ADCA III
SCA 11	SCA11	Unknown	Unknown	ADCA III
SCA 12	PPP2R2B	PPase2[8]	CAG_n	ADCA I
SCA 13	SCA13	Unknown	Unknown	[9]
SCA 14	SCA14	Unknown	Unknown	ADCA III
SCA 15	SCA15	Unknown	Unknown	ADCA III
SCA 16	SCA16	Unknown	Unknown	ADCA III
SCA17	TBP	TATA-binding protein	CAG_n	ADCA I

[1] FA, Friedreich's ataxia.

[2] XYZ_n, expanded XYZ trinucleotide repeat; $VWXYZ_n$, expanded VWXYZ pentanucleotide repeat.

[3] Childhood onset, ataxia, dysarthria, pyramidal signs, neuropathy, scoliosis, cardiomyopathy, diabetes.

[4] SCA, spinocerebellar ataxia.

[5] ADCA I includes ataxia, dysarthria, pyramidal signs, extrapyramidal signs, ophthalmoplegia and dementia; ADCA II includes ataxia, dysarthria, and pigmentary maculopathy; ADCA III includes ataxia, dysarthria, and sometimes mild pyramidal signs.

[6] MJD, Machado-Joseph disease (same as SCA3).

[7] P/Q-type voltage-gated calcium channel, α_{1A}-subunit.

[8] Protein phosphatase 2, regulatory subunit B, β isoform.

[9] Childhood onset, ataxia, and mental retardation.

arched feet with clawing of the toes caused by weakness and wasting of the intrinsic foot muscles) is a widely recognized sign, but it may also be an isolated finding in otherwise unaffected family members. It is also a classic feature of other neurologic disorders, notably certain hereditary peripheral neuropathies (eg, Charcot-Marie-Tooth disease). Severe progressive kyphoscoliosis contributes to functional disability and may lead to chronic restrictive lung disease. While cardiomyopathy is sometimes detectable only by echocardiography or vectorcar-diography, it may result in congestive heart failure and is a major cause of morbidity and death.

Other abnormalities include visual impairment (usually from optic atrophy), nystagmus, paresthesias, tremor, hearing loss, vertigo, spasticity, leg pains, and diabetes mellitus.

Differential Diagnosis

Friedreich's ataxia can usually be differentiated from other cerebellar and spinocerebellar degenerations (see

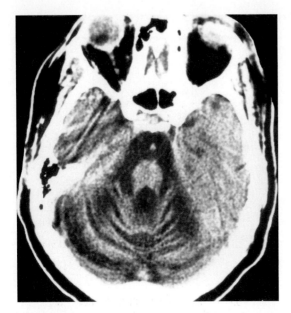

Figure 3–15. CT scan in spinocerebellar atrophy, showing an atrophic cerebellum and brainstem. (Courtesy of A Gean.)

above) by its early onset and the presence of prominent sensory impairment, areflexia, skeletal abnormalities, and cardiomyopathy. A somewhat similar disorder may result from vitamin E deficiency. Cerebellar ataxia that begins in childhood can also be caused by ataxia-telangiectasia; the clinical features that distinguish Friedreich's ataxia from ataxia-telangiectasia are discussed below.

Prognosis

No treatment is available, but orthopedic procedures such as tenotomy may help to correct foot deformities. Advances in antimicrobial therapy have altered the ultimate course of the disorder, so that cardiomyopathy has become more frequent and infection less frequent as a cause of death. Neurologic dysfunction typically results in the inability to walk unaided within 5 years after the onset of symptoms and in a bedridden state within 10–20 years. The average duration of symptomatic illness is about 25 years, with death occurring at a mean age of about 35 years.

8. Ataxia-Telangiectasia

Ataxia-telangiectasia (also known as Louis-Bar syndrome) is an inherited autosomal recessive disorder with its onset in infancy. The disease results from mutations in the *ATM* gene, which has been localized to chromosome 11q22.3. Deletions, insertions, and substitutions have all been described and are presumed to represent loss-of-function

mutations, consistent with the autosomal recessive inheritance of ataxia-telangiectasia. Although the abnormal gene product has not been identified, a defect in DNA repair is thought to be involved in pathogenesis. Ataxia-telangiectasia is characterized by progressive cerebellar ataxia, oculocutaneous telangiectasia, and immunologic deficiency. All patients suffer from progressive pancerebellar degeneration—characterized by nystagmus, dysarthria, and gait, limb, and trunk ataxia—that begins in infancy. Choreoathetosis, loss of vibration and position sense in the legs, areflexia, and disorders of voluntary eye movement are almost universal findings. Mental deficiency is commonly observed in the second decade; oculocutaneous telangiectasia usually appears in the teen years. The bulbar conjunctivae are typically affected first, followed by sun-exposed areas of the skin, including the ears, nose, face, and antecubital and popliteal fossae. The vascular lesions, which rarely bleed, spare the central nervous system. Immunologic impairment (decreased circulating IgA and IgE) usually becomes evident later in childhood and is manifested by recurrent sinopulmonary infections in more than 80% of patients.

Other common clinical findings are progeric changes of the skin and hair, hypogonadism, and insulin resistance. The characteristic laboratory abnormalities include those related to immunologic deficiency and elevation of α-fetoprotein and carcinoembryonic antigen levels.

Because the vascular and immunologic manifestations of ataxia-telangiectasia occur later than the neurologic symptoms, the condition may be confused with Friedreich's ataxia, which also manifests in childhood (see above). Ataxia-telangiectasia can be distinguished by its earlier onset (before age 4 years), associated choreoathetosis, and the absence of such skeletal abnormalities as kyphoscoliosis.

There is no specific treatment for ataxia-telangiectasia, but antibiotics are useful in the management of infections and x-rays should be avoided because of the abnormal cellular sensitivity to ionizing radiation in this disorder.

9. Wilson's Disease

Cerebellar symptoms may occur in Wilson's disease, a disorder of copper metabolism characterized by copper deposition in a variety of tissues. Wilson's disease is an inherited autosomal recessive disorder due to mutations in the *ATP7B* gene on chromosome 13q14.3–q21.1, which codes for the β polypeptide of a copper-transporting ATPase. Wilson's disease is discussed in more detail in Chapter 7.

10. Creutzfeldt-Jakob Disease

Creutzfeldt-Jakob disease is described in Chapter 1 as a prion disease that causes dementia. Cerebellar signs are present in about 60% of patients, and the patients present with ataxia in about 10% of cases. Cerebellar involvement is diffuse, but the vermis is often most severely affected. In contrast to most other cerebellar disorders, depletion of granule cells is frequently more striking than Purkinje cell loss.

Patients with cerebellar manifestations of Creutzfeldt-Jakob disease usually complain first of gait ataxia. Dementia is usually evident at this time, and cognitive dysfunction always develops eventually. Nystagmus, dysarthria, truncal ataxia, and limb ataxia are all present initially in about half the patients with the ataxic form of Creutzfeldt-Jakob disease. The course is characterized by progressive dementia, myoclonus, and extrapyramidal and pyramidal dysfunction. Death typically occurs within 1 year after onset.

11. Posterior Fossa Tumors

Tumors of the posterior fossa cause cerebellar symptoms when they arise in the cerebellum or compress it from without. The most common cerebellar tumors of childhood are astrocytomas and medulloblastomas. Metastases from primary sites outside the nervous system predominate in adults (Table 3–12).

Patients with cerebellar tumors present with headache from the increased intracranial pressure or with ataxia. Nausea, vomiting, vertigo, cranial nerve palsies, and hydrocephalus are common. The nature of the clinical findings varies with the location of the tumor. Most metastases are located in the cerebellar hemispheres, causing asymmetric cerebellar signs. Medulloblastomas and ependymomas, on the other hand, tend to arise in the midline, with early involvement of the vermis and hydrocephalus.

As in the case of most brain tumors, the CT scan or—especially—MRI is extremely useful in diagnoses but biopsy may be required for histologic characterization. Methods of treatment include surgical resection and irradiation. Corticosteroids are useful in controlling the associated edema.

Metastases—from the lung and breast and less often from other sites—are the most common tumors of the cerebellum, especially in adults. The site of the primary tumor may or may not be evident at the time the patient presents with central nervous system involvement. If the site is not evident, careful examination of the breasts and skin, chest x-ray, urinalysis, and tests for the presence of occult blood in the stool may lead to a diagnosis. The prognosis for patients with cerebellar metastases is usually worse than for patients with supratentorial lesions. Patients with carcinoma of the breast tend to survive longer than those with primary lung tumors.

Cerebellar astrocytomas usually occur between the ages of 2 and 20 years, but older patients can also be

Table 3–12. Tumors of the cerebellum.[1]

Type	Percentage of All Cerebellar Tumors	Percentage of Cerebellar Tumors in Adults (≥20 years)
Metastasis	36	56
Astrocytoma	28	10
Medulloblastoma	16	9
Schwannoma	4	7
Hemangioblastoma	4	5
Meningioma	4	5
Ependymoma	2	1
Other	6	7

[1]Data from Gilman S, Bloedel JR, Lechtenberg R: Page 334 in: *Disorders of the Cerebellum.* Vol 21 of *Contemporary Neurology Series.* Davis, 1981.

affected. These tumors are often histologically benign and cystic in appearance. Symptoms of increased intracranial pressure, including headache and vomiting, typically precede the onset of cerebellar dysfunction by several months. If complete surgical resection is possible, cerebellar astrocytoma is potentially curable.

Medulloblastoma is common in children but rare in adults. It is believed to originate from neuroectodermal rather than glial cells. In contrast to astrocytomas, medulloblastomas tend to be highly malignant. They often spread through the subarachnoid space and ventricles and may metastasize outside the nervous system. Whereas most childhood medulloblastomas are located in the midline, adult-onset tumors usually arise laterally. Headache, vomiting, ataxia, and visual deterioration are common presenting symptoms. Hemiataxia is a frequent finding in adults because of the hemispheric location of most tumors. Gait ataxia, papilledema, nystagmus, facial palsy, and neck stiffness are also common. Without treatment, medulloblastoma causes death within a few months after presentation. Treatment with partial surgical resection, decompression, and craniospinal irradiation may prolong survival for years. Developing the tumors in adulthood and being female are favorable prognostic factors.

Acoustic neuromas have been discussed previously as a cause of vestibular nerve dysfunction. Growth of these or other less common tumors of the cerebellopontine angle may result in compression of the ipsilateral cerebellar hemisphere, causing hemiataxia in addition to the earlier symptoms of vertigo and hearing loss. These tumors are histologically benign and often fully resectable. Unilateral acoustic neuromas can occur in **neurofibromatosis 1** (von Recklinghausen's disease), whereas bilateral acoustic neuromas are characteristic of **neurofibromatosis 2.** These disorders are discussed in more detail in the section on cerebellopontine angle tumors (above).

Hemangioblastoma is a rare benign tumor that usually affects adults. It can be an isolated abnormality or a feature of von Hippel-Lindau disease. In the latter case, associated features include retinal hemangioblastoma; cysts of the kidney, pancreas, or other viscera; and polycythemia. Patients typically present with headache, and common examination findings include papilledema, nystagmus, and ataxia. Treatment is by surgical resection.

Meningiomas of the posterior fossa constitute 9% of all meningiomas. They are benign tumors, derived from arachnoidal cap cells, and involve the cerebellum indirectly by compression. The locations of posterior fossa meningiomas (in decreasing order of frequency) include the posterior surface of the petrous bone, the tentorium cerebelli, the clivus, the cerebellar convexities, and the foramen magnum. Meningiomas grow slowly and usually present with headache, although tumors of the cerebellopontine angle or clivus may come to attention when they give rise to cranial nerve or brainstem symptoms. Where possible, complete surgical resection is curative.

Ependymomas most commonly arise from the walls or choroid plexus of the fourth ventricle. Like medulloblastomas, they are malignant tumors that seed through the ventricular system and usually occur in children. Because of their location they produce early hydrocephalus; cerebellar signs caused by compression are late or minor manifestations. Surgical resection, craniospinal irradiation, and shunting procedures to relieve hydrocephalus may prolong survival, but widespread dissemination of the tumors and postoperative recurrences are common.

12. Posterior Fossa Malformations

Developmental anomalies affecting the cerebellum and brainstem may present with vestibular or cerebellar symptoms in adulthood. This occurs most commonly with type I (adult) **Arnold-Chiari malformation,** which consists of downward displacement of the cerebellar tonsils through the foramen magnum. The clinical manifestations of this malformation are related to cerebellar involvement, obstructive hydrocephalus, brainstem compression, and syringomyelia. Type II Arnold-Chiari malformation is associated with meningomyelocele (protrusion of the spinal cord, nerve roots, and meninges

through a fusion defect in the vertebral column) and has its onset in childhood.

Cerebellar ataxia in the type I malformation usually affects the gait and is bilateral; in some cases it is asymmetric. Hydrocephalus leads to headache and vomiting. Compression of the brainstem by herniated cerebellar tissue may be associated with vertigo, nystagmus, and lower cranial nerve palsies. Syringomyelia typically produces a capelike distribution of defective pain and temperature sensation.

Arnold-Chiari malformation can be diagnosed by CT or MRI studies that demonstrate cerebellar tonsillar herniation. High cervical laminectomy with decompression of the posterior fossa may be of therapeutic benefit.

SENSORY ATAXIAS

Sensory ataxia results from impaired proprioceptive sensation at the level of peripheral nerves or roots, posterior

Table 3–13. Causes of sensory ataxia.

Polyneuropathy[1]
Autosomal dominant sensory ataxic neuropathy
Cisplatin (*cis*-platinum)
Dejerine-Sottas disease (HMSN[2] type III)
Diabetes
Diphtheria
Hypothyroidism
Immune-mediated neuropathies (GALOP syndrome, anti-MAG antibody syndrome, Miller Fisher syndrome, anti-GD1b antibody syndrome)
Isoniazid
Paraneoplastic sensory neuronopathy (anti-Hu antibodies)
Pyridoxine
Refsum's disease
Taxol
Myelopathy[3]
Acute transverse myelitis
AIDS (vacuolar myelopathy)
Multiple sclerosis
Tumor or cord compression
Vascular malformations
Polyneuropathy or myelopathy
Friedreich's ataxia
Neurosyphilis (tabes dorsalis)
Nitrous oxide
Vitamin B$_{12}$ deficiency
Vitamin E deficiency

[1] Involving large, myelinated sensory fibers.

[2] Hereditary motor and sensory neuropathy.

[3] Involving posterior columns.

zation is preserved (Figure 4–3). The central region of the visual field (**macula**) projects to the most posterior portion of the visual cortex, while the inferior and superior parts of the field are represented above and below the calcarine fissure, respectively.

Vascular Supply

The vascular supply of the visual system is derived from the ophthalmic, middle cerebral, and posterior cerebral arteries (Figure 4–4); thus, ischemia or infarction in the territory of any of these vessels can produce visual field defects.

A. Retina

The retina is supplied by the central retinal artery, a branch of the ophthalmic artery that, in turn, branches from the internal carotid artery. Because the central retinal artery subsequently divides into superior and inferior retinal branches, vascular disease of the retina tends to produce altitudinal (ie, superior or inferior) visual field deficits.

B. Optic Nerve

The optic nerve receives arterial blood primarily from the ophthalmic artery and its branches.

C. Optic Radiations

As the optic radiations course backward toward the visual cortex, they are supplied by branches of the middle cerebral artery. Ischemia or infarction in the distribution of the middle cerebral artery may thus cause loss of vision in the contralateral visual field.

D. Primary Visual Cortex

The principal source of arterial blood for the primary visual cortex is the posterior cerebral artery. Occlusion of one posterior cerebral artery produces blindness in the contralateral visual field, although the dual (middle and posterior cerebral) arterial supply to the macular region of the visual cortex (Figures 4–3 and 4–4) may spare central (macular) vision. Because the posterior cerebral arteries arise together from the basilar artery, occlusion at the tip of the basilar artery can cause bilateral occipital infarction and complete cortical blindness—although, in some cases, macular vision is spared.

FUNCTIONAL ANATOMY OF THE OCULAR MOTOR SYSTEM

Extraocular Muscles

Movement of the eyes is accomplished by the action of six muscles attached to each globe (Figure 4–5A). These muscles act to move the eye into each of six cardinal positions of gaze (Figure 4–5B and C). Equal and opposed actions of these six muscles in the resting state place the eye in mid or primary position, ie, looking directly forward. When the function of one extraocular muscle is disrupted, the eye is unable to move in the direction of action of the affected muscle (**ophthalmoplegia**) and may deviate in the opposite direction because of the unopposed action of other extraocular muscles. When the eyes are thus misaligned, visual images of perceived objects fall on a different region of each retina, creating the illusion of double vision, or **diplopia**.

Cranial Nerves

The extraocular muscles are innervated by the oculomotor (III), trochlear (IV), and abducens (VI) nerves. Because of this differential innervation of the ocular muscles, the pattern of their involvement in pathologic conditions can help to distinguish a disorder of the ocular muscles per se from a disorder that affects a cranial nerve. Cranial nerves that control eye movement traverse long distances to pass from the brainstem to the eye; they are thereby rendered vulnerable to injury by a variety of pathologic processes.

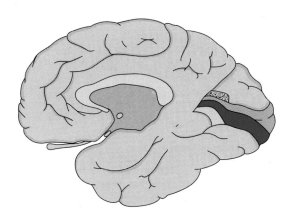

Upper peripheral quadrant of retina

Upper quadrant of macula

Lower quadrant of macula

Lower peripheral quadrant of retina

Figure 4–3. Representation of the visual field at the level of the primary visual cortex, midsagittal view, shows the medial surface of the right occipital lobe, which receives visual input from the left side of the visual field of both eyes.

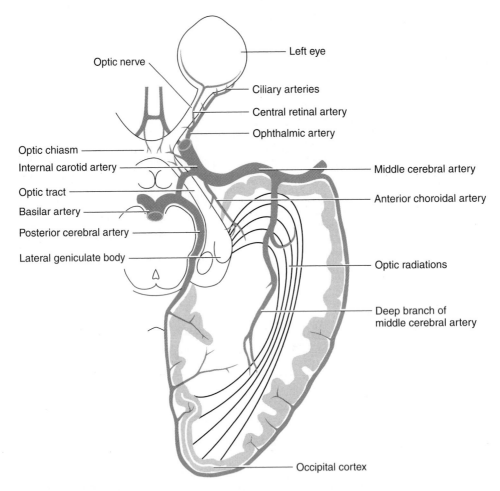

Figure 4–4. Arterial supply of the visual system, viewed from below.

A. NERVE III

The oculomotor nerve supplies the medial rectus, superior and inferior rectus, and inferior oblique muscles and carries fibers to the levator palpebrae (which raises the eyelid). It also supplies the parasympathetic fibers responsible for pupillary constriction. With a complete nerve III lesion, the eye is partially abducted and there is an inability to adduct, elevate, and depress the eye; the eyelid droops (ptosis), and the pupil is nonreactive.

B. NERVE IV

The trochlear nerve innervates the superior oblique muscle. Lesions of this nerve result in defective depression of the adducted eye.

C. NERVE VI

Lesions of the abducens nerve cause lateral rectus palsy, with impaired abduction of the affected eye.

Cranial Nerve Nuclei

The nuclei of the oculomotor and trochlear nerves are located in the dorsal midbrain, ventral to the cerebral aqueduct (of Sylvius), while the abducens nerve nucleus occupies a similarly dorsal and periventricular position in the pons.

Lesions involving these nuclei give rise to clinical abnormalities similar to those produced by involvement of their respective cranial nerves; in some cases, nuclear and nerve lesions can be distinguished.

A. NERVE III NUCLEUS

While each oculomotor nerve supplies muscles of the ipsilateral eye only, fibers to the superior rectus originate in the contralateral oculomotor nerve nucleus, and the levator palpebrae receives bilateral nuclear innervation. Thus, ophthalmoplegia affecting only one eye with ipsi-

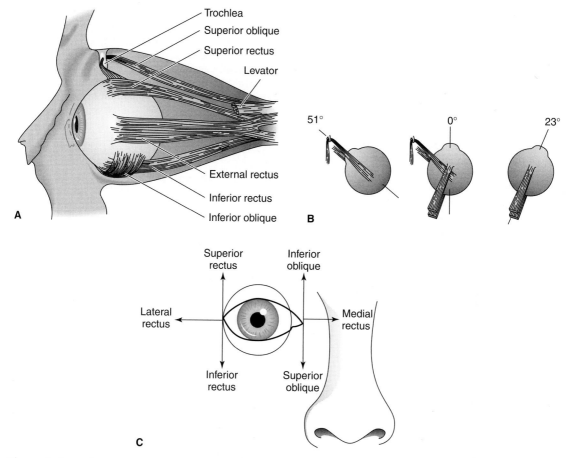

Figure 4–5. **A:** The origin and insertions of the extraocular muscles in the right orbit. **B:** An illustration of the right eye viewed from above in the primary position (**center figure**) showing the angle of attachment of the superior and inferior rectus muscles and the superior and inferior oblique muscles. With the eye directed to the right, the superior and inferior rectus muscles can now be examined as pure elevators and depressors of the globe (**right image**) and with the eye deviated to the left, the oblique muscles can now be examined as pure elevators and depressors of the globe as illustrated in **C. C:** The six cardinal positions of gaze for testing the function of the extraocular muscles. The eye is adducted by the medial rectus and abducted by the lateral rectus. The adducted eye is elevated by the inferior oblique and depressed by the superior oblique; the abducted eye is elevated by the superior rectus and depressed by the inferior rectus.

lateral ptosis or superior rectus palsy suggests oculomotor nerve disease, whereas ophthalmoplegia accompanied by bilateral ptosis or a contralateral superior rectus palsy is probably due to a nuclear lesion.

B. NERVE IV NUCLEUS

It is not possible to distinguish clinically between lesions of the trochlear nerve and those of its nucleus.

C. NERVE VI NUCLEUS

In disorders affecting the abducens nerve nucleus rather than the nerve itself, lateral rectus paresis is often associated with facial weakness, paresis of ipsilateral conjugate gaze, or a depressed level of consciousness. This is because of the proximity of the abducens nerve nucleus to the facial (VII) nerve fasciculus, pontine lateral gaze center, and ascending reticular activating system, respectively.

Supranuclear Control of Eye Movements

Supranuclear control of eye movements enables the two eyes to act in concert to produce **version** (**conjugate gaze**) or **vergence** (**convergence and divergence**) movements.

A. Brainstem Gaze Centers

Centers that control horizontal and vertical gaze are located in the pons and in the pretectal region of the midbrain, respectively, and receive descending inputs from the cerebral cortex that allow voluntary control of gaze (Figure 4–6). Each **lateral gaze center**, located in the paramedian pontine reticular formation (PPRF) adjacent to the abducens nerve nucleus, mediates ipsilateral conjugate horizontal gaze via its connections to the ipsilateral abducens and contralateral oculomotor nerve nucleus. A lesion in the pons affecting the PPRF therefore produces a **gaze preference** away from the side of the lesion—and toward the side of an associated hemiparesis, if present.

B. Cortical Input

The PPRF receives cortical input from the contralateral frontal lobe, which regulates rapid eye movements (**sac-** cades), and from the ipsilateral parietooccipital lobe, which regulates slow eye movements (**pursuits**). Therefore, a destructive lesion affecting the frontal cortex interferes with the mechanism for contralateral horizontal gaze and may result in a gaze preference toward the side of the lesion (and away from the side of associated hemiparesis). By contrast, an irritative (seizure) focus in the frontal lobe may cause gaze away from the side of the focus (see Figure 4–19).

HISTORY

Nature of Complaint

The first step in evaluating a neuroophthalmologic disorder is to obtain a clear description of the complaint. Patients often complain only of vague symptoms, such as blurred vision, which provide little diagnostic infor-

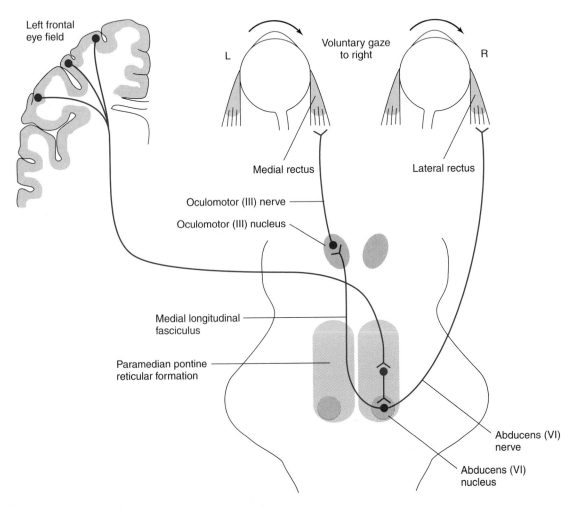

Figure 4–6. Neuronal pathways involved in horizontal gaze.

mation. An attempt must be made to determine exactly what the patient means to convey—decreased visual acuity in one or both eyes, loss of vision in part of the visual field, diplopia, an unstable visual image, pain in or about the eye, or some other problem.

Temporal Pattern of Symptoms

Once the nature of the complaint has been established, inquiries regarding its temporal pattern can provide clues to the underlying pathologic process.

A. SUDDEN ONSET

Vascular disorders that affect the eye or its connections in the brain tend to produce symptoms of sudden onset.

B. SLOW ONSET

With inflammatory or neoplastic disease, symptoms usually evolve over a longer period.

C. TRANSIENT, RECURRENT SYMPTOMS

Symptoms that are transient and recurrent suggest a select group of pathologic processes, including ischemia, demyelinating disease, and myasthenia gravis.

Associated Neurologic Abnormalities

The nature of any associated neurologic abnormalities, such as impaired facial sensation, weakness, ataxia, or aphasia, can be valuable in localizing the anatomic site of involvement.

Medical History

The history should be scrutinized for conditions that predispose the patient to neuroophthalmologic problems.

Multiple sclerosis often involves the optic nerve or brainstem, leading to a variety of neuroophthalmologic disorders. A history of disturbances that also involve other parts of the central nervous system should suggest this diagnosis.

Atherosclerosis, hypertension, and diabetes can be complicated by vascular disorders of the eye, cranial nerves, or visual or ocular motor pathways in the brain.

Endocrine disorders (eg, hyperthyroidism) can cause ocular myopathy.

Connective tissue disease and systemic cancer can affect the visual and ocular motor systems at a variety of sites in the brain or subarachnoid space.

Patients with nutritional deficiencies may present with neuroophthalmologic symptoms, as in the amblyopia (decreased visual acuity) associated with malnutrition and the ophthalmoplegia of Wernicke's encephalopathy.

Numerous drugs (eg, ethambutol, isoniazid, digi-

talis, clioquinol) are known to be toxic to the visual system, and others (sedative drugs, anticonvulsants) commonly produce ocular motor disorders.

NEUROOPHTHALMOLOGIC EXAMINATION

Visual Acuity

A. ASSESSMENT

To assess visual acuity from a neurologic standpoint, vision is tested under conditions that eliminate refractive errors. Therefore, patients who wear glasses should be examined while wearing them (a pinhole can be substituted if the corrective lenses usually worn are not available at the time of testing). Visual acuity must be assessed for each eye separately. Distant vision is tested using a Snellen eye chart, with the patient 6 m (20 ft) away. Near vision is tested with the Rosenbaum pocket eye chart held about 36 cm (14 in.) from the patient. In each case, the smallest line of print that can be read is noted.

B. RECORDING

Visual acuity is expressed as a fraction (eg, 20/20, 20/40, 20/200). The numerator is the distance (in feet) from the test figures at which the examination is performed, and the denominator is the distance (in feet) at which figures of a given size can be correctly identified by persons with normal vision. For example, if a patient standing 20 ft away from the eye chart is unable to identify figures that can normally be seen from that distance but can identify the larger figures that would be visible 40 ft away with normal acuity, the visual acuity is recorded as 20/40. If the patient can read most of a given line but makes some errors, acuity may be recorded as 20/40–1, for example, indicating that all but one letter on the 20/40 line were correctly identified. When visual acuity is markedly reduced, it can still be quantified, though less precisely, in terms of the distance at which the patient can count fingers (CF), discern hand movement (HM), or perceive light. If an eye is totally blind, the examination will reveal no light perception (NLP).

C. RED-GREEN COLOR VISION

Red-green color vision is often disproportionately impaired in optic nerve lesions and can be tested with colored objects such as pens or hatpins or with color vision plates.

Visual Fields

Evaluating the visual fields can be a lengthy and tedious procedure if conducted in an undirected fashion. Familiarity with the common types of visual field defects is important if testing is to be reasonably rapid and yield useful information. The most common visual field abnormalities are illustrated in Figure 4–7.

A. Extent of Visual Fields

The normal monocular visual field subtends an angle of about 160 degrees in the horizontal plane and about

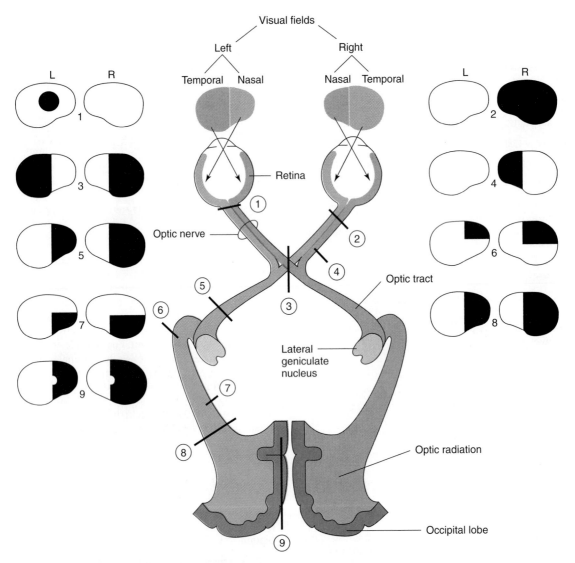

Figure 4–7. Common visual field defects and their anatomical bases. 1. **Central scotoma** caused by inflammation of the optic disk (optic neuritis) or optic nerve (retrobulbar neuritis). 2. **Total blindness of the right eye** from a complete lesion of the right optic nerve. 3. **Bitemporal hemianopia** caused by pressure exerted on the optic chiasm by a pituitary tumor. 4. **Right nasal hemianopia** caused by a perichiasmal lesion (eg, calcified internal carotid artery). 5. **Right homonymous hemianopia** from a lesion of the left optic tract. 6. **Right homonymous superior quadrantanopia** caused by partial involvement of the optic radiation by a lesion in the left temporal lobe (Meyer's loop). 7. **Right homonymous inferior quadrantanopia** caused by partial involvement of the optic radiation by a lesion in the left parietal lobe. 8. **Right homonymous hemianopia** from a complete lesion of the left optic radiation. (A similar defect may also result from lesion 9.) 9. **Right homonymous hemianopia (with macular sparing)** resulting from posterior cerebral artery occlusion.

135 degrees in the vertical plane (Figure 4–8). With binocular vision, the horizontal range of vision exceeds 180 degrees.

B. PHYSIOLOGIC BLIND SPOT

Within the normal field of each eye is a 5-degree blind spot, corresponding to the optic disk, which lacks receptor cells.

C. MEASUREMENT TECHNIQUES

Numerous techniques exist for measuring the visual field—which, like visual acuity, must be examined separately for each eye.

1. The simplest method for visual field testing is the **confrontation** technique (Figure 4–9). The examiner stands at about arm's length from the patient, with the eyes of both patient and examiner aligned in the horizontal plane. The eye not being tested is covered by the patient's hand or an eye patch. The examiner closes the eye opposite the patient's covered eye, and the patient is instructed to fix on the examiner's open eye. Now the monocular fields of patient and examiner are superim-posed, which allows comparison of the patient's field with the examiner's presumably normal field. The examiner uses the index fingers of either hand to locate the boundaries of the patient's field, moving them slowly inward from the periphery in all directions until the patient detects them. The boundaries are then defined more carefully by determining the farthest peripheral sites at which the patient can detect slight movements of the fingertips or the white head of a pin. The patient's blind spot can be located in the region of the examiner's own blind spot, and the sizes of these spots can be compared using a pin with a white head as the target. The procedure is then repeated for the other eye.

2. Subtle field defects may be detected by asking the patient to compare the brightness of colored objects presented at different sites in the field or by measuring the fields using a pin with a red head as the target.

3. In young children, the fields may be assessed by standing behind the child and bringing an attention-getting object, such as a toy, forward around the child's head in various directions until it is first noticed.

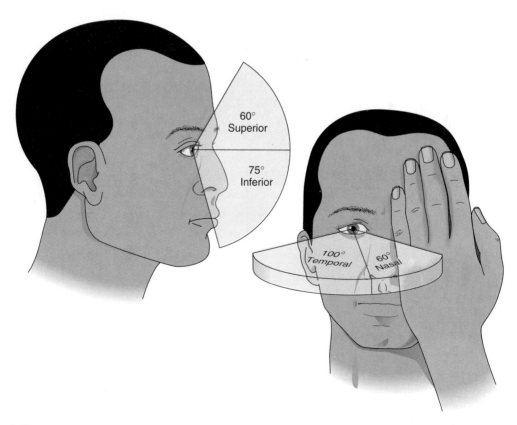

Figure 4–8. Normal limits of the visual field.

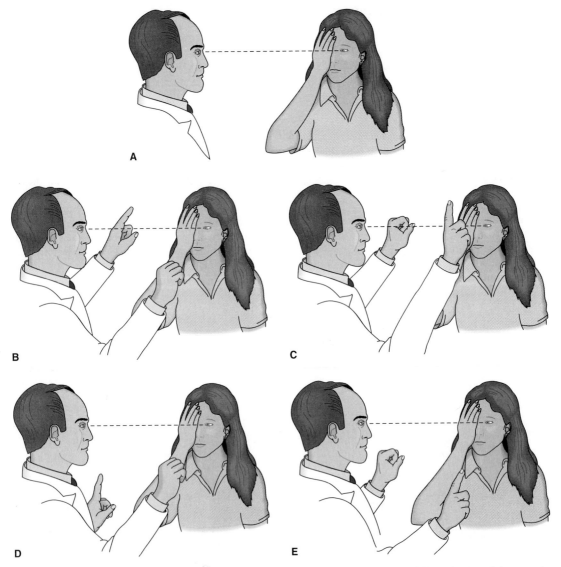

Figure 4–9. Confrontation testing of the visual field. **A:** The left eye of the patient and the right eye of the examiner are aligned. **B:** Testing the superior nasal quadrant. **C:** Testing the superior temporal quadrant. **D:** Testing the inferior nasal quadrant. The procedure is then repeated for the patient's other eye. **E:** Testing the inferior temporal quadrant.

4. A gross indication of visual field abnormalities may be obtained in obtunded patients by determining whether they blink in response to a visual threat—typically the examiner's finger—brought toward the patient's eye in various regions of the field.

5. Although many visual field deficits are detectable by these screening procedures, more precise mapping of the fields requires the use of one of many perimetry techniques: standard **tangent screen testing** or automated perimetry techniques.

Ophthalmoscopy

A. PREPARATION OF THE PATIENT

Ophthalmoscopic examination of the optic fundus is particularly important in evaluating neuroophthalmologic disorders that affect the retina or optic disk and in the evaluation of patients with a suspected increase in intracranial pressure. The examination should be conducted in a dark room so that the pupils are dilated; in some patients, the use of mydriatic (sympathomimetic or anticholinergic) eye drops is necessary. In the latter case, visual acuity and pupillary reflexes should always be assessed before instilling the drops. Mydriatic agents should be avoided in patients with glaucoma and in situations—such as impending or ongoing transtentorial herniation—in which the state of pupillary reactivity is an important guide to management.

B. Examination of the Fundus

Familiarity with the normal appearance of the optic fundus (Figure 4–10) is necessary if abnormalities are to be appreciated.

1. Optic disk

a. Normal appearance—The optic disk is usually easily recognizable as a yellowish, slightly oval structure situated nasally at the posterior pole of the eye. The temporal side of the disk is often paler than the nasal side. The disk margins should be sharply demarcated, though the nasal edge is commonly somewhat less distinct than the temporal edge. The disk is normally in the same plane as the surrounding retina.

b. Optic disk swelling—Among the many ophthalmoscopic findings that provide useful diagnostic information, the abnormality that most often requires prompt interpretation and attention is optic nerve swelling (**papilledema**). Although this condition implies increased intracranial pressure, it must be differentiated from swelling that is due to other causes, such as local inflammation (papillitis) and ischemic optic neuropathy. In making this distinction, it is most helpful to bear in mind that papilledema is almost always bilateral; it does not typically impair vi-

sion, except for enlargement of the blind spot, and it is not associated with eye pain. Papilledema can also be simulated by disk abnormalities such as drusen (colloid or hyaline bodies).

Increased intracranial pressure is thought to cause papilledema by the increased pressure blocking axonal transport in the optic nerve. Because this compartment communicates with the subarachnoid space, disorders associated with increased intracranial pressure that also obstruct the subarachnoid space, such as meningitis, are less likely to cause papilledema. The ophthalmoscopic changes in papilledema typically develop over days or weeks but may become apparent within hours following a sudden increase in intracranial pressure—as, for example, following intracranial hemorrhage. In early papilledema (Figure 4–11), the retinal veins appear engorged and spontaneous venous pulsations are absent. The disk may be hyperemic, and linear hemorrhages may be seen at its borders. The disk margins become blurred, with the temporal edge last to be affected. In fully developed papilledema, the optic disk is elevated above the plane of the retina.

c. Optic disk pallor—Optic disk pallor with impaired visual acuity, visual fields, or pupillary reactivity is associated with a wide variety of disorders that affect the optic nerve, including inflammatory conditions, nutritional deficiencies, and heredodegenerative diseases. Note that a pale optic disk with normal visual function can occur as a congenital variant.

2. Arteries and veins—To determine the caliber of the retinal arteries and veins, they are observed at the point where they arise from the disk and pass over its

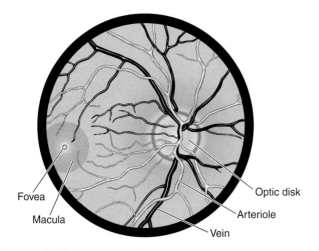

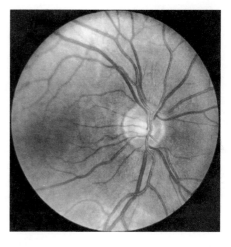

Fovea
Macula
Optic disk
Arteriole
Vein

Figure 4–10. The normal fundus. The diagram shows landmarks corresponding to the photograph. (Photo by Diane Beeston; reproduced with permission, from Vaughan D, Asbury T, Riordan-Eva P: *General Ophthalmology*, 15th ed. Appleton & Lange, 1992.)

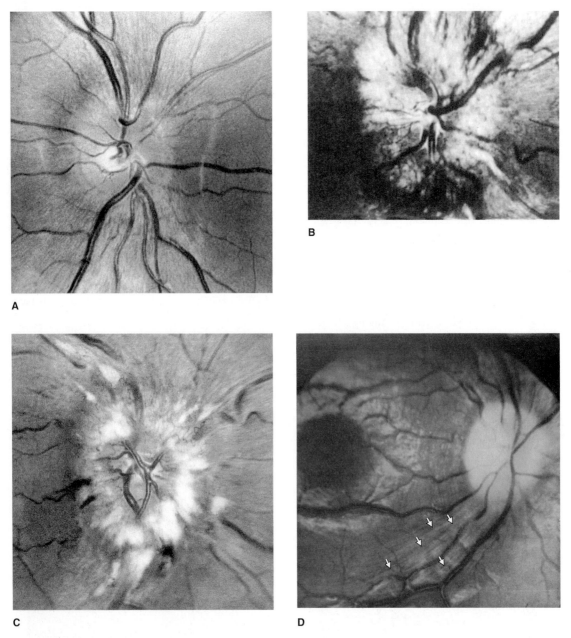

Figure 4–11. Appearance of the fundus in papilledema. **A:** In early papilledema, the superior and inferior margins of the optic disk are blurred by the thickened layer of nerve fibers entering the disk. **B:** Swollen nerve fibers (white patches) and hemorrhages can be seen. **C:** In fully developed papilledema, the optic disk is swollen, elevated, and congested, and the retinal veins are markedly dilated. **D:** In chronic atrophic papilledema, the optic disk is pale and slightly elevated, and its margins are blurred. The white areas surrounding the macula are reflected light from the vitreoretinal interface. The inferior temporal nerve fiber bundles are partially atrophic **(arrows)**. (Photos courtesy of WF Hoyt.)

edges onto the retina. Observations include whether they are easily visible throughout their course, whether they appear engorged, and whether spontaneous venous pulsations are present. The remainder of the visible retina is inspected, noting the presence of hemorrhages, exudates, or other abnormalities.

3. Macula—The macula, a somewhat paler area than the rest of the retina, is located about two disk diameters temporal to the temporal margin of the optic disk. It can be visualized quickly by having the patient look at the light from the ophthalmoscope. Ophthal-

moscopic examination of the macula can reveal abnormalities related to visual loss from age-related macular degeneration, from macular holes, or from hereditary cerebromacular degenerations.

Pupils

A. Size

Assessing the size and reactivity of the pupils provides an evaluation of nervous system pathways from the optic nerve to the midbrain (Figure 4–12). The normal pupil

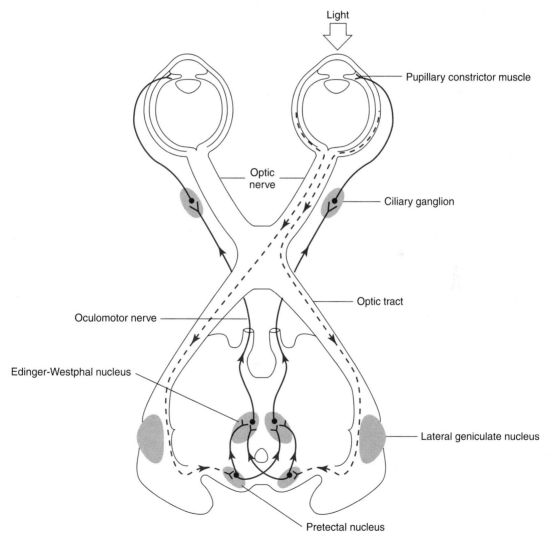

Figure 4–12. Anatomic basis of the pupillary light reflex. The afferent visual pathways from the retina to the pretectal nuclei of the midbrain are represented by dashed lines and the efferent pupilloconstrictor pathways from the midbrain to the retinas by solid lines. Note that illumination of one eye results in bilateral pupillary constriction.

is round, regular, and centered within the iris; its size varies with age and with the intensity of ambient light. In a brightly illuminated examining room, normal pupils are about 3 mm in diameter in adults. They are often smaller in the elderly and commonly 5 mm or more in diameter in children. Pupillary size may be asymmetric in as much as 20% of the population (physiologic **anisocoria**), but the difference in size is not more than 1 mm. Symmetrically rapid constriction in response to a bright light indicates that the size difference is not due to oculomotor nerve compression.

B. REACTION TO LIGHT

Direct (ipsilateral) and **consensual (contralateral)** pupillary constriction in response to a bright light shined in one eye demonstrates the integrity of the pathways shown in Figure 4–12. Normally, the direct response to light is slightly brisker and more pronounced than the consensual response.

C. REACTION TO ACCOMMODATION

When the eyes converge to focus on a nearer object, the pupils normally constrict. The reaction to accommodation is tested by having the patient focus alternately on a distant object and a finger held just in front of his or her nose.

D. PUPILLARY ABNORMALITIES

1. Nonreactive pupils—Unilateral disorders of pupillary constriction are seen with local disease of the iris (trauma, iritis, glaucoma), oculomotor nerve compression (tumor, aneurysm), and optic nerve disorders (optic neuritis, multiple sclerosis).

2. Light-near dissociation—Impaired pupillary reactivity to light with preserved constriction during accommodation (light-near dissociation) is usually bilateral and may result from neurosyphilis, diabetes, optic nerve disorders, and tumors compressing the midbrain tectum.

3. Argyll Robertson pupils—These pupils are small, poorly reactive to light, often irregular in shape, and frequently unequal in size; they show light-near dissociation (Table 4–1). Neurosyphilis is the classic cause but other lesions in the region of the Edinger-Westphal nucleus (eg, multiple sclerosis) are now more common.

4. Tonic pupil—The tonic (**Adie's**) pupil (see Table 4–1) is larger than the contralateral unaffected pupil and reacts sluggishly to changes in illumination or accommodation. Because the tonic pupil does eventually react, anisocoria becomes less marked during the time of the examination. This abnormality is most commonly a manifestation of a benign, often familial disorder that frequently affects young women (**Holmes-Adie syndrome**) and may be associated with depressed deep tendon reflexes (especially in the legs), segmental anhidrosis (localized lack of sweating), orthostatic hypotension, or cardiovascular autonomic instability. The condition may be bilateral. The pupillary abnormality may be caused by degeneration of the ciliary ganglion, followed by aberrant reinnervation of the pupilloconstrictor muscles.

5. Horner's syndrome—Horner's syndrome (Table 4–1 and Table 4–2) results from a lesion of the central or peripheral sympathetic nervous system and consists of a small (miotic) pupil associated with mild ptosis (Figure 4–13A) and sometimes loss of sweating (**anhidrosis**).

Table 4–1. Common pupillary abnormalities.

	Appearance	Response	Differential Diagnosis
Tonic (Adie's) pupil	Unilateral (rarely bilateral) dilated pupil	Reacts sluggishly and only to persistent bright light or 0.125% pilocarpine eye drops; accommodation less affected	Holmes-Adie syndrome, ocular trauma, autonomic neuropathy
Horner's syndrome	Unilateral small pupil and slight ptosis	Normal response to light and accommodation	Lateral medullary infarcts, cervical cord lesions, pulmonary apical or mediastinal tumors, neck trauma or masses, carotid artery thrombosis, intrapartum brachial plexus injury, cluster headache
Argyll Robertson pupil	Unequal irregular pupils less than 3 mm in diameter (usually bilateral)	Poorly reactive to light; more responsive to accommodation	Neurosyphilis; mimicked by diabetes, pineal region tumors

Table 4–2. Causes of Horner's syndrome in 100 hospitalized patients.[1]

	Percentage
Central (first) neuron	63
Brainstem infarction	36
Cerebral hemorrhage/infarction	12
Multiple sclerosis	3
Intracranial tumor	2
Trauma (including surgery)	2
Syrinx	2
Transverse myelopathy	2
Other or unknown	4
Preganglionic (second) neuron	21
Thoracic and neck tumor	14
Trauma	
Nonsurgical	4
Surgical	3
Other or unknown	0
Postganglionic (third) neuron	13
Intracranial tumor (cavernous sinus)	7
Trauma (including surgical)	2
Vascular headache	2
Other or unknown	2
Unknown localization	3

[1] Data from Keane JR: *Arch Neurol* 1979;36:13–16.

a. Oculosympathetic pathways—The sympathetic pathway controlling pupillary dilation (Figure 4–13B) consists of an uncrossed three-neuron arc: **hypothalamic neurons**, the axons of which descend through the brainstem to the intermediolateral column of the spinal cord at the T1 level; **preganglionic sympathetic neurons** projecting from the spinal cord to the superior cervical ganglion; and **postganglionic sympathetic neurons** that originate in the superior cervical ganglion, ascend in the neck along the internal carotid artery, and enter the orbit with the first (ophthalmic) division of the trigeminal (V) nerve. Horner's syndrome is caused by interruption of these pathways at any site.

b. Clinical features—The lesions—and the pupillary abnormality produced—are usually unilateral. The pupillary diameter on the involved side is typically reduced by 0.5–1 mm compared with the normal side. This inequality is most marked in dim illumination and in other situations in which the pupils are normally dilated, such as during a painful stimulus or startle. The pupillary abnormality is accompanied by mild to moderate ptosis (see below) of the upper lid (as opposed to the pronounced ptosis with oculomotor nerve lesions), often associated with elevation of the lower lid. When Horner's syndrome has been present since infancy, the ipsilateral iris is lighter and blue (**heterochromia iridis**).

Deficits in the pattern of sweating, which are most prominent in acute-onset Horner's syndrome, can help localize the lesion. If sweating is decreased on an entire half of the body and face, the lesion is in the central nervous system. Cervical lesions produce anhidrosis of the face, neck, and arm only. Sweating is unimpaired if the lesion is above the bifurcation of the carotid artery. The differential diagnosis of Horner's syndrome is presented in Table 4–2.

6. Relative afferent pupillary defect (Marcus Gunn pupil)—In this condition, one pupil constricts less markedly in response to direct illumination than to illumination of the contralateral pupil, whereas normally the direct response is greater than the consensual response. The abnormality is detected by rapidly moving a bright flashlight back and forth between the eyes while continuously observing the suspect pupil (**Gunn's pupillary test**). Relative afferent pupillary defect is commonly associated with disorders of the ipsilateral optic nerve, which interrupt the afferent limb and affect the pupillary light reflex (Figure 4–12). Such disorders also commonly impair vision (especially color vision) in the involved eye.

Optokinetic Response

Optokinetic nystagmus consists of eye movements elicited by sequential fixation on a series of targets passing in front of a patient's eyes, such as telephone poles seen from a moving train. For clinical testing, a revolving drum with vertical stripes or a vertically striped strip of cloth moved across the visual field is used to generate these movements. Testing produces a slow following phase in the direction of the target's movement, followed by a rapid return jerk in the opposite direction. The slow (pursuit) phase tests ipsilateral parietooccipital pathways; the rapid (saccadic) movement tests pathways originating in the contralateral frontal lobe. The presence of an optokinetic response reflects the ability to perceive movement or contour and is sometimes useful for documenting visual perception in newborns or in psychogenic blindness. Visual acuity required to produce the optokinetic response is minimal, however (20/400, or finger counting at 3–5 ft). Unilateral impairment of the optokinetic response may be found when targets are moved toward the side of a parietal lobe lesion.

Eyelids

The eyelids (**palpebrae**) should be examined with the patient's eyes open. The distance between the upper and lower lids (interpalpebral fissure) is usually about 10 mm and equal in both eyes, though physiologic asym-

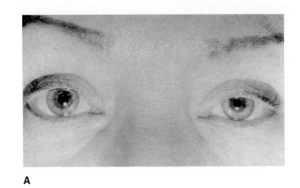

A

Hypothalamus

Ophthalmic division
of trigeminal nerve

Long ciliary nerve

To sweat glands of forehead

To smooth muscle of eyelid

To pupil

Internal carotid artery

To sweat glands of face

External carotid artery

C2

Third neuron

Superior cervical ganglion

First neuron

T1

Second neuron

Spinal cord

B

Figure 4–13. **A:** Left Horner's syndrome (ptosis and myosis) after an attempted intercostal nerve block complicated by pneumothorax. (Courtesy of JR Keane.) **B:** Oculosympathetic pathway involved in Horner's syndrome. This
three-neuron pathway projects from the hypothalamus to the intermediolateral column of the spinal cord, then to
the superior cervical (sympathetic) ganglion, and finally to the pupil, smooth muscle of the eyelid, and sweat glands
of the forehead and face.

metries do occur. The position of the inferior margin of the upper lid relative to the superior border of the iris should be noted in order to detect drooping (**ptosis**) or abnormal elevation of the eyelid (**lid retraction**). The upper lid normally covers 1–2 mm of the iris.

Unilateral ptosis is seen with paralysis of the levator palpebrae muscle itself, lesions of the oculomotor nerve or its superior branch, and Horner's syndrome. In the last condition, ptosis is customarily associated with miosis and may be momentarily overcome by effortful eye opening.

Bilateral ptosis suggests disease affecting the oculomotor nerve nucleus; a disorder of the neuromuscular junction, such as myasthenia gravis; or a disorder of muscle, such as myotonic, ocular, or oculopharyngeal dystrophy.

Lid retraction (abnormal elevation of the upper lid) is seen in hyperthyroidism; in **Parinaud's syndrome**, it is caused by tumors in the pineal region.

Exophthalmos

Abnormal protrusion of the eye from the orbit (**exophthalmos or proptosis**) is best detected by standing behind the seated patient and looking down at his or her eyes. The causes include hyperthyroidism, orbital tumor or pseudotumor, and carotid artery-cavernous sinus fistula. A bruit may be audible on auscultation over the proptotic eye in patients with carotid artery-cavernous sinus fistula or other vascular anomalies.

Eye Movements

A. OCULAR EXCURSION AND GAZE

Ocular palsies and gaze palsies are detected by having the patient gaze in each of the six cardinal positions (see Figure 4–5). If voluntary eye movement is impaired or the patient is unable to cooperate with the examination (eg, is comatose), reflex eye movements can be induced by one of two maneuvers (Figure 10–3). The **doll's head (oculocephalic) maneuver** is performed by rotating the head horizontally, to elicit horizontal eye movements, and vertically, to elicit vertical movements. The eyes should move in the direction opposite to that of head rotation. This may be an inadequate stimulus for inducing eye movements, however, and the reflex may be overridden in conscious patients. **Caloric (oculovestibular) stimulation** is a more potent stimulus and is performed by irrigating the tympanic membrane with cold (30°C) or warm (44°C) water. Otoscopic examination should always be undertaken before this maneuver is attempted: it is contraindicated if the tympanic membrane is perforated. In conscious patients, unilateral cold water irrigation produces nystagmus with the fast phase directed away from the irrigated side. Because this

procedure may produce discomfort and nausea or vomiting, only small volumes (eg, 1 mL) of water should be used in conscious patients. In comatose patients with intact brainstem function, unilateral cold water irrigation results in tonic deviation of the eyes toward the irrigated side. Bilateral irrigation with cold water causes tonic downward deviation, whereas bilateral stimulation with warm water induces tonic upward deviation. An absent or impaired response to caloric stimulation with large volumes (eg, 50 mL) of cold water is indicative of peripheral vestibular disease, a structural lesion in the posterior fossa (cerebellum or brainstem), or intoxication with sedative drugs. If limitations in movement are observed, the muscles involved are noted and the nature of the abnormality is determined according to the following scheme.

1. Ocular palsy—This weakness of one or more eye muscles results from nuclear or infranuclear (nerve, neuromuscular junction, or muscle) lesions. An ocular palsy cannot be overcome by caloric stimulation of reflex eye movement. Nerve lesions produce distinctive patterns of ocular muscle involvement.

a. Oculomotor (III) nerve palsy—A complete lesion of the oculomotor nerve produces closure of the affected eye because of impaired levator function. Passively elevating the paralyzed lid (Figure 4–14) shows the involved eye to be laterally deviated because of the unopposed action of the lateral rectus muscle, which is not innervated by the oculomotor nerve. Diplopia is present in all directions of gaze except for lateral gaze toward the side of involvement. The pupil's function may be normal (pupillary sparing) or impaired.

b. Trochlear (IV) nerve palsy—With trochlear nerve lesions, which paralyze the superior oblique muscle, the involved eye is elevated during primary (forward) gaze; the extent of elevation increases during adduction and decreases during abduction. Elevation is greatest when the head is tilted toward the side of the

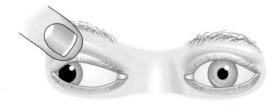

Figure 4–14. Clinical findings with oculomotor (III) nerve lesion. With the ptotic lid passively elevated, the affected (right) eye is abducted. On attempted downgaze, the unaffected superior oblique muscle, which is innervated by the trochlear (IV) nerve, causes the eye to turn inward.

involved eye and abolished by tilt in the opposite direction (Bielschowsky's head-tilt test; Figure 4–15). Diplopia is most pronounced when the patient looks downward with the affected eye adducted (as in looking at the end of one's nose). Spontaneous head tilting, intended to decrease or correct the diplopia, is present in about half the patients with unilateral palsies and in an even greater number with bilateral palsies.

c. Abducens (VI) nerve palsy—An abducens nerve lesion causes paralysis of the lateral rectus muscle, resulting in adduction of the involved eye at rest and failure of attempted abduction (Figure 4–16). Diplopia occurs on lateral gaze to the side of the affected eye.

2. Gaze palsy—Gaze palsy is the diminished ability of a pair of yoked muscles (muscles that operate in concert to move the two eyes in a given direction) to move the eyes in voluntary gaze; it is caused by supranuclear lesions in the brainstem or cerebral hemisphere. Gaze palsy, unlike ocular palsies, affects both eyes and can usually be overcome by caloric stimulation. Its pathophysiology and causes are discussed more fully in the section on gaze palsy. Mild impairment of upgaze is not uncommon in asymptomatic elderly subjects.

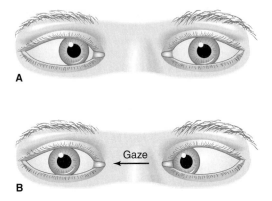

Figure 4–16. Clinical findings with abducens (VI) nerve lesion. The affected (right) eye is adducted at rest (**A**) and cannot be abducted (**B**).

3. Internuclear ophthalmoplegia—This disorder results from a lesion of the medial longitudinal fasciculus, an ascending pathway in the brainstem that projects from the abducens to the contralateral oculomotor

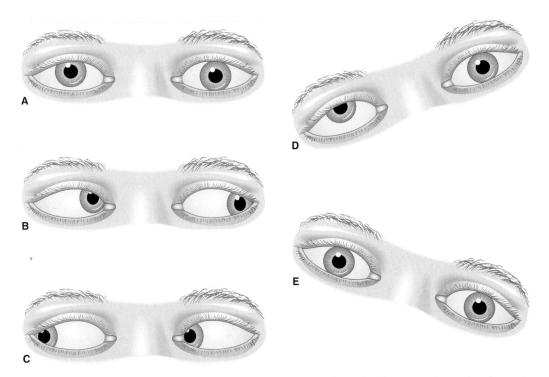

Figure 4–15. Clinical findings with trochlear (IV) nerve lesion. The affected (right) eye is elevated on forward gaze (**A**). The extent of elevation is increased with adduction (**B**) and decreased with abduction (**C**). Elevation increases with head tilting to the affected side (**D**) and decreases with head tilting in the opposite direction (**E**).

nerve nucleus. As a consequence, the actions of the abducens and oculomotor nerves during voluntary gaze or caloric-induced movement are uncoupled. Excursion of the abducting eye is full, but adduction of the contralateral eye is impaired (Figure 4–17). Internuclear ophthalmoplegia cannot be overcome by caloric stimulation; it can be distinguished from oculomotor nerve palsy by noting preservation of adduction with convergence. Its causes are discussed later (see *Internuclear Ophthalmoplegia*).

4. One-and-a-half syndrome—A pontine lesion affecting both the medial longitudinal fasciculus and the ipsilateral paramedian pontine reticular formation (lateral gaze center) produces a syndrome that combines internuclear ophthalmoplegia with an inability to gaze toward the side of the lesion (Figure 4–18). The ipsilateral eye is immobile in the horizontal plane and movement of the contralateral eye is restricted to abduction, which may be associated with nystagmus. The causes include pontine infarct, multiple sclerosis, and pontine hemorrhage.

B. DIPLOPIA TESTING

When the patient complains of diplopia, maneuvers to test eye movement should be used to determine its anatomic basis. The patient is asked to fix his or her vision on an object, such as a flashlight, in each of the six cardinal positions of gaze (see Figure 4–5). With normal conjugate gaze, light from the flashlight falls at the same spot on both corneas; a lack of such congruency confirms that gaze is disconjugate. When the patient notes diplopia in a given direction of gaze, each eye should be covered in turn and the patient is asked to report which of the two images disappears. The image displaced farther in the direction of gaze is always referable to the weak eye, because that image will not fall on the fovea. A variation of this procedure is the **red glass test**, in which one eye is covered with translucent red glass, plastic, or cellophane; this allows the eye responsible for each image to be identified.

C. NYSTAGMUS

Nystagmus is rhythmic oscillation of the eyes. **Pendular nystagmus**, which usually has its onset in infancy, occurs with equal velocity in both directions. **Jerk nystagmus** is characterized by a slow phase of movement followed by a fast phase in the opposite direction; the direction of jerk nystagmus is specified by stating the direction of the fast phase (eg, leftward-beating nystagmus). Jerk nystagmus usually increases in amplitude with gaze in the direction of the fast phase.

Nystagmus, a normal component of both the optokinetic response and the response to caloric stimulation of reflex eye movements, can also occur at the extremes of voluntary gaze in normal subjects. In other settings, however, it is commonly due to anticonvulsant or sedative drugs or is a sign of disease in the peripheral vestibular apparatus, central vestibular pathways, or cerebellum.

To detect nystagmus, the eyes are observed in the primary position and in each of the cardinal positions of gaze (see Figure 4 –5). Nystagmus is described in terms of the position of gaze in which it occurs, its direction and amplitude, precipitating factors such as changes in head position, and associated symptoms, such as vertigo.

Many forms of nystagmus and related ocular oscillations have been described, but two syndromes of acquired **pathologic jerk nystagmus** are by far the most common.

1. Gaze-evoked nystagmus—As its name implies, gaze-evoked nystagmus occurs when the patient attempts to gaze in one or more directions away from the primary position. The fast phase is in the direction of gaze. Nystagmus evoked by gaze in a single direction is a common sign of early or mild residual ocular palsy. Multidirectional gaze-evoked nystagmus is most often an adverse effect of anticonvulsant or sedative drugs, but it can also result from cerebellar or central vestibular dysfunction.

2. Vestibular nystagmus—Vestibular nystagmus increases with gaze toward the fast phase and is usually accompanied by vertigo when caused by a lesion of the **peripheral vestibular apparatus**. Vestibular nystagmus is characteristically unidirectional, horizontal, or horizontal and rotatory and is associated with severe vertigo. In contrast, **central vestibular nystagmus** may be bidirectional and purely horizontal, vertical, or rotatory, and the accompanying vertigo is typically mild. **Positional nystagmus**—elicited by changes in head

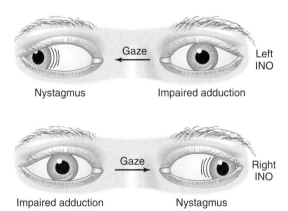

Figure 4–17. Eye movements in internuclear ophthalmoplegia (INO) resulting from a lesion of the medial longitudinal fasciculus bilaterally.

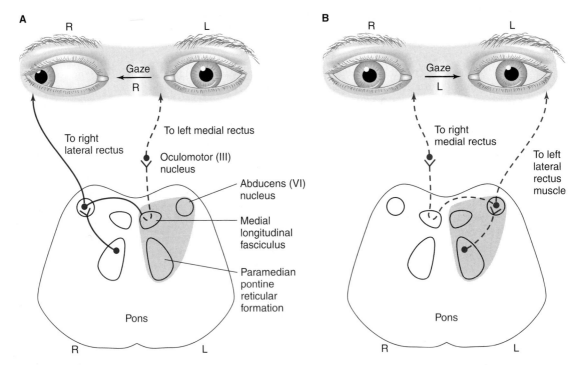

Figure 4–18. One-and-a-half syndrome. This results from a pontine lesion (shaded area) involving the paramedian pontine recticular formation (lateral gaze center) and medial longitudinal fasciculus, and sometimes also the abducens (VI) nucleus, and affecting the neuronal pathways indicated by dotted lines. Attempted gaze away from the lesion (**A**) activates the uninvolved right lateral gaze center and abducens (VI) nucleus; the right lateral rectus muscle contracts and the right eye abducts normally. Involvement of the medial longitudinal fasciculus interrupts the pathway to the left oculomotor (III) nucleus, and the left eye fails to adduct. On attempted gaze toward the lesion (**B**), the left lateral gaze center cannot be activated, and the eyes do not move. There is a complete (bilateral) gaze palsy in one direction (toward the lesion) and one-half (unilateral) gaze palsy in the other direction (away from the lesion), accounting for the name of the syndrome.

position—can occur with either peripheral or central vestibular lesions. The most helpful distinguishing features are the presence of hearing loss or tinnitus with peripheral lesions and of corticospinal tract or additional cranial nerve abnormalities with central lesions.

DISORDERS OF THE VISUAL SYSTEM

MONOCULAR DISORDERS

Common syndromes of monocular visual loss include two reversible and two irreversible disorders. **Transient monocular blindness** caused by optic nerve or retinal ischemia is sudden in onset and resolves rapidly. Sub-

acute, painful, unilateral visual loss with partial resolution is associated with **optic neuritis**. Less reversible visual loss of sudden onset occurs in idiopathic **ischemic optic neuropathy** and in **giant cell (temporal) arteritis**.

1. Transient Monocular Blindness

 This condition, sometimes called **amaurosis fugax**, is characterized by unilateral transient diminution or loss of vision that develops over seconds, remains maximal for 1–5 minutes, and resolves over 10–20 minutes. Although the cause of these episodes often remains uncertain, the presence of what appears to be embolic material in retinal arteries during episodes suggests that emboli are the cause. The major site of origin of such emboli appears to be atherosclerotic lesions at the carotid bifurcation. Mitral valve prolapse and other cardiac sources of emboli can produce a similar syndrome. The risk for subsequent hemispheric infarction is increased (14% within 7 years) in patients with a history of transient monocular blindness but is only about one-half that in patients with hemispheric transient ischemic attacks (TIAs).

Diagnostic evaluation and treatment of patients with transient monocular blindness resemble that recommended for patients with hemispheric TIAs (see Chapter 9). Recent studies have shown that in patients with transient monocular blindness or TIAs and high-grade (>70%) stenosis of the carotid artery at angiography, the combination of aspirin plus surgical removal of plaque (endarterectomy) is superior to aspirin alone.

2. Optic Neuritis

Inflammation of the optic nerve produces the syndrome of optic neuritis, which can be idiopathic; it is caused by demyelination or (rarely) parameningeal, meningeal, or intraocular inflammation or is associated with viral infections or post-viral-infection syndromes. Unilateral impairment of visual acuity occurs over hours to days, becoming maximal within 1 week. The visual loss is associated with headache, globe tenderness, or eye pain in over 90% of cases; the pain is typically exacerbated by eye movement.

On visual field testing, there is usually a central scotoma (blind spot) associated with decreased visual acuity. Examination of the fundus is normal in two-thirds of patients, since the inflammatory process is usually posterior to the optic disk (retrobulbar neuritis), but unilateral disk swelling may be seen. The pupils are equal in size but show a diminished reaction to illumination of the affected eye (relative afferent pupillary defect; discussed above). Visual acuity usually but not invariably improves over 2–3 weeks to normal. Intravenous methylprednisolone, 1 g/d for 3 days, followed by oral prednisone, 1 mg/kg/d for 11 days, has been shown to hasten recovery but does not alter the final outcome. Oral prednisone alone in lower doses was associated with a higher recurrence rate than occurred in patients treated with placebo. The frequency with which optic neuritis is the first sign of more widespread central nervous system demyelination (multiple sclerosis) remains uncertain and varies with the length of follow-up studies. Most prospective and retrospective series, however, report progression to definite multiple sclerosis in many of these patients (74% of women and 34% of men) over the subsequent 15 years. Rare causes of optic neuropathy include toxins (eg, methanol, ethambutol), neurosyphilis, and vitamin B_{12} deficiency. Evolving data support immunomodulatory treatment for presumed multiple sclerosis if demyelinating lesions are seen on a brain magnetic resonance imaging (MRI) scan (see Chapter 5).

3. Anterior Ischemic Optic Neuropathy (AION)

Idiopathic infarction of the anterior portion of the optic nerve is termed anterior ischemic optic neuropathy. Such visual loss is sudden in onset, usually painless, always monocular, and without premonitory ocular symptoms. Visual loss is usually maximal at onset and frequently subtotal, producing a field defect that is typically **altitudinal** (superior or inferior) in configuration; in one-third of cases the course is stuttering or progressive. Examination reveals ipsilateral disk swelling often with peripapillary hemorrhages. In the absence of this finding, the diagnosis is tenuous, and other causes, such as a rapidly expanding intracranial mass or neoplastic meningitis, should be sought. Although ischemic optic neuropathy is often assumed to be atherosclerotic in origin, there is no consistent association with other risk factors for cerebrovascular disease, such as hypertension, diabetes, or atherosclerotic carotid artery disease. Patients with AION have a structurally smaller than normal disc; 40% will go on to have the other eye affected within 2–4 years.

Attempts at treatment have been uniformly unsuccessful. As disk swelling resolves, ophthalmoscopic evaluation shows optic atrophy.

4. Giant Cell (Temporal) Arteritis

Arteritic infarction of the anterior portion of the optic nerve is the most devastating complication of giant cell, or temporal, arteritis. This disorder is usually accompanied by systemic symptoms such as fever, malaise, night sweats, weight loss, and headache (see Chapter 2) and often by **polymyalgia rheumatica**. Transient retinal ischemia, mimicking embolic events, may precede optic nerve infarction. The visual loss is sudden and often total. On examination, the optic disk appears swollen and pale. Immediate treatment with corticosteroids (methylprednisolone, 1000 mg/d intravenously, then prednisone, 60–80 mg/d orally) is urgently required to protect what vision remains. The prednisone may be gradually reduced over many months while monitoring the erythrocyte sedimentation rate.

Because giant cell arteritis is treatable, it is most important to distinguish it from idiopathic or nonarteritic anterior ischemic optic neuropathy as the cause of monocular visual loss. Patients with giant cell arteritis tend to be older (aged 70–80 years), and they may have premonitory symptoms. The most helpful differential features are the erythrocyte sedimentation rate, which is greater than 50 mm/h (Westergren) in most patients with giant cell arteritis, and the C-reactive protein.

BINOCULAR DISORDERS

1. Papilledema

Papilledema is the passive bilateral disk swelling that is associated with increased intracranial pressure. Less common causes include congenital cyanotic heart disease and disorders associated with increased cerebrospinal fluid (CSF) protein content, including spinal cord tumor and idiopathic inflammatory polyneuropathy (Guillain-Barré syndrome).

The speed with which papilledema develops is dictated by the underlying cause. When intracranial pressure increases suddenly, as in subarachnoid or intracerebral hemorrhage, disk swelling may be seen within hours, but it most often evolves over days. Papilledema may require 2–3 months to resolve following restoration of normal intracranial pressure. Associated nonspecific symptoms of raised intracranial pressure include headache, nausea, vomiting, and diplopia from abducens nerve palsy. Funduscopic examination (Figure 4–11) reveals (in order of onset) blurring of the nerve fiber layer, absence of venous pulsations (signifying intracranial pressure greater than approximately 200 mm Hg), hemorrhages in the nerve fiber layer, elevation of the disk surface with blurring of the margins, and disk hyperemia.

Papilledema requires urgent evaluation to search for an intracranial mass and to exclude papillitis from syphilis, carcinoma, or sarcoidosis, which may produce a similar ophthalmoscopic appearance. In the history and examination, attention should be directed at symptoms and signs of intracranial masses, such as hemiparesis, hemianopia or seizures, and signs of meningeal irritation.

If an intracranial mass lesion and the disorders listed in Table 2–4 are ruled out by the history, examination, and computed tomography (CT) scanning or MRI; if inflammatory meningeal processes are excluded by CSF examination; and if CSF pressure is elevated, a diagnosis of **pseudotumor cerebri** is established by exclusion. The idiopathic form, which is the most common, occurs most often in obese women during the childbearing years. Although this disorder is usually self-limited, prolonged elevation of intracranial pressure can lead to permanent visual loss (see discussion in Chapter 2).

2. Chiasmal Lesions

The major lesions that produce visual impairment at the level of the optic chiasm are tumors, especially those of pituitary origin. Other causes include trauma, demyelinating disease, and expanding berry aneurysms. The classic pattern of visual deficit caused by lesions of the optic chiasm is **bitemporal hemianopia** (Figure 4–7).

Chiasmal visual loss is gradual in onset, and the resulting impairment in depth perception or in the lateral visual fields may not be noted for some time. Associated involvement of the oculomotor, trochlear, trigeminal, or abducens nerve suggests tumor expansion laterally into the cavernous sinus. Nonophthalmologic manifestations of pituitary tumors include headache, acromegaly, amenorrhea, galactorrhea, and Cushing's syndrome.

Headache, endocrine abnormalities, and occasionally blurred or double vision may occur in patients with an enlarged sella turcica (shown on radiographic examination) but in whom neither tumor nor increased intracranial pressure is found. This **empty sella syndrome** is most common in women and occurs mainly between the fourth and seventh decades of life. Treatment is symptomatic.

3. Retrochiasmal Lesions

Optic Tract & Lateral Geniculate Body

Lesions of the optic tract and lateral geniculate body are usually due to infarction. The resulting visual field abnormality is typically a **noncongruous homonymous hemianopia**, ie, the field defect is not the same in the two eyes. Associated hemisensory loss may occur with thalamic lesions.

Optic Radiations

Lesions of the optic radiations produce field deficits that are congruous and homonymous (bilaterally symmetric). Visual acuity is normal in the unaffected portion of the field. With lesions in the **temporal lobe**, where tumors are the most common cause, the field deficit is denser superiorly than inferiorly, resulting in a **superior quadrantanopia** (pie in the sky deficit; Figure 4–7).

Lesions affecting the optic radiations in the **parietal lobe** may be due to tumor or vascular disease and are usually associated with contralateral weakness and sensory loss. Actually a gaze preference is common, with the eyes conjugately deviated to the side of the parietal lesion. The visual field abnormality is either complete **homonymous hemianopia** or **inferior quadrantanopia** (see Figure 4–7). The optokinetic response to a visual stimulus moved toward the side of the lesion is impaired, which is not the case with pure temporal or occipital lobe lesions.

Occipital Cortex

Lesions in the occipital cortex usually produce **homonymous hemianopias** affecting the contralateral visual field. The patient may be unaware of the visual deficit. Because the region of the occipital cortex in which the macula is represented is often supplied by branches of both the posterior and middle cerebral arteries (see Figure 4–4), visual field abnormalities caused by vascular lesions in the occipital lobe may show **sparing of macular vision** (see Figure 4–7). It has also been suggested that in some cases, macular sparing may result from bilateral cortical representation of the macular region of the visual field.

The most common cause of visual impairment in the occipital lobe is infarction in the posterior cerebral artery territory (90% of cases). Occipital lobe arteriovenous malformations (AVMs), vertebral angiography, and watershed infarction following cardiac arrest are less common causes. Additional symptoms and signs of basilar artery ischemia may occur. Tumors and occipital lobe AVMs are often associated with unformed visual hallucinations that are typically unilateral, stationary, or moving, and often brief or flickering; they can be colored or not colored.

Bilateral occipital lobe involvement produces **cortical blindness**. Pupillary reactions are normal, and bilateral macular sparing may preserve central (tunnel) vision. With more extensive lesions, denial of blindness may occur (**Anton's syndrome**).

DISORDERS OF OCULAR MOTILITY

GAZE PALSY

Lesions in the cortex or brainstem above the level of the oculomotor nuclei may impair conjugate (yoked) movement of the eyes, producing gaze disorders.

Hemispheric Lesions

Acutely, hemispheric lesions produce tonic deviation of both eyes toward the side of the lesion and away from the side of the hemiparesis (Figure 4–19A). This gaze deviation lasts for up to several days in alert patients—somewhat longer in comatose patients. Seizure discharges involving the frontal gaze centers can also produce gaze deviation by driving the eyes away from the discharging focus. When the ipsilateral motor cortex is also involved, producing focal motor seizures, the patient gazes toward the side of the motor activity (Figure 4–19B).

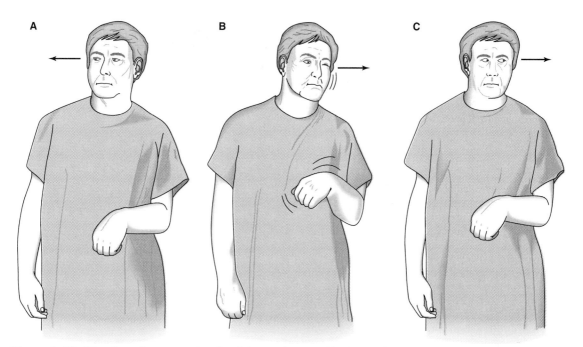

Figure 4–19. Disorders of gaze associated with hemispheric and brainstem lesions. **A:** Destructive lesion in the frontal lobe of the right cerebral hemisphere. **B:** Seizure arising from the frontal lobe of the right cerebral hemisphere. **C:** Destructive lesion in the right pons. Arrows indicate the direction of gaze preference (away from the hemiparetic side in **A** and toward the convulsing or hemiparetic side in **B** and **C**).

Midbrain Lesions

Lesions of the dorsal midbrain affect the center responsible for voluntary upward gaze and may therefore produce upgaze paralysis. In addition, all or some of the features of **Parinaud's syndrome** may occur. These include preserved reflex vertical eye movements with the doll's head maneuver or Bell's phenomenon (elevation of the eye with eyelid closure), nystagmus (especially on downward gaze and typically associated with retraction of the eyes), paralysis of accommodation, midposition pupils, and light-near dissociation.

Pontine Lesions

Brainstem lesions at the level of the pontine gaze centers produce disorders of conjugate horizontal gaze. Gaze palsies from pontine involvement (unlike those from hemispheric lesions) cause eye deviation toward—rather than away from—the side of the hemiparesis (Figure 4–19C). This occurs because, at this level of the brainstem, the corticobulbar pathways that regulate gaze have decussated but the descending motor pathways have not yet crossed. Brainstem gaze pareses are characteristically far more resistant to attempts to move the eyes (via the doll's eye maneuver or caloric stimulation) than are supratentorial gaze pareses and are commonly associated with abducens nerve dysfunction because of the involvement of the abducens nerve nucleus.

INTERNUCLEAR OPHTHALMOPLEGIA

Internuclear ophthalmoplegia results from lesions of the **medial longitudinal fasciculus** between the midpons and the oculomotor nerve nucleus that disconnect the abducens nerve nucleus from the contralateral oculomotor nucleus (see Figure 4–6). The site of the internuclear ophthalmoplegia is named according to the side on which oculomotor nerve function is impaired. There is a characteristic abnormality consisting of disconjugate gaze with impaired adduction and nystagmus of the abducting eye (Figure 4–17). Such a finding strongly supports a diagnosis of intrinsic brainstem disease. The most common cause, especially in young adults or in patients with bilateral involvement, is multiple sclerosis. In older patients and those with unilateral involvement, vascular disease is likely. These two diagnoses encompass 80% or more of all cases in reported series. Rarer causes include brainstem encephalitis, intrinsic brainstem tumors, syringobulbia, sedative drug intoxication, and Wernicke's encephalopathy. Because the oculomotor abnormalities of myasthenia gravis can closely mimic a lesion of the medial longitudinal fasciculus, myasthenia must be ruled out in patients with isolated internuclear ophthalmoplegia.

OCULOMOTOR (III) NERVE LESIONS

Lesions of the oculomotor nerve can occur at any of several levels. The most common causes are listed in Table 4–3; oculomotor disorders resulting from diabetes are discussed separately below.

Brainstem

Within the brainstem, associated neurologic signs permit localization of the lesion; associated contralateral hemiplegia (Weber's syndrome) and contralateral ataxia (Benedikt's syndrome) are the most common vascular syndromes.

Subarachnoid Space

As the oculomotor nerve exits the brainstem in the interpeduncular space, it is susceptible to injury from trauma and from aneurysms of the posterior communicating artery. The latter often cause acute oculomotor

Table 4–3. Causes of oculomotor (III), trochlear (IV), and abducens (VI) nerve lesions.[1]

Cause	Nerve III (%)	Nerve IV (%)	Nerve VI (%)
Unknown	23	29	26
Vasculopathy[2]	20	21	17
Aneurysm	19	1	3
Trauma	14	32	14
Neoplasm[3]	12	7	20
Syphilis	2	—	1
Multiple sclerosis	—	—	6
Other	10[4]	10[5]	13[6]

[1] Data are from several series, as compiled in Burde RM, Savino PJ, Trobe JD: *Clinical Decisions in Neuro-ophthalmology.* Mosby, 1984.

[2] Includes diabetes, hypertension, and atherosclerosis.

[3] Includes pituitary and parapituitary tumors, cavernous sinus meningioma, and primary and metastatic tumors of the brainstem.

[4] Includes sinusitis, Hodgkin's disease, herpes zoster, giant cell arteritis, meningitis, encephalitis, collagen vascular diseases, Paget's disease, and postoperative neurosurgical complications.

[5] Includes herpes zoster, collagen vascular disease, hypoxia, hydrocephalus, postoperative complications, and encephalitis.

[6] Includes raised intracranial pressure from any cause, Wernicke's encephalopathy, cervical manipulation, meningitis, sarcoidosis, post-lumbar-puncture complications, postoperative complications, migraine, and sinusitis.

palsy from aneurysmal expansion with a characteristic impairment of the pupillary light reflex.

Cavernous Sinus

In the cavernous sinus (Figure 4–20), the oculomotor nerve is usually involved along with the trochlear and abducens nerves and the first and sometimes the second division of the trigeminal nerve. Horner's syndrome

may occur. Oculomotor nerve lesions in the cavernous sinus tend to produce partial deficits that may or may not spare the pupil.

Orbit

Unlike cavernous sinus lesions, orbital lesions that affect the oculomotor nerve are often associated with optic nerve involvement and exophthalmos; however, disor-

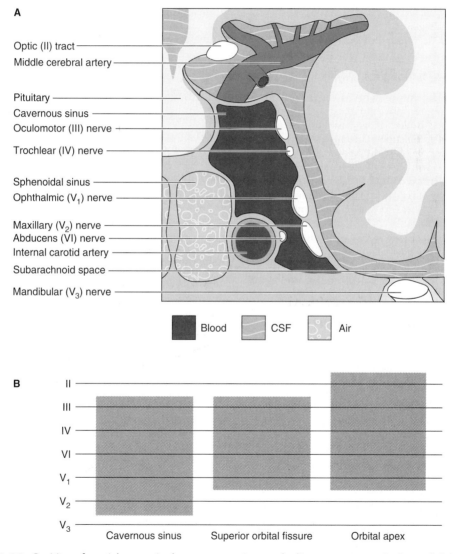

Figure 4–20. Position of cranial nerves in the cavernous sinus and adjacent structures. **A:** Coronal view through the cavernous sinus, with the midline at left and the temporal lobe at right. **B:** Location of cranial nerves as they course anteriorly **(left to right)** in relation to the cavernous sinus, superior orbital fissure, and orbital apex. Note that a lesion in the cavernous sinus spares the optic (II) and mandibular (V$_3$) nerves, a lesion in the superior orbital fissure additionally spares the maxillary (V$_2$) nerve, and a lesion in the orbital apex spares both V$_2$ and V$_3$ but may involve II.

ders of the orbit and cavernous sinus may be clinically indistinguishable except by CT scanning or MRI.

TROCHLEAR (IV) NERVE LESIONS

Head trauma, often minor, is the most common cause of an isolated trochlear nerve palsy (Table 4–3). Although trochlear palsies in middle-aged and elderly patients are also frequently attributed to vascular disease or diabetes, they often occur without obvious cause. For patients with isolated trochlear nerve palsies without a history of trauma, in whom diabetes, myasthenia, thyroid disease, and orbital mass lesions have been excluded, observation is the appropriate clinical approach.

ABDUCENS (VI) NERVE LESIONS

Patients with abducens nerve lesions complain of horizontal diplopia due to weakness of the lateral rectus muscle (Figure 4–16). Lateral rectus palsies can occur as a result of disorders of either the muscle itself or the abducens nerve, and each of these possibilities should be investigated in turn. The causes of abducens nerve lesions are summarized in Table 4–3. In elderly patients, abducens nerve involvement is most often idiopathic or caused by vascular disease or diabetes, but the erythrocyte sedimentation rate should be determined to exclude a rare presentation of giant cell arteritis. Radiographic investigation of the base of the skull is indicated to exclude nasopharyngeal carcinoma or other tumors. In painless abducens palsy—when the above studies are normal, other systemic and neurologic symptoms are absent, and intracranial pressure is not elevated—patients can be followed conservatively. A trial of prednisone (60 mg/d orally for 5 days) may produce dramatic relief in painful abducens nerve palsy, giving support to a tentative diagnosis of idiopathic inflammation of the superior orbital fissure (**superior orbital fissure syndrome**) or cavernous sinus (**Tolosa-Hunt syndrome**). Persistent pain despite treatment with steroids should prompt investigation of the cavernous sinus by CT scanning or MRI, followed, in some cases, by angiography.

DIABETIC OPHTHALMOPLEGIAS

An isolated oculomotor, trochlear, or abducens nerve lesion may occur in patients with diabetes mellitus, and noninvasive imaging procedures (CT scanning or MRI) reveal no abnormality. Such oculomotor nerve lesions are characterized by **pupillary sparing** with or without pain. Pain, when present, may be severe enough to suggest aneurysmal expansion as a likely diagnosis. The lack of pupillary involvement is commonly attributed to infarction of the central portion of the nerve with sparing of the more peripherally situated fibers that mediate pupillary constriction. Pupil-sparing oculomotor palsies can also be seen occasionally, however, with compressive, infiltrative, or inflammatory lesions of the oculomotor nerve or with infarcts, hemorrhages, or tumors that affect the oculomotor nucleus or fascicle within the midbrain.

In known diabetics, painful ophthalmoplegia with exophthalmos and metabolic acidosis requires urgent attention to determine the possibility of fungal infection in the paranasal sinus, orbit, or cavernous sinus by **mucormycosis** (see Chapter 1). The diagnosis is usually made by biopsy of the nasal mucosa. Failure to make a prompt diagnosis and to institute treatment at once with amphotericin B and surgical debridement of necrotic tissue may lead to a fatal outcome.

PAINFUL OPHTHALMOPLEGIAS

Dysfunction of one or more of the ocular motor nerves with accompanying pain may be produced by lesions located anywhere from the posterior fossa to the orbit (Table 4–4). The evaluation should consist of careful documentation of the clinical course, inspection and palpation of the globe for proptosis (localizing the process to the orbit or anterior cavernous sinus), auscultation over the globe to detect a bruit (which would strongly support a diagnosis of carotid artery-cavernous sinus fistula or another vascular anomaly), and evaluation for diabetes. Useful laboratory studies include an orbital CT scan or MRI, carotid arteriography, and orbital venography.

Therapy for these disorders is dictated by the specific diagnosis. Idiopathic inflammation of the orbit (orbital

Table 4–4. Causes of painful ophthalmoplegia.

Orbit
Orbital pseudotumor
Sinusitis
Tumor (primary or metastatic)
Infections (bacterial or fungal)
Cavernous sinus
Tolosa-Hunt syndrome (idiopathic granulomatous inflammation)
Tumor (primary or metastatic)
Carotid artery–cavernous sinus fistula or thrombosis
Aneurysm
Sella and posterior fossa
Pituitary tumor or apoplexy
Aneurysm
Metastatic tumor
Other
Diabetes
Migraine
Giant cell arteritis

pseudotumor) or cavernous sinus (Tolosa-Hunt syndrome) responds dramatically to corticosteroids (prednisone, 60–100 mg/d orally). However, the pain and ocular signs of some neoplasms may also improve transiently during corticosteroid therapy so that a specific etiologic diagnosis may depend on biopsy.

MYASTHENIA GRAVIS

Myasthenia eventually involves the ocular muscles in approximately 90% of patients; more than 60% present with ocular involvement. The syndrome is painless; pupillary responses are always normal, and there are no sensory abnormalities. The diagnosis is confirmed by a positive response to intravenous edrophonium (Tensilon). Details of this disorder are discussed in Chapter 5.

OCULAR MYOPATHIES

Ocular myopathies are painless syndromes that spare pupillary function and are usually bilateral. The most common is the myopathy of **hyperthyroidism**, a common cause of double vision beginning in midlife or later. Note that many patients are otherwise clinically euthyroid at the time of diagnosis. Double vision on attempted elevation of the globe is the most common symptom, but in mild cases there is lid retraction during staring or lid lag during rapid up-and-down movements of the eye. Exophthalmos is a characteristic finding, especially in advanced cases. The diagnosis can be confirmed by the forced duction test, which detects mechanical resistance to forced movement of the anesthetized globe in the orbit. This restrictive ocular myopathy is usually self-limited. The patient should be referred for testing of thyroid function and treated for hyperthyroidism as appropriate.

The **progressive external ophthalmoplegias** are a group of syndromes characterized by slowly progressive, symmetric impairment of ocular movement that cannot be overcome by caloric stimulation. Pupillary function is spared, and there is no pain; ptosis may be prominent. This clinical picture can be produced by **ocular** or **oculopharyngeal muscular dystrophy**. Progressive external ophthalmoplegia associated with myotonic contraction on percussion of muscle groups (classically, the thenar group in the palm) suggests the diagnosis of **myotonic dystrophy**. In **Kearns-Sayre-Daroff syndrome**, which has been associated with deletions in muscle mitochondrial DNA, progressive external ophthalmoplegia is accompanied by pigmentary degeneration of the retina, cardiac conduction defects, cerebellar ataxia, and elevated CSF protein. The muscle biopsy shows ragged red fibers that reflect the presence of abnormal mitochondria. Disorders that simulate progressive external ophthalmoplegia include progressive supranuclear palsy and Parkinson's disease, but in these conditions the impairment of (usually vertical) eye movements can be overcome by oculocephalic or caloric stimulation.

REFERENCES

Beck RW et al: A randomized, controlled trial of corticosteroids in the treatment of acute optic neuritis. N Engl J Med 1992; 326:581–588.

Beck RW et al: The effect of corticosteroids for acute optic neuritis on the subsequent development of multiple sclerosis. The Optic Neuritis Study Group. N Engl J Med 1993;329: 1764–1769.

Brazis PW: Localization of lesions of the oculomotor nerve: recent concepts. Mayo Clin Proc 1991;66:1029–1035.

Druschky A et al: Progression of optic neuritis to multiple sclerosis: an 8-year follow-up study. Clin Neurol Neurosurg 1999; 101:189–192.

Fisher CM: Some neuroophthalmological observations. J Neurol Neurosurg Psychiatry 1967;30:383–392.

Glaser JS: *Neuro-ophthalmology,* 2nd ed. Lippincott, 1990.

Hunt, WE, Brightman RP: The Tolosa-Hunt syndrome: a problem in differential diagnosis. Acta Neurochir 1988;Suppl 42:248–252.

Kapoor R et al: Effects of intravenous methylprednisolone on outcome in MRI-based prognostic subgroups in acute optic neuritis. Neurology 1998;50:230–237.

Keane JR: Acute bilateral ophthalmoplegia: 60 Cases. Neurology 1986;36:279–281.

Keane JR: The pretectal syndrome: 206 patients. Neurology 1990; 40:684–690.

Keane JR: Fourth nerve palsy: historical review and study of 215 inpatients. Neurology 1993;43:2439–2443.

Keane JR: Cavernous sinus syndrome. Analysis of 151 cases. Arch Neurol 1996;53:967–971.

Nadeau SE, Trobe JD: Pupil sparing in oculomotor palsy: a brief review. Ann Neurol 1983;13:143–148.

Newman NJ: Optic neuropathy. Neurology 1996;46:315–322.

Salvarani C et al: Polymyalgia rheumatica. Lancet 1997;350: 43–47.

Wall M, Wray SH: The one-and-a-half syndrome—a unilateral disorder of the pontine tegmentum: A study of 20 cases and review of the literature. Neurology 1983;33:971–980.

Motor Deficits

5

CONTENTS

KEY CONCEPTS

 The cause of weakness is best determined after the disorder has been localized to a particular level of the neuromuscular system by any associated symptoms and signs.

 It is important to record all medication that have been taken, as motor disorders at all levels of the neuromuscular system may be drug-related.

 Hereditary causes of weakness must be excluded, if necessary, by examination of other family members. A number of hereditary disorders have variable clinical expression and can be identified by genetic testing.

The distribution of weakness is helpful in distinguishing between a radiculopathy, plexopathy, and peripheral neuropathy, and between neurogenic and myopathic disorders.

 Weakness that is patchy, varies in severity with activity, and does not conform in distribution to the territory of a nerve or nerve root suggests a disorder of neuromuscular transmission.

APPROACH TO DIAGNOSIS

Motor function can be impaired by a lesion that involves the nervous system either centrally or peripherally. Several parts of the central nervous system are involved in the regulation of motor activity; these include the pyramidal and extrapyramidal systems, the cerebellum, and the lower motor neurons of the brainstem and spinal cord.

The **pyramidal system** consists of fibers that descend from the cerebral cortex through the internal capsule, traverse the medullary pyramid, and then mostly decussate, to descend in the lateral corticospinal tract on the side opposite that of their origin, where they synapse on lower motor neurons in the spinal cord. All other descending influences on lower motor neurons belong to the **extrapyramidal system** and originate primarily in the basal ganglia and cerebellum. Disorders of the basal ganglia (see Chapter 7) and cerebellum (see Chapter 3) are considered separately.

The motor fibers that make up the cranial and peripheral nerves have their origin in the **lower motor neurons** (Figure 5–1). A disturbance of function at any point in the peripheral nervous system (anterior horn cell, nerve root, limb plexus, peripheral nerve, or neuromuscular junction) can disturb motor function, as can disease that primarily affects the muscles themselves.

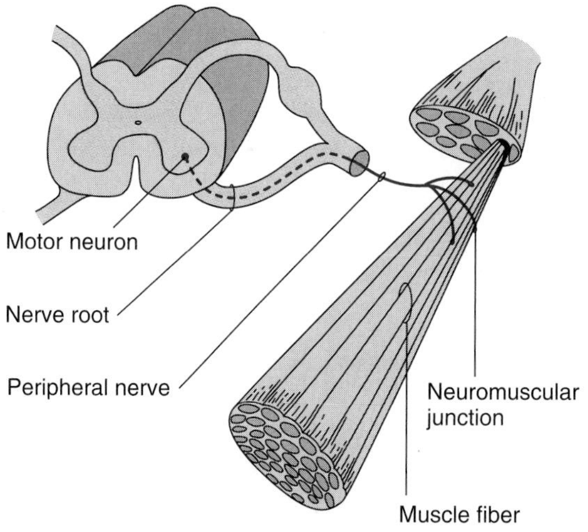

HISTORY & EXAMINATION

Patients with motor deficits generally complain of weakness, heaviness, stiffness, clumsiness, impaired muscular control, or difficulty in executing movements. The term *weakness* is sometimes used in a nonspecific way to denote fatigue or loss of energy, drive, or enthusiasm, and care must be taken to clarify what the patient means. The word is properly used to mean loss of muscle power, and it is in this sense that it is employed here.

History of Present Illness

Several aspects of the present complaint must be documented.

A. MODE OF ONSET

An abrupt onset suggests a vascular disturbance, such as a stroke, or certain toxic or metabolic disturbances, whereas subacute onset of days to weeks is commonly associated with a neoplastic, infective, or inflammatory process (Table 5–1). Weakness that evolves slowly over several months or years often has a hereditary, degenerative, endocrinologic, or neoplastic basis.

B. COURSE

A progressive increase in the motor deficit from its onset suggests continuing activity of the underlying process. Episodic progression suggests a vascular or inflammatory origin; a steadily progressive course is more suggestive of neoplastic disorder or such degenerative conditions as motor neuron disease. Rapid fluctuation of symptoms over short periods (eg, activity leads to fatigue and an exacerbation of weakness; rest is followed by recovery of strength) is characteristic of myasthenia gravis.

C. ASSOCIATED SYMPTOMS

The distribution of weakness and the presence of associated symptoms may indicate the approximate site of the lesion. For example, weakness in the right arm and leg may result from a

Figure 5–1. Anatomic components of the motor unit.

Motor neuron

Nerve root

Peripheral nerve

Neuromuscular junction

Muscle fiber

Table 5–1. Causes of weakness of acute or subacute onset.

Supraspinal lesions
  Stroke
  Other structural lesions
Spinal cord lesions
  Infective: poliomyelitis, coxsackievirus infection
  Inflammatory: transverse myelitis, multiple sclerosis
  Compressive: tumor, disk protrusion, abscess
  Vascular: infarction, hematomyelia
Peripheral neuropathy
  Guillain-Barré syndrome
  Diphtheria
  Shellfish poisoning
  Porphyria
  Arsenic poisoning
  Organophosphate toxicity
Disorders of neuromuscular transmission
  Myasthenia gravis
  Botulism
  Aminoglycoside toxicity
Muscle disorders
  Necrotizing myopathies
  Acute hypo- or hyperkalemia
  Periodic paralyses

lesion of the contralateral motor cortex or the corticospinal pathway at any point above the fifth cervical segment of the spinal cord. Associated right facial weakness indicates that the lesion must be above the level of the facial (VII) nerve nucleus in the brainstem, and an accompanying aphasia (see Chapter 1) or visual field defect (see Chapter 4) localizes it to the cerebral hemisphere.

The character of the associated symptoms may suggest the nature of the lesion at any given site in the nervous system. Thus, progressive leg weakness caused by myelopathy is often preceded or accompanied by pain in the back or legs when the myelopathy is due to a compressive lesion—but not when it has a metabolic or hereditary basis.

D. Severity of Symptoms

An attempt must be made to evaluate the functional severity of any motor deficit by determining whether there has been any restriction of daily activities, difficulty in performing previously easy tasks, or reduction in exercise tolerance. The nature of the functional disturbance depends on the muscles involved.

Weakness of proximal muscles in the legs leads to difficulty in climbing or descending stairs or in getting up from a squatting position, whereas weakness in the arms leads to difficulty with such tasks as combing the hair. Distal weakness in the arms may lead to clumsi-

ness, difficulty with such fine motor tasks as doing up buttons or tying shoelaces, and eventually the inability to pick up or grasp objects with the hands, so that even eating becomes difficult or impossible.

Involvement of the muscles supplied by the cranial nerves may lead to diplopia (oculomotor [III], trochlear [IV], and abducens [VI] cranial nerves; see Chapter 4); difficulty in chewing (trigeminal [V] nerve) or sucking, blowing, or using the facial muscles (facial [VII] nerve); and difficulty in swallowing, with nasal regurgitation and dysarthria (glossopharyngeal [IX], vagus [X], and hypoglossal [XII] nerves).

Weakness of the respiratory muscles leads to tachypnea, the use of accessory muscles of respiration, and anxiety at a stage when arterial blood gases are usually still normal. A vital capacity of less than 1 L in an adult generally calls for ventilatory support, especially if weakness is increasing.

Medical History

The importance of the history depends upon the patient's present complaint and the nature of any previous illnesses. For example, in a patient with known carcinoma of the lung, limb weakness may be due to metastasis or to a remote (nonmetastatic) complication of cancer. Leg weakness in a diabetic may reflect peripheral nerve, plexus, or multiple root involvement, and hand weakness in a myxedematous patient may be associated with carpal tunnel syndrome.

The history should include careful note of all drugs taken by the patient. Drugs can cause peripheral neuropathy, impair neuromuscular transmission, or lead to myopathy (Table 5–2).

Developmental History

When symptoms develop during infancy, childhood, or early adult life, it is particularly important to obtain a full developmental history, including details of the delivery, birth weight, the patient's condition in the neonatal period, and the dates at which motor milestones were attained. Congenital or perinatal cerebral disease accounts for most causes of infantile diplegia (weakness of all four limbs, with the legs more severely affected than the arms).

Family History

Hereditary factors may be important, and the patient's family background must therefore be explored. Some types of myopathy, motor neuron disease, and peripheral neuropathy have a genetic basis, as do some spinocerebellar degenerations, hereditary spastic paraparesis, and certain other neurologic disorders. In certain instances, it may be necessary to

Table 5–2. Motor disorders associated with drugs.

Drugs that cause motor (or predominantly motor) peripheral neuropathy[1]
Dapsone
Imipramine
Certain sulfonamides

Drugs that can impair neuromuscular transmission

ACTH	Penicillamine
Aminoglycoside antibiotics	Phenothiazines
β-Blockers	Phenytoin
Chloroquine	Polymyxin
Colistin	Procainamide
Corticosteroids	Quinidine, quinine
Lithium	Tetracycline
Magnesium-containing cathartics	

Drugs associated with myopathy

β-Blockers

Chloroquine	ε-Aminocaproic acid
Clofibrate	HMG-CoA reductase inhibitors
Corticosteroids	
Drugs causing hypokalemia	Zidovudine
Emetine	Penicillamine

[1]A number of drugs cause mixed sensory and motor neuropathies, as shown in Table 6–2.

examine other family members to determine whether the patient's disorder has a hereditary basis.

Examination of the Motor System

In examining the motor system, a systematic approach will help to avoid overlooking important abnormalities. A sequential routine for the examination should be developed.

A. MUSCLE APPEARANCE

Wasting, or muscle **atrophy,** suggests that weakness is due to a lesion of the lower motor neurons or of the muscle itself.

The distribution of wasting may help to localize the underlying disorder. Upper motor neuron disorders are not usually accompanied by muscle wasting, though muscle atrophy may occasionally occur with prolonged disuse. **Pseudohypertrophy** of muscles occurs in certain forms of myopathy, but the apparently enlarged muscles are weak and flabby.

The presence of **fasciculations**—visible irregular flickerings over the surface of the affected muscle caused by spontaneous contractions of individual motor units—suggests that weakness is due to a lower motor neuron lesion. Fasciculations are most apt to be seen in anterior horn cell disorders, but also occur in normal individuals. Although such activity does not occur with upper motor neuron disorders, **flexor or extensor spasms** of the limbs are sometimes seen in these latter conditions as a result of impaired supraspinal control of reflex activity.

B. MUSCLE TONE

For clinical purposes, tone can be defined as the resistance of muscle to passive movement of a joint. Tone depends on the degree of muscle contraction and on the mechanical properties of muscle and connective tissue. The degree of muscle contraction depends, in turn, on the activity of anterior horn cells, which is governed by spinal and supraspinal mechanisms. Tone is assessed by observing the position of the extremities at rest, by palpating the muscle belly, and particularly by determining the resistance to passive stretch and movement. Postural abnormalities may result from the increased activity of certain muscle groups caused by disturbances of reflex function, as exemplified by the typical hemiplegic posture—flexion of the upper limb and extension of the ipsilateral lower limb—of many patients who have had a stroke. To assess resistance to passive movement, the patient is asked to relax while each limb is examined in turn by passively taking the major joints through their full range of movement at different speeds and estimating whether the force required is more or less than normal.

1. Hypertonia—Two types of increased tone can be distinguished.

a. Spasticity—consists of an increase in tone that affects different muscle groups to different extents. In the arms, tone is increased to a greater extent in the flexor muscles than in the extensors; in the legs, tone is increased to a greater extent in the extensor muscles than in the flexors. Moreover, the resistance of affected muscle is not the same throughout the range of movement but tends to be most marked when passive movement is initiated and then diminishes as the movement continues (the **clasp-knife phenomenon**). The increase in tone is velocity dependent, so that passive movement at a high velocity—but not at lower velocities—may be met with increased resistance. Spasticity is caused by an upper motor neuron lesion, such as a stroke that involves the supplementary motor cortex or corticospinal tract. Spasticity may not become apparent for several days following the onset of an acute lesion, however.

b. Rigidity—consists of increased resistance to passive movement that is independent of the direction of the movement—ie, it affects agonist and antagonist muscle groups equally. The term **lead-pipe rigidity** is sometimes used for descriptive purposes, whereas **cogwheel rigidity** is used when there are superimposed ratchetlike interruptions in the passive movement, which probably relate to underlying tremor. In general, rigidity indicates extrapyramidal dysfunction and is due to a lesion of the basal ganglia (eg, Parkinson's disease).

2. Hypotonia (flaccidity)—This is characterized by excessive floppiness—a reduced resistance to passive movement—so that the distal portion of the limb is easily waved to and fro when the extremity is passively shaken. In hypotonic limbs it is often possible to hyperextend the joints, and the muscle belly may look flattened and feel less firm than usual. Although hypotonia usually relates to pathologic involvement of the lower motor neuron supply to the affected muscles, it can also occur with primary muscle disorders, disruption of the sensory (afferent) limb of the reflex arc, cerebellar disease, and certain extrapyramidal disorders such as Huntington's disease, as well as in the acute stage of a pyramidal lesion.

3. Paratonia—Some patients give the impression of being unable to relax and will move the limb being examined as the physician moves it, despite instructions to the contrary. In more advanced cases, there seems to be rigidity when the examiner moves the limb rapidly but normal tone when the limb is moved slowly. This phenomenon—paratonia—is particularly apt to occur in patients with frontal lobe or diffuse cerebral disease.

C. MUSCLE POWER

When muscle power is to be tested, the patient is asked to resist pressure exerted by the examiner. Selected individual muscles are tested in turn, and strength on the two sides is compared so that minor degrees of weakness can be recognized. Weakness can result from a disturbance in function of the upper or the lower motor neurons; the distribution of weakness is of paramount importance in distinguishing between these two possibilities. Upper motor neuron lesions (eg, stroke) lead to weakness that characteristically involves the extensors and abductors more than the flexors and adductors of the arms—and the flexors more than the extensors of the legs. Lower motor neuron lesions produce weakness of the muscles supplied by the affected neurons; the particular distribution of the weakness may point to lower motor neuron involvement at the spinal cord, nerve root, plexus, or peripheral nerve level.

On the basis of the history and other findings, muscles that are particularly likely to be affected are selected for initial evaluation, and other muscles are subsequently examined to determine the distribution of the weakness more fully and to shorten the list of diagnostic possibilities. For instance, if an upper motor neuron (pyramidal) lesion is suspected, the extensors and abductors of the upper extremity and the flexors of the lower extremity are tested in the most detail, since these muscles will be the most affected.

Weakness may also result from a primary muscle disorder (myopathy) or from a disorder of neuromuscular transmission. In patients with a motor deficit in all limbs that is not due to an upper motor neuron lesion, proximal distribution of weakness suggests a myopathic disorder, whereas predominantly distal involvement suggests a lower motor neuron disturbance. Marked variability in the severity and distribution of weakness over short periods of time suggests myasthenia gravis, a disorder of neuromuscular transmission. Apparent weakness that is not organic in nature also shows a characteristic variability; it is often more severe on formal testing than is consistent with the patient's daily activities. Moreover, palpation of antagonist muscles commonly reveals that they contract each time the patient is asked to activate the agonist.

For practical and comparative purposes, power is best graded in the manner shown in Table 5–3. **Monoplegia** denotes paralysis or severe weakness of the muscles in one limb, and **monoparesis** denotes less severe weakness in one limb, although the two words are often used interchangeably. **Hemiplegia** or **hemiparesis** is weakness in both limbs (and sometimes the face) on one side of the body; **paraplegia** or **paraparesis** is weakness of both legs; and **quadriplegia** or **quadriparesis** (also **tetraplegia, tetraparesis**) is weakness of all four limbs.

D. COORDINATION

The coordination of motor activity can be impaired by weakness, sensory disturbances, or cerebellar disease and requires careful evaluation.

Voluntary activity is observed with regard to its accuracy, velocity, range, and regularity, and the manner in which individual actions are integrated to produce a smooth complex movement. In the finger-nose test, the patient moves the index finger to touch the tip of his or

Table 5–3. Grading of muscle power according to the system suggested by the Medical Research Council.[1]

Grade	Muscle Power
5	Normal power
4	Active movement against resistance and gravity
3	Active movement against gravity but not resistance
2	Active movement possible only with gravity eliminated
1	Flicker or trace of contraction
0	No contraction

[1] Reproduced, with permission, from *Aids to the Investigation of Peripheral Nerve Injuries*. HMSO, 1943.

her nose and then the tip of the examiner's index finger; the examiner can move his or her own finger about during the test to change the location of the target and should position it so that the patient's arm must extend fully to reach it. In the heel-knee-shin test, the recumbent patient lifts one leg off the bed, flexes it at the knee, places the heel on the other knee, and runs the heel down the shin as smoothly as possible.

The patient should also be asked to tap repetitively with one hand on the back of the other; to tap alternately with the palm and back of one hand on the back of the other hand or on the knee; to screw an imaginary light bulb into the ceiling with each arm in turn; and to rub the fingers of one hand in a circular polishing movement on the back of the other hand. Other tests of rapid alternating movement include tapping on the ball of the thumb with the tip of the index finger or tapping the floor as rapidly as possible with the sole while keeping the heel of the foot in place. During all these tests, the examiner looks for irregularities of rate, amplitude, and rhythm and for precision of movements. With pyramidal lesions, fine voluntary movements are performed slowly. With cerebellar lesions, the rate, rhythm, and amplitude of such movements are irregular.

If loss of sensation may be responsible for impaired coordination, the maneuver should be repeated both with eyes closed and with visual attention directed to the limb; with visual feedback the apparent weakness or incoordination will improve. In patients with cerebellar disease, the main complaint and physical finding are often of incoordination, and examination may reveal little else. Further discussion of the ataxia of cerebellar disease and the various terms used to describe aspects of it will be found in Chapter 3.

E. TENDON REFLEXES

Changes in the tendon reflexes may accompany disturbances in motor (or sensory) function and provide a guide to the cause of the motor deficit. The tendon is tapped with a reflex hammer to produce a sudden brisk stretch of the muscle and its contained spindles. The clinically important stretch reflexes and the nerves, roots, and spinal segments subserving them are indicated in Table 5–4. When the reflexes are tested, the limbs on each side should be placed in identical positions and the reflexes elicited in the same manner.

1. Areflexia—Apparent loss of the tendon reflexes in a patient may merely reflect a lack of clinical expertise on the part of the examiner. Performance of Jendrassik's maneuver (an attempt by the patient to pull apart the fingers of the two hands when they are hooked together) or some similar action (such as making a fist with the hand that is not being tested) may elicit the reflex response when it is otherwise unobtainable. A reflex may be lost or depressed by any lesion that interrupts

Table 5–4. Muscle stretch reflexes.[1]

Reflex	Segmental Innervation	Nerve
Jaw	Pons	Mandibular branch, trigeminal
Biceps	C5, C6	Musculocutaneous
Brachioradialis	C5, C6	Radial
Triceps	C7, C8	Radial
Finger	C8, T1	Median
Knee	L3, L4	Femoral
Ankle	S1, S2	Tibial

[1] At the National Institutes of Health, the reflexes are graded on the following scale: 0, absent; 1, reduced, trace response, or present only with reinforcement; 2 and 3, in lower and upper half of normal range, respectively; 4, enhanced, with or without clonus.

the structural or functional continuity of its reflex arc, as in a root lesion or peripheral neuropathy. In addition, reflexes are often depressed during the acute stage of an upper motor neuron lesion, in patients who are deeply comatose, and in patients with cerebellar disease.

2. Hyperreflexia—Increased reflexes occur with upper motor neuron lesions, but they may also occur with symmetric distribution in certain healthy subjects and in patients under emotional tension. The presence of reflex asymmetry is therefore of particular clinical significance. **Clonus** consists of a series of rhythmic reflex contractions of a muscle that is suddenly subjected to sustained stretch, with each beat caused by renewed stretch of the muscle during relaxation from its previous contracted state. Sustained clonus—more than three or four beats in response to sudden sustained stretch—is always pathologic and is associated with an abnormally brisk reflex. In hyperreflexic states, there may be spread of the region from which a particular reflex response can be elicited. For example, elicitation of the biceps reflex may be accompanied by reflex finger flexion, or eliciting the finger flexion reflex may cause flexion of the thumb (Hoffmann's sign).

3. Reflex asymmetry—Although the intensity of reflex responses varies considerably among subjects, reflexes should be symmetric in any individual. Several general points can be made regarding reflex asymmetries.

a. Lateralized asymmetries of response—ie, reflexes that are brisker on one side of the body than on the other—usually indicate an upper motor neuron disturbance, but sometimes reflect a lower motor neuron lesion on the side with the depressed reflexes.

b. Focal reflex deficits often relate to root, plexus, or peripheral nerve lesions. For example, unilateral depression of the ankle jerk commonly reflects an S1 radiculopathy resulting from a lumbosacral disk lesion.

c. Loss of distal tendon reflexes (especially ankle jerks), with preservation of more proximal ones, is common in polyneuropathies.

F. SUPERFICIAL REFLEXES

1. The polysynaptic superficial abdominal reflexes, which depend on the integrity of the T8–12 spinal cord segments, are elicited by gently stroking each quadrant of the abdominal wall with a blunt object such as a wooden stick. A normal response consists of contraction of the muscle in the quadrant stimulated, with a brief movement of the umbilicus toward the stimulus. Asymmetric loss of the response may be of diagnostic significance.

a. The response may be depressed or lost on one side in patients with an upper motor neuron disturbance from a lesion of the contralateral motor cortex or its descending pathways.

b. Segmental loss of the response may relate to local disease of the abdominal wall or its innervation, as in a radiculopathy.

c. The cutaneous abdominal reflexes are frequently absent bilaterally in the elderly, in the obese, in multiparous women, and in patients who have had abdominal surgery.

2. The **cremasteric reflex,** mediated through the L1 and L2 reflex arcs, consists of retraction of the ipsilateral testis when the inner aspect of the thigh is lightly stroked; it is lost in patients with a lesion involving these nerve roots. It is also lost in patients with contralateral upper motor neuron disturbances.

3. Stimulation of the lateral border of the foot in a normal adult leads to plantar flexion of the toes and dorsiflexion of the ankle. The **Babinski response** consists of dorsiflexion of the big toe and fanning of the other toes in response to stroking the lateral border of the foot, which is part of the S1 dermatome; flexion at the hip and knee may also occur. Such an extensor plantar response indicates an upper motor neuron lesion involving the contralateral motor cortex or the corticospinal tract. It can also be found in anesthetized or comatose subjects, in patients who have had a seizure, and in normal infants. An extensor plantar response can also be elicited, though less reliably, by such maneuvers as pricking the dorsal surface of the big toe with a pin (Bing's sign), firmly stroking down the anterior border of the tibia from knee to ankle (Oppenheim's maneuver), squeezing the calf muscle (Gordon's maneuver) or Achilles tendon (Schafer's maneuver), flicking the little toe (Gonda's maneuver), or stroking the back of the foot just below the lateral malleolus (Chaddock's maneuver). In interpreting responses, attention must be focused only on the direction in which the big toe first moves.

G. GAIT

In evaluating gait, the examiner first observes the patient walking at a comfortable pace. Attention is directed at the stance and posture; the facility with which the patient starts and stops walking and turns to either side; the length of the stride; the rhythm of walking; the presence of normally associated movements, such as swinging of the arms; and any involuntary movements. Subtle gait disorders become apparent only when the patient is asked to run, walk on the balls of the feet or the heels, hop on either foot, or walk heel-to-toe along a straight line. Gait disorders occur in many neurologic disturbances and in other contexts that are beyond the scope of this chapter. A motor or sensory disturbance may lead to an abnormal gait whose nature depends upon the site of pathologic involvement. Accordingly, the causes and clinical types of gait disturbance are best considered together.

1. Apraxic gait—Apraxic gait occurs in some patients with disturbances, usually bilateral, of frontal lobe function, such as may occur in hydrocephalus or progressive dementing disorders. There is no weakness or incoordination of the limbs, but the patient is unable to stand unsupported or to walk properly—the feet seem glued to the ground. If walking is possible at all, the gait is unsteady, uncertain, and short-stepped, with marked hesitation ("freezing"), and the legs are moved in a direction inappropriate to the center of gravity.

2. Corticospinal lesions—A corticospinal lesion, irrespective of its cause, can lead to a gait disturbance that varies in character depending on whether there is unilateral or bilateral involvement. In patients with hemiparesis, the selective weakness and spasticity lead to a gait in which the affected leg must be **circumducted** to be advanced. The patient tilts at the waist toward the normal side and swings the affected leg outward as well as forward, thus compensating for any tendency to drag or catch the foot on the ground because of weakness in the hip and knee flexors or the ankle dorsiflexors. The arm on the affected side is usually held flexed and adducted. In mild cases, there may be no more than a tendency to drag the affected leg, so that the sole of that shoe tends to be excessively worn.

With severe bilateral spasticity, the legs are brought stiffly forward and adducted, often with compensatory movements of the trunk. Such a gait is commonly described as **scissorslike.** This gait is seen in its most extreme form in children with spastic diplegia from perinatally acquired static encephalopathy. In patients with mild spastic paraparesis, the gait is shuffling, slow, stiff, and awkward, with the feet tending to drag.

3. Frontal disorders—Some patients with frontal lobe or white matter lesions have a gait characterized by short, shuffling steps; hesitation in starting or turning; unsteadiness; and a wide or narrow base. Sometimes referred to as **marche à petit pas,** this abnormality may be mistaken for a parkinsonian gait, but the wide base, preserved arm swing, absence of other signs of parkinsonism, and accompanying findings of cognitive impairment, frontal release signs, pseudobulbar palsy, pyramidal deficits, and sphincter disturbances are helpful in indicating the correct diagnosis. In patients with frontotemporal dementia, however, a parkinsonian gait and other extrapyramidal findings may be present.

4. Extrapyramidal disorders—Extrapyramidal disorders can produce characteristic gait disturbances.

a. In advanced parkinsonism, the patient is often stooped and has difficulty in beginning to walk. Indeed, the patient may need to lean farther and farther forward while walking in place in order to advance; once in motion, there may be unsteadiness in turning and difficulty in stopping. The gait itself is characterized by small strides, often taken at an increasing rate until the patient is almost running (**festination**), and by loss of the arm swinging that normally accompanies locomotion. In mild parkinsonism, a mildly slowed or unsteady gait, flexed posture, or reduced arm swinging may be the only abnormality found.

b. Abnormal posturing of the limbs or trunk is a feature of dystonia; it can interfere with locomotion or lead to a distorted and bizarre gait.

c. Chorea can cause an irregular, unpredictable, and unsteady gait, as the patient dips or lurches from side to side. Choreiform movements of the face and extremities are usually well in evidence.

d. Tremor that occurs primarily on standing (orthostatic tremor) may lead to an unsteady, uncertain gait, with hesitancy in commencing to walk.

5. Cerebellar disorders—In cerebellar disorders (see Chapter 3), the gait may be disturbed in several ways.

a. Truncal ataxia results from involvement of midline cerebellar structures, especially the vermis. The gait is irregular, clumsy, unsteady, uncertain, and broadbased, with the patient walking with the feet wide apart for additional support. Turning and heel-to-toe walking are especially difficult. There are often few accompanying signs of a cerebellar disturbance in the limbs. Causes include midline cerebellar tumors and the cerebellar degeneration that can occur with alcoholism or hypothyroidism, as a nonmetastatic complication of cancer, and with certain hereditary disorders.

b. In extreme cases, with gross involvement of midline cerebellar structures (especially the vermis), the patient cannot stand without falling.

c. A lesion of one cerebellar hemisphere leads to an unsteady gait in which the patient consistently falls or lurches toward the affected side.

6. Impaired sensation—Impaired sensation, especially disturbed proprioception, also leads to an unsteady gait, which is aggravated by walking in the dark or with the eyes closed, since visual input cannot then compensate for the sensory loss. Because of their defective position sense, many patients lift their feet higher than necessary when walking, producing a **steppage gait.** Causes include tabes dorsalis, sensory neuropathies, vitamin B_{12} deficiency, and certain hereditary disorders (discussed in Chapter 6).

7. Anterior horn cell, peripheral motor nerve, or striated muscle disorders—These disorders lead to gait disturbances if the muscles involved in locomotion are affected. Weakness of the anterior tibial muscles leads to **foot drop;** to avoid catching or scuffing the foot on the ground, the patient must lift the affected leg higher than the other, in a characteristic steppage gait. Weakness of the calf muscles leads to an inability to walk on the balls of the feet. Weakness of the trunk and girdle muscles, such as occurs in muscular dystrophy, other myopathic disorders, and Kugelberg-Welander syndrome, leads to a **waddling gait** because the pelvis tends to slump toward the non-weight-bearing side.

8. Unsteady gait in the elderly—Many elderly persons complain of unsteadiness when walking and a fear of falling, but neurologic examination reveals no abnormality. Their symptoms have been attributed to reduced sensory input from several different afferent systems and impaired central processing of sensory input; an impairment of vestibular function may also be important.

CLINICAL LOCALIZATION OF THE LESION

The findings on examination should indicate whether the weakness or other motor deficit is due to an upper or lower motor neuron disturbance, a disorder of neuromuscular transmission, or a primary muscle disorder. In the case of an upper or lower motor neuron disturbance, the clinical findings may also help to localize the lesion more precisely to a single level of the nervous system. Such localization helps to reduce the number of diagnostic possibilities.

Upper Motor Neuron Lesions

A. SIGNS

- Weakness or paralysis.
- Spasticity.
- Increased tendon reflexes.
- An extensor plantar (Babinski) response.
- Loss of superficial abdominal reflexes.
- Little, if any, muscle atrophy.

Such signs occur with involvement of the upper motor neuron at any point, but further clinical findings depend upon the actual site of the lesion. Note that it may not be possible to localize a lesion by its motor signs alone.

B. LOCALIZATION OF UNDERLYING LESION

1. A parasagittal intracranial lesion produces an upper motor neuron deficit that characteristically affects both legs and may later involve the arms.

2. A discrete lesion of the cerebral cortex or its projections may produce a focal motor deficit involving, for example, the contralateral hand. Weakness may be restricted to the contralateral leg in patients with anterior cerebral artery occlusion or to the contralateral face and arm if the middle cerebral artery is involved. A more extensive cortical or subcortical lesion will produce weakness or paralysis of the contralateral face, arm, and leg and may be accompanied by aphasia, a visual field defect, or a sensory disturbance of cortical type.

3. A lesion at the level of the internal capsule, where the descending fibers from the cerebral cortex are closely packed, commonly results in a severe hemiparesis that involves the contralateral limbs and face.

4. A brainstem lesion commonly—but not invariably—leads to bilateral motor deficits, often with accompanying sensory and cranial nerve disturbances, and disequilibrium. A more limited lesion involving the brainstem characteristically leads to a cranial nerve disturbance on the ipsilateral side and a contralateral hemiparesis; the cranial nerves affected depend on the level at which the brainstem is involved.

5. A unilateral spinal cord lesion above the fifth cervical segment (C5) causes an ipsilateral hemiparesis that spares the face and cranial nerves. Lesions between C5 and the first thoracic segment (T1) affect the ipsilateral arm to a variable extent as well as the ipsilateral leg; a lesion below T1 will affect only the ipsilateral leg. Because, in practice, both sides of the cord are commonly involved, quadriparesis or paraparesis usually results. If there is an extensive but unilateral cord lesion, the motor deficit is accompanied by ipsilateral impairment of vibration and position sense and by contralateral loss of pain and temperature appreciation (**Brown-Séquard syndrome**). With compressive and other focal lesions that involve the anterior horn cells in addition to the fiber tracts traversing the cord, the muscles innervated by the affected cord segment weaken and atrophy. Therefore, a focal lower motor neuron deficit exists at the level of the lesion and an upper motor neuron deficit exists below it—in addition to any associated sensory disturbance.

Lower Motor Neuron Lesions

A. SIGNS

- Weakness or paralysis.
- Wasting and fasciculations of involved muscles.

- Hypotonia (flaccidity).
- Loss of tendon reflexes when neurons subserving them are affected.
- Normal abdominal and plantar reflexes—unless the neurons subserving them are directly involved, in which case reflex responses are lost.

B. LOCALIZATION OF THE UNDERLYING LESION

In distinguishing weakness from a root, plexus, or peripheral nerve lesion, the distribution of the motor deficit is of particular importance. Only those muscles supplied wholly or partly by the involved structure are weak (Tables 5–5 and 5–6). The distribution of any accompanying sensory deficit similarly reflects the location of the underlying lesion (see Figure 6–1). It may be impossible to distinguish a radicular (root) lesion from discrete focal involvement of the spinal cord. In the latter situation, however, there is more often a bilateral motor deficit at the level of the lesion, a corticospinal or sensory deficit below it, or a disturbance of bladder, bowel, or sexual function. Certain disorders selectively affect the anterior horn cells of the spinal cord diffusely (see *Anterior Horn Cell Diseases*) or the motor nerves; the extensive lower motor neuron deficit without sensory changes helps to indicate the site and nature of the pathologic involvement.

Cerebellar Dysfunction

A. SIGNS

- Hypotonia.
- Depressed or pendular tendon reflexes.
- Ataxia.
- Gait disorder.
- Imbalance of station.
- Disturbances of eye movement.
- Dysarthria.

Ataxia is a complex movement disorder caused, at least in part, by impaired coordination. It occurs in the limbs on the same side as a lesion affecting the cerebellar hemisphere. With midline lesions, incoordination may not be evident in the limbs at all, but there is marked truncal ataxia that becomes evident on walking. The term **dysmetria** is used when movements are not adjusted accurately for range, so that—for example—a moving finger overshoots a target at which it is aimed. **Dysdiadochokinesia** denotes rapid alternating movements that are clumsy and irregular in terms of rhythm and amplitude. **Asynergia** or **dyssynergia** denotes the breakdown of complex actions into the individual movements composing them; when asked to touch the tip of the nose with a finger, for example, the patient may first flex the elbow and then bring the hand up to the nose instead of com-

Table 5–5. Innervation of selected muscles of upper limbs.

Muscle	Main Root	Peripheral Nerve	Main Action
Supraspinatus	C5	Suprascapular	Abduction of arm
Infraspinatus	C5	Suprascapular	External rotation of arm at shoulder
Deltoid	C5	Axillary	Abduction of arm
Biceps	C5, C6	Musculocutaneous	Elbow flexion
Brachioradialis	C5, C6	Radial	Elbow flexion
Extensor carpi radialis longus	C6, C7	Radial	Wrist extension
Flexor carpi radialis	C6, C7	Median	Wrist flexion
Extensor carpi ulnaris	C7	Radial	Wrist extension
Extensor digitorum	C7	Radial	Finger extension
Triceps	C8	Radial	Extension of elbow
Flexor carpi ulnaris	C8	Ulnar	Wrist flexion
Abductor pollicis brevis	T1	Median	Abduction of thumb
Opponens pollicis	T1	Median	Opposition of thumb
First dorsal interosseous	T1	Ulnar	Abduction of index finger
Abductor digiti minimi	T1	Ulnar	Abduction of little finger

Table 5–6. Innervation of selected muscles of lower limbs.

Muscle	Main Root	Peripheral Nerve	Main Action
Iliopsoas	L2, L3	Femoral	Hip flexion
Quadriceps femoris	L3, L4	Femoral	Knee extension
Adductors	L2, L3, L4	Obturator	Adduction of thigh
Gluteus maximus	L5, S1, S2	Inferior gluteal	Hip extension
Gluteus medius and minimus, tensor fasciae latae	L4, L5, S1	Superior gluteal	Hip abduction
Hamstrings	L5, S1	Sciatic	Knee flexion
Tibialis anterior	L4, L5	Peroneal	Dorsiflexion of ankle
Extensor digitorum longus	L5, S1	Peroneal	Dorsiflexion of toes
Extensor digitorum brevis	S1	Peroneal	Dorsiflexion of toes
Peronei	L5, S1	Peroneal	Eversion of foot
Tibialis posterior	L4	Tibial	Inversion of foot
Gastrocnemius	S1, S2	Tibial	Plantar flexion of ankle
Soleus	S1, S2	Tibial	Plantar flexion of ankle

bining the maneuvers into one action. **Intention tremor** occurs during activity and is often most marked as the target is neared. The **rebound phenomenon** is the overshooting of the limb when resistance to a movement or posture is suddenly withdrawn.

The gait becomes unsteady in patients with disturbances of either the cerebellar hemispheres or midline structures, as discussed in Chapter 3.

Jerk nystagmus, which is commonly seen in patients with a unilateral lesion of the cerebellar hemisphere, is slowest and of greatest amplitude when the eyes are turned to the side of the lesion. Nystagmus is not present in patients with lesions of the anterior cerebellar vermis.

Speech becomes dysarthric and takes on an irregular and explosive quality in patients with lesions that involve the cerebellar hemispheres. Speech is usually unremarkable when only the midline structures are involved.

B. Localization of the Underlying Lesion

The relationship of symptoms and signs to lesions of different parts of the cerebellum is considered in Chapter 3.

Neuromuscular-Transmission Disorders

A. Signs

- Normal or reduced muscle tone.
- Normal or depressed tendon and superficial reflexes.
- No sensory changes.
- Weakness, often patchy in distribution, not conforming to the distribution of any single anatomic structure; frequently involves the cranial muscles and may fluctuate in severity over short periods, particularly in relation to activity.

B. Localization of the Underlying Lesion

Pathologic involvement of either the pre- or postsynaptic portion of the neuromuscular junction may impair neuromuscular transmission. Disorders affecting neuromuscular transmission are discussed later.

Myopathic Disorders

A. Signs

- Weakness, usually most marked proximally rather than distally.
- No muscle wasting or depression of tendon reflexes until at least an advanced stage of the disorder.
- Normal abdominal and plantar reflexes.
- No sensory loss or sphincter disturbances.

B. Differentiation

In distinguishing the various myopathic disorders, it is important to determine whether the weakness is congenital or acquired, whether there is a family history of a similar disorder, and whether there is any clinical evidence that a systemic disease may be responsible. The distribution of affected muscles is often especially important in distinguishing the various hereditary myopathies (see *Myopathic Disorders,* later, and Table 5–13).

INVESTIGATIVE STUDIES

Investigative studies of patients with weakness from focal cerebral deficits are considered in Chapter 11. The investigations discussed here may be helpful in evaluating patients with weakness from other causes (Table 5–7).

Imaging

A. Plain X-Rays of the Spine

Congenital abnormalities and degenerative, inflammatory, neoplastic, or traumatic changes may be revealed by plain x-rays of the spine, which should therefore be undertaken in the evaluation of patients with suspected cord or root lesions.

B. CT Scan or MRI

A computed tomography (CT) scan of the spine, especially when performed after instilling water-soluble contrast material into the subarachnoid space, may also reveal disease involving the spinal cord or nerve roots. Magnetic resonance imaging (MRI) is superior to CT scanning in this regard (see Chapter 11).

C. Myelography

Radiologic study of the spinal subarachnoid space with injection of a contrast medium is an important means of visualizing intramedullary tumors and extramedullary lesions that compress the spinal cord or nerve roots, and certain vascular malformations. It can also permit detection of congenital or acquired structural abnormalities, especially in the region of the foramen magnum. For most purposes, however, spinal MRI is superior to myelography (see Chapter 11).

Electrodiagnostic Studies

The function of the normal motor unit, which consists of a lower motor neuron and all of the muscle fibers it innervates, may be disturbed at any of several sites in patients with weakness. A lesion may, for example, affect the anterior horn cell or its axon, interfere with neuromuscular transmission, or involve the muscle fibers directly so that they cannot respond normally to neural activation. In each circumstance, characteristic changes

Table 5–7. Investigation of patients with weakness.

Test	Spinal Cord	Anterior Horn Cell Disorders	Peripheral Nerve or Plexus	Neuromuscular Junction	Myopathy
Serum enzymes	Normal	Normal	Normal	Normal	Normal or increased
Electromyography	Reduced number of motor units under voluntary control; with lesions causing axonal degeneration, abnormal spontaneous activity (eg, fasciculations, fibrillations) may be present if sufficient time has elapsed after onset; with reinnervation, motor units may be large, long, and polyphasic			Often normal, but individual motor units may show abnormal variability in size	Small, short, abundant polyphasic motor unit potentials; abnormal spontaneous activity may be conspicuous in myositis
Nerve conduction velocity	Normal	Normal	Slowed, especially in demyelinative neuropathies. May be normal in axonal neuropathies	Normal	Normal
Muscle response to repetitive motor nerve stimulation	Normal	Normal, except in active stage of disease	Normal	Abnormal decrement or increment depending on stimulus frequency and disease	Normal
Muscle biopsy	May be normal in acute stage but subsequently suggestive of denervation			Normal	Changes suggestive of myopathy
Myelography or spinal MRI	May be helpful	Helpful in excluding other disorders	Not helpful	Not helpful	Not helpful

in the electrical activity can be recorded from affected muscle by a needle electrode inserted into it and connected to an oscilloscope (electromyography). Depending on the site of pathology, nerve conduction studies or the muscle responses to repetitive nerve stimulation may also be abnormal. See Chapter 11 for further details.

Serum Enzymes

Damage to muscle fibers may lead to the release of certain enzymes [creatine kinase (CK), aldolase, lactic acid dehydrogenase, and the transaminases] that can then be detected in increased amounts in serum. Serum CK shows the greatest increase and is the most useful for following the course of muscle disease. It is also present in high concentrations in the heart and brain, however, and damage to these structures can lead to increased serum CK levels. Fractionation of serum CK into isoenzyme forms is useful for determining the tissue of origin. In patients with weakness, elevated serum CK levels are generally indicative of a primary myopathy, especially one that is evolving rapidly. A moderately elevated serum CK may also occur in motor neuron disease, however, and more marked elevations can follow trauma, surgery, intramuscular injections, EMG, or vigorous activity.

Muscle Biopsy

Histopathologic examination of a specimen of weak muscle can be important in determining whether the underlying weakness is neurogenic or myopathic in origin. With neurogenic disorders, muscle biopsy specimens show atrophied fibers occurring in groups, with adjacent groups of larger, uninvolved fibers. In myopathies, atrophy occurs in a random pattern; nuclei of muscle cells may be centrally situated, in contrast to their normal peripheral location; and fibrosis or fatty infiltration may be seen. In addition, examination of a muscle biopsy specimen may permit recognition of certain inflammatory muscle diseases (eg, polymyositis) for which specific treatment is available—helping to differentiate them from muscle disorders that have no specific treatment.

SPINAL CORD DISORDERS

Cord lesions can lead to motor, sensory, or sphincter disturbances or to some combination of these deficits. Depending upon whether it is unilateral or bilateral, a lesion above C5 may cause either an ipsilateral hemiparesis or quadriparesis. With lesions located lower in the cervical cord, involvement of the upper limbs is partial, and a lesion below T1 affects only the lower limbs on one or both sides. Disturbances of sensation are considered in detail in Chapter 6, but it should be noted here that unilateral involvement of the posterior columns of the cord leads to ipsilateral loss of position and vibration sense. In addition, any disturbance in function of the spinothalamic tracts in the anterolateral columns impairs contralateral pain and temperature appreciation below the level of the lesion.

Spasticity is a common accompaniment of upper motor neuron lesions and may be especially troublesome below the level of the lesion in patients with myelopathies. When the legs are weak, the increased tone of spasticity may help to support the patient in the upright position. Marked spasticity, however, may lead to deformity, interfere with toilet functions, and cause painful flexor or extensor spasms. Pharmacologic management includes treatment with diazepam, baclofen, dantrolene, or tizanidine, as discussed below under *Traumatic Myelopathy*, but reduction in tone may lead to increased disability from underlying leg weakness.

TRAUMATIC MYELOPATHY

Although cord damage may result from whiplash (recoil) injury, severe injury to the cord usually relates to fracture-dislocation in the cervical, lower thoracic, or upper lumbar region.

Clinical Findings

A. TOTAL CORD TRANSECTION

Total transection results in immediate permanent paralysis and loss of sensation below the level of the lesion. Although reflex activity is lost for a variable period after the injury, a persistent increase in reflex function follows.

1. In the acute stage, there is flaccid paralysis with loss of tendon and other reflexes, accompanied by sensory loss and by urinary and fecal retention. This is the stage of **spinal shock.**

2. Over the following weeks, as reflex function returns, the clinical picture of a spastic paraplegia or quadriplegia emerges, with brisk tendon reflexes and extensor plantar responses; however, a flaccid, atrophic (lower motor neuron) paralysis may affect muscles innervated by spinal cord segments at the level of the lesion, where anterior horn cells are damaged. The bladder and bowel now regain some reflex function, so that urine and feces are expelled at intervals.

3. Flexor or extensor spasms of the legs may become increasingly troublesome and are ultimately elicited by even the slightest cutaneous stimulus, especially in the presence of bedsores or a urinary tract infection. Eventually, the patient assumes a posture with the legs in flexion or extension, the former being especially likely with cervical or complete cord lesions.

B. LESS SEVERE INJURY

With lesser degrees of injury, the neurologic deficit is less severe and less complete, but patients may be left with a mild paraparesis or quadriparesis or a distal sensory disturbance. Sphincter function may also be impaired—urinary urgency and urgency incontinence are especially common. Hyperextension injuries of the neck can lead to focal cord ischemia that causes bibrachial paresis (weakness of both arms) with sparing of the legs and variable sensory signs.

Treatment

A. IMMOBILIZATION

Initial treatment consists of immobilization until the nature and extent of the injury are determined. If there is cord compression, urgent decompressive surgery will be necessary. An unstable spine may require surgical fixation, and vertebral dislocation may necessitate spinal traction.

B. CORTICOSTEROIDS

Corticosteroids (eg, methylprednisolone, 30 mg/kg intravenous bolus, followed by intravenous infusion at 5.4 mg/kg/h for 24 hours) can improve motor and sensory function at 6 months when treatment is begun within 8 hours of traumatic spinal cord injury. The mechanism of the action is unknown, but it may involve the inhibition of lipid peroxidation and the improvement of blood flow to the injured spinal cord.

C. PAINFUL SPASMS

Painful flexor or extensor spasms can be treated with drugs that enhance spinal inhibitory mechanisms (baclofen, diazepam) or uncouple muscle excitation from contraction (dantrolene). Baclofen should be given 5 mg orally twice daily, increasing up to 30 mg four times daily; diazepam, 2 mg orally twice daily up to as high as 20 mg three times daily; and dantrolene, 25 mg/d orally to 100 mg four times daily. Tizanidine, a central α_2-agonist, may also be helpful but its precise mechanism of action is unclear. The daily dose is built up gradually, usually to 8 mg three times daily. Side effects include dryness of the mouth, somnolence, and hypotension, but the drug is usually well tolerated. Patients who fail to benefit from or who cannot tolerate sufficient doses of oral medications may respond to intrathecal infusion of baclofen.

All these drugs may increase functional disability by reducing tone. Dantrolene may also increase weakness and should be avoided in patients with severely compromised respiratory function.

D. Skin Care

Particular attention must be given to skin care, avoiding continued pressure on any single area.

E. Bladder and Bowel Disorders

Depending on the severity of the injury, catheterization may be necessary initially. Subsequently, the urgency and frequency of the spastic bladder may respond to a parasympatholytic drug such as oxybutinin, 5 mg three times daily. Suppositories and enemas will help maintain regular bowel movements and may prevent or control fecal incontinence.

DEMYELINATING MYELOPATHIES

1. Multiple Sclerosis

Epidemiology

Multiple sclerosis is one of the most common neurologic disorders, affecting about 300,000 patients in the United States, and its highest incidence is in young adults. It is defined clinically by the involvement of different parts of the central nervous system at different times—provided that other disorders causing multifocal central dysfunction have been excluded. Initial symptoms generally commence before the age of 55 years, with a peak incidence between ages 20 and 40; women are affected nearly twice as often as men.

Epidemiologic studies show that the prevalence of the disease rises with increasing distance from the equator, and no population with a high risk for the disease exists between latitudes 40°N and 40°S. A genetic predisposition is suggested by twin studies, the occasional familial incidence, and the strong association between the disease and specific HLA antigens (HLA DR2). Present evidence supports the belief that the disease has an autoimmune basis.

Pathology

The disorder is characterized pathologically by the development of focal—often perivenular—scattered areas of demyelination followed by a reactive gliosis; there may be axonal damage as well. These lesions occur in the white matter of the brain and cord and in the optic (II) nerve.

Pathophysiology

The cause of multiple sclerosis is unknown, but tissue damage and neurologic symptoms are thought to result from an immune mechanism directed against myelin antigens. Viral infection or other inciting factors may promote the entry of T cells and antibodies into the central nervous system by disrupting the blood–brain barrier. This leads to increased expression of cell-adhesion molecules, matrix metalloproteinases, and proinflammatory cytokines, which work in concert to attract additional immune cells, break down the extracellular matrix to aid their migration, and activate autoimmune responses against antigens such as myelin basic protein, myelin-associated glycoprotein, myelin oligodendrocyte glycoprotein, proteolipid protein, α B-crystallin, phosphodiesterases, and S-100. Binding of these target antigens by antigen-presenting cells triggers an autoimmune response that may involve cytokines, macrophages, and complement. Immune attack on myelin denudes axons, which slows nerve conduction and leads to neurologic symptoms.

Clinical Findings

A. Initial or Presenting Symptoms

Patients can present with any of a variety of symptoms (Table 5–8). Common initial complaints are focal weakness, numbness, tingling, or unsteadiness in a limb; sudden loss or blurring of vision in one eye (optic neuritis); diplopia; disequilibrium; or a bladder-function disturbance (urinary urgency or hesitancy). Such symptoms are often transient, disappearing after a few days or weeks, even though some residual deficit may be found on careful neurologic examination. Other patients present with an acute or gradually progressive spastic paraparesis and sensory deficit; this should raise concern about the possibility of an underlying structural lesion unless there is evidence on clinical examination of more widespread disease.

B. Subsequent Course

There may be an interval of months or years after the initial episode before further neurologic symptoms appear. New symptoms may then develop, or the original ones may recur and progress. Relapses may be triggered by infection and, in women, are more likely in the 3 months or so following childbirth. A rise in body temperature can cause transient deterioration in patients with a fixed and stable deficit. With time—and after a number of relapses and usually incomplete remissions—the patient may become increasingly disabled by weakness, stiffness, sensory disturbances, unsteadiness of the limbs, impaired vision, and urinary incontinence.

Based on its course, the disease is divided into a **relapsing-remitting** form (85% of cases) in which progression does not occur between attacks; a **secondary**

Table 5–8. Symptoms and signs of multiple sclerosis.[1]

	Percentage of Patients
Symptoms (at presentation)	
Paresthesia	37
Gait disorder	35
Lower extremity weakness or incoordination	17
Visual loss	15
Upper extremity weakness or incoordination	10
Diplopia	10
Signs	
Absent abdominal reflexes	81
Hyperreflexia	76
Lower extremity ataxia	57
Extensor plantar responses	54
Impaired rapid alternating movements	49
Impaired vibratory sense	47
Optic neuropathy	38
Nystagmus	35
Impaired joint position sense	33
Intention tremor	32
Spasticity	31
Impaired pain or temperature sense	22
Dysarthria	19
Paraparesis	17
Internuclear ophthalmoplegia	11

[1] Adapted from Swanson JW: Multiple sclerosis: Update in diagnosis and review of prognostic factors. Mayo Clin Proc 1989;64:577–586.

progressive form (80% of cases after 25 years) characterized by a gradually progressive course after an initial relapsing-remitting pattern; and a **primary progressive** form (10% of cases) in which there is gradual progression of disability from clinical onset. A **progressive-relapsing** form occurs rarely, with acute relapses being superimposed on a primary progressive course.

Examination in advanced cases commonly reveals optic atrophy, nystagmus, dysarthria, and upper motor neuron, sensory, or cerebellar deficits in some or all of the limbs (see Table 5–8). Note that the diagnosis cannot be based on any single symptom or sign but only on a total clinical picture that indicates involvement of different parts of the central nervous system at different times.

Diagnosis

The diagnosis of multiple sclerosis requires evidence that at least two different regions of the central white matter have been affected at different times. Clinically definite disease can be diagnosed in patients with a relapsing-remitting course and signs of at least two lesions involving different regions of the central white matter. Probable multiple sclerosis is diagnosed when patients have evidence of multifocal white matter disease but have had only one clinical attack, or have a history of at least two clinical episodes but signs of only a single lesion.

Investigative Studies

These may help to support the clinical diagnosis and exclude other disorders but do not themselves justify a definitive diagnosis of multiple sclerosis.

The cerebrospinal fluid (CSF) is commonly abnormal, with mild lymphocytosis or a slightly increased protein concentration, especially if examined soon after an acute relapse. CSF protein electrophoresis shows the presence of discrete bands in the immunoglobulin G (IgG) region (**oligoclonal bands**) in 90% of patients. The antigens responsible for these antibodies are not known.

If clinical evidence of a lesion exists at only one site in the central nervous system, a diagnosis of multiple sclerosis cannot properly be made unless other regions have been affected subclinically, as detected by the electrocerebral responses evoked by one or more of the following: monocular visual stimulation with a checkerboard pattern (**visual evoked potentials**); monaural stimulation with repetitive clicks (**brainstem auditory evoked potentials**); and electrical stimulation of a peripheral nerve (**somatosensory evoked potentials**).

MRI may also detect subclinical lesions and has become nearly indispensible in confirming the diagnosis (Figure 5–2A,B).

In patients presenting with the spinal form of the disorder and no evidence of disseminated disease, spinal MRI or myelography may be necessary to exclude the possibility of a single congenital or acquired surgically treatable lesion. The region of the foramen magnum must be visualized to exclude the possibility of a lesion such as Arnold-Chiari malformation, in which part of the cerebellum and the lower brainstem are displaced into the cervical canal, producing mixed pyramidal and cerebellar deficits in the limbs.

Treatment

In patients with relapsing-remitting disease, treatment with interferon β-1a given intramuscularly once weekly or interferon β-1b given subcutaneously on alternate days reduces the relapse rate. Glatiramer acetate (formerly copolymer 1, a mixture of random polymers simulating the amino acid composition of myelin basic protein) given by daily subcutaneous injection is also

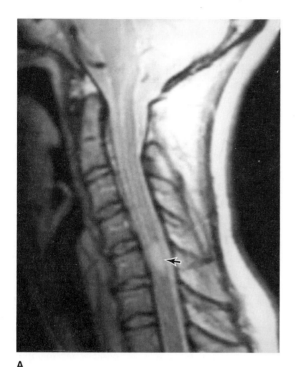

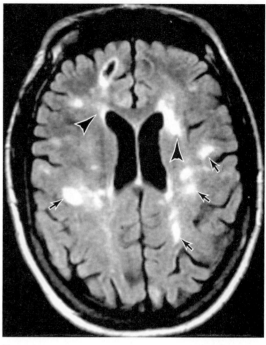

A   B

Figure 5–2. **A:** A mid-sagittal T2-weighted MRI of the cervical spinal cord in a young woman with multiple sclerosis. An abnormal region of high signal intensity **(arrow)** is seen. (Courtesy of RA Heyman.) **B:** Axial T2-weighted MR brain images of a patient with multiple sclerosis showing multiple, primarily punctate, white matter plaques **(arrows)**; note the typical location in the periventricular region **(arrowheads)**. (Courtesy of RA Heyman.)

effective. In addition to their effect on relapses, interferon β-1a and glatiramer acetate may also delay the onset of significant disability in patients with relapsing disease. Intravenous immunoglobulin (IVIg) infusions may also reduce the relapse rate in relapsing-remitting disease, but treatment recommendations are premature.

The most common side effects of interferons are a flu-like syndrome and (in the case of interferon β-1b) injection site reactions. Glatiramer acetate is generally tolerated well, but it may produce erythema at the sites of injection, and about 15% of patients experience transient episodes of flushing, dyspnea, chest tightness, palpitations, and anxiety after injections. All three of these agents are approved for use in relapsing-remitting multiple sclerosis and are available by prescription. They are expensive, but their cost must be balanced against the reduced need for medical care and reduced time lost from work that follows their use.

Corticosteroids may hasten recovery from acute relapses, but the extent of the recovery itself is unchanged. Long-term steroid administration does not prevent relapses and should not be used because of unacceptable side effects. There is no standard schedule

of treatment with corticosteroids, but the regimen most commonly used is intravenous methylprednisolone (1 g daily) for 3–5 days, followed by an oral prednisone taper (1 mg/kg/d for 1 week, with rapid reduction over the ensuing 1–2 weeks). For mild attacks, some clinicians prefer oral treatment with prednisone 60 or 80 mg/d, or dexamethasone 16 mg/d, given for a week and tapered rapidly over the following 2 weeks. ACTH (corticotropin) is no longer used.

Appropriate treatment of primary or secondary progressive multiple sclerosis is less well established. Recent studies suggest that interferon β-1b (and probably interferon β-1a) are effective in reducing the progression rate as determined clinically and by MRI in secondary progressive disease, but there is only limited experience with glatiramer acetate in this setting. Treatment with cyclophosphamide, azathioprine, methotrexate, cladribine, or mitoxandrone may help to arrest the course of secondary progressive disease, but studies are inconclusive. Pulse therapy with high-dose intravenous methylprednisolone (1 g/d once a month) is also sometimes effective and may carry a lower risk of long-term complications than the cytotoxic drugs.

No specific immunomodulatory therapy has been shown to be effective in primary progressive multiple sclerosis, and management is with symptomatic measures.

Maintenance of general health and symptomatic treatment should not be neglected in the comprehensive management of multiple sclerosis. Exercise and physical therapy are important, but excessive exertion must be avoided, particularly during periods of acute relapse. Fatigue is a serious problem for many patients, and sometimes responds to amantadine or one of the selective serotonin reuptake inhibitor antidepressants. Treatment for spasticity (discussed earlier) is often needed, as is aggressive bladder and bowel management. Treatment for other aspects of advanced multiple sclerosis such as cognitive deficits, pain, tremor, and ataxia is generally less successful.

Prognosis

At least partial recovery from an acute episode can be anticipated, but it is impossible to predict when the next relapse will occur. Features that tend to imply a more favorable prognosis include female sex, onset before age 40, and presentation with visual or somatosensory, rather than pyramidal or cerebellar, dysfunction. Although some degree of disability is likely to result eventually, about half of all patients are only mildly or moderately disabled 10 years after the onset of symptoms.

2. Acute Disseminated Encephalomyelitis

This occurs as a single episode of neurologic symptoms and signs that develop over a few days in association with a viral infection, especially measles or chickenpox. The neurologic deficit resolves, at least in part, over the succeeding few weeks. Pathologically, perivascular areas of demyelination are scattered throughout the brain and spinal cord, with an associated inflammatory reaction. A similar disorder may also occur independently, with no apparent infection; it may then represent the initial manifestation of multiple sclerosis.

The initial symptoms often consist of headache, fever, and confusion; seizures may also occur, and examination reveals signs of meningeal irritation. Flaccid weakness and sensory disturbance of the legs, extensor plantar responses, and urinary retention are common manifestations of cord involvement. Other neurologic signs may indicate involvement of the optic nerves, cerebral hemispheres, brainstem, or cerebellum.

Examination of the CSF may show an increased mononuclear cell count, with normal protein and glucose concentrations.

Corticosteroids are often prescribed, but there is little evidence of benefit. Treatment with intravenous immunoglobulins or plasmapheresis has been helpful in small series of cases. A mortality rate of 5–30% is reported, and survivors often have severe residual deficits.

OTHER INFECTIVE OR INFLAMMATORY MYELOPATHIES

Epidural Abscess

Epidural abscess may occur as a sequel to skin infection, septicemia, vertebral osteomyelitis, intravenous drug abuse, back trauma or surgery, or lumbar puncture. Predisposing factors include acquired immunodeficiency syndrome (AIDS) and iatrogenic immunosuppression. The most common causative organisms are *Staphylococcus aureus,* streptococci, gram-negative bacilli, and anaerobes. Fever, backache and tenderness, pain in the distribution of a spinal nerve root, headache, and malaise are early symptoms, followed by rapidly progressive paraparesis, sensory disturbances in the legs, and urinary and fecal retention.

Spinal epidural abscess is a neurologic emergency that requires prompt diagnosis and treatment. MRI with gadolinium enhancement is the imaging study of choice and should be sufficient to determine the extent of the abscess. A block may be found at myelography. Laboratory investigations reveal a peripheral leukocytosis and increased erythrocyte sedimentation rate. A spinal tap should not be performed at the site of a suspected abscess as it may disseminate the infection from the epidural to subarachnoid space. Typically the CSF shows a mild pleocytosis with increased protein but normal glucose concentrations.

Treatment involves surgery and antibiotics. In the absence of cord compression, treatment with intravenous antibiotics alone has been successful. Nafcillin or vancomycin is administered to cover staphylococcal or streptococcal infection, and other agents are added or substituted based on the results of Gram's stain of excised material. The results of culture of the necrotic material that makes up the abscess may subsequently alter the antibiotic regimen. The antibiotic dosages are those used to treat bacterial meningitis, as given in Chapter 1. Intravenous antibiotics are usually continued for 3–4 weeks, but longer treatment is required in the presence of vertebral osteomyelitis.

Syphilis

Syphilis can produce meningovasculitis of the cord, resulting in spinal cord infarction. Vascular myelopathies are discussed later in this chapter.

Tuberculosis

Tuberculosis may lead to vertebral disease (**Pott's disease**) with secondary compression of the cord, to meningitis with secondary arteritis and cord infarction, or to cord compression by a tuberculoma. Such complications assume great importance in certain parts of the world, especially Asia and Africa, and among such groups as the homeless and intravenous drug users. Tuberculous meningitis is considered in more detail in Chapter 1.

AIDS

A disorder of the spinal cord, **vacuolar myelopathy,** is found at autopsy in about 20% of patients with AIDS. This disorder is characterized by vacuolation of white matter in the spinal cord, which is most pronounced in the lateral and posterior columns of the thoracic cord. Direct involvement of the spinal cord by human immunodeficiency virus-1 (HIV-1), the etiologic agent in AIDS, is thought to be the cause, but the correlation between presence and extent of HIV-1 infection and spinal pathology is poor. A metabolic basis has therefore been suggested. Vacuolar myelopathy in AIDS resembles myelopathy caused by vitamin B_{12} deficiency, but it tends to produce earlier incontinence and less conspicuous sensory abnormalities. Myelopathy in patients with AIDS may also be caused by lymphoma, cryptococcal infection, or herpesviruses.

Most patients with vacuolar myelopathy have coexisting AIDS dementia complex (see Chapter 1). Symptoms progress over weeks to months and include leg weakness, ataxia, incontinence, erectile dysfunction, and paresthesias. Examination shows paraparesis, lower extremity monoparesis, or quadriparesis; spasticity; increased or decreased tendon reflexes; Babinski signs; and diminished vibration and position sense. Sensation over the trunk is usually normal and a sensory level is difficult to define. MRI of the spinal cord is typically normal. Therapy is generally with antiretroviral drug combinations, but whether this helps to arrest the myelopathy is not clear.

Other Viral Infections

A retrovirus, human T-lymphotropic virus type I (HTLV-I), appears to be the cause of **tropical spastic paraparesis,** a disorder found especially in the Caribbean, off the Pacific coast of Colombia, and in the Seychelles. Transmission of the virus occurs in breast milk, during sexual intercourse, and by exposure to contaminated blood products. Clinical features of the disorder include spastic paraparesis, impaired vibration and joint position sense, and bowel and bladder dysfunction. Recent reports indicate that a clinically similar myelopathy may also follow infection with human T-lymphotropic virus type II (HTLV-II). Specific therapy is lacking, and treatment is symptomatic.

Herpesviruses can also produce myelopathy, which commonly affects spinal nerve roots as well as the cord (**radiculomyelopathy**), especially in immunocompromised patients, such as those with AIDS. Cytomegalovirus causes a myelopathy characterized by demyelination of the posterior columns of the spinal cord and by cytomegalic cells that contain Cowdry's type A inclusion bodies. The value of treatment with antiviral drugs such as ganciclovir and foscarnet is still uncertain. Herpes zoster and herpes simplex types 1 and 2 can also cause myelopathy, which may respond to treatment with acyclovir (see Chapter 1).

Tetanus

Tetanus is a disorder of neurotransmission associated with infection by *Clostridium tetani.* The organism typically becomes established in a wound, where it elaborates a toxin that is transported retrogradely along motor nerves into the spinal cord or, with wounds to the face or head, the brainstem. The toxin is also disseminated through the bloodstream to skeletal muscle, where it gains access to additional motor nerves. In the spinal cord and brainstem, tetanus toxin interferes with the release of inhibitory neurotransmitters, including glycine and GABA, resulting in motor nerve hyperactivity. Autonomic nerves are also disinhibited.

After an incubation period of up to 3 weeks, tetanus usually presents with **trismus** (lockjaw), difficulty in swallowing, or spasm of the facial muscles that resembles a contorted smile (**risus sardonicus**). Painful muscle spasms and rigidity progress to involve both axial and limb musculature and may give rise to hyperextended posturing (**opisthotonos**). Laryngospasm and autonomic instability are potential life-threatening complications.

Although the diagnosis is usually made on clinical grounds, the presence of continuous motor unit activity or absence of the normal silent period in the masseter muscle following elicitation of the jaw-jerk reflex is a helpful electromyographic finding. The serum CK may be elevated, and myoglobinuria may occur. The organisms can be cultured from a wound in only a minority of cases.

Tetanus is preventable through immunization with tetanus toxoid. Tetanus toxoid is usually administered routinely to infants and children in the United States, in combination with pertussis vaccine and diphtheria toxoids. In children under age 7 years, three doses of tetanus toxoid are administered at intervals of at least 1 month, followed by a booster dose 1 year later. For older children and adults, the third dose is delayed for at least 6 months after the second, and no fourth dose is required. Immunization lasts for 5–10 years.

Debridement of wounds is an important preventive measure. Patients with open wounds should receive an additional dose of tetanus toxoid if they have not received a booster dose within 10 years—or if the last booster dose was more than 5 years ago and the risk of infection with *C tetani* is moderate or high. A moderate likelihood of infection is associated with wounds that penetrate muscle, those sustained on wood or pavement, human bites, and nonabdominal bullet wounds. High-risk wounds include those acquired in barnyards, near sewers or other sources of waste material, and abdominal bullet wounds. Patients with moderate- or high-risk wounds should also be given tetanus immune globulin.

The treatment of tetanus includes hospitalization in an intensive care unit to monitor respiratory and circulatory function, tetanus immune globulin to neutralize the toxin, and penicillin for the infection itself. Diazepam, 10–20 mg intravenously or intramuscularly every 4–6 hours, and chlorpromazine, 25–50 mg intravenously or intramuscularly every 8 hours, are useful for treating painful spasms and rigidity. Neuromuscular blockade with curare or pancuronium may be required when these measures fail; if so, mechanical ventilation must be used.

Fatality rates of 10–60% are reported. Lower fatality rates are most likely to be achieved by early diagnosis, prompt institution of appropriate treatment before the onset of spasms, and the use of intrathecal—in addition to intramuscular—tetanus immune globulin. Among patients who recover, about 95% do so without long-term sequelae.

Chronic Adhesive Arachnoiditis

This inflammatory disorder is usually idiopathic but can follow subarachnoid hemorrhage; meningitis; intrathecal administration of penicillin, radiologic contrast materials, and certain forms of spinal anesthetic; trauma; and surgery.

The usual initial complaint is of constant radicular pain, but in other cases there is lower motor neuron weakness because of the involvement of anterior nerve roots. Eventually, a spastic ataxic paraparesis develops, with sphincter involvement. CSF protein is elevated, and the cell count may be increased. Myelography shows a characteristic fragmentation of the contrast material into pockets; MRI may disclose inflammation.

Treating this aseptic inflammatory leptomeningeal process with steroids or with nonsteroidal antiinflammatory analgesics may be helpful. Surgery may be indicated in cases with localized cord involvement.

VASCULAR MYELOPATHIES

Infarction of the Spinal Cord

This rare event generally occurs only in the territory of the anterior spinal artery (Figure 5–3). This artery, which supplies the anterior two-thirds of the cord, is itself supplied by only a limited number of feeding vessels,

whereas the paired posterior spinal arteries are supplied by numerous feeders at many different levels. Thus, anterior spinal artery syndrome usually results from interrupted flow in one of its feeders. Causes include trauma, dissecting aortic aneurysm, aortography, polyarteritis nodosa, and hypotensive crisis. Since the anterior spinal artery is particularly well supplied in the cervical region, infarcts almost always occur more caudally.

The typical clinical presentation is with the acute onset of a flaccid, areflexic paraparesis that, as spinal shock wears off after a few days or weeks, evolves into a spastic paraparesis with brisk tendon reflexes and extensor plantar responses. In addition, there is dissociated sensory impairment—pain and temperature appreciation are lost, but there is sparing of vibration and position sense because the posterior columns are supplied by the posterior spinal arteries. Treatment is symptomatic.

Hematomyelia

Hemorrhage into the spinal cord is rare; it is caused by trauma, a vascular anomaly, a bleeding disorder, or anticoagulant therapy. A severe cord syndrome develops acutely and is usually associated with blood in the CSF. The prognosis depends on the extent of the hemorrhage and the rapidity with which it occurs.

Epidural or Subdural Hemorrhage

Spinal epidural or subdural hemorrhage can occur in relation to trauma or tumor and as a complication of anticoagulation, aspirin therapy, thrombocytopenia, coagulopathy, epidural catheters, or lumbar puncture. It occasionally occurs spontaneously. The likelihood of hemorrhage following lumbar puncture—usually epidural in location—is increased when a disorder of coagulation is present. Therefore, the platelet count, prothrombin time, and partial thromboplastin time should be determined before lumbar puncture is performed, and if anticoagulant therapy is to be instituted, it should be delayed for at least 1 hour following the procedure. Patients with less than 20,000 platelets/mm^3 or those with rapidly falling counts (as high as 50,000) should be transfused prior to lumbar puncture. Spinal epidural hemorrhage usually presents with back pain that may radiate in the distribution of one or more spinal nerve roots; it is occasionally painless. Paraparesis or quadriparesis, sensory disturbances in the lower limbs, and bowel and bladder dysfunction may develop rapidly, necessitating urgent CT scan, MRI, or myelography, and surgical evacuation of the hematoma.

Arteriovenous Malformation (AVM)

This may present with subarachnoid hemorrhage or with myelopathy. Most of these lesions involve the lower part

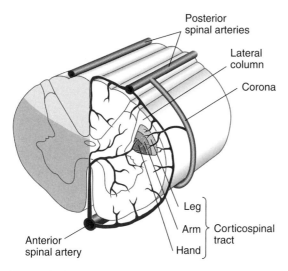

Figure 5–3. Blood supply to the cervical spinal cord (shown in transverse section). **Left:** Major territories supplied by the anterior spinal artery (dark shading) and the posterior spinal artery (light shading). **Right:** Pattern of supply by intramedullary arteries. From the pial vessels (around the circumference of the cord), radially oriented branches supply much of the white matter and the posterior horns of the gray matter. The remaining gray matter and the innermost portion of the white matter are supplied by the central artery (located in the anterior median fissure), which arises from the anterior spinal artery. The descending corticospinal tract is supplied by both the anterior and posterior spinal arteries.

of the cord. Symptoms include motor and sensory disturbances in the legs and disorders of sphincter function. Pain in the legs or back is often conspicuous. On examination, there may be an upper, a lower, or a mixed motor deficit in the legs, while sensory deficits are usually extensive but occasionally radicular; the signs indicate an extensive lesion in the longitudinal axis of the cord. In patients with cervical lesions, symptoms and signs may also be present in the arms. A bruit is sometimes audible over the spine, and there may be a cutaneous angioma. The diagnosis is suggested by the MRI appearance and the myelographic finding of serpiginous filling defects caused by enlarged vessels, and it is confirmed by selective spinal arteriography. Spinal MRI is sometimes normal despite the presence of an AVM and therefore cannot be relied upon to exclude this diagnosis.

Most lesions are extramedullary and posterior to the cord; they can be treated by embolization or by ligation of feeding vessels and excision of the anomalous arteriovenous nidus of the malformation, which is usually dural in location. Left untreated, the patient is likely to become increasingly disabled until chair-bound or bed-bound.

DEFICIENCY DISORDERS

Subacute combined degeneration of the cord as a result of vitamin B_{12} deficiency is characterized by an upper motor neuron deficit in the limbs that is usually preceded by sensory symptoms and signs caused by posterior column involvement (see Chapter 6). In addition to the myelopathy, there may be optic atrophy, mental changes, or peripheral neuropathy.

CERVICAL SPONDYLOSIS

Cervical spondylosis is characterized by any or all of the following: pain and stiffness in the neck; pain in the arms, with or without a segmental motor or sensory deficit in the arms; and an upper motor neuron deficit in the legs. It results from chronic cervical disk degeneration, with herniation of disk material, secondary calcification, and associated osteophytic outgrowths. It can lead to involvement of one or more nerve roots on either or both sides and to myelopathy related to compression, vascular insufficiency, or recurrent minor trauma to the cord.

Clinical Findings

Patients often present with neck pain and limitation of head movement or with occipital headache. In some cases, radicular pain and other sensory disturbances occur in the arms, and there may be weakness of the arms or legs. Examination commonly reveals restricted lateral flexion and rotation of the neck. There may be a segmental pattern of weakness or dermatomal sensory loss in one or both arms, along with depression of those tendon reflexes mediated by the affected root(s). Cervical spondylosis tends to affect particularly the C5 and C6 nerve roots, so there is commonly weakness of muscles (eg, deltoid, supra- and infraspinatus, biceps, brachioradialis) supplied from these segments, pain or sensory loss about the shoulder and outer border of the arm and forearm, and depressed biceps and brachioradialis reflexes. If there is an associated myelopathy, upper motor neuron weakness develops in one or both legs, with concomitant changes in tone and reflexes. There may also be posterior column or spinothalamic sensory deficits.

Investigative Studies

Plain x-rays show osteophyte formation, narrowing of disk spaces, and encroachment on the intervertebral foramina. MRI, CT scanning, or even myelography may be necessary to confirm the diagnosis and exclude other structural causes of myelopathy. The CSF obtained at the time of myelography is usually normal, but the protein concentration may be increased, especially if there is a block in the subarachnoid space. Electrophysiologic studies, especially needle electromyography, are helpful in identifying a radiculopathy and in determining whether degenerative anatomic abnormalities of the cervical spine are of any clinical relevance.

Differential Diagnosis

Spondylotic myelopathy may resemble myelopathy caused by such disorders as multiple sclerosis, motor neuron disease, subacute combined degeneration, cord tumor, syringomyelia, or hereditary spastic paraplegia. Moreover, degenerative changes in the spine are common in the middle-aged and elderly and may coincide with one of these other disorders.

Treatment

Treatment with a cervical collar to restrict neck movements may relieve any pain. Operative treatment may be necessary to prevent further progression if there is a significant neurologic deficit; it may also be required if the root pain is severe, persistent, and unresponsive to conservative measures.

CONGENITAL ANOMALIES

A combination of corticospinal and cerebellar signs may be found in the limbs of patients with congenital skeletal abnormalities such as **platybasia** (flattening of the base of the skull) or **basilar invagination** (an upward bulging of the margins of the foramen magnum). **Syringomyelia** (cavitation of the cord), which can be congenital or acquired, may lead to a lower motor neuron deficit, a dissociated sensory loss in the arms, and upper motor neuron signs in the legs. Because the sensory findings are so characteristic, this disorder, which is frequently associated with Arnold-Chiari malformation, is discussed in detail in Chapter 6.

TUMORS & CORD COMPRESSION

Common causes of cord compression are disk protrusion, trauma, and tumors; in certain parts of the world, tuberculous disease of the spine is also a frequent cause. Rare but important causes include epidural abscess and hematoma. The present section will be restricted to a consideration of tumors, and other causes will be considered elsewhere.

Classification

Tumors can be divided into two groups: **intramedullary** (10%) and extramedullary (90%). **Ependymomas** are the most common type of intramedullary tumor, and the various types of **gliomas** make up the remainder. Extramedullary tumors can be either extradural or intradural in location. Among the primary extramedullary tumors, **neurofibromas** and **meningiomas** are relatively common and are benign; they can be intra- or extradural. Carcinomatous metastases (especially from bronchus, breast, or prostate), lymphomatous or leukemic deposits, and myeloma are usually extradural.

Clinical Findings

Irrespective of its nature, a tumor can lead to cord dysfunction and a neurologic deficit by direct compression, ischemia secondary to arterial or venous obstruction, or, in the case of intramedullary lesions, by invasive infiltration.

A. Symptoms

Symptoms may develop insidiously and progress gradually or—as is often the case with spinal cord compression from metastatic carcinoma—exhibit a rapid course.

Pain is a conspicuous feature—and usually the initial abnormality—in many patients with extradural lesions; it can be radicular, localized to the back, or experienced diffusely in an extremity and is characteristically aggravated by coughing or straining (Table 5–9).

Motor symptoms (heaviness, weakness, stiffness, or focal wasting of one or more limbs) may develop, or there may be paresthesias or numbness, especially in the legs. When sphincter disturbances occur, they usually are particularly disabling.

B. Signs

Examination sometimes reveals localized spinal tenderness. Involvement of anterior roots leads to an appropriate lower motor neuron deficit, and involvement of posterior roots leads to dermatomal sensory changes at the level of the lesion. Involvement of pathways traversing the cord may cause an upper motor neuron deficit below the level of the lesion and a sensory deficit with an upper level on the trunk. The distribution of signs varies with the level of the lesion and may take the form of Brown-Séquard or central cord syndrome (see Figures 6–5 and 6–7).

Investigative Studies

The CSF is often xanthochromic, with a greatly increased protein concentration, a normal or elevated white blood cell count, and normal or depressed glucose concentration; Queckenstedt's test at lumbar puncture may reveal a partial or complete block. A plain x-ray of the spine may or may not be abnormal, and myelography, CT scanning, or MRI is necessary to delineate the lesion and localize it accurately.

Table 5-9. Clinical features of spinal cord compression by extradural metastasis.[1]

Sign or Symptom	Initial Feature (%)	Present at Diagnosis (%)
Pain	96	96
Weakness	2	76
Sensory disturbance	0	51
Sphincter dysfunction	0	57

[1] Adapted from Byrne TN, Waxman SG: *Spinal Cord Compression.* Vol 33 of: *Contemporary Neurology Series.* Davis, 1990.

Treatment

Treatment depends upon the nature of the lesion. Extradural metastases must be treated urgently. Depending upon the nature of the primary neoplasm, they are best managed by analgesics, corticosteroids, radiotherapy, and hormonal treatment; decompressive laminectomy is often unnecessary. Intradural (but extramedullary) lesions are best removed if possible. Intramedullary tumors are treated by decompression and surgical excision when feasible and by radiotherapy.

Prognosis

The prognosis depends upon the cause and severity of the cord compression before it is relieved. Cord compression by extradural metastasis is usually manifested first by pain alone and may progress rapidly to cause permanent impairment of motor, sensory, and sphincter function. Therefore, the diagnosis must be suspected early in any patient with cancer and spinal or radicular pain, who must be investigated immediately. Reliance on motor, sensory, or sphincter disturbances to make the diagnosis will unnecessarily delay treatment and worsen the outcome.

ANTERIOR HORN CELL DISORDERS

Disorders that predominantly affect the anterior horn cells are characterized clinically by wasting and weakness of the affected muscles without accompanying sensory changes. Electromyography shows changes that are characteristic of chronic partial denervation, with abnormal spontaneous activity in resting muscle and a reduction in the number of motor units under voluntary control; signs of reinnervation may also be present. Motor conduction velocity is usually normal but may be slightly reduced, and sensory conduction studies are normal. Muscle biopsy shows the histologic changes of denervation. Serum CK may be mildly elevated, but it never reaches the extremely high values seen in some muscular dystrophies.

IDIOPATHIC ANTERIOR HORN CELL DISORDERS

The clinical features and outlook depend in part on the patient's age at onset. The cause of these disorders is unknown, but the genetic basis for some of them is being clarified.

1. *Motor Neuron Disease in Children*

Three forms of spinal muscular atrophy (SMA-I, II, and III) have been described in infants and children, and the responsible gene has been mapped to chromosome 5q11.12–13.3, an area that contains the survival motor neuron (SMN) gene, the neuronal apoptosis inhibitory protein (NAIP) gene, and the BTF2p44 gene. Abnormalities of the SMN gene have been identified in 95% of all patients with SMA, and of the NAIP gene in 45% of patients with SMA-I and 18% of those with SMA-II and SMA-III. The NAIP gene may modify disease severity.

Infantile Spinal Muscular Atrophy (Werdnig-Hoffmann Disease or SMA-I)

This autosomal recessive disorder usually manifests itself within the first 3 months of life. The infant is floppy and may have difficulty with sucking, swallowing, or ventilation. In established cases, examination reveals impaired swallowing or sucking, atrophy and fasciculation of the tongue, and muscle wasting in the limbs that is sometimes obscured by subcutaneous fat. The tendon reflexes are normal or depressed, and the plantar responses may be absent. There is no sensory deficit. The disorder is rapidly progressive, generally leading to death from respiratory complications by about age 3 years.

The cause is unknown, and there is no effective treatment.

Intermediate Spinal Muscular Atrophy (Chronic Werdnig-Hoffmann Disease or SMA-II)

This also has an autosomal recessive mode of inheritance but usually begins in the latter half of the first year of life. Its main clinical features are wasting and weakness of the extremities; bulbar weakness occurs less commonly. The disorder progresses slowly, ultimately leading to severe disability with kyphoscoliosis and contractures, but its course is more benign than the infantile variety described above, and many patients survive into adulthood.

Treatment is essentially supportive and directed particularly at the prevention of scoliosis and other deformities.

Juvenile Spinal Muscular Atrophy (Kugelberg-Welander Disease or SMA-III)

Generally this disorder develops in childhood or early adolescence, on either a hereditary or sporadic basis. The usual mode of inheritance is autosomal recessive. It particularly tends to affect the proximal limb muscles, with generally little involvement of the bulbar musculature. It follows a gradually progressive course, leading to disability in early adult life. The proximal weakness may lead to a mistaken diagnosis of muscular dystrophy, but serum CK determination, electromyography, and muscle biopsy will differentiate the disorders.

There is no effective treatment.

2. Motor Neuron Disease in Adults

Motor neuron disease in adults generally begins between the ages of 30 and 60 years and has an annual incidence in the order of 2 per 100,000, with a male predominance. It is characterized by degeneration of anterior horn cells in the spinal cord, motor nuclei of the lower cranial nerves in the brainstem, and corticospinal and corticobulbar pathways. The disorder usually occurs sporadically but may be familial in 5–10% of cases. An autosomal dominant familial motor neuron disease (with upper and lower motor neuron signs) has been related in some cases to mutations of the copper/zinc superoxide dismutase gene on the long arm of chromosome 21 (21q22.1–22.2) whereas an autosomal recessive form maps to 2q33–q35. Additional loci for autosomal dominant, autosomal recessive, and X-linked forms have also been identified, as have sporadic cases with apparently new mutations in neurofilament heavy chain (22q12). The cause of the sporadic disorder is unknown but no robust environmental risk factors have emerged.

How hereditary or sporadic motor neuron disease produces symptoms is uncertain, but one or more of four proposed pathophysiologic mechanisms may be involved. These include oxidative injury by reactive oxygen species that escape scavenging by defective copper/zinc superoxide dismutase, aggregation of abnormal superoxide dismutase proteins, strangulation of axonal transport by protein aggregates or mutant neurofilament proteins, and excitotoxicity due to defective glutamate uptake into astrocytes through the excitatory amino acid (glutamate) transporter, EAAT2.

Five varieties of the disorder can be distinguished by their predominant distribution (limb or bulbar muscu-

lature) and the nature of their clinical deficits (upper or lower motor neuron).

Classification

A. PROGRESSIVE BULBAR PALSY

Bulbar involvement predominates and is due to lesions affecting the motor nuclei of cranial nerves (ie, lower motor neurons) in the brainstem.

B. PSEUDOBULBAR PALSY

This term is used when bulbar involvement predominates and is due primarily to upper motor neuron disease, ie, to bilateral involvement of corticobulbar pathways. A pseudobulbar palsy can occur in any disorder that causes bilateral corticobulbar disease, however, and the use of the term must not be taken to imply that the underlying cause is *necessarily* motor neuron disease.

C. PROGRESSIVE SPINAL MUSCULAR ATROPHY

There is primarily a lower motor neuron deficit in the limbs, caused by anterior horn cell degeneration in the spinal cord. Familial forms have been recognized.

D. PRIMARY LATERAL SCLEROSIS

In this rare disorder, a purely upper motor neuron (corticospinal) deficit is found in the limbs.

E. AMYOTROPHIC LATERAL SCLEROSIS

A mixed upper and lower motor neuron deficit is found in the limbs. There may also be bulbar involvement of the upper or lower motor neuron type.

Clinical Findings

In about 20% of patients with amyotrophic lateral sclerosis, the initial symptoms are related to weakness of bulbar muscles. Bulbar involvement is generally characterized by difficulty in swallowing, chewing, coughing, breathing, and speaking (dysarthria). In progressive bulbar palsy, examination may reveal drooping of the palate, a depressed gag reflex, a pool of saliva in the pharynx, a weak cough, and a wasted and fasciculating tongue. The tongue is contracted and spastic in pseudobulbar palsy and cannot be moved rapidly from side to side.

Weakness of the upper extremity muscles is the presenting complaint in about 40% of patients; lower extremity muscles are first affected in a similar proportion of patients. Limb involvement is characterized by easy fatigability, weakness, stiffness, twitching, wasting, and muscle cramps, and there may be vague sensory complaints and weight loss. Examination reveals no sensory deficit but only upper or lower motor neuron signs, as indicated above.

Diagnostic criteria for amyotrophic lateral sclerosis have been established by the World Federation of Neurology. Criteria vary depending on the level of certainty of the diagnosis, as shown in Table 5–10. Definitive diagnosis requires the presence of upper and lower motor neuron signs in the bulbar region and at least two other spinal regions (cervical, thoracic, or lumbosacral), or in three spinal regions.

There is generally no involvement of extraocular muscles or sphincters. The CSF is normal.

Treatment

There is no specific treatment for the idiopathic disorder, although therapeutic trials of various nerve growth factors are in progress. Riluzole (100 mg daily) may reduce mortality and slow progression of amyotrophic lateral sclerosis, possibly because it blocks glutamatergic transmission in the central nervous system (CNS). Adverse effects include fatigue, dizziness, gastrointestinal disorders, reduced pulmonary function, and a rise in liver enzymes. Symptomatic measures may include anticholinergic drugs (eg, glycopyrrolate, trihexyphenidyl, amitriptyline, transdermal hyoscine, atropine) if drooling of saliva is troublesome. Braces or a walker may improve mobility, and physical therapy may prevent contractures.

A semiliquid diet or feeding via nasogastric tube may be required for severe dysphagia. Percutaneous endoscopic gastroscopy (PEG) is indicated for dysphagia with accelerated weight loss due to insufficient caloric intake, dehydration, or choking on food. For optimal safety, it should be offered when the patient's vital

Table 5–10. Clinical diagnosis of amyotrophic lateral sclerosis: El Escorial Criteria of the World Federation of Neurology.

Diagnostic Certainty	Clinical Features
Definite	Upper and lower motor neuron signs in the bulbar and two spinal regions *or* in three spinal regions
Probable	Upper and lower motor neuron signs in two or more regions; the regions may differ, but some upper motor neuron signs must be rostral to the lower motor neuron deficit
Possible	Upper and lower motor neuron signs in only one region *or* upper motor neuron signs alone in two or more regions *or* lower motor neuron signs rostral to upper motor neuron signs
Suspected	Lower (but not upper) motor neuron signs in at least two regions

capacity is more than 50% of predicted. Noninvasive or invasive ventilation may be necessary as hypoventilation develops. In these circumstances, however, palliative care to relieve distress without prolonging life becomes an important consideration and requires detailed discussion with the patient and family. Such discussions are best initiated early in the course of the disease, with continuing discussion as the disease advances.

Prognosis

Motor neuron disease is progressive and usually has a fatal outcome within 3–5 years, most commonly from pulmonary infections. In general, patients with bulbar involvement have a poorer prognosis than those in whom dysfunction is limited to the extremities.

OTHER NONINFECTIVE DISORDERS OF ANTERIOR HORN CELLS

Bulbospinal neuronopathy (Kennedy's syndrome) is a sex-linked recessive disorder associated with an expanded trinucleotide repeat sequence on the androgen receptor gene. It has a more benign prognosis than the other motor neuron diseases. Its clinical characteristics include tremor (resembling essential tremor), cramps, fasciculations, proximal weakness, and twitching movements of the chin that are precipitated by pursing of the lips.

Juvenile spinal muscular atrophy can occur in patients with **hexosaminidase deficiency.** Rectal biopsy may be abnormal, and reduced hexosaminidase A is found in serum and leukocytes.

Patients with **monoclonal gammopathy** may present with pure motor syndromes. Plasmapheresis and immunosuppressive drug treatment (with dexamethasone and cyclophosphamide) may be beneficial in such cases.

Anterior horn cell disease may occur as a rare complication of **lymphoma.** Both men and women are affected, and the symptoms typically have their onset after the diagnosis of lymphoma has been established. The principal manifestation is weakness, which primarily affects the legs, may be patchy in its distribution, and spares bulbar and respiratory muscles. The reflexes are depressed, and sensory abnormalities are minor or absent. Neurologic deficits usually progress over months, followed by spontaneous improvement and, in some cases, resolution.

INFECTIVE DISORDERS OF ANTERIOR HORN CELLS

Poliomyelitis—still common in certain parts of the world—has become rare in developed countries since the introduction of immunization programs. It is caused by an RNA virus of the picornavirus group. The usual route of infection is fecal-oral, and the incubation period varies between 5 and 35 days.

Neurologic involvement follows a prodromal phase of fever, myalgia, malaise, and upper respiratory or gastrointestinal symptoms in a small number of cases. This involvement may consist merely of aseptic meningitis but in some instances leads to weakness or paralysis. Weakness develops over the course of one or a few days, sometimes in association with recrudescence of fever, and is accompanied by myalgia and signs of meningeal irritation. The weakness is asymmetric in distribution and can be focal or unilateral; the bulbar and respiratory muscles may be affected either alone or in association with limb muscles. Tone is reduced in the affected muscles, and tendon reflexes may be lost. There is no sensory deficit.

CSF pressure is often mildly increased, and spinal fluid analysis characteristically shows an increased number of cells, a slightly elevated protein concentration, and a normal glucose level. Diagnosis may be confirmed by virus isolation from the stool or nasopharyngeal secretions—and less commonly from the CSF. A rise in viral antibody titer in convalescent-phase serum, compared with serum obtained during the acute phase of the illness, is also diagnostically helpful. A clinically similar disorder is produced by coxsackievirus infection.

There is no specific treatment, and management is purely supportive, with attention directed particularly to the maintenance of respiratory function. With time, there is often useful recovery of strength even in severely weakened muscles.

The **postpolio syndrome** is characterized by the occurrence some years after the original illness of increasing weakness in previously involved or seemingly uninvolved muscles. Muscle pain and ease of fatigue are common. Slow progression occurs and may lead to increasing restriction of daily activities. It probably relates to loss of anterior horn cells with aging from a pool that was depleted by the original infection. There is no specific treatment.

NERVE ROOT LESIONS

ACUTE INTERVERTEBRAL DISK PROLAPSE

Lumbar Disk Prolapse

Acute prolapse of a lumbar disk (Figure 5–4C and Table 5–11) generally leads to pain in the back and in a radicular distribution (L5 or S1) in the leg, where it is often accompanied by numbness and paresthesias. A motor deficit may also be found; this depends on the root affected. An L5 radiculopathy causes weakness of dorsiflexion of the foot and toes, whereas S1 root involve-

ment produces weakness of plantar flexion of the foot and a depressed ankle jerk. Movement of the spine is restricted, and there is local back tenderness and palpable spasm of the paraspinous muscles. Straight-leg raising in the supine position is restricted, often to about 20 or 30 degrees of hip flexion, from a normal value of about 80 or 90 degrees, because of reflex spasm of the hamstring muscles (**Lasègue's sign**). A centrally prolapsed disk can lead to bilateral symptoms and signs and to sphincter involvement.

The symptoms and signs of a prolapsed lumbar intervertebral disk can be either sudden or insidious in onset and may follow trauma. Pelvic and rectal examination and plain x-rays of the spine help to exclude lesions such as tumors.

Bed rest on a firm mattress for 1–2 weeks often permits symptoms to settle, but persisting pain, an increasing neurologic deficit, or any evidence of sphincter dysfunction should lead to CT, MRI, or myelography (Figure 11–5) followed by surgical treatment. Drug treatment for pain includes aspirin or acetaminophen with 30 mg of codeine, two doses three or four times daily, or other nonsteroidal analgesics such as ibuprofen or naproxen. Muscle spasm may respond to cyclobenzaprine, 10 mg orally three times daily or as needed and tolerated, or diazepam, 5–10 mg orally three times daily or as tolerated.

Cervical Disk Prolapse

Acute protrusion of a cervical disk can occur at any age, often with no preceding trauma, and leads to pain in the neck and radicular pain in the arm. The pain is exacerbated by head movement. With lateral herniation of the disk, a motor, sensory, or reflex deficit may be found in a radicular (usually C6 or C7) distribution on the affected side (Table 5–11); with more centrally directed herniations, the spinal cord may also be involved (Figure 5–4B), leading to a spastic paraparesis and sensory disturbance in the legs, sometimes accompanied by impaired sphincter function. The diagnosis is confirmed by CT scanning, MRI, or myelography. Surgical treatment may be needed.

CERVICAL SPONDYLOSIS

This disorder has been described on p 173.

TRAUMATIC AVULSION OF NERVE ROOTS

Erb-Duchenne Paralysis

Traumatic avulsion of the C5 and C6 roots can occur at birth as a result of traction on the head during delivery

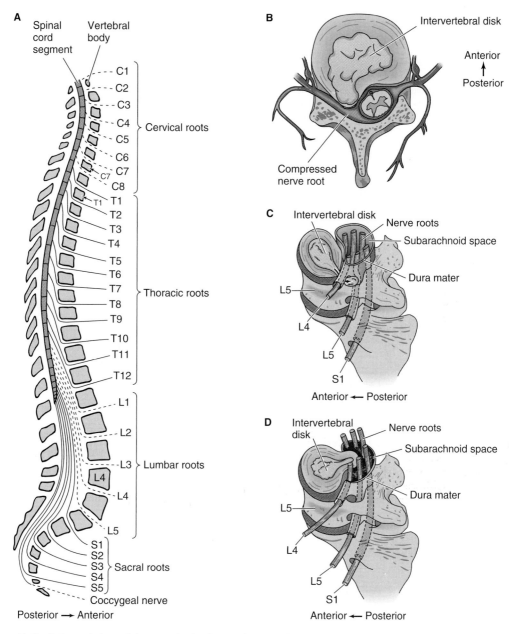

Figure 5–4. **A:** Lateral view of the vertebral column, showing the levels at which the various nerve roots exit; nerves exit above their numbered vertebral body in the cervical spine but below in the lumbar spine. **B:** Lateral disk prolapse in cervical spine, causing compression of exiting nerve root and compressing cervical cord. **C:** Lateral disk prolapse in lumbar spine, causing compression of the root existing at the next lower vertebral level (eg, L4 disk compresses the L5 nerve root). **D:** Central disk prolapse in lumbar spine, causing bilateral root compression.

of the shoulder. It can also be the result of injuries causing excessive separation of the head and shoulder. It leads to loss of shoulder abduction and elbow flexion. In consequence, the affected arm is held internally rotated

at the shoulder, with a pronated forearm and extended elbow. The biceps and brachioradialis jerks are lost, but sensory impairment is usually inconspicuous, since it is confined to a small area overlying the deltoid muscle.

Table 5–11. The most common patterns of weakness, sensory symptoms, and reflex changes in nerve root lesions.[1]

	C5	C6	C7	C8	L4	L5	S1
Weak muscle(s)	Deltoids > biceps	Biceps	Triceps, finger extensors	Finger extensors plus abductors of index and fifth fingers	Quadriceps	Great toe extension	Plantar flexion (tested standing-"get up on toes")
Pattern of sensory changes	Lateral upper arm	Thumb	Middle finger(s)	Little finger	Medial shin	Medial foot, great toe	Lateral foot, small toe
Depressed reflex		Biceps	Triceps		Knee		Ankle

[1] Overlap and individual variation occur. In some cases this summary table does not distinguish root from single nerve lesions. If a peripheral nerve lesion is suspected see Appendix C or Tables 5–5 and 5–6, p 163.

Klumpke's Paralysis

Involvement of the C8 and T1 roots causes paralysis and wasting of the small muscles of the hand and of the long finger flexors and extensors. Horner's syndrome is sometimes an associated finding. This kind of lower plexus paralysis often follows a fall that has been arrested by grasping a fixed object with one hand or may result from traction on the abducted arm.

NEURALGIC AMYOTROPHY (IDIOPATHIC BRACHIAL PLEXOPATHY)

This disorder typically begins with severe pain about the shoulder followed within a few days by weakness, reflex changes, and sensory disturbances in the arm, often involving the C5 and C6 segments especially. Symptoms and signs are usually unilateral but may be bilateral, and wasting of the affected muscles is often profound. The motor deficit sometimes corresponds to the territory of an individual nerve, especially the axillary, suprascapular, or radial nerve, but in other instances appears to arise in the brachial plexus. Its precise cause is unknown. It sometimes occurs shortly after minor injury, injections, inoculations, or minor systemic infections, but whether these are of etiologic relevance is unclear. Familial cases occur occasionally, as an autosomal dominant disorder characterized by recurrent symptoms. The disorder has been mapped to a genetic locus on chromosome 17q25 in some but not other cases.

Treatment is symptomatic. Recovery over the ensuing weeks and months is the rule—but it is sometimes incomplete.

CERVICAL RIB SYNDROME

The C8 and T1 roots or the lower trunk of the brachial plexus may be compressed by a cervical rib or band arising from the seventh cervical vertebra. This leads to weakness and wasting of intrinsic hand muscles, especially those in the thenar eminence, accompanied by pain and numbness in the appropriate dermatomal distribution (often like that of an ulnar nerve lesion but extending up the medial border of the forearm). The subclavian artery may also be compressed; this forms the basis of **Adson's test** for diagnosing the disorder. The radial pulse decreases in amplitude when the seated patient turns the head to the affected side and inhales deeply. A positive Adson's test, however, can also be seen in normal subjects; a supraclavicular bruit during the maneuver supports the diagnosis of subclavian artery compromise.

X-rays may show the cervical rib or a long transverse process of the seventh cervical vertebra, but normal findings do not exclude the possibility of a cervical band. Electromyography shows evidence of chronic partial denervation in the hand—in a territory beyond that of any individual peripheral nerve. Nerve conduction studies show no evidence of peripheral nerve disease, but there is a small or absent ulnar sensory nerve action potential on stimulation of the little finger.

Treatment is by surgical excision of the rib or band.

DISORDERS OF PERIPHERAL NERVES

The term **peripheral neuropathy** designates a disturbance in function of one or more peripheral nerves. Several types of peripheral neuropathy are distinguishable by the extent of involvement.

Depending upon the underlying cause, there may be selective involvement of motor, sensory, or autonomic fibers or more diffuse involvement of all fibers in the peripheral nerve.

The clinical deficit is usually a mixed one, and sensory symptoms and signs are often the initial—and most conspicuous—feature of peripheral nerve involvement. Further discussion of these disorders and their treatment is therefore deferred to Chapter 6, except in those instances in which presentation is typically with acute motor deficits. For convenience, however, the root and peripheral nerve supply of the major limb muscles is set forth in Tables 5–5 and 5–6. Reference to the tables should facilitate evaluation of patients presenting with focal weakness of lower motor neuron type.

POLYNEUROPATHY

In polyneuropathy, because there is symmetric and simultaneous involvement of various nerves, the deficits resulting from individual nerves cannot be recognized clinically. Polyneuropathies are discussed in Chapter 6, but brief mention is made here of those neuropathies in which patients present with acute weakness.

Acute Inflammatory Polyradiculoneuropathy (Guillain-Barré Syndrome)

This disorder commonly presents with weakness that is often symmetric and most commonly begins in the legs. The speed and extent of progression vary, but in severe cases there is marked weakness of all limbs in addition to bilateral facial weakness. There may also be subjective sensory complaints, although objective sensory disturbances are usually far less conspicuous than motor deficits. Autonomic involvement is common and may lead to a fatal outcome, as may aspiration pneumonia or impaired respiration from weakness. Further details about this disorder are given in Chapter 6.

Critical Illness Polyneuropathy

Patients with sepsis and multiorgan failure may develop a polyneuropathy that often first comes to attention when unexpected difficulty is encountered in weaning the patients from a mechanical ventilator. In more advanced cases, wasting and weakness of the extremities

are present and the tendon reflexes are lost. Sensory abnormalities are overshadowed by the motor deficit. Electrophysiologic studies reveal an axonal neuropathy. The underlying pathogenesis is obscure. Treatment is supportive, with the long-term outlook being good in patients who recover from the underlying critical illness.

Diphtheritic Polyneuritis

Infection with *Corynebacterium diphtheriae* can occur either in the upper respiratory tract or by infection of a skin wound, and neuropathy results from a neurotoxin that is released by the organism. Palatal weakness may develop 2–3 weeks after infection of the throat, and cutaneous diphtheria may be followed by focal weakness of neighboring muscles after a similar interval. Impaired pupillary responses to accommodation may occur about 4–5 weeks after infection and a generalized sensorimotor polyneuropathy after 1–3 months. The weakness may be asymmetric and is often more marked proximally than distally. Respiratory paralysis occurs in severe cases. Recovery usually occurs over the following 2–3 months but may take longer in severe cases.

In patients with polyneuropathy, CSF protein content is usually increased, and there may be a mild pleocytosis. Electrophysiologic studies show a slowing of nerve conduction velocity, but this is often not manifest until the patient has begun to improve clinically. Treatment consists of early administration of equine diphtheria antitoxin without awaiting the results of bacterial culture, provided the patient is not hypersensitive to horse serum. A 2-week course of penicillin or erythromycin will usually eradicate the infection but does not alter the incidence of serious complications. In patients with marked weakness, supportive measures, including ventilatory support, are necessary.

Paralytic Shellfish Poisoning

Mussels and clams found on the East and West Coasts of the United States may be dangerous to eat, especially in the summer months. They feed on poisonous varieties of plankton and come to contain saxitoxin, which blocks sodium channels—and therefore action potentials—in motor and sensory nerves and in muscle. A rapidly progressive acute peripheral neuropathy, with sensory symptoms and a rapidly ascending paralysis, begins within 30 minutes after eating affected shellfish and may lead to respiratory paralysis and death. There is no available antitoxin, but with proper supportive care (including mechanical ventilation if necessary) the patient recovers completely. A cathartic or enema may help remove unabsorbed toxin.

Porphyria

Acute polyneuropathy may occur with the hereditary hepatic porphyrias. Attacks can be precipitated by drugs (eg, barbiturates, estrogens, sulfonamides, griseofulvin, phenytoin, succinimides) that can induce the enzyme δ-aminolevulinic acid synthetase, or by infection, a period of fasting, or, occasionally, menses or pregnancy. Colicky abdominal pain frequently precedes neurologic involvement, and there may also be acute confusion or delirium and convulsions. Weakness is the major neurologic manifestation and is due to a predominantly motor polyneuropathy that causes a symmetric disturbance that is sometimes more marked proximally than distally. It may begin in the upper limbs and progress to involve the lower limbs or trunk. Progression occurs at a variable rate and can lead to complete flaccid quadriparesis with respiratory paralysis over a few days. Sensory loss occurs also but is less conspicuous and extensive. The tendon reflexes may be depressed or absent. The disorder may be accompanied by fever, persistent tachycardia, hypertension, hyponatremia, and peripheral leukocytosis. The CSF may show a slight increase in protein concentration and a slight pleocytosis. The diagnosis is confirmed by demonstrating increased levels of porphobilinogen and δ-aminolevulinic acid in the urine or deficiency of uroporphyrinogen I synthetase in red blood cells (**acute intermittent porphyria**) or of coproporphyrinogen oxidase in lymphocytes (**hereditary coproporphyria**).

Treatment is with intravenous dextrose to suppress the heme biosynthetic pathway and propranolol to control tachycardia and hypertension. Hematin, 4 mg/kg by intravenous infusion over 15 minutes once or twice daily, is also effective in improving the clinical state. The best index of progress is the heart rate. The abdominal and mental symptoms (but not the neuropathy) may be helped by chlorpromazine or another phenothiazine. Respiratory failure may necessitate tracheostomy and mechanical ventilation. Preventing acute attacks by avoiding known precipitants is important.

Acute Arsenic or Thallium Poisoning

Acute arsenic or thallium poisoning can produce a rapidly evolving sensorimotor polyneuropathy, often with an accompanying or preceding gastrointestinal disturbance. Arsenic may also cause a skin rash, with increased skin pigmentation and marked exfoliation, together with the presence of Mees lines (transverse white lines) on the nails in long-standing cases. Thallium can produce a scaly rash and hair loss. Sensory symptoms are often the earliest manifestation of polyneuropathy; this is followed by symmetric motor impairment, which is usually more marked distally than proximally and occurs in the legs rather than the arms. The CSF protein may be increased, with little or no change in cell content, and the electrophysiologic findings sometimes resemble those of Guillain-Barré syndrome, especially in the acute phase of the disorder. The diagnosis of arsenic toxicity is best estab-

lished by measuring the arsenic content of hair protected from external contamination (eg, hair from the pubic region). Urine also contains arsenic in the acute phase. The diagnosis of thallium poisoning is made by finding thallium in body tissues or fluids, especially in urine. The degree of neurologic recovery depends upon the severity of the intoxication.

Chelating agents are of uncertain value.

Organophosphate Polyneuropathy

Organophosphate compounds are widely used as insecticides and are also the active principles in the nerve gas of chemical warfare. They have a variety of acute toxic effects, particularly manifestations of cholinergic crisis caused by inhibition of acetylcholinesterase. Some organophosphates, however, also induce a delayed polyneuropathy that generally begins about 1–3 weeks after acute exposure. Cramping muscle pain in the legs is usually the initial symptom of neuropathy, sometimes followed by distal numbness and paresthesias. Progressive leg weakness then occurs, along with depression of the tendon reflexes. Similar deficits may develop in the upper limbs after several days. Sensory disturbances also develop in some instances, initially in the legs and then in the arms, but these disturbances are often mild or inconspicuous. Examination shows a distal symmetric, predominantly motor polyneuropathy, with wasting and flaccid weakness of distal leg muscles. In some patients, involvement may be severe enough to cause quadriplegia, whereas in others the weakness is much milder. Mild pyramidal signs may also be present. Objective evidence of sensory loss is usually slight. The acute effects of organophosphate poisoning may be prevented by the use of protective masks and clothing or by pretreatment with pyridostigmine, a short-acting acetylcholinesterase inhibitor. Treatment after exposure includes decontamination of the skin with bleach or soap and water and administration of atropine, 2–6 mg every 5 minutes, and pralidoxime, 1 g every hour for up to 3 hours, both given intramuscularly or intravenously. There is no treatment for the neuropathy other than supportive care. Recovery of peripheral nerve function may occur with time, but central deficits are usually permanent and may govern the extent of ultimate functional recovery.

MONONEUROPATHY MULTIPLEX

This term signifies that there is involvement of various nerves but in an asymmetric manner and at different times, so that the individual nerves involved can usually be identified until the disorder reaches an advanced stage. Comment here will be restricted to two disorders characterized by motor involvement in the absence of sensory symptoms and signs.

Lead Toxicity

Lead toxicity is common among persons involved in the manufacture or repair of storage batteries or other lead-containing products, the smelting of lead or lead-containing ores, and the shipbreaking industry. It may also occur in persons using lead-containing paints or those who ingest contaminated alcohol. Inorganic lead can produce dysfunction of both the central and peripheral nervous systems. In children, who can develop toxicity by ingesting lead-containing paints that flake off old buildings or furniture, acute encephalopathy is the major neurologic feature. The peripheral neuropathy is predominantly motor, and in adults it is more severe in the arms than in the legs. It typically affects the radial nerves, although other nerves may also be affected, leading to an asymmetric progressive motor disturbance. Sensory loss is usually inconspicuous or absent. There may be loss or depression of tendon reflexes. Systemic manifestations of lead toxicity include anemia, constipation, colicky abdominal pain, gum discoloration, and nephropathy. The extent to which exposed workers develop minor degrees of peripheral nerve damage as a result of lead toxicity is not clear. Similarly, there is no agreement about the lowest concentration of blood lead that is associated with damage to the peripheral nerves.

The optimal approach to treatment is not known, but intravenous or intramuscular edetate calcium disodium (EDTA) and oral penicillamine have been used, as has dimercaprol (BAL).

Multifocal Motor Neuropathy

This disorder is characterized by progressive asymmetric wasting and weakness, electrophysiologic evidence of multifocal motor demyelination with partial motor conduction block but normal sensory responses, and the presence of antiglycolipid (usually anti-GM1 IgM) antibodies in the serum of many patients. Cramps and fasciculations sometimes occur and may lead to an erroneous diagnosis of motor neuron disease unless electrophysiologic studies are performed. Treatment with prednisone and plasmapheresis has been disappointing, but patients may improve after treatment with cyclophosphamide, 1 g/m^2 intravenously once a month for 6 months, or in response to human immunoglobulin, 2 g/kg intravenously, given over 3–5 days. Improvement is sometimes associated with a decrease in anti-GM1 antibody levels.

MONONEUROPATHY SIMPLEX

In mononeuropathy simplex there is involvement of a single peripheral nerve. Most of the common mononeuropathies entail both motor and sensory involvement (as discussed in Chapter 6). Accordingly, only Bell's palsy, which leads primarily to a motor deficit, is discussed here.

Bell's Palsy

Facial weakness of the lower motor neuron type caused by idiopathic facial nerve involvement outside the central nervous system, without evidence of aural or more widespread neurologic disease, has been designated Bell's palsy. The cause is unclear, but the disorder occurs more commonly in pregnant women and diabetics. Increasing evidence suggests that reactivation of herpes simplex virus type 1 infection in the geniculate ganglion may injure the facial nerve and is responsible for Bell's palsy in at least some patients.

Facial weakness is often preceded or accompanied by pain about the ear. Weakness generally comes on abruptly but may progress over several hours or even a day or so. Depending upon the site of the lesion, there may be associated impairment of taste, lacrimation, or hyperacusis. There may be paralysis of all muscles supplied by the affected nerve (**complete palsy**) or variable weakness in different muscles (**incomplete palsy**). Clinical examination reveals no abnormalities beyond the territory of the facial nerve. Most patients recover completely without treatment, but this may take several days in some instances and several months in others. A poor prognosis for complete recovery is suggested by severe pain at onset and complete palsy when the patient is first seen. Even if recovery is incomplete, permanent disfigurement or some other complication affects only about 10% of patients. It is not clear whether treatment with acyclovir or other antiviral agents confers any benefit, as the results of methodologically dissimilar studies have been conflicting. Treatment with corticosteroids (prednisone, 60 mg/d orally for 3 days, tapering over the next 7 days), beginning within 5 days after the onset of palsy, is said to increase the proportion of patients who recover completely. It should therefore be prescribed in patients who have a poor prognosis. However, the evidence that corticosteroids are indeed beneficial is incomplete, and they may have unpleasant side effects. Other conditions that can produce facial palsy include tumors, herpes zoster infection of the geniculate ganglion (Ramsay Hunt syndrome), Lyme disease, AIDS, and sarcoidosis.

DISORDERS OF NEUROMUSCULAR TRANSMISSION

MYASTHENIA GRAVIS

Myasthenia gravis can occur at any age and is sometimes associated with thymic tumor, thyrotoxicosis, rheumatoid arthritis, or disseminated lupus erythematosus. More common in females than males, it is characterized by fluctuating weakness and easy fatigability of voluntary muscles; muscle activity cannot be maintained, and initially powerful movements weaken readily. There is a predilection for the external ocular muscles and certain other cranial muscles, including the masticatory, facial, pharyngeal, and laryngeal muscles. Respiratory and limb muscles may also be affected. Weakness is due to a variable block of neuromuscular transmission related to an immune-mediated decrease in the number of functioning acetylcholine receptors (Figure 5–5). In approximately 80% of cases, antibodies to the muscle nicotinic acetylcholine receptor are present and lead to loss of receptor function. In patients seronegative for these antibodies, the disease is probably also immune mediated; many of these patients have antibodies against the muscle-specific receptor tyrosine kinase (MuSK) that is involved in the clustering of acetylcholine receptors during development and is also expressed in mature neuromuscular junctions.

A similar disorder in patients receiving penicillamine for rheumatoid arthritis frequently remits when the drug is discontinued.

Clinical Findings

Although the onset of the disease is usually insidious, the disorder is sometimes unmasked by a concurrent infection, which leads to an exacerbation of symptoms. Exacerbations may also occur in pregnancy or before menses. Symptoms may be worsened by quinine, quinidine, procainamide, propranolol, phenytoin, lithium, tetracycline, and aminoglycoside antibiotics, which should therefore be avoided in such patients. Myasthenia follows a slowly progressive course. Patients present with ptosis, diplopia, difficulty in chewing or swallowing, nasal speech, respiratory difficulties, or weakness of the limbs (Table 5–12). These symptoms often fluctuate in intensity during the day, and this diurnal variation is superimposed on longer-term spontaneous relapses and remissions that may last for weeks.

Clinical examination confirms the weakness and fatigability of affected muscles. The weakness does not conform to the distribution of any single nerve, root, or level of the central nervous system. In more than 90% of cases the extraocular muscles are involved, leading to often asymmetric ocular palsies and ptosis. Pupillary responses are not affected. The characteristic feature of the disorder is that sustained activity of affected muscles leads to temporarily increased weakness. Thus, sustained upgaze for 2 minutes can lead to increased ptosis, with power in the affected muscles improving after a brief rest. In advanced cases, there may be some mild atrophy of affected muscles. Sensation is normal, and there are usually no reflex changes.

Diagnosis

The diagnosis of myasthenia gravis can generally be confirmed by the benefit that follows administration of anticholinesterase drugs; the power of affected muscles is influenced at a dose that has no effect on normal muscles and slight, if any, effect on muscles weakened by other causes.

The most commonly used pharmacological test is the **edrophonium** (**Tensilon**) **test.** Edrophonium is given intravenously in a dose of 10 mg (1 mL), of which 2 mg is given initially and the remaining 8 mg about 30 seconds later if the test dose is well tolerated. In myasthenic patients, there is an obvious improvement in the strength of weak muscles that lasts for about 5 minutes.

Alternatively, 1.5 mg of **neostigmine** can be given intramuscularly, with a response that lasts for about 2 hours; atropine sulfate (0.6 mg) should be available to counteract the muscarinic cholinergic side effects of increased salivation, diarrhea, and nausea. Atropine does not affect nicotinic cholinergic function at the neuromuscular junction. The longer-acting neostigmine reduces the incidence of false-negative evaluations.

Investigative Studies

X-rays and CT scans of the chest may reveal a coexisting thymoma. Impaired neuromuscular transmission can be detected electrophysiologically by a decremental response of muscle to repetitive supramaximal stimulation (at 2 or 3 Hz) of its motor nerve, but normal findings do not exclude the diagnosis. Single-fiber electromyography shows increased variability in the interval between two muscle fiber action potentials from the same motor unit in clinically weak muscles. Measuring serum acetylcholine receptor antibody levels is often helpful, since increased values are found in 80–90% of patients with generalized myasthenia gravis.

Treatment

Medications (referred to earlier) that impair neuromuscular transmission should be avoided. The following approaches to treatment are recommended.

A. ANTICHOLINESTERASE DRUGS

Treatment with these drugs provides symptomatic benefit without influencing the course of the underlying disease. The mainstay of treatment is pyridostigmine, at doses individually determined but usually between 30 and 180 mg (average, 60 mg) four times daily. The older drug neostigmine may still be used, in rare instances, by parenteral administration. Small doses of atropine may attenuate side effects such as bowel hypermotility or hypersalivation. Overmedication can lead to increased weakness, which, unlike myasthenic weakness, is unaffected or enhanced by intravenous edrophonium. Such a **cholinergic crisis** may be accompanied by pallor, sweating, nausea, vomiting, salivation, colicky abdominal pain, and miosis.

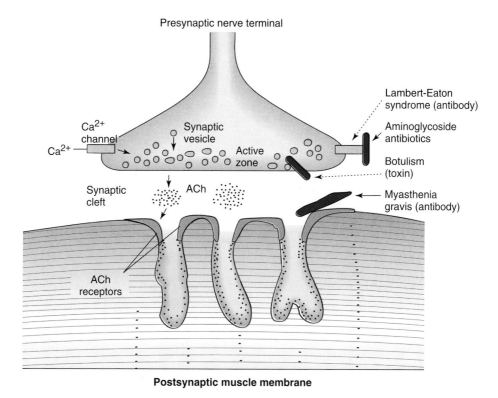

Presynaptic nerve terminal

Postsynaptic muscle membrane

Figure 5–5. Sites of involvement in disorders of neuromuscular transmission. At left, normal transmission involves depolarization-induced influx of calcium (Ca) through voltage-gated channels. This stimulates release of acetylcholine (ACh) from synaptic vesicles at the active zone and into the synaptic cleft. ACh binds to ACh receptors and depolarizes the postsynaptic muscle membrane. At right, disorders of neuromuscular transmission result from blockage of Ca channels (Lambert-Eaton syndrome or aminoglycoside antibiotics), impairment of Ca-mediated ACh release (botulinum toxin), or antibody-induced internalization and degradation of ACh receptors (myasthenia gravis).

Table 5–12. Presenting symptoms in myasthenia gravis.[1]

Symptom	Percentage of Patients
Diplopia	41
Ptosis	25
Dysarthria	16
Lower extremity weakness	13
Generalized weakness	11
Dysphagia	10
Upper extremity weakness	7
Masticatory weakness	7

[1] Adapted from Herrmann C Jr: Myasthenia gravis—Current concepts. West J Med 1985;142:797–809.

B. THYMECTOMY

Thymectomy should be performed in patients under 60 years of age, and considered in those older, with weakness that is not restricted to the extraocular muscles. Although thymectomy usually leads to symptomatic benefit or remission, the mechanism by which it confers benefit is unclear, and its beneficial effect may not be evident immediately.

C. CORTICOSTEROIDS

Corticosteroids are indicated for patients who have responded poorly to anticholinesterase drugs and have already undergone thymectomy. Treatment is initiated with the patient in the hospital, as weakness may initially be exacerbated. An initial high dose of prednisone (60–100 mg/d orally) can gradually be tapered to a relatively low maintenance level (5–15 mg/d) as improvement occurs. Alternate-day treatment is helpful in reducing the incidence of side effects, which are described (as clinical findings) in the section on hyperadrenalism in Chapter 1.

D. AZATHIOPRINE

This drug can be used in patients with severe or progressive disease despite thymectomy and treatment with anticholinesterases and corticosteroids. It can also be given in place of high doses of corticosteroids to patients who show no sustained benefit with low doses. The usual dose is 2–3 mg/kg/d, increased from a lower initial dose.

E. PLASMAPHERESIS

Plasmapheresis may be used to achieve temporary improvement in patients deteriorating rapidly or in myasthenic crisis, and in certain special circumstances, such as prior to surgery that is likely to produce postoperative respiratory compromise.

F. INTRAVENOUS IMMUNOGLOBULINS

Intravenous immunoglobulins have also been used to provide temporary benefit in circumstances similar to those in which plasmapheresis is used.

G. MYCOPHENOLATE MOFETIL

This agent selectively inhibits proliferation of T and B lymphocytes and has been used as an immunosuppressant with only modest side effects, including diarrhea, nausea, abdominal pain, fever, leukopenia, and edema. Preliminary studies indicate that many patients with myasthenia gravis improve or are able to lower their steroid intake in response to this medication (1 g twice daily by mouth), but usually after a delay of several months.

Prognosis

Most patients can be managed successfully with drug treatment. The disease may have a fatal outcome because of respiratory complications such as aspiration pneumonia.

MYASTHENIC SYNDROME (LAMBERT-EATON SYNDROME)

This disorder has a well-recognized association with an underlying neoplasm and may occasionally be associated with such autoimmune diseases as pernicious anemia; occasionally no cause is found. In the paraneoplastic disorder, antibodies directed against tumor antigens cross-react with voltage-gated calcium channels involved in acetylcholine release, leading to a disturbance of neuromuscular transmission (see Figure 5–5).

Clinically there is weakness, especially of the proximal muscles of the limbs. Unlike myasthenia gravis, however, the extraocular muscles are characteristically spared, and power steadily increases if a contraction is maintained. Autonomic disturbances, such as dry mouth, constipation, and impotence, may also occur.

The diagnosis is confirmed electrophysiologically by the response to repetitive nerve stimulation. There is a remarkable increase in the size of the muscle response to stimulation of its motor nerve at high rates—even in muscles that are not clinically weak. The presence of autoantibodies to the P/Q subtype of voltage-gated calcium channels, found on the presynaptic membrane of the neuromuscular junction, is highly sensitive and specific to the Lambert-Eaton syndrome of any etiology.

Immunosuppressive drug therapy (corticosteroids and azathioprine as described earlier for myasthenia gravis) and plasmapheresis or intravenous immunoglobulin therapy may lead to improvement. Guanidine hydrochloride, 25–50 mg/kg/d in three or four divided doses, is sometimes helpful in seriously disabled patients, but adverse effects of the drug include bone marrow suppression and renal failure. The response to treatment with anticholinesterase drugs such as pyridostigmine or neostigmine, alone or in combination with guanidine, is variable. 3,4-Diaminopyridine (investigational in the United States), at doses up to 25 mg orally four times daily, may improve weakness and autonomic dysfunction; paresthesia is a common side effect, and seizures may occur. The disease improves with treatment of the underlying condition.

BOTULISM

The toxin of *Clostridium botulinum* can cause neuromuscular paralysis. It acts by preventing the release of acetylcholine at neuromuscular junctions and autonomic synapses (Figure 5–5). Botulism occurs most commonly following ingestion of home-canned food that is contaminated with the toxin; it occurs rarely from infected wounds. The shorter the latent period between ingestion of the toxin and the onset of symptoms, the greater the dose of toxin and the risk for further involvement of the nervous system.

Clinical Findings

Fulminating weakness begins 12–72 hours after ingestion of the toxin and characteristically is manifested by diplopia, ptosis, facial weakness, dysphagia, nasal speech, and then difficulty with respiration; weakness usually appears last in the limbs. In addition to the motor deficit, blurring of vision is characteristic, and there may be dryness of the mouth, paralytic ileus, and postural hypotension. There is no sensory deficit, and the tendon reflexes are usually unchanged unless the involved muscles are quite weak. Symptoms can progress for several days after their onset.

The **periodic paralysis syndromes,** which may be familial (dominant inheritance), are characterized by episodes of flaccid weakness or paralysis that may be associated with abnormalities of the plasma potassium level. Strength is normal between attacks. In the **hypokalemic form,** sometimes associated with **thyrotoxicosis,** attacks tend to occur on awakening, after exercise, or after a heavy meal—and may last for several days. The disorder is due to a mutation in the gene encoding the dihydropyridine receptor on chromosome 1q32. The clinical disorder is genetically heterogeneous and has also been associated with mutations at 11q13–q14 and at 17q23.1–q25.3.

Acetazolamide or oral potassium supplements often prevent attacks, and ongoing attacks may be aborted by potassium chloride given orally or even intravenously. If hyperthyroidism is associated, its treatment may prevent recurrences. Attacks associated with **hyperkalemia** also tend to come on after exercise but are usually much briefer, lasting less than 1 hour. Severe attacks may be terminated by intravenous calcium gluconate, intravenous diuretics (furosemide, 20–40 mg), or glucose, while daily acetazolamide or chlorothiazide may help prevent further episodes. Many families with this disorder have a defect in the sodium channel gene (SCN4A) for the α-subunit on chromosome 17q23.1–q25.3; several allelic mutations have been recognized and account for some phenotypic variation, such as the presence of myotonia or paramyotonia. **Paramyotonia congenita** is a dominantly inherited disorder, related to mutation of the SCN4A gene, in which weakness and myotonia are provoked by cold and worsened by exercise; attacks of hyperkalemic periodic paralysis may also occur. **Normokalemic** periodic paralysis is sometimes unresponsive to treatment; in severe attacks, it may be impossible to move the limbs, but respiration and swallowing are rarely affected.

Proximal muscle weakness may also occur in **osteomalacia,** often with associated bone pain and tenderness, mild hypocalcemia, and elevated serum alkaline phosphatase. Strength improves following treatment with vitamin D.

ENDOCRINE MYOPATHIES

Myopathy may occur in association with hyper- or hypothyroidism, hyper- or hypoparathyroidism, hyper- or hypoadrenalism, hypopituitarism, and acromegaly. Treatment is that of the underlying endocrine disorder.

ALCOHOLIC MYOPATHIES

Acute Necrotizing Myopathy

Heavy binge drinking may result in an acute necrotizing myopathy that develops over 1 or 2 days. Presenting symptoms include muscle pain, weakness, and sometimes dysphagia. On examination, the affected muscles are swollen, tender, and weak. Weakness is proximal in distribution and may be asymmetric or focal. Serum CK is moderately to severely elevated, and myoglobinuria may occur. As hypokalemia and hypophosphatemia can produce a similar syndrome in alcoholic patients, serum potassium and phosphorus concentrations should be determined. With abstinence from alcohol and a nutritionally adequate diet, recovery can be expected over a period of weeks to months.

Chronic Myopathy

Chronic myopathy characterized by proximal weakness of the lower limbs may develop insidiously over weeks to months in alcoholic patients. Muscle pain is not a prominent feature. Cessation of drinking and an improved diet are associated with clinical improvement over several months in most cases.

DRUG-INDUCED MYOPATHIES

Myopathy can occur in association with administration of corticosteroids, chloroquine, clofibrate, emetine, aminocaproic acid, certain β-blockers, bretylium tosylate, colchicine, HMG-CoA reductase inhibitors, zidovudine, or drugs that cause potassium depletion.

MYOGLOBINURIA

This can result from muscle injury or ischemia (irrespective of its cause) and leads to a urine that is dark red. The following causes are important:

- Excessive unaccustomed exercise, leading to muscle necrosis (rhabdomyolysis) and thus to myoglobinuria, sometimes on a familial basis.
- Crush injuries.
- Muscle infarction.
- Prolonged tonic-clonic convulsions.
- Polymyositis.
- Chronic potassium depletion.
- An acute alcoholic binge.
- Certain viral infections associated with muscle weakness and pain.
- Hyperthermia.
- Metabolic myopathies (eg, McArdle's disease).

Serum CK levels are elevated, often greatly. Myoglobin can be detected in the urine by the dipstick test for heme pigment; a positive test indicates the presence of myoglobin in the urine unless red blood cells are present. In severe cases, myoglobinuria may lead to renal failure, and peritoneal dialysis or hemodialysis may then be necessary. Otherwise, treatment consists of increasing the urine volume by hydration. The serum potassium level must be monitored, as it may rise rapidly.

MOTOR-UNIT HYPERACTIVITY STATES

Disorders affecting the central or peripheral nervous system at a variety of sites can produce abnormal, increased activity in the motor unit (Table 5–17).

CENTRAL DISORDERS

Stiff-Person Syndrome

This is a rare, usually sporadic, and slowly progressive disorder manifested by tightness, stiffness, and rigidity of axial and proximal limb muscles with superimposed painful spasms that may be accompanied by hyperhidrosis and an increase in blood pressure. Examination may show tight muscles, a slow or cautious gait, and hyperreflexia. The disorder sometimes has an autoimmune basis and it may be associated with other autoimmune disorders. Many patients have diabetes. Stiff-person syndrome can be distinguished from tetanus by its more gradual onset and by the absence of trismus (lockjaw). In some cases, the blood contains autoantibodies against glutamic acid decarboxylase, which is involved in synthesis of the neurotransmitter γ-aminobutyric acid (GABA), and is concentrated in pancreatic β-cells and in GABAergic neurons of the central nervous system. A defect in central GABAergic transmission has been proposed as the cause of the disorder, and treatment is with drugs that enhance GABAergic transmission, such as diazepam, 5–75 mg orally four times daily. Baclofen, vigabatrin, sodium valproate, and gabapentin may also be helpful for relieving symptoms in some patients. Treatment with intravenous immunoglobulins is sometimes effective in refractory cases.

Table 5–17. Motor-unit hyperactivity states.

Site of Pathology	Syndrome	Clinical Features	Treatment
Central nervous system	Stiff-person syndrome	Rigidity, spasms	Diazepam Baclofen Sodium valproate Vigabatrin Gabapentin Immunosuppression
	Tetanus	Rigidity, spasms	Diazepam
Peripheral nerve	Cramps	Painful contraction of single muscle relieved by passive stretch	Quinine Phenytoin Carbamazepine
	Neuromyotonia	Stiffness, myokymia, delayed relaxation	Phenytoin Carbamazepine
	Tetany	Chvostek's sign	Calcium
		Trousseau's sign Carpopedal spasm	Magnesium Correction of alkalosis
	Hemifacial spasm	Involuntary hemifacial contraction	Carbamazepine Botulinum toxin Decompressive surgery
Muscle	Myotonia	Delayed relaxation, percussion myotonia	Phenytoin Carbamazepine Procainamide Quinine Tocainide Mexilitene
	Malignant hyperthermia	Rigidity, fever	Dantrolene

Tetanus

Tetanus, a disorder of central inhibitory neurotransmission caused by a toxin produced by *Clostridium tetani*, is discussed earlier in this chapter.

PERIPHERAL NERVE DISORDERS

Cramps

These involuntary and typically painful contractions of a muscle or portion of a muscle are thought to arise distally in the motor neuron. Palpable knotlike hardening of the muscle may occur. Cramps are characteristically relieved by passive stretching of the affected muscle. They usually represent a benign condition and are common at night or during or after exercise. However, cramps may also be a manifestation of motor neuron disease or polyneuropathy, metabolic disturbances (pregnancy, uremia, hypothyroidism, adrenal insufficiency), or fluid or electrolyte disorders (dehydration, hemodialysis). If a reversible underlying cause cannot be found, daytime cramps may respond to treatment with phenytoin, 300–400 mg/d orally, or carbamazepine, 200–400 mg orally three times a day. Nocturnal cramps may respond to a single oral bedtime dose of quinine sulfate (325 mg), phenytoin (100–300 mg), carbamazepine (200–400 mg), or diazepam (5–10 mg).

Neuromyotonia

Neuromyotonia (**Isaacs' syndrome**) is a rare, sporadic disorder that produces continuous muscle stiffness, rippling muscle movements (**myokymia**), and delayed relaxation following muscle contraction. Some cases have an autosomal dominant mode of inheritance; in others, the neuromyotonia occurs as a paraneoplastic disorder, or in association with other autoimmune diseases or with hereditary motor and sensory neuropathies. It may also follow irradiation of the nervous system. In acquired neuromyotonia, antibodies against voltage-gated potassium channels are often found in the serum and CSF.

Symptoms may be controlled with phenytoin, 300–400 mg/d orally, or carbamazepine, 200–400 mg orally three times a day.

Tetany

Tetany—not to be confused with tetanus (see above)—is a hyperexcitable state of peripheral nerves usually associated with hypocalcemia, hypomagnesemia, or alkalosis. Signs of tetany (Chvostek's sign, Trousseau's sign, carpopedal spasm) are described in the section on hypocalcemia in Chapter 1. Treatment is by correction of the underlying electrolyte disorder.

Hemifacial Spasm

Hemifacial spasm is characterized by repetitive, involuntary contractions of some or all of the muscles supplied by one facial nerve. Symptoms often commence in the orbicularis oculi and then spread to the cheek and levator anguli oris muscles. The contractions initially are brief but become more sustained as the disorder progresses; they may be provoked by blinking or voluntary activity. Slight facial weakness may also be found on examination. The disorder commonly relates to the presence of an anomalous blood vessel compressing the intracranial facial nerve, but MRI should be performed to exclude other structural lesions. The involuntary movements have been attributed to ephaptic transmission and ectopic excitation of demyelinated fibers in the compressed segment, to altered excitability of the facial nerve nucleus in the brainstem, or to both mechanisms. Treatment with carbamazepine or phenytoin is sometimes helpful, and injection of botulinum toxin into the affected muscles suppresses the contractions temporarily. Microvascular decompressive procedures are often curative.

MUSCLE DISORDERS

Myotonia

Disorders that produce myotonia are discussed on p 190.

Malignant Hyperthermia

This disorder, which is often inherited in autosomal dominant fashion, is due to a defect of the ryanodine receptor gene on the long arm of chromosome 19. The clinical abnormality is thought to result from abnormal excitation-contraction coupling in skeletal muscle. Symptoms are usually precipitated by administration of neuromuscular blocking agents (eg, succinylcholine) or inhalational anesthetics. Clinical features include rigidity, hyperthermia, metabolic acidosis, and myoglobinuria. Mortality rates as high as 70% have been reported. Treatment includes prompt cessation of anesthesia; administration of the excitation-contraction uncoupler dantrolene, 1–2 mg/kg intravenously every 5–10 minutes as needed, to a maximum dose of 10 mg/kg; reduction of body temperature; and correction of acidosis with intravenous bicarbonate. Patients who require surgery and are known or suspected to have malignant hyperthermia should be pretreated with dantrolene (four 1-mg/kg oral doses) on the day prior to surgery. Preoperative administration of atropine (which can also cause hyperthermia) should be avoided, and the anesthetics used should be restricted to those known to be safe in this condition (nitrous oxide, opiates, barbiturates, droperidol).

REFERENCES

General

Ackerman MJ, Clapham DE: Ion channels—basic science and clinical disease. N Engl J Med 1997;336:1575–1586.

Aminoff MJ: *Electromyography in Clinical Practice,* 3rd ed. Churchill Livingstone, 1998.

Aminoff MJ (editor): *Neurology and General Medicine,* 3rd ed. Churchill Livingstone, 2001.

Argov Z, Lofberg M, Arnold DL: Insights into muscle diseases gained by phosphorus magnetic resonance spectroscopy. Muscle Nerve 2000;23:1316–1334.

Brown P: Pathophysiology of spasticity. J Neurol Neurosurg Psychiatry 1994;57:773–777.

Critchley E, Eisen A (editors): *Spinal Cord Disease.* Springer, 1997.

Dalakas MC: Intravenous immunoglobulin in the treatment of autoimmune neuromuscular diseases: present status and practical therapeutic guidelines. Muscle Nerve 1999;22:1479–1497.

Engel AG, Franzini-Armstrong C (editors): *Myology: Basic and Clinical.* McGraw-Hill, 1994.

Engel AG (editor): *Myasthenia Gravis and Myasthenic Disorders.* Oxford University Press, 1999.

Fife TD, Baloh RW: Disequilibrium of unknown cause in older people. Ann Neurol 1993;34:694–702.

Griggs RC et al: *Evaluation and Treatment of Myopathies.* Davis, 1995.

Hallett M: NINDS myotatic reflex scale. Neurology 1993;43:2723.

Kokontis L, Gutmann L: Current treatment of neuromuscular diseases. Arch Neurol 2000;57:939–943.

Layzer RB: *Neuromuscular Manifestations of Systemic Disease.* Vol 25 of: *Contemporary Neurology Series.* Davis, 1984.

Lieberman AP, Fischbeck KH: Triplet repeat expansion in neuromuscular disease. Muscle Nerve 2000;23:843–850.

Nutt JG, Marsden CD, Thompson PD: Human walking and higher-level gait disorders, particularly in the elderly. Neurology 1993;43:268–279.

Rudnicki SA, Dalmau J: Paraneoplastic syndromes of the spinal cord, nerve, and muscle. Muscle Nerve 2000;23:1800–1818.

Schapira AV, Griggs RC: *Muscle Diseases.* Butterworth-Heinemann, 1999.

Smyth MD, Peacock WJ: The surgical treatment of spasticity. Muscle Nerve 2000;23:153–163.

Spencer PS, Schaumburg HH (editors): *Experimental and Clinical Neurotoxicology,* 2nd ed. Oxford University Press, 2000.

Spinner RJ, Kline DG: Surgery for peripheral nerve and brachial plexus injuries or other nerve lesions. Muscle Nerve 2000;23:680–695.

Strober JB: Genetics of pediatric neuromuscular disease. Curr Opin Pediatr 2000;12:549–553.

Sudarsky L: Geriatrics: Gait disorders in the elderly. N Engl J Med 1990;322:1441–1446.

Wulff EA, Simpson DM: Neuromuscular complications of HIV-1 infection. Curr Infect Dis Rep 1999;1:192–197.

Spinal Cord Disorders

Achiron A et al: Intravenous immunoglobulin treatment in multiple sclerosis: effect on relapses. Neurology 1998;50:398–402.

Aminoff MJ: Spinal vascular disease. Pages 423–442 in: *Spinal Cord Disease.* Critchley E, Eisen A (editors). Springer, 1997.

Balestri P et al: Plasmapheresis in a child with acute disseminated encephalomyelitis. Brain Dev 2000;22:123–126.

Bitsch A et al: Acute axonal injury in multiple sclerosis: correlation with demyelination and inflammation. Brain 2000;123:1174–1183.

Bracken MB et al: A randomized, controlled trial of methylprednisolone or naloxone in the treatment of acute spinal-cord injury. N Engl J Med 1990;322:1405–1411.

Byrne TN, Waxman SG: Spinal Cord Compression. Vol 33 of: *Contemporary Neurology Series.* Davis, 1990.

Chabert E et al: Intramedullary cavernous malformations. J Neuroradiol 1999;26:262–268.

Cheshire WP et al: Spinal cord infarction: etiology and outcome. Neurology 1996;47:321–330.

Darouiche RO et al: Bacterial spinal epidural abscess: review of 43 cases and literature survey. Medicine 1992;71:369–385.

DiRocco A: Diseases of the spinal cord in human immunodeficiency virus infection. Semin Neurol 1999;19:151–155.

Dittuno JF, Formal CS: Chronic spinal cord injury. N Engl J Med 1994;330:550–556.

Engstrom JW: HTLV-I infection and the nervous system. Pages 777–788 in: *Neurology and General Medicine,* 3rd ed. Aminoff MJ (editor). Churchill Livingstone, 2001.

Forsyth PA, Roa WH: Primary central nervous system tumors in adults. Curr Treat Options Neurol 1999;1:377–394.

Geraci A et al: AIDS myelopathy is not associated with elevated HIV viral load in cerebrospinal fluid. Neurology 2000;55:440–442.

Gezen F et al: Review of 36 cases of spinal cord meningioma. Spine 2000;25:727–731.

Goodin DS et al: The relationship of MS to physical trauma and psychological stress: report of the Therapeutics and Technology Assessment Subcommittee of the American Academy of Neurology. Neurology 1999;52:1737–1745.

Harrington WJJ et al: Spastic ataxia associated with human T-cell lymphotropic virus type II infection. Ann Neurol 1993;33:411–414.

Houser OW et al: Cervical spondylotic stenosis and myelopathy: evaluation with computed tomographic myelography. Mayo Clin Proc 1994;69:557–563.

IFNB Multiple Sclerosis Study Group and the University of British Columbia MS/MRI Analysis Group: Interferon beta-1b in the treatment of multiple sclerosis: final outcome of the randomized controlled trial. Neurology 1995;45:1277–1285.

Jacobs LD et al: Intramuscular interferon beta-1a therapy initiated during a first demyelinating event in multiple sclerosis. N Engl J Med 2000;343:898–904.

Jacobson S et al: Isolation of HTLV-II from a patient with chronic, progressive neurological disease clinically indistinguishable from HTLV-I-associated myelopathy/tropical spastic paraparesis. Ann Neurol 1993;33:392–396.

Johnson KP et al: Copolymer 1 reduces relapse rate and improves disability in relapsing-remitting multiple sclerosis. Neurology 1995;45:1268–1276.

Johnson KP et al: Extended use of glatiramer acetate (Copaxone) is well tolerated and maintains its clinical effects on multiple sclerosis relapse rate and degree of disability. Neurology 1998;50:701–708.

Lonjon MM et al: Nontraumatic spinal epidural hematoma: report of four cases and review of the literature. Neurosurgery 1997;41:483–486.

Lucchinetti C et al: Heterogeneity of multiple sclerosis lesions: implications for the pathogenesis of demyelination. Ann Neurol 2000;47:707–717.

Miller DH et al: Effect of interferon-1b on magnetic resonance imaging outcomes in secondary progressive multiple sclerosis: results of a European multicenter, randomized, double-blind, placebo-controlled trial. Ann Neurol 1999;46:850–859.

Nishikawa M et al: Intravenous immunoglobulin therapy in acute disseminated encephalomyelitis. Pediatr Neurol 1999;21:583–586.

Noseworthy JH, Lucchinetti C, Rodriguez M, Weinshenker BG: Multiple sclerosis. N Engl J Med 2000;343:938–952.

Once Weekly Interferon for MS Study Group: Evidence of interferon beta-1a dose response in relapsing-remitting MS. Neurology 1999;53:679–686.

Panitch HS: Influence of infection on exacerbations of multiple sclerosis. Ann Neurol 1994;36:S25–S28.

Petito CK et al: Vacuolar myelopathy pathologically resembling subacute combined degeneration in patients with the acquired immunodeficiency syndrome. N Engl J Med 1985;312:874–879.

Rodichok LD et al: Early diagnosis of spinal epidural metastases. Am J Med 1981;70:1181–1188.

Rudick RA et al: Management of multiple sclerosis. N Engl J Med 1997;337:1604–1611.

Sahlas DJ et al: Treatment of acute disseminated encephalomyelitis with intravenous immunoglobulin. Neurology 2000;54:1370–1372.

Sampath P et al: Outcome of patients treated for cervical myelopathy. A prospective, multicenter study with independent clinical review. Spine 2000;25:670–676.

Sandson TA, Friedman JH: Spinal cord infarction: report of 8 cases and review of the literature. Medicine 1989;68:282–292.

Sorensen PS et al: Intravenous immunoglobulin G reduces MRI activity in relapsing multiple sclerosis. Neurology 1998;50:1273–1281.

Staudinger R, Henry K: Remission of HIV myelopathy after highly active antiretroviral therapy. Neurology 2000;54:267–268.

Sypert GW, Cole HO: Management of multilevel cervical spondylosis with myelopathy. Surg Neurol 1999;51:4–5.

Taylor GP: Pathogenesis and treatment of HTLV-I associated myelopathy. Sex Transm Infect 1998;74:316–322.

Trapp BD et al: Axonal transection in the lesions of multiple sclerosis. N Engl J Med 1998;338:278–285.

Wagstaff AJ, Bryson HM: Tizanidine. Drugs 1997;53:435–452.

Yonenobu K: Cervical radiculopathy and myelopathy: when and what can surgery contribute to treatment? Eur Spine J 2000;9:1–7.

Zevgaridis D et al: Cavernous haemangiomas of the spinal cord. A review of 117 cases. Acta Neurochir 1999;141:237–245.

Anterior Horn Cell Disease

Al-Chalabi A, Leigh PN: Recent advances in amyotrophic lateral sclerosis. Curr Opin Neurol 2000;13:397–405.

Aminoff MJ, Olney R, So YT: X-linked recessive bulbospinal neuronopathy: distinction from other motor neuron diseases. Pages 31–37 in: *ALS—From Charcot to the Present and into the Future.* Rose FC (editor). Smith-Gordon, 1994.

Armon C: Environmental risk factors for amyotrophic lateral sclerosis. Neuroepidemiology 2001;20:2–6.

Biros I, Forrest S: Spinal muscular atrophy: untangling the knot? J Med Genet 1999;36:1–8.

Festoff BW: Amyotrophic lateral sclerosis. Drugs 1996;51:28–44.

Gelanis DF: Respiratory failure or impairment in amyotrophic lateral sclerosis. Curr Treat Options Neurol 2001;3:133–138.

Jablonka S et al: The role of SMN in spinal muscular atrophy. J Neurol 2000;247(Suppl 1):37–42

Julien JP: Amyotrophic lateral sclerosis: unfolding the toxicity of the misfolded. Cell 2001;104:581–591.

Meriggioli MN, Rowin J, Sanders DB: Distinguishing clinical and electrodiagnostic features of X-linked bulbospinal neuronopathy. Muscle Nerve 1999;22:1693–1697.

Miller RG et al: Practice parameter: the care of the patient with amyotrophic lateral sclerosis (an evidence-based review). Report of the Quality Standards Subcommittee of the American Academy of Neurology. Neurology 1999;52:1311–1323.

Naka D, Mills KR: Further evidence for corticomotor hyperexcitability in amyotrophic lateral sclerosis. Muscle Nerve 2000;23:1044–1050.

Ringel SP et al: The natural history of amyotrophic lateral sclerosis. Neurology 1993;43:1316–1322.

Siddique T et al: Linkage of a gene causing familial amyotrophic lateral sclerosis to chromosome 21 and evidence of genetic-locus heterogeneity. N Engl J Med 1991;324:1381–1384.

Williams DB, Windebank AJ: Motor neuron disease (amyotrophic lateral sclerosis). Mayo Clin Proc 1991;66:54–82.

Wokke J: Riluzole. Lancet 1996;348:795–799.

World Federation of Neurology Research Group on Neuromuscular Diseases: El Escorial World Federation of Neurology criteria for the diagnosis of amyotrophic lateral sclerosis. J Neurol Sci 1994;124(Suppl):96–107.

Younger DS: Motor neuron disease and malignancy. Muscle Nerve 2000;23:658–660.

Nerve Root or Plexus Lesions

Tsairis P, Dyck PJ, Mulder DW: Natural history of brachial plexus neuropathy: Report on 99 patients. Arch Neurol 1972;27:109–117.

Watts GD et al: Evidence for genetic heterogeneity in hereditary neuralgic amyotrophy. Neurology 2001;56:675–678.

Disorders of Peripheral Nerves

Adour KK et al: Bell's palsy treatment with acyclovir and prednisone compared with prednisone alone: a double-blind, randomized, controlled trial. Ann Otol Rhinol Laryngol 1996;105:371–378.

Amato AA, Collins MP: Neuropathies associated with malignancy. Semin Neurol 1998;18:125–144.

Bolton CF, Young GB: Neurological complications in critically ill patients. Pages 861–877 in: *Neurology and General Medicine,* 3rd ed. Aminoff MJ (editor). Churchill Livingstone, 2001.

De Diego JI et al: Idiopathic facial paralysis: a randomized, prospective, and controlled study using single-dose prednisone versus acyclovir three times daily. Laryngoscope 1998;108:573–575.

Dyck PJ et al: *Peripheral Neuropathy,* 3rd ed. Saunders, 1993.

Federico P et al: Multifocal motor neuropathy improved by IVIg: randomized, double-blind, placebo-controlled study. Neurology 2000;55:1256–1262.

Kaji R et al: Activity-dependent conduction block in multifocal motor neuropathy. Brain 2000;123:1602–1611.

Kuwabara S et al: Intravenous immunoglobulin therapy for Guillain-Barré syndrome with IgG anti-GM1 antibody. Muscle Nerve 2001;24:54–58.

Leger JM et al: Intravenous immunoglobulin therapy in multifocal motor neuropathy: a double-blind, placebo-controlled study. Brain 2001;124:145–153.

Manji H: Neuropathy in HIV infection. Curr Opin Neurol 2000; 13:589–592.

Marra CM: Bell's palsy and HSV-1 infection. Muscle Nerve 1999; 22:1476–1478.

Ouvrier RA, McLeod JG, Pollard JD: *Peripheral Neuropathy in Childhood.* MacKeith Press, 1999.

Quarles RH, Weiss MD: Autoantibodies associated with peripheral neuropathy. Muscle Nerve 1999;22:800–822.

Ramsay MJ et al: Corticosteroid treatment for idiopathic facial nerve paralysis: a meta-analysis. Laryngoscope 2000;110: 335–341.

Robinson LR: Traumatic injury to peripheral nerves. Muscle Nerve 2000;23:863–873.

Ropper AH, Gorson KC: Neuropathies associated with paraproteinemia. N Engl J Med 1998;338:1601–1607.

Rosenbaum R: Neuromuscular complications of connective tissue disease. Muscle Nerve 2001;24:154–169.

Said G: Vasculitic neuropathy. Curr Opin Neurol 1999;12: 627–629.

Schaumburg HH, Berger AK, Thomas PK: *Disorders of Peripheral Nerves,* 2nd ed. Vol 36 of: *Contemporary Neurology Series.* Davis, 1992.

Taylor BV et al: Natural history of 46 patients with multifocal motor neuropathy with conduction block. Muscle Nerve 2000; 23:900 –908.

Van den Berg-Vos RM et al: Multifocal motor neuropathy: diagnostic criteria that predict the response to immunoglobulin treatment. Ann Neurol 2000;48:919–926.

Van der Meche FG, Van Doorn PA: Guillain-Barré syndrome. Curr Treat Options Neurol 2000;2: 507–516.

Disorders of Neuromuscular Transmission

Bain PG et al: Effects of intravenous immunoglobulin on muscle weakness and calcium-channel autoantibodies in the Lambert-Eaton myasthenic syndrome. Neurology 1996;47:678–683.

Chaudhry V et al: Mycophenolate mofetil: a safe and promising immunosuppressant in neuromuscular diseases. Neurology 2001;56:94–96.

Ciafaloni E et al: Mycophenolate mofetil for myasthenia gravis: an open-label pilot study. Neurology 2001;56:97–99.

Drachman DB: Myasthenia gravis. N Engl J Med 1994;330: 1797–1810.

Engel AG (editor): *Myasthenia Gravis and Myasthenic Disorders.* Oxford University Press, 1999.

Finley JC, Pascuzzi RM: Rational therapy of myasthenia gravis. Semin Neurol 1990;10:70–82.

Gronseth GS, Barohn RJ: Practice parameter: thymectomy for autoimmune myasthenia gravis (an evidence-based review): report of the Quality Standards Subcommittee of the American Academy of Neurology. Neurology 2000;55:7–15.

Hoch W et al: Auto-antibodies to the receptor tyrosine kinase MuSK in patients with myasthenia gravis withour acetylcholine receptor antibodies. Nat Med 2001;7:365–368.

Howard JF Jr: Adverse drug effects on neuromuscular transmission. Semin Neurol 1990;10:89–102.

Hughes JM et al: Clinical features of types A and B food-borne botulism. Ann Intern Med 1981;95:442–445.

Lennon VA et al: Calcium-channel antibodies in the Lambert-Eaton syndrome and other paraneoplastic syndromes. N Engl J Med 1995;332:1467–1474.

Lindstrom JM: Acetylcholine receptors and myasthenia. Muscle Nerve 2000;23:453–477.

Maddison P et al: Long term outcome in Lambert-Eaton myasthenic syndrome without lung cancer. J Neurol Neurosurg Psychiatry 2001;70:212–217.

McEvoy KM et al: 3,4-Diaminopyridine in the treatment of Lambert-Eaton myasthenic syndrome. N Engl J Med 1989;321: 1567–1571.

Newsom-Davis J: Lambert-Eaton myasthenic syndrome. Curr Treat Options Neurol 2001;3:127–131.

Oh SJ et al: Diagnostic sensitivity of the laboratory tests in myasthenia gravis. Muscle Nerve 1992;15:720–724.

Sanders DB: Clinical neurophysiology of disorders of the neuromuscular junction. J Clin Neurophysiol 1993;10:167–180.

Vincent A, Beeson D, Lang B: Molecular targets for autoimmune and genetic disorders of neuromuscular transmission. Eur J Biochem 2000;267:6717–6728.

Myopathic Disorders

Amato AA, Barohn RJ: Idiopathic inflammatory myopathies. Neurol Clin 1997;15:615–648.

Angelini C et al: The clinical spectrum of sarcoglycanopathies. Neurology 1999;52:176–179.

Bonifati MD et al: A multicenter, double-blinded, randomized trial of deflazacort versus prednisone in Duchenne muscular dystrophy. Muscle Nerve 2000;23:1344–1347.

Buckley AE, Dean J, Mahy IR: Cardiac involvement in Emery Dreifuss muscular dystrophy: a case series. Heart 1999;82: 105–108.

Bunch TW: Polymyositis: A case history approach to the differential diagnosis and treatment. Mayo Clin Proc 1990;65: 1480–1497.

Bushby KMD: Making sense of the limb-girdle muscular dystrophies. Brain 1999;122:1403–1420.

Chariot P et al: Acute rhabdomyolysis in patients infected by human immunodeficiency virus. Neurology 1994;44:1692–1696.

Charness ME, Simon RP, Greenberg DA: Ethanol and the nervous system. N Engl J Med 1989;321:442–454.

Chuang TY et al: Polymyalgia rheumatica: a 10-year epidemiologic and clinical study. Ann Intern Med 1982;97:672–680.

Cohn RD, Campbell KP: Molecular basis of muscular dystrophies. Muscle Nerve 2000;23:1456–1471.

Dalakas MC: Polymyositis, dermatomyositis, and inclusion-body myositis. N Engl J Med 1991;325:1487–1498.

Dalakas MC et al: Mitochondrial myopathy caused by long-term zidovudine therapy. N Engl J Med 1990;322:1098–1105.

Dalakas MC: Molecular immunology and genetics of inflammatory muscle diseases. Arch Neurol 1998;55:1509–1512.

Dalakas MC et al: A controlled study of intravenous immunoglobulin combined with prednisone in the treatment of IBM. Neurology 2001;56:323–327.

Evans JM, Hunder GG: Polymyalgia rheumatica and giant cell arteritis. Rheum Dis Clin North Am 2000;26:493–515.

Feero WG et al: Hyperkalemic periodic paralysis: rapid molecular diagnosis and relationship of genotype to phenotype in 12 families. Neurology 1993;43:668–673.

Fischbeck KH, Garbern JY: Facioscapulohumeral muscular dystrophy defect identified. Nature Genet 1992;2:3–4.

Fontaine B et al: Hyperkalemic periodic paralysis and the adult muscle sodium channel alpha-subunit gene. Science 1990;250:1000–1002.

Fontaine B et al: Mapping of the hypokalaemic periodic paralysis (HypoPP) locus to chromosome 1q31-32 in three European families. Nature Genet 1994;6:267–272.

Griggs RC et al: Inclusion body myositis and myopathies. Ann Neurol 1995;38:705–713.

Hirano M, Pavlakis SG: Mitochondrial myopathy, encephalopathy, lactic acidosis, and strokelike episodes (MELAS): current concepts. J Child Neurol 1994;9:4–13.

Karpati G, Acsadi G: The potential for gene therapy in Duchenne muscular dystrophy and other genetic muscle diseases. Muscle Nerve 1993;16:1141–1153.

Lacomis D, Zochodne DW, Bird SJ: Critical illness myopathy. Muscle Nerve 2000;23:1875–1878.

Leff RL et al: The treatment of inclusion body myositis: A retrospective review and a randomized, prospective trial of immunosuppressive therapy. Medicine 1993;72:225–235.

Mastaglia FL, Ojeda VJ: Inflammatory myopathies. (2 parts.) Ann Neurol 1985;17:215–227, 317–323.

Mastaglia FL: Treatment of autoimmune inflammatory myopathies. Curr Opin Neurol 2000;13:507–509.

Meola G: Clinical and genetic heterogeneity in myotonic dystrophies. Muscle Nerve 2000;23:1789–1799.

Ozawa E et al: From dystrophinopathy to sarcoglycanopathy: evolution of a concept of muscular dystrophy. Muscle Nerve 1998;21:421–438.

Peng A et al: Disease progression in sporadic inclusion body myositis: observations in 78 patients. Neurology 2000;55:296–298.

Petty RKH, Harding AE, Morgan-Hughes JA: The clinical features of mitochondrial myopathy. Brain 1986;109:915–938.

Phillips BA et al: Frequency of relapses in patients with polymyositis and dermatomyositis. Muscle Nerve 1998;21:1668–1672.

Ptacek L: The familial periodic paralyses and nondystrophic myotonias. Am J Med 1998;104:58–70.

Ranum LPW et al: Genetic mapping of a second myotonic dystrophy locus. Nature Genet 1998;19:196–198.

Rosenbaum R: Neuromuscular complications of connective tissue disease. Muscle Nerve 2001;24:154–169.

Schapira AV, Griggs RC: Muscle Diseases. Butterworth-Heinemann, 1999.

Serratrice GT et al: Bent spine syndrome. J Neurol Neurosurg Psychiatry 1996;60:51–54.

Simpson DM, Bender AN: Human immunodeficiency virus-associated myopathy: analysis of 11 patients. Ann Neurol 1988;24:79–84.

Simpson DM et al: Myopathies associated with human immunodeficiency virus and zidovudine: can their effects be distinguished? Neurology 1993;43:971–976.

Thornton CA et al: Myotonic dystrophy with no trinucleotide repeat expansion. Ann Neurol 1994;35:269–272.

Urbano-Marquez A et al: The effects of alcoholism on skeletal and cardiac muscle. N Engl J Med 1989;320:409–415.

Walter MC et al: Creatine monohydrate in muscular dystrophies: a double-blind, placebo-controlled clinical study. Neurology 2000;54:1848–1850.

Walter MC et al: High-dose immunoglobulin therapy in sporadic inclusion body myositis: a double-blind, placebo-controlled study. J Neurol 2000;247:22–28.

Motor-Unit Hyperactivity States

Auger RG: Diseases associated with excess motor unit activity. Muscle Nerve 1994;17:1250–1263.

Brown P, Marsden CD: The stiffman and stiffman-plus syndromes. J Neurol Neurosurg Psychiatry 1999;246:648–652.

Dalakas MC et al: The clinical spectrum of anti-GAD antibody-positive patients with stiff-person syndrome. Neurology 2000;55:1531–1535.

Dinkel K et al: Inhibition of gamma-aminobutyric acid synthesis by glutamic acid decarboxylase autoantibodies in stiff-man syndrome. Ann Neurol 1998;44:194–201.

Floeter MK et al: Physiologic studies of spinal inhibitory circuits in patients with stiff-person syndrome. Neurology 1998;51:85–93.

Grimaldi LME et al: Heterogeneity of autoantibodies in stiff-man syndrome. Ann Neurol 1993;34:57–64.

Hart IK: Acquired neuromyotonia: a new autoantibody-mediated neuronal potassium channelopathy. Am J Med Sci 2000;319:209–216.

Khanlou H, Eiger G: Long-term remission of refractory stiff-man syndrome after treatment with intravenous immunoglobulins. Mayo Clin Proc 1999;74:1231–1232.

Layzer RB et al (editors): Motor Unit Hyperactivity States. Raven Press, 1993.

McEvoy KM: Stiff-man syndrome. Semin Neurol 1991; 11:197–205.

Newsom-Davis J: Autoimmune neuromyotonia (Isaacs' syndrome): an antibody-mediated channelopathy. Ann NY Acad Sci 1997;835:111–119.

Vincent A: Understanding neuromyotonia. Muscle Nerve 2000;23:655–657.

Disorders of Somatic Sensation

6

CONTENTS

KEY CONCEPTS

 Sensory symptoms commonly precede sensory signs; the absence of signs in a patient with sensory symptoms does not imply a psychogenic basis of symptoms.

 The distribution of sensory symptoms and signs often suggests their site of origin in the neuraxis, and their temporal profile may suggest their cause.

 In patients with neck or back pain, structural abnormalities revealed by imaging studies must be interpreted cautiously as they may be an incidental finding unrelated to the presenting complaint.

 A dissociated sensory loss—with abnormalities of some but not other sensory modalities—may occur with lesions of the central or peripheral nervous system.

APPROACH TO DIAGNOSIS

An appreciation of the functional anatomy of the sensory components of the nervous system is essential for properly interpreting the history and clinical signs of patients with disorders of **somatic sensation.** As used here, the term includes sensations of touch or pressure, vibration, joint position, pain, temperature, and more complex functions that rely on these primary sensory modalities (eg, two-point discrimination, stereognosis, graphesthesia); it excludes special senses such as smell, vision, taste, and hearing.

FUNCTIONAL ANATOMY OF THE SOMATIC SENSORY PATHWAYS

The sensory pathway between the skin and deeper structures and the cerebral cortex involves three neurons, with two synapses occurring centrally. The cell body of the first sensory neuron of the spinal nerve is in the dorsal root ganglion (Figure 6–1). Each cell located there sends a peripheral process that terminates in a free nerve ending or encapsulated sensory receptor and a central process that enters the spinal cord. Sensory receptors are relatively specialized for particular sensations and, in addition to free nerve endings (pain), include Meissner's corpuscles, Merkel's corpuscles, and hair cells (touch); Krause's end-bulbs (cold); and Ruffini's corpuscles (heat). The location of the first central synapse depends upon the type of sensation but is either in the posterior gray column of the spinal cord or in the upward extension of this column in the lower brainstem. The second synapse is located in the anterior part of the anterolateral nucleus of the thalamus, from which there is sensory radiation to the cerebral cortex. In the spinal cord, fibers mediating touch, pressure, and postural sensation ascend in the posterior white columns to the medulla, where they synapse in the gracile and cuneate nuclei (see Figure 6–1). From these nuclei, fibers cross the midline and ascend in the medial lemniscus to the thalamus. Other fibers that mediate touch and those subserving pain and temperature appreciation synapse on neurons in the posterior horns of the spinal cord, particularly in the substantia gelatinosa. The fibers from these neurons then cross the midline and ascend in the anterolateral part of the cord; fibers mediating touch pass upward in the anterior spinothalamic tract, whereas pain and temperature fibers generally travel in the lateral spinothalamic tract (see Figure 6–1). Fibers from this anterolateral system pass to the thalamic relay nuclei and to nonspecific thalamic projection nuclei and the mesencephalic reticular formation. Fibers from the lemniscal and anterolateral systems are joined in the brainstem by fibers subserving sensation from the head. Cephalic pain and temperature sensation are dependent upon the spinal nucleus of the trigeminal (V) nerve; touch, pressure, and postural sensation are conveyed mostly by the main sensory and mesencephalic nuclei of this nerve.

HISTORY

Sensory disturbances may consist of loss of sensation, abnormal sensations, or pain.

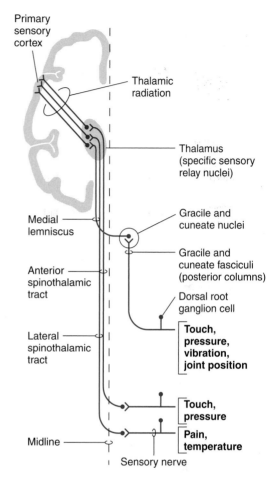

Figure 6–1. Sensory pathways conveying touch, pressure, vibration, joint position, pain, and temperature sensation.

The term **paresthesia** is used to denote abnormal spontaneous sensations, such as burning, tingling, or pins and needles. The term **dysesthesia** denotes any unpleasant sensation produced by a stimulus that is usually painless. The term **numbness** is often used by patients to describe a sense of heaviness, weakness, or deadness in the affected part of the body—and sometimes to signify any sensory impairment; its meaning must be clarified whenever the word is used.

In obtaining a history of sensory complaints, it is important to determine the location of the symptoms; the mode of onset and progression of the symptoms; whether the symptoms are constant or episodic in nature; whether any factors specifically produce, enhance, or relieve symptoms; and whether there are any accompanying symptoms.

The **location** of symptoms may provide a clue to their origin. For example, sensory disturbances involving all the limbs suggest peripheral neuropathy, a cervical cord or brainstem lesion, or a metabolic disturbance such as hyperventilation syndrome. Involvement of one entire limb—or of one side of the body—suggests a central (brain or spinal cord) lesion. A hemispheric or brainstem lesion may lead to lateralized sensory symptoms, but the face is also commonly affected. In addition, there may be other symptoms and signs, such as aphasia, apraxia, and visual field defects with hemispheric disease, or dysarthria, weakness, vertigo, diplopia, disequilibrium, and ataxia with brainstem disorders. Involvement of part of a limb or a discrete region of the trunk raises the possibility of a nerve or root lesion, depending upon the precise distribution. With a root lesion, symptoms may show some relationship to neck or back movements, and pain is often conspicuous.

The **course** of sensory complaints provides a guide to their cause. Intermittent or repetitive transient symptoms may represent sensory seizures, ischemic phenomena, or metabolic disturbances such as those accompanying hyperventilation. Intermittent localized symptoms that occur at a consistent time may suggest the diagnosis or an exogenous precipitating factor. For example, the pain and paresthesias of carpal tunnel syndrome (median nerve compression at the wrist) characteristically occur at night and awaken the patient from sleep.

SENSORY EXAMINATION

In the investigation of sensory complaints, various modalities are tested in turn, and the distribution of any abnormality is plotted with particular reference to the normal root and peripheral nerve territories. Complete loss of touch appreciation is **anesthesia,** partial loss is **hypesthesia,** and increased sensitivity is **hyperesthesia.** The corresponding terms for pain appreciation are **analgesia, hypalgesia,** and **hyperalgesia** or **hyperpathia; allodynia** refers to the misperception of a trivial tactile sensation as pain.

1. Primary Sensory Modalities

Light Touch

The appreciation of light touch is evaluated with a wisp of cotton wool, which is brought down carefully on a small region of skin. The patient lies quietly, with the eyes closed, and makes a signal each time the stimulus is felt. The appreciation of light touch depends on fibers that traverse the posterior column of the spinal cord in the gracile (leg) and cuneate (arm) fasciculi ipsilaterally

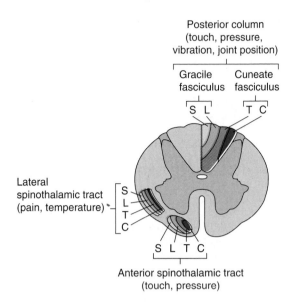

Figure 6–2. Location and lamination of sensory pathways in the spinal cord. C (cervical), T (thoracic), L (lumbar), and S (sacral) indicate the level of origin of fibers within each tract.

(Figures 6–1 and Figure 6–2), passing to the medial lemniscus of the brainstem (Figure 6–3), and on fibers in the contralateral anterior spinothalamic tract.

Pinprick & Temperature

Pinprick appreciation is tested by asking the patient to indicate whether the point of a pin (not a hypodermic needle, which is likely to puncture the skin and draw blood) feels sharp or blunt. Appreciation of pressure or touch by the pinpoint must not be confused with the appreciation of sharpness. Temperature appreciation is evaluated by application to the skin of containers of hot or cold water. Pinprick and temperature appreciation depend upon the integrity of the lateral spinothalamic tracts (see Figures 6–1 and 6–2). The afferent fibers cross in front of the central canal after ascending for two or three segments from their level of entry into the cord.

Deep Pressure

Deep pressure sensibility is evaluated by pressure on the tendons, such as the Achilles tendon at the ankle.

Vibration

Vibration appreciation is evaluated with a tuning fork (128 Hz) that is set in motion and then placed over a bony prominence; the patient is asked to indicate

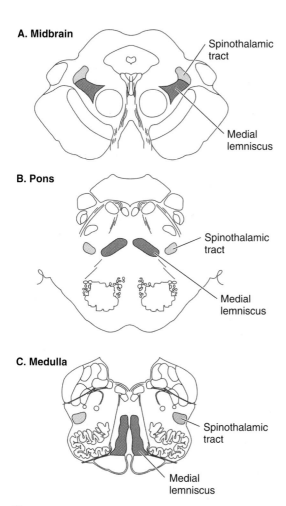

A. Midbrain

Spinothalamic tract

Medial lemniscus

B. Pons

Spinothalamic tract

Medial lemniscus

C. Medulla

Spinothalamic tract

Medial lemniscus

Figure 6–3. Sensory pathways in the brainstem. In the medulla, spinothalamic fibers conveying pain and temperature sensation are widely separated from medial lemniscal fibers mediating touch and pressure; these pathways converge as they ascend in the pons and midbrain.

whether vibration, rather than simple pressure, is felt. Many healthy elderly patients have impaired appreciation of vibration below the knees.

Joint Position

Joint position sense is tested by asking the patient to indicate the direction of small passive movements of the terminal interphalangeal joints of the fingers and toes. Patients with severe impairment of joint position sense may exhibit slow, continuous movement of the fingers (**pseudoathetoid movement**) when attempting to hold the hands outstretched with the eyes closed. For clinical

purposes, both joint position sense and the ability to appreciate vibration are considered to depend on fibers carried in the posterior columns of the cord, although there is evidence that this is not true for vibration.

2. Complex Sensory Functions

Romberg's Test

The patient is asked to assume a steady stance with feet together, arms outstretched, and eyes closed and is observed for any tendency to sway or fall. The test is positive (abnormal) if unsteadiness is markedly increased by eye closure—as occurs, for example, in tabes dorsalis. A positive test is indicative of grossly impaired joint position sense in the legs.

Two-Point Discrimination

The ability to distinguish simultaneous touch at two neighboring points depends upon the integrity of the central and peripheral nervous system, the degree of separation of the two points, and the part of the body that is stimulated. The patient is required to indicate whether he or she is touched by one or two compass points, while the distance between the points is varied in order to determine the shortest distance at which they are recognized as different points. The threshold for two-point discrimination approximates 4 mm at the fingertips and may be several centimeters on the back. When peripheral sensory function is intact, impaired two-point discrimination suggests a disorder affecting the sensory cortex.

Graphesthesia, Stereognosis, & Barognosis

Agraphesthesia, the inability to identify a number traced on the skin of the palm of the hand despite normal cutaneous sensation, implies a lesion involving the contralateral parietal lobe. The same is true of inability to distinguish between various shapes or textures by touch (**astereognosis**) or impaired ability to distinguish between different weights (**abarognosis**).

Bilateral Sensory Discrimination

In some patients with apparently normal sensation, simultaneous stimulation of the two sides of the body reveals an apparent neglect of (or inattention to) sensation from one side, usually because of some underlying contralateral cerebral lesion.

SENSORY CHANGES & THEIR SIGNIFICANCE

It is important to determine the nature and distribution of any sensory change. Failure to find clinical evidence of sensory loss in patients with sensory symptoms must *never* be taken to imply that the symptoms have a psychogenic basis. Sensory symptoms often develop well before the onset of sensory signs.

Peripheral Nerve Lesions

A. MONONEUROPATHY

In patients with a lesion of a single peripheral nerve, sensory loss is usually less than would have been predicted on anatomic grounds because of overlap from adjacent nerves. Moreover, depending upon the type of lesion, the fibers in a sensory nerve may be affected differently. Compressive lesions, for example, tend to affect preferentially the large fibers that subserve touch.

B. POLYNEUROPATHY

In patients with polyneuropathies, sensory loss is generally symmetric and is greater distally than proximally—as suggested by the term **stocking-and-glove sensory loss.** As a general rule the loss will have progressed almost to the knees before the hands are affected. Certain metabolic disorders (such as **Tangier disease,** a recessive trait characterized by the near absence of high-density lipoproteins) preferentially involve small nerve fibers that subserve pain and temperature appreciation. Sensory loss may be accompanied by a motor deficit and reflex changes.

Root Involvement

Nerve root involvement produces impairment of cutaneous sensation in a segmental pattern (Figures 6–4A and 6–4B), but because of overlap there is generally no loss of sensation unless two or more adjacent roots are affected. Pain is often a conspicuous feature in patients with compressive root lesions. Depending on the level affected, there may be loss of tendon reflexes (C5–6, biceps and brachioradialis; C7–8, triceps; L3–4, knee; S1, ankle), and if the anterior roots are also involved, there may be weakness and muscle atrophy (see Table 5–11).

Cord Lesion

In patients with a cord lesion, there may be a transverse sensory level. Physiologic areas of increased sensitivity do occur, however, at the costal margin, over the breasts, and in the groin, and these must not be taken as abnormal. Therefore, the level of a sensory deficit affecting the trunk is best determined by careful sensory testing over the back rather than the chest and abdomen.

A. CENTRAL CORD LESION

With a central cord lesion—such as occurs in syringomyelia, following trauma, and with certain cord tumors—

there is characteristically a loss of pain and temperature appreciation with sparing of other modalities. This loss is due to the interruption of fibers conveying pain and temperature that cross from one side of the cord to the spinothalamic tract on the other. Such a loss is usually bilateral, may be asymmetric, and involves only the fibers of the involved segments. It may be accompanied by lower motor neuron weakness in the muscles supplied by the affected segments and sometimes by a pyramidal and posterior column deficit below the lesion (Figure 6–5).

B. ANTEROLATERAL CORD LESION

Lesions involving the anterolateral portion of the spinal cord (lateral spinothalamic tract) can cause contralateral impairment of pain and temperature appreciation in segments below the level of the lesion. The spinothalamic tract is laminated, with fibers from the sacral segments the outermost. Intrinsic cord (intramedullary) lesions often spare the sacral fibers, whereas extramedullary lesions, which compress the cord, tend to involve these fibers as well as those arising from more rostral levels.

C. ANTERIOR CORD LESION

With destructive lesions involving predominantly the anterior portion of the spinal cord, pain and temperature appreciation are impaired below the level of the lesion from lateral spinothalamic tract involvement. In addition, weakness or paralysis of muscles supplied by the involved segments of the cord results from damage to motor neurons in the anterior horn. With more extensive disease, involvement of the corticospinal tracts in the lateral funiculi may cause a pyramidal deficit below the lesion. There is relative preservation of posterior column function (Figure 6–6). Ischemic myelopathies caused by occlusion of the anterior spinal artery take the form of anterior cord lesions.

D. POSTERIOR COLUMN LESION

A patient with a posterior column lesion may complain of a tight or bandlike sensation in the regions corresponding to the level of spinal involvement and sometimes also of paresthesias (like electric shocks) radiating down the extremities on neck flexion (**Lhermitte's sign**). There is loss of vibration and joint position sense below the level of the lesion, with preservation of other sensory modalities. The deficit may resemble that resulting from involvement of large fibers in the posterior roots.

E. CORD HEMISECTION

Lateral hemisection of the cord leads to **Brown-Séquard's syndrome.** Below the lesion, there is an ipsilateral pyramidal deficit and disturbed appreciation of vibration and joint position sense, with contralateral loss of pain and temperature appreciation that begins two or three segments below the lesion (Figure 6–7).

Peripheral nerve

Nerve root

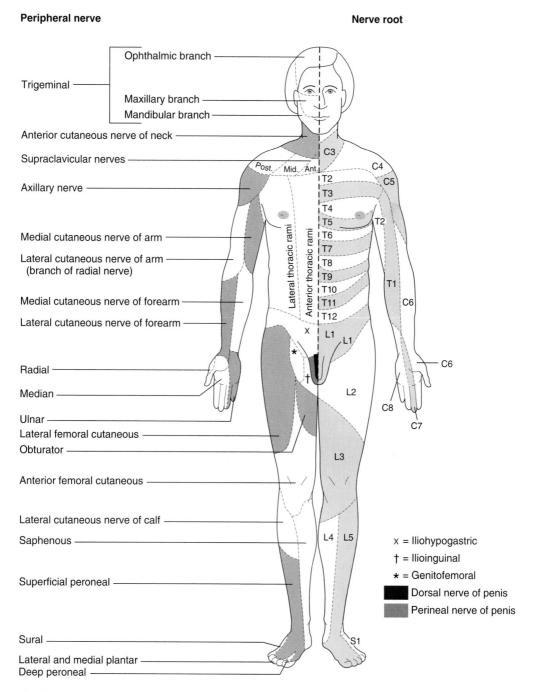

Figure 6–4A. Cutaneous innervation (anterior view). The segmental or radicular (nerve root) distribution is shown on the left side of the body, and the peripheral nerve distribution on the right side of the body. *(continued)*

Nerve root

Peripheral nerve

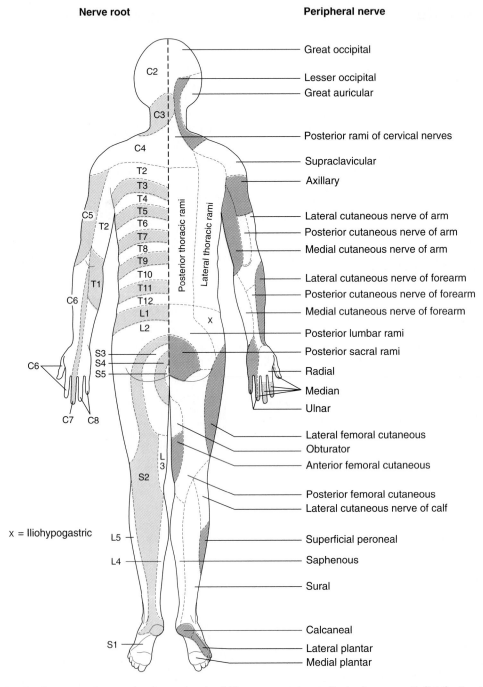

Great occipital

Lesser occipital
Great auricular

Posterior rami of cervical nerves

Supraclavicular

Axillary

Lateral cutaneous nerve of arm
Posterior cutaneous nerve of arm
Medial cutaneous nerve of arm

Lateral cutaneous nerve of forearm
Posterior cutaneous nerve of forearm
Medial cutaneous nerve of forearm

Posterior lumbar rami

Posterior sacral rami

Radial

Median

Ulnar

Lateral femoral cutaneous
Obturator
Anterior femoral cutaneous

Posterior femoral cutaneous
Lateral cutaneous nerve of calf

Superficial peroneal

Saphenous

Sural

Calcaneal
Lateral plantar
Medial plantar

x = Iliohypogastric

Figure 6–4B. Cutaneous innervation (posterior view). The segmental or radicular (nerve root) distribution is shown on the left side of the body, and the peripheral nerve distribution on the right side of the body. For details of radial median, ulnar, peroneal, and femoral nerves, see Appendix C.

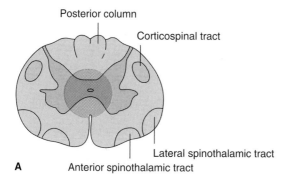

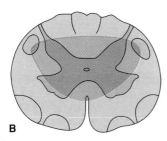

Figure 6–5. Central cord lesions (blue) of moderate **(A)** or marked **(B)** extent. Less extensive lesions impair pain and temperature appreciation by interrupting incoming sensory fibers as they cross to the contralateral spinothalamic tract; involvement of anterior horn cells causes lower motor neuron weakness. These deficits are restricted to dermatomes and muscles innervated by the involved spinal cord segments. More extensive lesions also produce disturbances of touch, pressure, vibration, and joint position sense because of involvement of the posterior columns and cause pyramidal signs because of corticospinal tract involvement, especially involving the arms (see lamination of corticospinal tract in Figure 5–3). These deficits occur below the level of the lesion.

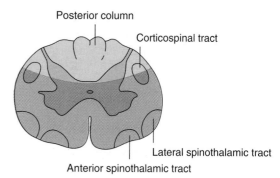

Figure 6–6. Anterior cord lesion (blue) associated with occlusion of the anterior spinal artery. Clinical features are similar to those seen with severe central cord lesions (Figure 6–5B), except that posterior column sensory functions are spared and the defect in pain and temperature sensation extends to sacral levels.

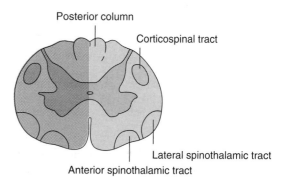

Figure 6–7. Cord lesion (blue) in Brown-Séquard syndrome. Hemisection of the cord causes ipsilateral pyramidal dysfunction and impairment of posterior column sensory function below the level of the lesion and contralateral impairment of pain and temperature sensation with an upper limit slightly below the level of the lesion.

Brainstem Lesion

Sensory disturbances may be accompanied by a motor deficit, cerebellar signs, and cranial nerve palsies when the lesion is in the brainstem.

In patients with lesions involving the spinothalamic tract in the dorsolateral medulla and pons, pain and temperature appreciation are lost in the limbs and trunk on the opposite side of the body. When such a lesion is located in the medulla, it also typically involves the spinal trigeminal nucleus, impairing pain and temperature sensation on the same side of the face as the lesion. The result is a crossed sensory deficit that affects the ipsilateral face and contralateral limbs. In contrast, spinothalamic lesions above the spinal trigeminal nucleus affect the face, limbs, and trunk contralateral to the lesion. With lesions affecting the medial lemniscus, there is loss of touch and proprioception on the opposite side of the body. In the upper brainstem, the spinothalamic tract and medial lemniscus run together so that a single lesion may cause loss of all superficial and deep sensation over the contralateral side of the body (see Figure 6–3).

Thalamic Lesions

Thalamic lesions may lead to loss or impairment of all forms of sensation on the contralateral side of the body.

Spontaneous pain, sometimes with a particularly unpleasant quality, may occur on the affected side. Patients may describe it as burning, tearing, knifelike, or stabbing, but often have difficulty characterizing it. Any form of cutaneous stimulation can lead to painful or unpleasant sensations. Such a thalamic syndrome (**Dejerine-Roussy syndrome**) can also occasionally result from lesions of the white matter of the parietal lobe or from cord lesions.

Lesions of the Sensory Cortex

Disease limited to the sensory cortex impairs discriminative sensory function on the opposite side of the body. Thus, patients may be unable to localize stimuli on the affected side or to recognize the position of different parts of the body. They may not be able to recognize objects by touch or to estimate their size, weight, consistency, or texture. Cortical sensory disturbances are usually more conspicuous in the hands than in the trunk or proximal portions of the limbs.

DISTINCTION OF ORGANIC & PSYCHOGENIC SENSORY DISTURBANCES

Psychogenic disturbances of sensation may be associated with such psychiatric disturbances as conversion disorder. They may take any form but most often are restricted to loss of cutaneous sensation. There may be several characteristic features.

Nonorganic sensory loss does not conform in its distribution to any specific neuroanatomic pattern. It may surround a bony landmark or involve an area defined by surface landmarks rather than innervation. Indeed, it is not uncommon for there to be an apparent loss of sensation in one or more extremities, with the margin occurring circumferentially in the axilla or groin; organic sensory loss with such a margin is unusual. Organic peripheral sensory loss over the trunk or face does not usually extend to the midline but stops 3–5 cm before it, because of overlap in the innervation on the two sides; with nonorganic disturbances, apparent sensory loss commonly stops precisely at the midline.

There is often a sudden transition between areas of nonorganic sensory loss and areas with normal sensation. By contrast, with organic disturbances, there is usually an area of altered sensation between insensitive areas and adjacent areas with normal sensibility.

In nonorganic disturbances, there may be a dissociated loss that is difficult to interpret on an anatomic basis. For example, there may be a total loss of pinprick appreciation but preserved temperature sensation. Moreover, despite the apparent loss of posterior column function, the patient may be able to walk normally or maintain the arms outstretched without difficulty or pseudoathetoid movements.

In nonorganic sensory disturbances, appreciation of vibration may be impaired on one side but not the other side of a bony midline structure, such as the skull or sternum. The vibrations are in fact conducted to both sides by the bone, so that even if there is a hemisensory disturbance, the vibrations are appreciated on either side in patients with organic sensory disorders.

Finally, it should be noted that sensory disturbances are often suggested to the patient by the examiner's own expectations. Such findings can be particularly misleading because they may be neuroanatomically correct. One helpful approach is to have the patient outline on the body the extent of any perceived sensory disturbance before formal sensory testing is undertaken.

PERIPHERAL NERVE LESIONS

Sensory symptoms are usually a conspicuous feature in patients with peripheral nerve lesions (Table 6–1). Sensory impairment may be in a distal stocking-and-glove pattern in patients with polyneuropathies or may follow the pattern of individual peripheral nerves in patients with mononeuropathies.

Classification

A. MONONEUROPATHY SIMPLEX

This term signifies involvement of a single peripheral nerve.

B. MONONEUROPATHY MULTIPLEX

In this disorder, several individual nerves are affected, usually at random and noncontiguously. Clinical examination reveals a clinical deficit attributable to involvement of one or more isolated peripheral nerves, except when mononeuropathy multiplex is extensive and the resulting deficits become confluent.

C. POLYNEUROPATHY

This term denotes a disorder in which the function of numerous peripheral nerves is affected at the same time. This leads to a predominantly distal and symmetric deficit, with loss of tendon reflexes except when small fibers are selectively involved. Polyneuropathies are sometimes subclassified according to the primary site at which the nerve is affected. In **distal axonopathies,** the axon is the principal pathologic target; most polyneuropathies fall into this category. **Myelinopathies** are conditions that involve the myelin sheath surrounding the axon. These disorders include acute idiopathic polyneuropathy (Guillain-Barré syndrome), chronic inflammatory demyelinating neuropathy, diphtheria,

Table 6–1. Causes of peripheral neuropathy.

Idiopathic inflammatory neuropathies	Toxins
Acute idiopathic polyneuropathy (Guillain-Barré syndrome)	Organic compounds
Chronic inflammatory demyelinating polyneuropathy	Hexacarbons
Metabolic and nutritional neuropathies	Organophosphates
Diabetes	Heavy metals
Other endocrinopathies	Arsenic
Hypothyroidism	Lead
Acromegaly	Thallium
Uremia	Gold
Liver disease	Platinum
Vitamin B_{12} deficiency	Tryptophan (contaminant)
Infective and granulomatous neuropathies	**Hereditary neuropathies**
AIDS	Idiopathic
Leprosy	Hereditary motor and sensory neuropathies
Diphtheria	Hereditary sensory neuropathies
Sarcoidosis	Friedreich's ataxia
Sepsis and multiorgan failure	Familial amyloidosis
Vasculitic neuropathies	Metabolic
Polyarteritis nodosa	Porphyria
Rheumatoid arthritis	Metachromatic leukodystrophy
Systemic lupus erythematosus	Krabbe's disease
Neoplastic and paraproteinemic neuropathies	Abetalipoproteinemia
Compression and infiltration by tumor	Tangier's disease
Paraneoplastic syndromes	Refsum's disease
Paraproteinemias	Fabry's disease
Amyloidosis	**Entrapment neuropathies**
Drug-induced and toxic neuropathies	
Alcohol	
Other drugs (see Table 6–2)	

certain paraneoplastic and paraproteinemic states, and various hereditary conditions including metachromatic leukodystrophy, Krabbe's disease, and types 1 and 3 Charcot-Marie-Tooth hereditary motor and sensory neuropathy (CMT1 and 3). Finally, certain disorders—termed **neuronopathies**—principally affect nerve cell bodies in the anterior horn of the spinal cord or dorsal root ganglion. Examples are type 2 Charcot-Marie-Tooth hereditary motor and sensory neuropathy, pyridoxine-induced neuropathy, and some paraneoplastic syndromes.

Clinical Findings

A. SENSORY DISTURBANCES

Involvement of sensory fibers can lead to numbness and impaired sensation. It can also lead to abnormal spontaneous sensations, such as pain and paresthesias, and to perverted sensations such as hyperpathia.

1. Pain is a conspicuous feature of certain neuropathies, especially if small fibers within the nerves are affected. The precise mechanism of its genesis is unclear. Polyneuropathies associated with prominent pain include those related to diabetes, alcoholism, porphyria, Fabry's disease, amyloidosis, rheumatoid arthritis, and acquired immunodeficiency syndrome (AIDS), as well as dominantly inherited sensory neuropathy and paraneoplastic sensory neuronopathy. Pain is also a feature of many entrapment neuropathies and of idiopathic brachial plexopathy.

2. Dissociated sensory loss is impairment of some sensory modalities, such as pain and temperature, with preservation of others, such as light touch, vibration, and joint position sense. Although the presence of a dissociated sensory loss often indicates a spinal cord lesion, it also occurs in peripheral neuropathies when there is selective involvement of peripheral nerve fibers of a certain size, such as occurs in amyloid neuropathy, leprous neuritis, or hereditary sensory neuropathy. In such cases, preferential involvement of small fibers is commonly associated with disproportionate impairment of pain and temperature appreciation, spontaneous pain, and autonomic dysfunction. Large-fiber disease, on the other hand, results in defective touch, vibration, and joint position sense, early loss of tendon reflexes, and prominent motor symptoms.

B. MOTOR DEFICITS

The motor deficit that occurs with a peripheral nerve lesion consists of weakness of muscles innervated by the nerve, accompanied in severe cases by wasting and fasciculation. There may be difficulty in the performance of fine tasks; this is compounded by any accompanying sensory loss. The clinical findings reflect a lower motor neuron deficit, and it is the distribution of these signs and the presence of accompanying sensory and reflex changes that suggest they may be due to peripheral nerve involvement.

C. TENDON REFLEXES

These are impaired or lost if reflex arcs are interrupted on either the afferent or efferent side (C5 –6, biceps and brachioradialis; C7–8, triceps; L3–4, knee; S1, ankle). The ankle reflexes are usually the first to be lost in patients with polyneuropathies, but may be absent in healthy elderly subjects.

D. AUTONOMIC DISTURBANCES

Autonomic disturbances may be particularly conspicuous in some peripheral neuropathies—especially Guillain-Barré syndrome and neuropathies related to diabetes, renal failure, porphyria, or amyloidosis. Symptoms include postural hypotension, coldness of the extremities, impaired thermoregulatory sweating, disturbances of bladder and bowel function, and impotence.

E. ENLARGED NERVES

Palpably enlarged peripheral nerves raise the possibility of leprosy, amyloidosis, hereditary motor and sensory neuropathies, Refsum's disease, acromegaly, or chronic inflammatory demyelinating polyneuropathy.

Evaluation of Patients

A. TIME COURSE

Polyneuropathy that develops acutely over a few days usually relates to an inflammatory process, as in the Guillain-Barré syndrome. It may also relate to an underlying neoplasm, to infections such as diphtheria, to metabolic disorders such as acute intermittent porphyria, or to exposure to such toxic substances as thallium or triorthocresyl phosphate. A chronic course with a gradual evolution over several years is typical of many hereditary or metabolic polyneuropathies but also characterizes chronic inflammatory demyelinating polyneuropathy.

Mononeuropathy of acute onset is likely to be traumatic or ischemic in origin, whereas one evolving gradually is more likely to relate to entrapment (ie, compression by neighboring anatomic structures) or to recurrent minor trauma.

B. AGE AT ONSET

Polyneuropathies that develop during childhood or early adult life often have a hereditary basis, but they may also relate to an underlying inflammatory disorder. Those developing in later life are more likely to be due to a metabolic, toxic, or inflammatory disorder or to an underlying neoplasm.

Mononeuropathy presenting in the neonatal period is likely to be developmental in origin or related to birth injury; one developing in later life may relate to entrapment or injury that is often occupationally determined.

C. OCCUPATIONAL HISTORY

Various industrial substances can lead to peripheral neuropathy, including carbon disulfide, *n*-hexane, ethylene oxide, methyl bromide, acrylamide, triorthocresyl phosphate and certain other organophosphates, DDT, arsenic, lead, and thallium. A mononeuropathy is sometimes the first clinical manifestation of an occupationally related polyneuropathy, but it may also develop in response to entrapment or recurrent minor occupational trauma. For example, carpal tunnel syndrome is more common in persons who do heavy manual labor or develop repetitive motion injury as a result of computer terminal use, and a lesion of the deep palmar branch of the ulnar nerve may relate to repeated pressure on the palm of the hand by, for example, punching down heavily on a stapler or using heavy equipment such as a pneumatic road drill.

D. MEDICAL HISTORY

1. Peripheral neuropathy may relate to **metabolic disorders** such as diabetes mellitus, uremia, liver disease, myxedema, acromegaly, metachromatic leukodystrophy, or Fabry's disease. That caused by diabetes is especially important and may take the form of an entrapment mononeuropathy, acute ischemic mononeuritis, distal sensorimotor polyneuropathy, subacute proximal motor polyradiculopathy (diabetic amyotrophy), thoracoabdominal radiculopathy, or autonomic neuropathy.

2. A peripheral neuropathy may also relate to an underlying malignant **neoplasm.** The peripheral nerves, spinal nerves, and limb plexuses may be compressed or infiltrated by extension of primary tumors or metastatic lymph nodes. Neoplastic disease can also lead to a nonmetastatic (paraneoplastic) sensory or sensorimotor polyneuropathy or to Lambert-Eaton syndrome, a disorder of neuromuscular transmission discussed in Chapter 5.

3. Certain **connective tissue disorders,** especially polyarteritis nodosa, rheumatoid arthritis, Churg-Strauss syndrome, and Wegener's granulomatosis, may be associated with mononeuropathy multiplex or, less commonly, polyneuropathy or cranial neuropathy. Polyneuropathy is more common in systemic lupus erythematosus. Patients with rheumatoid arthritis are particularly likely to develop focal entrapment or compressive mononeuropathies in the vicinity of the affected joints.

4. AIDS is commonly associated with a distal, symmetric, primarily sensory polyneuropathy. Peripheral nerve involvement in AIDS less frequently takes the form of an acute or chronic inflammatory demyelinating polyneuropathy, polyradiculopathy, mononeuropathy multiplex, or autonomic neuropathy. Neuropathies are also seen in patients with AIDS-related complex, asymptomatic human immunodeficiency virus-1 (HIV-1) infection, and HIV-1 seroconversion.

E. Drug and Alcohol History

Some of the drugs that cause peripheral neuropathy are shown in Table 6–2; there may be selective involvement of motor or sensory fibers with some drugs.

Table 6–2. Drugs inducing peripheral neuropathy.[1]

Sensory neuropathy
Chloramphenicol
Cisplatin
Pyridoxine
Taxol
Taxotere
Predominantly sensory neuropathy
Ethambutol
Hydralazine
Misonidazole
Metronidazole
Motor neuropathy
Dapsone
Imipramine
Certain sulfonamides
Mixed sensory and motor neuropathy
Amiodarone
Chloroquine
Disulfiram
Gold
Indomethacin
Isoniazid
Nitrofurantoin
Penicillamine
Perhexilene
Phenytoin
Thalidomide
Tryptophan (contaminant)
Vincristine

[1] Selected drugs.

F. Family Background

Certain polyneuropathies have a hereditary basis. These are discussed later in this chapter in the section on hereditary neuropathies.

Differential Diagnosis

Peripheral neuropathies can lead to a motor or sensory deficit or both. The preservation of sensation and tendon reflexes distinguishes the motor deficit that results from pure pyramidal lesions or is associated with spinal muscular atrophies, myopathies, or disorders of neuromuscular transmission from that caused by peripheral nerve involvement. Other distinguishing features are discussed in Chapter 5.

Myelopathies are characterized by a pyramidal deficit below the level of the lesion as well as by distal sensory loss.

In tabes dorsalis, there is often a history of syphilitic infection, and examination reveals other stigmas of syphilis. In addition, tactile sensation is preserved.

Radiculopathies are distinguished from peripheral neuropathies by the distribution of motor or sensory deficits (Figures 6–4A and 6–4B). The presence of neck or back pain that radiates to the extremities in a radicular distribution also suggests a root lesion.

Investigative Studies

Laboratory studies in patients with peripheral neuropathy are directed at confirming the diagnosis and revealing any underlying cause. Electromyography may reveal evidence of denervation in the affected muscles and can be used to determine whether any motor units remain under voluntary control. Nerve conduction studies permit conduction velocity to be measured in motor and sensory fibers. On the basis of electrodiagnostic or histopathologic studies, peripheral neuropathies can be divided into demyelinating or axonal neuropathies. In the former, electromyography typically reveals little or no evidence of denervation, but there is conduction block or marked slowing of maximal conduction velocity in affected nerves. In the axonal neuropathies, electromyography shows that denervation has occurred, especially distally in the extremities, but maximal nerve conduction velocity is normal or slowed only slightly.

In patients with electrophysiologically confirmed peripheral neuropathy, laboratory studies should include a complete blood count; erythrocyte sedimentation rate; serum urea nitrogen and creatinine, fasting blood glucose, and serum vitamin B_{12}; serum protein, protein electrophoresis, and immunoelectrophoresis; liver and thyroid function blood tests; serologic tests for syphilis (FTA or MHA-TP), rheumatoid factor, and antinuclear antibody; and chest x-ray. Depending on the clinical circumstances, serologic tests for Lyme disease, hepatitis, or infection with human immunodeficiency virus may be required. Genetic studies may also be necessary after appropriate genetic counseling. If toxic causes are suspected, a 24-hour urine collection followed by analysis for heavy metals may be necessary, and hair and fingernail clippings can be analyzed for arsenic. Examination of a fresh specimen of urine for porphobilinogen and δ-aminolevulinic acid is necessary if porphyria is suspected.

Treatment

Treatment of the underlying cause may limit the progression of or even reverse the neuropathy. Nursing care is important in patients with severe motor or sensory deficits to prevent decubitus ulcers, joint contractures, and additional compressive peripheral nerve damage. Respiratory function must also be monitored carefully—particularly in acute idiopathic polyneuropathy (Guillain-Barré syndrome), chronic inflammatory demyelinating polyneuropathy, and diphtheritic neuropathy—and preparations must be made to assist ventilation if the vital capacity falls below about 1 L. In patients with severe dysesthesia, a cradle (inverted metal bar frame) can be used to keep the bedclothes from touching sensitive areas of the skin. Treatment with phenytoin, 300 mg/d, carbamazepine, up to 1200 mg/d, or mexiletine, 600–900 mg/d is sometimes helpful in relieving the lancinating pain of certain neuropathies. If the pain is more constant, burning, or dysesthetic, amitriptyline 25–100 mg at bedtime is often helpful as are other tricyclic agents. Gabapentin (300 mg three times daily, with subsequent increments depending on response and tolerance) is effective in treating various neuropathic pain disorders; pain relief may similarly occur with lamotrigine or topiramate, but this has been documented less well. Topical capsaicin is also helpful in neuropathic pain syndromes.

Extremities with sensory loss must be protected from repeated minor trauma, such as thermal injury, that can destroy tissues. The temperature of hot surfaces should be checked with a part of the body in which sensation is preserved, and the setting of water heaters must be reduced to prevent scalding. The skin and nails must be cared for meticulously.

Dysautonomic symptoms may be troublesome, especially in diabetic or alcoholic polyneuropathy. Waist-high elastic hosiery, dietary salt supplementation, and treatment with fludrocortisone, 0.1–1 mg/d orally, may help relieve postural hypotension, but the patient must be monitored carefully to prevent recumbent hypertension. Instructing the patient to sleep in a semierect rather than a recumbent position is helpful because dysautonomic patients are often unable to conserve salt and water when recumbent at night.

POLYNEUROPATHIES

IDIOPATHIC INFLAMMATORY NEUROPATHIES

Acute Idiopathic Polyneuropathy (Guillain-Barré Syndrome)

Guillain-Barré syndrome is an acute or subacute polyneuropathy that can follow minor infective illnesses, inoculations, or surgical procedures—or may occur without obvious precipitants. Clinical and epidemiologic evidence suggests an association with preceding *Campylobacter jejuni* infection. Its precise cause is unclear, but it appears to have an immunologic basis. Both demyelinating and axonal forms have been recognized, with distinctive clinical and electrophysiologic features. The demyelinative form is more common in the United States, but an axonal variant is encountered occasionally (**acute motor sensory axonal neuropathy**). In northern China a related axonal form occurs frequently and has been designated **acute motor axonal neuropathy.**

A. CLINICAL FEATURES

The features useful for diagnosing Guillain-Barré syndrome are summarized in Table 6–3. Patients generally present with weakness that is symmetric, usually begins in the legs, is often more marked proximally than distally, and is sometimes so severe that it is life-threatening, especially if the muscles of respiration or swallowing are involved. Muscle wasting develops if axonal degeneration has occurred. Sensory complaints, while usually less marked than motor symptoms, are also frequent. The deep tendon reflexes are typically absent. There may be marked autonomic dysfunction, with tachycardia, cardiac irregularities, labile blood pressure, disturbed sweating, impaired pulmonary function, sphincter disturbances, paralytic ileus, and other abnormalities.

B. INVESTIGATIVE STUDIES

The CSF often shows a characteristic abnormality, with increased protein concentration but a normal cell count; abnormalities may not be found in the first week, however. Electrophysiologic studies may reveal marked slowing of motor and sensory conduction velocity, or evidence of denervation and axonal loss. The time course of the electrophysiologic changes does not necessarily parallel any clinical developments. When HIV-1 infection is suspected because of the clinical context in which the neuropathy has developed or the presence of high-risk factors, appropriate serologic studies should be performed.

C. TREATMENT

Plasmapheresis appears to reduce the time required for recovery and may decrease the likelihood of residual neu-

Table 6–3. Diagnostic criteria for Guillain-Barré syndrome.[1]

Required for diagnosis
 Progressive weakness of more than one limb
 Distal areflexia with proximal areflexia or hyporeflexia
Supportive of diagnosis
 Progression for up to 4 weeks
 Relatively symmetric deficits
 Mild sensory involvement
 Cranial nerve (especially VII) involvement
 Recovery beginning within 4 weeks after progression stops
 Autonomic dysfunction
 No fever at onset
 Increased CSF protein after 1 week
 CSF white blood cell count ≤10/μl
 Nerve conduction slowing or block by several weeks
Against diagnosis
 Markedly asymmetric weakness
 Bowel or bladder dysfunction (at onset or persistent)
 CSF white blood cell count >50 or PMN count >O/μL
 Well-demarcated sensory level
Excluding diagnosis
 Isolated sensory involvement
 Another polyneuropathy that explains clinical picture

[1] Adapted from Asbury AK, Cornblath DR: Assessment of current diagnostic criteria for Guillain-Barré syndrome. Ann Neurol 1990;27(Suppl):S21–S24.

rologic deficits. It is best instituted early, and it is indicated especially in patients with a severe or rapidly progressive deficit or respiratory compromise. Intravenous immunoglobulin (400 mg/kg/d for 5 days) appears to be equally effective and should be used in preference to plasmapheresis in adults with cardiovascular instability and in children; the two therapies are not additive.

Therapy is otherwise symptomatic, the aim being to prevent such complications as respiratory failure or vascular collapse. For this reason, patients who are severely affected are best managed in intensive care units, where facilities are available for monitoring and assisted respiration if necessary (eg, if the vital capacity falls below about 1 L, the patient is short of breath, or the blood oxygen saturation declines). Volume replacement or treatment with pressor agents is sometimes required to counter hypotension, and low-dose heparin may help to prevent pulmonary embolism. Corticosteroids may affect the outcome adversely or delay recovery, and are not indicated.

D. Prognosis

Symptoms and signs cease to progress by about 4 weeks into the illness. The disorder is self-limiting, and improvement occurs over the weeks or months follow-

ing onset. About 70–75% of patients recover completely, 25% are left with mild neurologic deficits, and 5% die, usually as a result of respiratory failure. The prognosis is poorer when there is evidence of preceding *Campylobacter jejuni* infection, and a more protracted course and less complete recovery are also likely when axonal degeneration rather than demyelination is the primary pathology. Advanced age, the need for ventilatory support, or more rapid onset of symptoms may also predict a poorer prognosis.

Chronic Inflammatory Demyelinating Polyneuropathy

Chronic inflammatory demyelinating polyneuropathy is clinically similar to Guillain-Barré syndrome except that it follows a chronic progressive course—or a course characterized by relapses—and no improvement is apparent within the 6 months after onset. Its cause is not known. Its clinical features are summarized in Table 6–4. Examination of the CSF reveals findings resembling those in Guillain-Barré syndrome. The electrophysiologic findings indicate a demyelinative neuropa-

Table 6–4. Clinical features of chronic inflammatory demyelinating polyneuropathy.[1]

	Percentage of Patients
Weakness hyporeflexia or areflexia	94
Distal upper extremity	85
Distal lower extremity	85
Proximal upper extremity	74
Proximal lower extremity	68
Respiratory muscles	11
Neck	4
Face	2
Sensory deficit on examination	
Distal lower extremity	83
Distal upper extremity	68
Paresthesia	
Upper extremity	79
Lower extremity	72
Face	6
Pain	
Lower extremity	17
Upper extremity	15
Dysarthria	9
Dysphagia	9
Impotence	4
Incontinence	2

[1] Adapted from Dyck PJ et al: Chronic inflammatory polyradiculopathy. Mayo Clin Proc 1975;50:621–637.

thy with superimposed axonal degeneration. The disorder is often responsive to treatment with corticosteroids (prednisone, 60–100 mg/d for 2–4 weeks, then gradually tapered to 5–20 mg every other day), which may have to be continued on a long-term basis. Treatment with intravenous immunoglobulin (1 g/kg daily for 2 days with a single additional infusion at 3 weeks, or 400 mg/kg/d for 5 consecutive days for a total of 2 g, with subsequent courses as needed to maintain benefit) is also effective as initial or later therapy. When used as the initial therapy, it has the advantage of fewer side effects (but greater expense) than prednisone. Its precise mode of action is unknown. Plasma exchange is another effective immunomodulator therapy, but is more difficult to administer. In nonresponsive patients, treatment with azathioprine or cyclophosphamide may be helpful.

METABOLIC & NUTRITIONAL NEUROPATHIES

Diabetes Mellitus

Peripheral nerve involvement in diabetes is common and may be characterized by polyneuropathy, which is of mixed (sensory, motor, and autonomic) character in about 70% of cases and predominantly sensory in about 30%; mononeuropathy multiplex; or mononeuropathy simplex (Table 6–5). Such clinical manifestations can

Table 6–5. Neuropathies associated with diabetes.

Type	Distribution
Polyneuropathy	
Mixed sensory, motor, and autonomic	Symmetric, distal, lower > upper limbs
Primarily sensory	
Mononeuropathy multiplex	Variable
Polyradiculopathy/plexopathy	
(Diabetic amyotrophy)	Asymmetric, proximal (pelvic girdle and thighs)
Thoracoabdominal radiculopathy	Chest, abdomen
Mononeuropathy simplex	
Peripheral	Ulnar, median, radial, lateral femoral cutaneous, sciatic, peroneal, other nerves
Cranial	Oculomotor (III) > abducens (VI) > trochlear Facial (IV) nerve

occur in isolation or in any combination. The incidence of peripheral nerve involvement may be influenced by the adequacy of diabetes control, which should, in any event, be optimal.

A. CLINICAL FEATURES

The most common manifestation is a distal sensory or mixed **polyneuropathy,** which is sometimes diagnosed, before it becomes symptomatic, from the presence of depressed tendon reflexes and impaired appreciation of vibration in the legs. Symptoms are generally more common in the legs than in the arms and consist of numbness, pain, or paresthesias. In severe cases, there is distal sensory loss in all limbs and some accompanying motor disturbance. Diabetic dysautonomia leads to many symptoms, including postural hypotension, disturbances of cardiac rhythm, impaired thermoregulatory sweating, and disturbances of bladder, bowel, gastric, and sexual function. Diabetic **mononeuropathy multiplex** is usually characterized by pain and weakness and often has a vascular basis. The clinical deficit will depend on the nerves that are affected. Diabetic **amyotrophy** is due to radiculoplexopathy, polyradiculopathy, or polyradiculoneuropathy. Pain, weakness, and atrophy of pelvic girdle and thigh muscles are typical, with absent quadriceps reflexes and little sensory loss. Diabetic **mononeuropathy simplex** is typically abrupt in onset and often painful. Cerebrospinal fluid (CSF) protein is typically increased in diabetic polyneuropathy and mononeuropathy multiplex.

B. TREATMENT AND PROGNOSIS

No specific treatment exists for the peripheral nerve complications of diabetes except when the patient has an entrapment neuropathy and may benefit from a decompressive procedure. Pain is troublesome in some patients and responds to the measures outlined earlier (p. 212).

Postural hypotension may respond to treatment with salt supplementation; sleeping in an upright position; wearing waist-high elastic hosiery; fludrocortisone, 0.1–1 mg/d; and midodrine (an α-agonist), 10 mg three times daily. Treatment is otherwise symptomatic. Diabetic amyotrophy and mononeuropathy simplex usually improve or resolve spontaneously.

Other Endocrinopathies

Hypothyroidism is a rare cause of polyneuropathy. More commonly, hypothyroidism is associated with entrapment neuropathy, especially carpal tunnel syndrome (see later, under *Median Nerve*). Polyneuropathy may be mistakenly diagnosed in patients with proximal limb weakness caused by hypothyroid myopathy or in patients with delayed relaxation of tendon reflexes, a classic manifestation of hypothyroidism that is independent of neuropathy. Other neurologic manifestations of hypothyroidism such as acute confusional state (see Chapter 1), dementia (see Chapter 1), and cerebellar degeneration (see Chapter 3) are discussed elsewhere.

Acromegaly also frequently produces carpal tunnel syndrome and, less often, polyneuropathy. Because many acromegalic patients are also diabetic, it may be difficult to determine which disorder is primarily responsible for polyneuropathy in a given patient.

Uremia

A symmetric sensorimotor polyneuropathy, predominantly axonal in type, may occur in uremia. It tends to affect the legs more than the arms and is more marked distally than proximally. Restless legs, muscle cramps, and burning feet have been associated with it. The extent of any disturbance in peripheral nerve function appears to relate to the severity of impaired renal function. The neuropathy itself may improve markedly with renal transplantation. Carpal tunnel syndrome (see later) has also been described in patients with renal disease and may develop distal to the arteriovenous fistulas placed in the forearm for access during hemodialysis. In patients on chronic hemodialysis, it often relates to amyloidosis and the accumulation of β_2-microglobulin.

Liver Disease

Primary biliary cirrhosis may lead to a sensory neuropathy that is probably of the axonal type. A predominantly demyelinative polyneuropathy can occur in patients with chronic liver disease. There does not appear to be any correlation between the neurologic findings and the severity of the hepatic dysfunction.

Vitamin B$_{12}$ Deficiency

Vitamin B$_{12}$ deficiency is associated with many features that are characteristic of polyneuropathy, including symmetric distal sensory and mild motor impairment and loss of tendon reflexes. Because controversy exists about the relative importance of polyneuropathy and myelopathy in producing this syndrome, vitamin B$_{12}$ deficiency is considered in more detail below in the section on myelopathies.

INFECTIVE & GRANULOMATOUS NEUROPATHIES

AIDS

Neuropathy is a common complication of HIV-1 infection (Table 6–6); involvement of peripheral nerves is seen at autopsy in about 40% of patients with AIDS.

Distal symmetric **sensorimotor polyneuropathy** is the most common neuropathy associated with HIV-1 infection. Axons, rather than myelin, are primarily affected. The cause is unknown, but in some patients vitamin B$_{12}$ deficiency or exposure to neurotoxic drugs may be responsible in part. HIV-1 is rarely identified in the affected nerves. Sensory symptoms predominate and include pain and paresthesias that affect the feet especially. Weakness is a minor or late feature. Ankle and sometimes knee reflexes are absent. The course is typically progressive and no treatment is available, but pain may be controlled pharmacologically, as described earlier on p. 212. Plasmapheresis is of no benefit.

Inflammatory demyelinating polyneuropathy may occur early in HIV-1 infection and may follow an acute or chronic course. The neuropathy may be immune mediated, but sometimes results from direct, secondary viral infection, as from cytomegalovirus. It is characterized by proximal, and sometimes distal, weakness with less pronounced sensory disturbances and areflexia or hyporeflexia. The CSF is abnormal, with an elevated protein concentration and often a lymphocytic pleocytosis (unlike the findings in Guillain-Barré syn-

Table 6–6. Neuropathies associated with AIDS.

Type	Stage of HIV-1 Infection	Immune Status	Distribution
Sensorimotor polyneuropathy	Early or late	Competent or suppressed	Symmetric, distal, lower > upper limbs
Inflammatory demyelinating polyneuropathy	Early	Competent	Proximal > distal limbs
Lumbosacral polyradiculopathy	Late	Suppressed	Proximal lower limbs, sphincters
Mononeuropathy multiplex	Early or late	Competent or suppressed	Cranial (eg, facial), peripheral (eg, peroneal)
Mononeuropathy simplex	Early	Competent	Cranial (eg, facial), peripheral (eg, peroneal)
Autonomic neuropathy	Early or late	Competent or suppressed	Not applicable

drome or chronic inflammatory demyelinating polyneuropathy in patients without HIV-1 infection). Some patients improve spontaneously or stabilize, and others may respond to corticosteroids, plasmapheresis, or intravenous immunoglobulins.

Lumbosacral polyradiculopathy occurs late in the course of HIV-1 infection, usually in patients with prior opportunistic infections. Cytomegalovirus infection is thought to be the cause, at least in some instances. Clinical features usually develop over several weeks and include diffuse, progressive leg weakness, back pain, painful paresthesias of the feet and perineum, lower extremity areflexia, and early urinary retention. The course may be fulminant, with ascending paralysis leading to respiratory failure. The course is more benign in some patients, however, especially when the etiology is unclear. CSF findings include mononuclear or polymorphonuclear pleocytosis, elevated protein, and decreased glucose. It is always important to exclude meningeal lymphomatosis, cord compression, or syphilis as the underlying cause, as these require specific treatment and affect the prognosis. Patients with cytomegalovirus infection may respond to ganciclovir, 2.5 mg/kg intravenously every 8 hours for 10 days, then 7.5 mg/kg/d 5 days per week.

Mononeuropathy multiplex affects multiple cranial and peripheral nerves, resulting in focal weakness and sensory loss. Some cases may have an autoimmune basis, whereas others result from neoplastic or infectious causes (eg, cytomegalovirus infection) or from vasculopathy. In early HIV-1 infection, mononeuropathy multiplex may be a self-limited disorder restricted to a single limb, with spontaneous stabilization or improvement. Late in AIDS, multiple limbs may be affected in a progressive fashion.

Mononeuropathy simplex tends to occur acutely in early HIV-1 infection and improve spontaneously. A vascular cause is probable.

Autonomic neuropathy tends to occur late in the course of HIV-1 infections and may lead to syncopal episodes, orthostatic hypotension, disturbances of sphincter or sexual function, impaired thermoregulatory sweating, and diarrhea. The dysautonomia may relate to central or peripheral pathology. Treatment is symptomatic (as discussed earlier under diabetic neuropathy).

Leprosy

Leprosy is one of the most frequent causes of peripheral neuropathy worldwide. In turn, neuropathy is the most disabling manifestation of leprosy. *Mycobacterium leprae* affects the skin and peripheral nerves because its growth is facilitated by the cooler temperatures present at the body surface.

In **tuberculoid leprosy,** the immune response is adequate to confine the infection to one or more small patches of skin and their associated cutaneous and subcutaneous nerves. This produces a hypopigmented macule or papule over which sensation is impaired, with pain and temperature appreciation most affected. Anhidrosis occurs as a result of local involvement of autonomic fibers. Sensory deficits occur most often in the distribution of the digital, sural, radial, and posterior auricular nerves, whereas motor findings usually relate to involvement of the ulnar or peroneal nerve. Involved nerves are often enlarged.

Lepromatous leprosy is a more widespread disorder that results in a symmetric, primarily sensory polyneuropathy that disproportionately affects pain and temperature sense. Its distribution is distinctive in that exposed areas of the body—especially the ears; nose; cheeks; dorsal surfaces of the hands, forearms, and feet; and lateral aspects of the legs—are preferentially involved. Unlike most polyneuropathies, that caused by leprosy tends to spare the tendon reflexes. Associated findings include resorption of the digits, trophic ulcers, and cyanosis and anhidrosis of the hands and feet.

Treatment depends on the type of leprosy, but typically involves dapsone, rifampin, and clofazimine. The most recent guidelines of the World Health Organization should be followed. In the United States, further information can be obtained from the Gillis W. Long Hansen's Disease Center, in Carville, Louisiana.

Diphtheria

Corynebacterium diphtheriae infects tissues of the upper respiratory tract and produces a toxin that causes demyelination of peripheral nerves. Within about 1 month after infection, patients may develop a cranial motor neuropathy with prominent impairment of ocular accommodation. Blurred vision is the usual presenting complaint. Extraocular muscles and the face, palate, pharynx, and diaphragm may also be affected, but the pupillary light reflex is preserved. Recovery typically occurs after several weeks. A more delayed syndrome that commonly has its onset 2–3 months following the primary infection takes the form of a symmetric distal sensorimotor polyneuropathy. Most patients recover completely. Diphtheritic neuropathy is discussed in more detail in Chapter 5.

Sarcoidosis

Sarcoidosis can produce mononeuropathy or, rarely, polyneuropathy. The mononeuropathy commonly involves cranial nerves, especially the facial nerve, in which case the resulting syndrome may be indistinguishable from idiopathic facial paralysis (Bell's palsy). X-rays of the lungs and bones and determination of serum levels of angiotensin-converting enzyme are helpful in establishing the diagnosis. Treatment with prednisone, 60 mg/d orally followed by tapering doses, may speed recovery.

Sepsis

Patients with sepsis and multiorgan failure may develop a **critical illness polyneuropathy.** This is manifest primarily by weakness and is therefore discussed in Chapter 5.

NEUROPATHIES IN VASCULITIS & COLLAGEN VASCULAR DISEASE

Systemic vasculitides and collagen vascular diseases can produce polyneuropathy, mononeuropathy simplex, mononeuropathy multiplex, or entrapment neuropathy (Table 6–7).

Systemic necrotizing vasculitis includes polyarteritis nodosa and allergic angiitis and granulomatosis (Churg-Strauss syndrome). Neuropathy occurs in about 50% of patients, most often as mononeuropathy multiplex, which may manifest itself with the acute onset of pain in one or more cranial or peripheral nerves. Distal symmetric sensorimotor polyneuropathy is less common. Treatment should begin as soon as the diagnosis is made; it includes prednisone, 60–100 mg/d orally, and cyclophosphamide, 2–3 mg/d orally. Plasmapheresis may also be helpful.

Wegener's granulomatosis is associated with mononeuropathy multiplex or polyneuropathy in up to 30% of cases. Treatment is the same as for systemic necrotizing vasculitis.

Giant cell arteritis is considered in detail in Chapter 2. Mononeuropathy affecting cranial nerves innervating the extraocular muscles can occur.

Rheumatoid arthritis produces entrapment neuropathy (most commonly involving the median nerve) in about 45% of patients and distal symmetric sensorimotor polyneuropathy in about 30%. Mononeuropathy multiplex is a frequent feature in cases complicated by necrotizing vasculitis.

Systemic lupus erythematosus is discussed in Chapter 1 as a cause of acute confusional states. Neuropathy occurs in up to 20% of patients. The most common pattern is a distal, symmetric sensorimotor polyneuropathy. An ascending, predominantly motor polyneuropathy (Guillain-Barré syndrome, see earlier) can also occur, as may mononeuropathy simplex or multiplex, which often affects the ulnar, radial, sciatic, or peroneal nerve.

Sjögren's syndrome involves the peripheral nerves in about 20% of cases. Distal symmetric sensorimotor polyneuropathy is most common, entrapment neuropathy (affecting especially the median nerve) is also frequent, and mononeuropathy multiplex can occur.

Progressive systemic sclerosis (scleroderma) and **mixed connective tissue disease** may produce cranial mononeuropathy, which most often involves the trigeminal (V) nerve.

NEOPLASTIC & PARAPROTEINEMIC NEUROPATHIES

Compression & Infiltration by Tumor

Nerve compression is a common complication of multiple myeloma, lymphoma, and carcinoma. Tumorous invasion of the epineurium may occur with leukemia, lymphoma, and carcinoma of the breast or pancreas.

Table 6–7. Neuropathies associated with vasculitis and collagen vascular disease.

Disease	Polyneuropathy	Mononeuropathy Simplex or Multiplex[1]	Entrapment Neuropathy[1]
Vasculitis			
Systemic necrotizing vasculitis[2]	+	+	−
Wegener's granulomatosis	+	+	−
Giant cell arteritis	−	+ (III, VI, IV)	−
Collagen vascular disease			
Rheumatoid arthritis	+	+	+ (M, U, R)
Systemic lupus erythematosus	+	+	−
Sjögren's syndrome	+	+ (V, III, VI)	+ (M)
Progressive systemic sclerosis	−	+ (V)	−
Mixed connective-tissue disease	+	+ (V)	−

[1] Commonly affected nerves: III, oculomotor; IV, trochlear; V, trigeminal; VI, abducens; M, median; R, radial; U, ulnar.

[2] Includes polyarteritis nodosa and Churg-Strauss syndrome.

+, present; −, absent.

Paraneoplastic Syndromes

Carcinoma (especially oat-cell carcinoma of the lung) and lymphoma may be associated with neuropathies that are thought to be immunologically mediated, based on the detection of autoantibodies to neuronal antigens in several cases.

Sensory or sensorimotor polyneuropathy occurs with both carcinoma and lymphoma. This can be either an acute or chronic disorder; it is sometimes asymmetric and may be accompanied by prominent pain.

Carcinoma can also cause **sensory neuronopathy,** which primarily affects the cell bodies of sensory neurons in the dorsal root ganglion and is associated with the presence of anti-Hu (or ANNA-1) antibodies (see Chapter 3). This rare condition may be the presenting manifestation of cancer. Initial symptoms of pain and numbness usually begin distally but sometimes begin proximally or in the face. The disorders often progress over days or several weeks, leading to marked sensory ataxia and impairment of all sensory modalities. Motor involvement is late, and autonomic dysfunction is uncommon. The CSF may have an inflammatory formulation. Treatment, even of the underlying tumor, is usually unrewarding.

Lymphoma may be complicated by **motor neuronopathy,** a disorder of anterior horn cells, which is discussed in Chapter 5. Hodgkin's disease and angioimmunoblastic lymphadenopathy are sometimes associated with Guillain-Barré syndrome.

Paraproteinemias

Polyneuropathy is a common complication of **multiple myeloma.** Patients affected by lytic myeloma are usually men. The clinical picture is of a distal symmetric sensorimotor polyneuropathy. All sensory modalities are affected, pain is a frequent feature, and the reflexes are depressed. The disorder is usually progressive and leads to death within 2 years. **Sclerotic myeloma** may be accompanied by a chronic demyelinating polyneuropathy. Motor involvement predominates, but vibration and position sense may also be impaired, and the reflexes are depressed. Pain is less common than in the neuropathy of lytic myeloma, and symptoms may improve with treatment of the underlying cancer or by plasmapheresis. The **POEMS syndrome** (polyneuropathy, organomegaly, endocrinopathy, M protein, and skin changes) may complicate plasma cell dyscrasias, especially osteosclerotic myeloma. The sensorimotor polyneuropathy may respond to treatment with corticosteroids or cyclophosphamide; irradiation of solitary osteosclerotic lesions may also be worthwhile.

A sensorimotor polyneuropathy similar to that observed with lytic myeloma may also occur in **Waldenström's macroglobulinemia** or **benign monoclonal gammopathy.** Treatment with immunosuppressant drugs and plasmapheresis is sometimes helpful.

Amyloidosis

Nonhereditary amyloidosis occurs as an isolated disorder (primary generalized amyloidosis) or in patients with multiple myeloma and may be associated with polyneuropathy. Polyneuropathy is also a feature of hereditary amyloidosis. Amyloid neuropathies are considered below in the section on hereditary neuropathies.

DRUG-INDUCED & TOXIC NEUROPATHIES

Alcoholism

Polyneuropathy is one of the most common neurologic complications of chronic alcoholism; it can occur alone or in combination with other alcohol-related neurologic disorders, such as Wernicke's encephalopathy (see Chapter 1) or the Korsakoff amnestic syndrome (see Chapter 1). Controversy exists concerning the relative contributions of direct neurotoxicity of alcohol and associated nutritional (especially thiamine) deficiency in producing polyneuropathy.

Alcoholic polyneuropathy is typically a symmetric distal sensorimotor neuropathy. The legs are particularly likely to be affected, resulting in defective perception of vibration and touch and depressed or absent ankle reflexes. In some cases, distal weakness is also pronounced and autonomic dysfunction may occur. When pain is a prominent feature, it may respond to the same treatment described on p. 212 for painful neuropathy.

Abstinence from alcohol and thiamine repletion can halt the progression of symptoms.

Other Drugs

As indicated in Table 6–2, a large number of drugs have been reported to cause neuropathies. A few merit brief comment.

Dapsone, a drug used to treat leprosy, can produce a primarily motor polyneuropathy that is reversible.

Hydralazine, an antihypertensive drug, is associated on rare occasions with a predominantly sensory polyneuropathy that has been attributed to drug-induced pyridoxine deficiency and that resolves after the drug is discontinued.

Isoniazid is a widely used antituberculous agent that interferes with pyridoxine metabolism and produces a polyneuropathy that principally affects the sensory neurons. High doses, hereditary variations in drug metabolism, and malnutrition predispose to this complication. Spontaneous recovery is the rule when administration of the drug is halted. Isoniazid-induced neuropathy can be prevented by concurrent administration of pyridoxine, 100 mg/d orally.

Phenytoin is often mentioned as a cause of polyneuropathy, but evidence for phenytoin treatment as a cause of symptomatic neuropathy is sparse.

Pyridoxine (vitamin B_6) toxicity has been implicated as the cause of a sensory neuronopathy that disproportionately impairs vibration and position sense. This disorder usually occurs in patients taking at least 200 mg of pyridoxine daily—about 100 times the minimum daily requirement. Sensory ataxia, Romberg's sign, Lhermitte's sign, and ankle areflexia are common findings. Pain is less common, and motor involvement is unusual. Symptoms are usually reversible over months to years if the abuse ceases, but an irreversible syndrome has also been reported following intravenous administration of high doses of pyridoxine.

Vincristine produces a polyneuropathy in most patients who receive the drug for treatment of (usually hematologic) cancer. The earliest manifestations are distal sensory symptoms and loss of reflexes. Motor deficits may predominate later in the course, however. Constipation is a common finding and may be due to autonomic involvement. Discontinuing the drug or administering it at a reduced dosage often leads to improvement.

Toxins

Organic compounds implicated as causes of polyneuropathy include hexacarbons present in solvents and glues (eg, *n*-hexane, methyl *n*-butyl ketone) and organophosphates used as plasticizers or insecticides (eg, triorthocresyl phosphate). Sensory involvement is most striking in *n*-hexane neuropathy, whereas neuropathy caused by triorthocresyl phosphate primarily affects motor nerves. Organophosphate neuropathy is discussed in more detail in Chapter 5.

Heavy metals may also be responsible for polyneuropathy. Neuropathy caused by lead, arsenic, and thallium is discussed in Chapter 5. Gold, which is used to treat rheumatoid arthritis, may cause a symmetric polyneuropathy, and cisplatin (a platinum analogue with anticancer activity) may produce a sensory neuropathy.

Eosinophilia-myalgia syndrome was first identified in 1989 in patients taking L-tryptophan who developed disabling myalgias with blood eosinophil counts above 1,000/μL. About 85% of patients are women. The cause appears to be 1,1′-ethylidenebis [tryptophan], a contaminant in certain commercial preparations of L-tryptophan, which have since been withdrawn. Symptoms include myalgia, arthralgia, dyspnea, cough, rash, fever, and sclerodermiform skin changes. Neurologic findings include weakness of distal and proximal limb and bulbar muscles, distal sensory loss, and areflexia. Eosinophilia, leukocytosis, and elevated liver enzymes are typical.

Nerve conduction studies and electromyography may show evidence of polyneuropathy, myopathy, or both. Inflammation is prominent in skin biopsy specimens, but less so in nerve and muscle, which show primarily axonal degeneration and muscle fiber atrophy. Treatment is discontinuation of L-tryptophan and administration of corticosteroids, nonsteroidal antiinflammatory drugs, and analgesics. Most patients improve or recover fully, but deaths have been reported.

HEREDITARY NEUROPATHIES

Hereditary Motor and Sensory Neuropathies

These are designated **Charcot-Marie-Tooth** (**CMT**) hereditary neuropathies. They constitute a genetically heterogeneous group of disorders having the same clinical phenotype. There is weakness and wasting of distal muscles in the limbs, with or without sensory loss; pes cavus and reduced or absent tendon reflexes also occur. They are divided into demyelinating (CMT1) and neuronal (CMT2) types, the latter sparing sensory neurons and resembling progressive spinal muscular atrophy (see Chapter 5). Both types have an autosomal dominant pattern of inheritance although "sporadic" cases occur.

CMT1 has its onset in the first decade, follows a slowly progressive course, and is of variable severity. The nerves are palpably thickened in about 50% of cases. Nerve conduction velocities are markedly reduced. CMT1 is subdivided on the basis of the genetic findings (Table 6–8). An X-linked dominant form (CMTX) and autosomal recessive types (CMT4) have also been described.

Dejerine-Sottas disease has its onset by 2 years of age with delayed motor milestones and is characterized by a severe sensorimotor neuropathy that frequently extends to the proximal muscles and is associated with skeletal abnormalities such as scoliosis. There is severe demyelination of the nerves. It was previously thought to have an autosomal recessive mode of inheritance, but it is now accepted that it is inherited in an autosomal dominant manner and the responsible mutations have involved the same genes as are associated with CMT1.

Hereditary Sensory and Autonomic Neuropathies (HSAN)

These neuropathies also take a variety of forms. In **HSAN type I,** there is a dominant inheritance, a gradually progressive course from onset in early adulthood, and symmetric loss of distal pain and temperature perception, with relative preservation of light touch. Perforating ulcers over pressure points and painless infections of the extremities are common. The tendon reflexes are depressed, but there is little, if any, motor disturbance. The gene maps to chromosome 9q22. In **HSAN type**

Table 6–8. Hereditary motor and sensory neuropathies of the Charcot-Marie-Tooth (CMT) type.

Disease	Inheritance[1]	Gene	Locus
CMT1A	AD	*PMP-22*	17p11.2
CMT1B	AD	*MPZ*	1q22–q23
CMT1C	AD	?	?
CMTX	XD	*GJB1*	Xq13–q22
CMT2A	AD	?	1p36–p35
CMT2B	AD	?	3q13–q22
CMT2C	AD	*MPD2*	5q
CMT2D	AD	?	7p14
CMT2E	AD	*NEFL*	8p21
Dejerine-Sottas	AD	*MPZ*	1q22–q23
		PMP-22	17p11.2
		EGR2	10q21–q22
		?	8q23–q24
CMT4A	AR	?	8q13–q21.1
CMT4B	AR	*MTMR2*	11q22
			11p15
CMT4C	AR	?	5q23–q33
CMT4D	AR	?	8q24
CMT4E	AR	?	10q21–q22
CMT4F	AR	?	19q13

[1] AD, autosomal dominant; AR, autosomal recessive; XD, X-linked dominant.

II, inheritance is recessive, onset is in infancy or early childhood, all sensory modalities are affected, and tendon reflexes are lost. **HSAN type III (Riley-Day syndrome, familial dysautonomia)** is a recessive disorder that commences in infancy and is characterized by conspicuous autonomic dysfunction (absent tearing, labile temperature and blood pressure), accompanied by absent taste sensation, impaired pain and temperature sensation, and areflexia. The disorder is linked to chromosome 9q31. **HSAN type IV** is associated with congenital insensitivity to pain and absent sweating, and has been related to recessive mutations in the gene encoding a receptor tyrosine kinase for nerve growth factor at chromosome 1q21–q22.

Amyloidosis

Polyneuropathy can occur in both the hereditary and nonhereditary forms of amyloidosis. Because small-diameter sensory and autonomic nerve fibers are especially likely to be involved, pain and temperature sensation and autonomic functions are prominently affected. Clinical presentation is commonly with distal paresthesias, dysesthesias, and numbness; postural hypotension; impaired thermoregulatory sweating; and disturbances of bladder, bowel, or sexual function. Distal weakness and wasting eventually occur. The tendon reflexes are often preserved until a relatively late stage. Entrapment neuropathy—especially carpal tunnel syndrome—may develop as a consequence of amyloid deposits. There is no specific treatment.

Friedreich's Ataxia

Friedreich's ataxia usually has a recessive mode of inheritance but occasionally occurs with dominant inheritance. It is caused in many cases by a triplet repeat expansion in a noncoding region of the frataxin gene (X25) on chromosome 9q13–q21.1, but there is some heterogeneity of phenotype and variation in age of onset among patients with this expansion. This expansion has not been found in all cases, suggesting that other genetic or environmental factors are sometimes responsible. An ataxic gait develops, followed by clumsiness of the hands and other signs of cerebellar dysfunction. Involvement of peripheral sensory fibers leads to sensory deficits of the limbs, with depressed or absent tendon reflexes. There may also be leg weakness and extensor plantar responses from central motor involvement. This condition is considered in detail in Chapter 3.

Hereditary Neuropathy with Liability to Pressure Palsies

This is a genetically heterogeneous disorder that relates most commonly to deletion of the PMP-22 gene on chromosome 17. Inheritance is as an autosomal dominant trait with variable expression. Patients present with simple or multiple mononeuropathies that occur after mild pressure or stretch of nerves, and electrophysiologic studies reveal that abnormalities are more widespread than is evident clinically.

Metabolic Disorders

In **acute intermittent porphyria**, which is transmitted by recessive inheritance, the initial neurologic manifestation is often a polyneuropathy that (usually) involves motor more than sensory fibers. Sensory symptoms and signs may be predominantly proximal or distal. The peripheral nerves may also be affected in **variegate porphyria**. Neuropathy caused by porphyria is considered in greater detail in Chapter 5.

Two recessive lipidoses are associated with polyneuropathy with a typical onset in infancy or childhood. These are **metachromatic leukodystrophy**, which results from deficiency of the enzyme arylsulfatase A, and **Krabbe's disease**, which is due to galactocerebroside β-galactosidase deficiency. Both are inherited in an autosomal recessive fashion.

Lipoprotein deficiencies that cause polyneuropathy include **abetalipoproteinemia,** which is associated with acanthocytosis, malabsorption, retinitis pigmentosa, and cerebellar ataxia; and **Tangier disease,** which produces cataract, orange discoloration of the tonsils, and hepatosplenomegaly. These are autosomal recessive conditions.

Refsum's disease is an autosomal recessive disorder related to impaired metabolism of phytanic acid. It produces polyneuropathy, cerebellar ataxia, retinitis pigmentosa, and ichthyosis. It can be treated by restricting dietary intake of phytol. Plasmapheresis to reduce body stores of phytanic acid may also be helpful at the initiation of treatment.

Fabry's disease is an X-linked recessive deficiency of the enzyme α-galactosidase-A. It results in a painful sensory and autonomic neuropathy, angiokeratomas, renal disease, and an increased incidence of stroke. The responsible gene has been localized to the long arm of the X chromosome; mutations causing the disease have been recognized and include gene rearrangements, an RNA-splicing defect, and various exonic lesions. Pharmacologic measures (p 212) may be helpful in treating the pain that characterizes the disorder. Enzyme replacement therapy is under investigation.

ENTRAPMENT NEUROPATHIES

Certain peripheral nerves are particularly susceptible to mechanical injury at vulnerable sites. The term **entrapment neuropathy** is used when the nerve is compressed, stretched, or angulated by adjacent anatomic structures to such an extent that dysfunction occurs. There are numerous entrapment neuropathies, and in many the initial or most conspicuous clinical complaints are of sensory symptoms or pain. Some of the more common syndromes are described below.

ENTRAPMENT SYNDROMES OF UPPER LIMBS

Median Nerve Compression

Compression of the median nerve can occur in the carpal tunnel at the wrist. **Carpal tunnel syndrome** is common during pregnancy and can occur as a complication of trauma, degenerative arthritis, tenosynovitis, myxedema, and acromegaly. Early symptoms are pain and paresthesias confined to a median nerve distribution in the hand, ie, involving primarily the thumb, index, and middle fingers and the lateral half of the ring finger (see Appendix C). There may be pain in the forearm and, in occasional patients, even in the upper arm, shoulder, and neck. Symptoms are often particularly troublesome at night and may awaken the patient from sleep. As the neuropathy advances, weakness and atrophy may eventually develop in the thenar muscles. Examination reveals impaired cutaneous sensation in the median nerve distribution in the hand and, with motor involvement, weakness and wasting of the abductor pollicis brevis and opponens pollicis muscles (see Appendix C). There may be a positive **Tinel sign** (percussion of the nerve at the wrist causes paresthesias in its distribution) or a positive response to **Phalen's maneuver** (flexion of the wrist for 1 minute exacerbates or reproduces symptoms). The diagnosis can generally be confirmed by electrophysiologic studies, showing sensory or motor conduction velocity to be slowed at the wrist; there may be signs of chronic partial denervation in median-supplied muscles of the hand.

If the symptoms fail to respond to local corticosteroid injections or simple maneuvers such as wearing a nocturnal wrist splint, surgical decompression of the carpal tunnel may be necessary.

Interdigital Neuropathy

Interdigital neuropathy may lead to pain in one or two fingers, and examination reveals hyperpathia or impaired cutaneous sensation in the appropriate distribution of the affected nerve or nerves. Such a neuropathy may result from entrapment in the intermetacarpal tunnel of the hand, direct trauma, tenosynovitis, or arthritis.

Treatment by local infiltration with corticosteroids is sometimes helpful, but in severe cases neurolysis may be necessary.

Ulnar Nerve Dysfunction

Ulnar nerve dysfunction at the **elbow** leads to paresthesias, hypesthesia, and nocturnal pain in the little finger and ulnar border of the hand. Pain may also occur about the elbow. Symptoms are often intensified by elbow flexion or use of the arm. Examination may reveal sensory loss on the ulnar aspect of the hand (see Appendix C) and weakness of the adductor pollicis, the deep flexor muscles of the fourth and fifth digits, and the intrinsic hand muscles (see Appendix C). The lesion may result from external pressure, from entrapment within the cubital tunnel, or from cubitus valgus deformity causing chronic stretch injury of the nerve. Electrodiagnostic studies may be helpful in localizing the lesion.

Avoiding pressure on or repetitive flexion and extension of the elbow, combined in some instances with splinting the elbow in extension, is sometimes sufficient to arrest progression and alleviate symptoms. Surgical decompression or ulnar nerve transposition to the flexor surface of the arm may also be helpful, depending on the cause and severity of the lesion and the duration of symptoms.

An ulnar nerve lesion may develop in the **wrist** or **palm** of the hand in association with repetitive trauma, arthritis, or compression from ganglia or benign tumors. Involvement of the deep terminal branch in the palm leads to a motor deficit in ulnar-innervated hand muscles other than the hypothenar group, whereas a more proximal palmar lesion affects the latter muscles as well; there is no sensory deficit. With lesions at the wrist involving either the ulnar nerve itself or its deep and superficial branches, both sensory and motor changes occur in the hand. Sensation over the dorsal surface of the hand is unaffected, however, because the cutaneous branch to this region arises proximal to the wrist. Surgical treatment is helpful in relieving compression from a ganglion or benign tumor.

Radial Nerve Compression

The radial nerve may be compressed in the axilla by pressure from crutches or other causes; this is frequently seen in alcoholics and drug addicts who have fallen asleep with an arm draped over some hard surface. The resulting deficit is primarily motor, with weakness or paralysis occurring in the muscles supplied by the nerve (see Appendix C), but sensory changes may also occur, especially in a small region on the back of the hand between the thumb and index finger (see Appendix C).

Treatment involves preventing further compression of the nerve. Recovery usually occurs spontaneously and completely except when a very severe injury has resulted in axonal degeneration. Physical therapy and a wrist splint may be helpful until recovery occurs.

Thoracic Outlet Syndrome

In thoracic outlet syndrome, a cervical rib or band or other anatomic structure may compress the lower part of the brachial plexus. Symptoms include pain, paresthesias, and numbness in a C8–T1 distribution (Figure 6–4). There may be diffuse weakness of the intrinsic hand muscles, often particularly involving the muscles in the thenar eminence and thereby simulating carpal tunnel syndrome. See the section on cervical rib syndrome in Chapter 5 for further details.

ENTRAPMENT SYNDROMES OF LOWER LIMBS

Peroneal Nerve Lesions

Peroneal nerve lesions can occur secondary to trauma or to pressure about the knee at the head of the fibula. The resulting weakness or paralysis of foot and toe extension—and foot eversion (see Appendix C)—is accompanied by impaired sensation over the dorsum of the foot and the lower anterior aspect of the leg (see Appendix C). The ankle reflex is preserved, as is foot inversion.

Treatment is purely supportive. It is important to protect the nerve from further injury or compression. Patients with foot drop may require a brace until recovery occurs. Recovery occurs spontaneously with time and is usually complete unless the injury was severe enough to cause marked axonal degeneration.

Tarsal Tunnel Syndrome

The posterior tibial nerve or its branches can be compressed between the floor and the ligamentous roof of the tarsal tunnel, which is located at the ankle immediately below and behind the medial malleolus. The usual complaint is of burning in the foot—especially at night—sometimes accompanied by weakness of the intrinsic foot muscles. The diagnosis can usually be confirmed electrophysiologically.

If treatment with local injection of steroids is not helpful, surgical decompression may be necessary.

Femoral Neuropathy

Isolated femoral neuropathy may occur in association with diabetes mellitus, vascular disease, bleeding diatheses (eg, hemophilia, treatment with anticoagulant drugs), or retroperitoneal neoplasms. The most conspicuous symptoms and signs relate to weakness of the quadriceps muscle, with reduced or absent knee reflex, but there may also be sensory disturbances in the anterior and medial aspects of the thigh and the medial part of the lower leg.

Treatment is of the underlying cause.

Saphenous Nerve Injury

The saphenous nerve is the terminal sensory branch of the femoral nerve and supplies cutaneous sensation to the medial aspect of the leg about and below the knee (see Figure 6–4). Mechanical injury to the nerve can occur at several points along its course; patients then complain of pain or impaired sensation in the distribution of the nerve. Weakness in quadriceps function (ie, extension at the knee; see Appendix C) reflects femoral nerve involvement.

There is no specific treatment, but the nerve should be protected from further injury.

Lateral Femoral Cutaneous Nerve Dysfunction

The lateral femoral cutaneous nerve supplies sensation to the outer border of the thigh (see Appendix C). Its function can be impaired by excessive angulation or compression by neighboring anatomic structures, especially in pregnancy or other conditions that cause exaggerated lumbar lordosis. This leads to pain and paresthesias in the lateral thigh, and examination reveals impaired sensation in this region. This syndrome, known as **meralgia paresthetica,** is best treated with symptomatic measures, as its course is often self-limited.

Obturator Nerve Injury

Trauma to the obturator nerve—eg, by pelvic fracture or a surgical procedure—can lead to pain radiating from the groin down the inner aspect of the thigh. An obturator hernia or osteitis pubis may cause a similar disorder; there is accompanying weakness of the adductor thigh muscles (see Appendix C).

ROOT & PLEXUS LESIONS

COMPRESSIVE & TRAUMATIC LESIONS

The clinical disturbances resulting from acute intervertebral disk prolapse, cervical spondylosis, traumatic plexopathy, cervical rib syndrome, and neuralgic amyotrophy were discussed in Chapter 5. In addition to these conditions, patients with metastatic cancer may develop root or plexus lesions from compression by tumor or as a result of trauma induced by radiation therapy. Root lesions are typically compressive in nature and usually occur in the setting of neoplastic meningitis, which is discussed in Chapter 1. Tumors (especially lung and breast cancer) can also infiltrate the brachial plexus, causing severe arm pain and sometimes dysesthesia. Because involvement of the lower trunk of the plexus is most common, symptoms usually occur within the C8 and T1 dermatomes, and Horner's syndrome (see Chapter 4) is present in about 50% of cases. Radiation injury—rather than direct invasion by tumor—should be suspected as the cause when the upper trunk of the brachial plexus (C5 and C6 nerve roots) is involved, weakness is a prominent presenting symptom, arm swelling occurs, or symptoms develop within 1 year after completion of radiation therapy with a total dose of more than 6000 R. Lumbosacral plexopathy is usually seen in patients with colorectal, cervical, uterine, or ovarian carcinoma or sarcoma. Clinical features that suggest tumor invasion in this setting include early and severe pain, unilateral involvement, leg swelling, and a palpable rectal mass. Radiation injury is more commonly associated with early prominent leg weakness and bilateral symptoms.

TABES DORSALIS

This type of neurosyphilis, now rare, is characterized mainly by sensory symptoms and signs that indicate marked involvement of the posterior roots, especially in the lumbosacral region, with resulting degeneration in the posterior columns of the spinal cord. Common complaints are of unsteadiness, sudden lancinating somatic pains, and urinary incontinence. Visceral crises characterized by excruciating abdominal pain also occur. Examination reveals marked impairment of vibration and joint position sense in the legs, together with an ataxic gait and Romberg's sign. Deep pain sensation is impaired, but superficial sensation is generally preserved. The bladder is often palpably enlarged; because it is flaccid and insensitive, there is overflow incontinence. Tendon reflexes are lost, and the limbs are hypotonic. Sensory loss and hypotonicity may lead to the occurrence of hypertrophic (Charcot) joints. In many patients there are other signs of neurosyphilis, including Argyll Robertson pupils, optic atrophy, ptosis, a variable ophthalmoplegia, and, in some cases, pyramidal and mental changes from cerebral involvement (taboparesis), as discussed in Chapter 1. Treatment is of the underlying infection.

LYME DISEASE

Lyme disease, like syphilis, is a spirochetal infection that produces both central and peripheral nervous system disease. Central nervous system involvement is manifested by meningitis or meningoencephalitis, as discussed in Chapter 1. Lyme disease is also associated with inflammatory mono- or polyradiculopathy, brachial plexopathy (see Chapter 5), mononeuropathy (including facial palsy), and mononeuropathy multiplex. The radiculopathy results in pain, sensory loss, or dysesthesia in affected dermatomes; it also causes focal weakness. One or more cervical, thoracic, or lumbar nerve roots may be involved. Electromyography can confirm the presence of radiculopathy, and serologic testing establishes Lyme disease as the cause. Treatment is described in Chapter 1.

MYELOPATHIES

Myelopathies may present with pain or with a variety of sensory complaints and with motor disturbances. The clinical findings should suggest the level of the lesion, but further investigation is necessary to delineate it more fully and determine its nature. Compressive, ischemic, inflammatory, demyelinative, and traumatic myelopathies were discussed in Chapter 5.

SYRINGOMYELIA

Syringomyelia is cavitation of the spinal cord. Communicating syringomyelia—with communication between the central canal of the cord and the cavity—is a hydrodynamic disorder of the CSF pathways. In noncommunicating syringomyelia, there is cystic dilation of the cord, which is not in communication with the CSF pathways. The precise clinical disturbance that results depends upon the site of cavitation. Typically, there is a dissociated sensory loss at the level of the lesion; pinprick and temperature appreciation are impaired, but light touch sensation is preserved. The sensory loss may be reflected by the presence of painless skin ulcers, scars, edema, hyperhidrosis, neuropathic joints, resorption of the terminal phalanges, and other disturbances. Weakness and wasting of muscles occur at the level of the lesion because of the involvement of the anterior horns of the cord. A pyramidal deficit and sphincter disturbances sometimes occur below the level of the lesion because of gliosis or compression of the corticospinal pathways in the lateral columns of the cord. The tendon reflexes may be depressed at the level of the lesion—because of interruption of their afferent, central, or efferent pathways—and increased below it. Scoliosis is a common accompaniment of cord cavitation. Cavitation commonly occurs in the cervical region; this can cause a capelike distribution of sensory loss over one or both shoulders, diffuse pain in the neck, and radicular pain in the arms; involvement of the T1 segment frequently leads to ipsilateral Horner's syndrome. If the cavitation involves the lower brainstem (**syringobulbia**), there may also be ipsilateral tongue wasting, palatal weakness, vocal cord paralysis, dissociated trigeminal sensory loss, and other evidence of brainstem involvement.

Communicating syringomyelia is often associated with developmental anomalies of the brainstem and foramen magnum region (such as Arnold-Chiari malformation; see Chapter 3) or with chronic arachnoiditis of the basal cisterns. Arnold-Chiari malformation can lead to hydrocephalus, cerebellar ataxia, pyramidal and sensory deficits in the limbs, and abnormalities of the lower cranial nerves, alone or in any combination. Myelography, magnetic resonance imaging (MRI), or computed tomographic (CT) scanning of the foramen magnum region confirms the diagnosis. Treatment is surgical.

Noncommunicating syringomyelia is often due to trauma, intramedullary tumors, or spinal arachnoiditis. Posttraumatic syringomyelia generally occurs in patients with preexisting, severe neurologic deficits from spinal trauma after an interval of several years, although rarely it may develop only a few months after the original injury. Presentation is with increase in a previously stable deficit; weakness, impaired sensation, and spasticity are often conspicuous, and radicular pain may be distressing.

Treatment depends upon the underlying cause. Decompression of a distended syrinx may provide transient benefit. In the case of communicating syringomyelia associated with Arnold-Chiari malformation, removal of the posterior rim of the foramen magnum and amputation of the cerebellar tonsils are sometimes helpful. The cord cavity should be drained, and, if necessary, an outlet should be made for the fourth ventricle. Posttraumatic syringomyelia is treated by surgery if it is causing a progressive neurologic deficit or intolerable pain. A variety of surgical approaches have been used, including various draining procedures from the cord cavity, myelotomy, and formation of surgical meningocele. Radicular pain and sensory disturbances are usually helped, whereas spasticity responds less satisfactorily.

SUBACUTE COMBINED DEGENERATION (VITAMIN B$_{12}$ DEFICIENCY)

Vitamin B$_{12}$ deficiency may result from impaired absorption by the gastrointestinal tract such as occurs in pernicious anemia or because of gastrointestinal surgery, sprue, or infection with fish tapeworm; it can also be caused by a strictly vegetarian diet. It may affect the spinal cord, giving rise to the syndrome of subacute combined degeneration. Onset is with distal paresthesias and weakness in the extremities (involvement of the hands occurs relatively early), followed by the development of spastic paraparesis, with ataxia from the impairment of postural sensation in the legs. Lhermitte's sign may be present, and examination reveals a combined posterior column (vibration and joint position sense) and pyramidal deficit in the legs. Plantar responses are extensor, but tendon reflexes may be increased or depressed, depending on the site and severity of the involvement. Signs of cord involvement can be accompanied by centrocecal scotoma or optic atrophy from optic (II) nerve involvement, by behavioral or psychiatric changes (see Chapter 1), or by peripheral neuropathy. The neurologic manifestations are often accompanied by macrocytic megaloblastic anemia, but this is not invariably present.

The serum vitamin B$_{12}$ level is low in untreated cases. If malabsorption of vitamin B$_{12}$ is the cause, the Schilling test is abnormal, and there is usually gastric achlorhydria with pernicious anemia. Hematologic findings may be normal, however, especially if folic acid supplements have been given.

Treatment is with vitamin B$_{12}$ given by intramuscular injection daily (50–1000 μg) for 2 weeks, then weekly (100 μg) for 2 months, and monthly (100 μg) thereafter. Note that folic acid supplements do not help the neurologic disorder; in addition, they may mask associated anemia.

CEREBRAL DISEASE

Sensory symptoms may relate to diverse diseases involving the brainstem or cerebral hemispheres. The clinical features of the sensory deficit have been described earlier in this chapter and, together with the nature and extent of any accompanying neurologic signs, should suggest the probable site of the lesion. The differential diagnosis of such lesions is considered separately in Chapter 9.

PAIN SYNDROMES

Pain from infective, inflammatory, or neoplastic processes is a feature of many visceral diseases and may be a conspicuous component of certain neurologic or psychiatric diseases. It can also occur with no obvious cause.

In evaluating patients with pain, it is important to determine the level of the nervous system at which the pain arises and whether it has a primary neurologic basis. In taking the history, attention should be focused on the mode of onset, duration, nature, severity, and location of the pain; any associated symptoms; and factors that precipitate or relieve the pain.

Treatment depends on the underlying cause and clinical context of the pain and is discussed below. A brief comment is necessary, however, about stimulation-produced analgesia and, in particular, about spinal cord stimulation (previously known as dorsal column stimulation) and peripheral nerve stimulation. These approaches were based on principles encapsulated by the Gate Control theory, in which activation of large myelinated fibers was held to interrupt nociceptive transmission in the spinal cord, but their precise mechanism of action is uncertain. Spinal cord stimulation is known to affect certain neurotransmitter systems, particularly substance P and γ-aminobutyric acid (GABAergic) sytems.

PERIPHERAL NERVE PAIN

Pain arising from peripheral nerve lesions is usually localized to the region that is affected pathologically or confined to the territory of the affected nerve. It may have a burning quality, and when mixed (motor and sensory) nerves are involved, there may be an accompanying motor deficit. Painful peripheral neuropathies include those caused by diabetes, polyarteritis, alcoholic-nutritional deficiency states, and the various entrapment neuropathies. Treatment of pain associated with peripheral neuropathies is discussed earlier. The term **causalgia** correctly is used for the severe persistent pain, often burning in quality, that results from nerve trauma. Such pain often radiates to a more extensive territory than is supplied by the affected nerve and is associated with exquisite tenderness. Onset of pain may be at any time within the first 6 weeks or so after nerve injury. The cause is uncertain, but it has been attributed to ephaptic transmission between efferent sympathetic and afferent somatic fibers at the site of injury. Pain may be accompanied by increased sweating and vasoconstriction of the affected extremity, which is commonly kept covered up and still by the patient. **Reflex sympathetic dystrophy** is a more general term that denotes sympathetically mediated pain syndromes precipitated by a wide variety of tissue injuries, including soft tissue trauma, bone fractures, and myocardial infarction. Medical approaches to treatment include sympathetic blockade by injection of local anesthetics into the sympathetic chain or by regional infusion of reserpine or guanethidine. One such procedure may produce permanent cessation of pain—or repeated sympathetic blocks may be required. Surgical sympathectomy is beneficial in up to 75% of cases. Spinal cord stimulation has also been successful in some instances for the treatment of reflex sympathetic dystrophy or causalgia.

RADICULAR PAIN

Radicular pain is localized to the distribution of one or more nerve roots and is often exacerbated by coughing, sneezing, and other maneuvers that increase intraspinal pressure. It is also exacerbated by maneuvers that stretch the affected roots. Passive straight leg raising leads to stretching of the sacral and lower lumbar roots, as does passive flexion of the neck. Spinal movements that narrow the intervertebral foramina can aggravate root pain. Extension and lateral flexion of the head to the affected side may thus exacerbate cervical root symptoms. In addition to pain, root lesions can cause paresthesias and numbness in a dermatomal distribution (see Figure 6–4); they can also cause segmental weakness and reflex changes, depending upon the level affected (see Table 5–11). Useful modes of treatment include immobilization, nonsteroidal antiinflammatory drugs or other analgesics, and surgical decompression.

THALAMIC PAIN

Depending upon their extent and precise location, thalamic lesions may lead to pain in all or part of the contralateral half of the body. The pain is of a burning nature with a particularly unpleasant quality that patients have difficulty describing. It is aggravated by emotional stress and tends to develop during partial recovery from a sensory deficit caused by the underlying thalamic lesion. Mild cutaneous stimulation may produce very unpleasant and painful sensations. This combination of sensory loss, spontaneous pain, and perverted cutaneous sensation has come to be called **Dejerine-Roussy** syndrome. Similar pain can be produced by a lesion that involves the parietal lobe or the sensory pathways at any point in the cord (posterior columns or spinothalamic tract) or in the brainstem. Treatment with analgesics, anticonvulsants (carbamazepine or phenytoin), or antidepressants and phenothiazines in combination is occasionally helpful.

BACK & NECK PAIN

Spinal disease occurs most commonly in the neck or low back and can cause local or root pain or both. It can also lead to pain that is referred to other parts of the involved dermatomes. Pain from the lower lumbar spine, for example, is often referred to the buttocks. Conversely, pain may be referred to the back from the viscera, especially the pelvic organs. Local pain may lead to protective reflex muscle spasm, which in turn causes further pain and may result in abnormal posture, limitation of movement, and local spinal tenderness.

The history may provide clues to the underlying cause, and physical examination will define any neurologic involvement.

Diagnostic studies that can help in evaluating patients include x-rays of the affected region and a complete blood count and erythrocyte sedimentation rate (especially if infective or inflammatory disorders or myeloma is suspected); determination of serum protein and protein electrophoresis; and measurement of serum calcium, phosphorus, alkaline and acid phosphatase, and uric acid. Electromyography may be helpful in determining the extent and severity of root involvement; it also provides a guide to prognosis. A CT scan, MRI of the spine, or a myelogram may be necessary, especially if neoplasm is suspected, neurologic deficits are progressive, pain persists despite conservative treatment measures, or there is evidence of cord involvement. At myelography, CSF can be obtained for laboratory examination.

1. Low Back Pain

Low back pain is a common cause of time lost from work. It has many causes.

Trauma

Unaccustomed exertion or activity—or lifting heavy objects without adequate bracing of the spine—can cause musculoskeletal pain that improves with rest. Clinical examination commonly reveals spasm of the lumbar muscles and restricted spinal movements. Management includes local heat, bed rest on a firm mattress, nonsteroidal antiinflammatory drugs or other analgesics, and muscle-relaxant drugs, eg, diazepam, 2 mg three times daily, increased gradually until symptoms are relieved (or to the highest dose tolerated). Vertebral fractures that follow more severe injury and lead to local pain and tenderness can be visualized at radiography. If cord involvement is suspected—eg, because of leg weakness following injury—the patient must be immobilized

until radiographed to determine whether fracture dislocation of the vertebral column has occurred.

Prolapsed Lumbar Intervertebral Disk

This most commonly affects the L5–S1 or the L4–5 disk. The prolapse may relate to injury, but in many patients it commonly follows minor strain or normal activity. Protruded disk material may press on one or more nerve roots and thus produce radicular pain, a segmental motor or sensory deficit, or a sphincter disturbance in addition to a painful stiff back. The pain may be reproduced by percussion over the spine or sciatic nerve, by passive straight leg raising, or by extension of the knee while the hip is flexed. The presence of bilateral symptoms and signs suggests that disk material has protruded centrally, and this is more likely to be associated with sphincter involvement than is lateral protrusion. An L5 radiculopathy causes weak dorsiflexion of the foot and toes, while an S1 root lesion leads to a depressed ankle reflex and weakness of plantar flexion of the foot (see Table 5–11). In either case, spinal movements are restricted, there is local tenderness, and Lasègue's sign (reproducing the patient's pain on stretching the sciatic nerve by straight leg raising) is positive. The L4 root is occasionally affected, but involvement of a higher lumbar root should arouse suspicion of other causes of root compression. Pelvic and rectal examination and plain x-rays of the spine help to exclude other diseases, such as local tumors or metastatic neoplastic deposits. Symptoms often resolve with simple analgesics, diazepam, and bed rest on a firm mattress for 2–3 days, followed by gradual mobilization. Bed rest for longer than 2-3 days provides no additional benefit. Nonsteroidal antiinflammatory drugs may be helpful for acute back pain but are often ineffective or provide only minor or transient benefits in patients with symptoms or signs of root compression. The utility of epidural steroid injection is uncertain.

Persisting pain, an increasing neurologic deficit, or any evidence of sphincter dysfunction should lead to MRI, CT scanning, or myelography, and surgical treatment if indicated by the results of these procedures. The detection of structural abnormalities by these imaging procedures does not mandate surgical treatment unless the clinical circumstances are appropriate—degenerative abnormalities are common in asymptomatic subjects, especially with advancing age, and may therefore be of no clinical relevance.

The persistence of low back and root pain despite surgery may have several causes including inadequate decompression, recurrent herniation of disk material, root compression or damage as a result of the operative procedure, surgery at the wrong level, infective or inflammatory complications of surgery, or spinal instability. In many instances, however, no specific cause can be identified and most patients do not require further surgery. Chronic pain in this setting may, however, respond to spinal cord stimulation. There is a high risk that patients will not return to work.

Lumbar Osteoarthropathy

This tends to occur in later life and may cause low back pain that is increased by activity. Radiologic abnormalities vary in severity. In patients with mild symptoms, a surgical corset is helpful, whereas in more severe cases operative treatment may be necessary. Even minor changes may cause root or cord dysfunction in patients with a congenitally narrowed spinal canal (**spinal stenosis**), leading to the syndrome of **intermittent claudication of the cord or cauda equina.** This is characterized by pain—sometimes accompanied by weakness or radicular sensory disturbances in the legs—that occurs with activity or with certain postures and is relieved by rest. In such circumstances, spinal decompression is indicated.

Ankylosing Spondylitis

Backache and stiffness, followed by progressive limitation of movement, characterize this disorder, which occurs predominantly in young men. Characteristic early radiologic findings consist of sclerosis and narrowing of the sacroiliac joints. Treatment is with nonsteroidal anti-inflammatory agents, especially indomethacin or aspirin. Physical therapy, including postural exercises, is also important.

Neoplastic Disease

Extradural malignant tumors are an important cause of back pain and should be suspected if there is persistent pain that worsens despite bed rest. They may eventually lead to cord compression or a cauda equina syndrome, depending upon the level of involvement. There may initially be no change on plain radiographs of the spine, but a bone scan is sometimes revealing. Benign osteogenic tumors also produce back pain, and plain x-rays then show a lytic lesion; treatment is by excision.

Infections

Tuberculous and pyogenic infections of the vertebrae or intervertebral disks can cause progressive low back pain and local tenderness. Although there are sometimes no systemic signs of infection, the peripheral white cell count and erythrocyte sedimentation rate are raised. X-rays may show disk space narrowing and a soft tissue mass, but they are frequently normal initially.

The osteomyelitis requires long-term antimicrobial

therapy; surgical debridement and drainage may also be needed. Spinal epidural abscess (see Chapter 5) similarly presents with localized pain and tenderness, sometimes associated with osteomyelitis. Cord compression may occur with the onset of a rapidly progressive flaccid paraplegia. MRI, CT scanning, or myelography and operative treatment are undertaken urgently if there is evidence of cord compression. In early cases without neurologic involvement, treatment with antibiotics alone may be sufficient.

Osteoporosis

Low back pain is a common complaint in patients with osteoporosis, and vertebral fractures may occur spontaneously or after trivial trauma. Pain may be helped by a brace to support the back. It is important that patients keep active and take a diet containing adequate amounts of calcium, vitamin D, and protein. Estrogen therapy may be helpful in postmenopausal women. In special circumstances, calcitonin, sodium fluoride, or phosphate supplements are helpful.

Paget's Disease of the Spine

Paget's disease, which is characterized by excessive bone destruction and repair, is of unknown cause but may have a familial basis. Pain is commonly the first symptom. Vertebral involvement may also lead to evidence of cord or root compression. The serum calcium and phosphorus levels are normal, but the alkaline phosphatase is markedly increased. Urinary hydroxyproline and calcium are increased when the disease is active. X-rays show expansion and increased density of the involved bones, and fissure fractures may be evident in the long bones.

Treatment includes prescription of a high-protein diet with vitamin C supplements. Calcium intake should be high in active patients and restricted in immobilized patients. Vitamin D supplements—50,000 units three times a week—and anabolic hormones may also be helpful. In active, progressive disease, treatment with calcitonin, diphosphonates, or mithramycin reduces osteoclastic activity.

Congenital Anomalies

Minor spinal anomalies can cause pain because of altered mechanics or alignment or because reduction in the size of the spinal canal renders the cord or roots more liable to compression by degenerative or other changes. Children or young adults with congenital defects in spinal fusion (**spinal dysraphism**) occasionally present with pain, a neurologic deficit in one or both legs, or sphincter disturbances. Treatment is of the underlying disorder.

Congenital **spinal stenosis** may lead to the syndrome of neurogenic claudication, but symptoms usually develop only in later life when minor degenerative changes have come to be superimposed on the congenital anomaly, as discussed on p 227.

Arachnoiditis

Severe pain in the back and legs can result from inflammation and fibrosis of the arachnoid layer of the spinal meninges (arachnoiditis), which may be idiopathic or causally related to previous surgery, infection, myelography, or long-standing disk disease. There is no adequate treatment, but operation may be possible if the arachnoiditis is localized. Spinal cord stimulation may provide symptomatic relief. This condition is considered in more detail in Chapter 5.

Referred Pain

Disease of the hip joints may cause pain in the back and thighs that is enhanced by activity; examination reveals limitation of movement at the joint with a positive **Patrick sign** (hip pain on external rotation of the hip), and x-rays show degenerative changes. Aortic aneurysms, cardiac ischemia, visceral and genitourinary disease (especially pelvic disorders in women), and retroperitoneal masses also cause back pain. There are often other symptoms and signs that suggest the underlying disorder. Moreover, there is no localized spinal tenderness or restriction of motility.

Treatment is of the underlying cause.

Nonspecific Chronic Back Pain

In many patients whose chronic back pain poses a difficult management problem, there are no objective clinical signs or obvious causes of pain despite detailed investigations. In some cases, the pain may have a postural basis; in others, it may be a somatic manifestation of a psychiatric disorder. Pain that initially had an organic basis is often enhanced or perpetuated by nonorganic factors and leads to disability out of proportion to the symptoms.

Nonsteroidal antiinflammatory drugs may provide short-term symptomatic relief. There is some controversy about the chronic use of narcotic analgesics in patients with persisting low back pain, but such agents are generally best avoided. Treatment with tricyclic antidepressant drugs is sometimes helpful, and psychiatric evaluation may be worthwhile. Unnecessary surgical procedures must be avoided.

2. Neck Pain

Neck pain is a common problem in the general population; surveys indicate that approximately one-third of the adult population have experienced it over the previous year and in many instances it lasts for more than 6 months.

Congenital abnormalities of the cervical spine, such as hemivertebrae or fused vertebrae, basilar impression, and instability of the atlantoaxial joint, can cause neck pain. The traumatic, infective, and neoplastic disorders mentioned above as causes of low back pain can also affect the cervical spine and then produce pain in the neck. Rheumatoid arthritis may involve the spine, especially in the cervical region, leading to pain, stiffness, and reduced mobility; cord compression may result from displacement of vertebrae or atlantoaxial subluxation and can be life-threatening if not treated by fixation.

Cervical injuries are an important cause of neck pain. **Whiplash** flexion-extension injuries have become especially common as a result of automobile accidents. Other occult cervical injuries such as disk clefts and fissures may be responsible for symptoms in some instances, but are difficult to recognize. Management of persistent symptoms following whiplash injuries is controversial. Conservative therapeutic measures are appropriate. Other approaches sometimes advocated include block of cervical facet joints with bupivacaine and injection into the joints of depot corticosteroids, but the response is variable and often short-lived. Subluxed cervical facet joints are another well-recognized complication of automobile accidents. Even minor trauma may lead to cervical fractures in an apparently ankylosed region in patients with diffuse idiopathic skeletal hyperostosis, but major neurologic deficits are common in such circumstances.

Acute Cervical Disk Protrusion

Patients may present with neck and radicular arm pain that is exacerbated by head movement. The mechanism responsible for the pain is unclear; pressure on nerve roots is unlikely to be the sole cause because pain may resolve with time and conservative measures despite persisting compression. With lateral herniation of the disk, there may also be segmental motor, sensory, or reflex changes, usually at the C6 or C7 level, on the affected side. With more centrally directed herniations, spastic paraparesis and a sensory disturbance in the legs, sometimes accompanied by impaired sphincter function, can occur as a result of cord involvement. The diagnosis is confirmed by CT scan, MRI, or myelography. However, these imaging studies may show abnormalities in asymptomatic subjects in middle or later life, so that any disk protrusion may be incidental and unrelated to patients' symptoms. Electromyography may help to establish that anatomic abnormalities are of functional relevance.

In mild cases, bed rest or intermittent neck traction, followed by immobilization of the neck in a collar for several weeks, often helps. If these measures fail or if there is a significant neurologic deficit, surgical treatment may be necessary.

Cervical Spondylosis

This is an important cause of pain in the neck and arms, sometimes accompanied by a segmental motor or sensory deficit in the arms or by spastic paraparesis. It is discussed in Chapter 5.

3. *Herpes Zoster (Shingles)*

This viral disorder becomes increasingly common with advancing age, causing an inflammatory reaction in one or more of the dorsal root or cranial nerve ganglia, in the affected root or nerve itself, and in the CSF. There seems to be spontaneous reactivation of varicella virus that remained latent in sensory ganglia after previous infection. Herpes zoster is common in patients with lymphoma, especially following regional radiotherapy. The initial complaint is of a burning or shooting pain in the involved dermatome, followed within 2–5 days by the development of a vesicular erythematous rash. The pain may diminish in intensity as the rash develops. The rash becomes crusted and scaly after a few days and then fades, leaving small anesthetic scars. Secondary infection is common. The pain and dysesthesias may last for several weeks or, in some instances, may persist for many months (**postherpetic neuralgia**) before subsiding, especially in the elderly. The increased incidence and severity of postherpetic neuralgia with age may reflect an age-related reduction in virus-specific cell-mediated immunity. It is not clear whether immunocompromise secondary to HIV infection or connective tissue disease predisposes to postherpetic neuralgia. Pain is exacerbated by touching the involved area. Superficial sensation is often impaired in the affected dermatome, and focal weakness and atrophy can also occur. Signs are usually limited to one dermatome, but more are occasionally involved. Mild pleocytosis and an increased protein concentration sometimes occur in the CSF. The most commonly involved sites are the thoracic dermatomes, but involvement of the first division of the fifth cranial nerve, also common, is especially distressing and may lead to corneal scarring and anesthesia, as well as to a variety of other ocular complications. Facial (VII) nerve palsy occurring in association with a herpetic eruption that involves the ear, palate, pharynx, or neck is called **Ramsay Hunt syndrome.** Other rare complications of herpes zoster include other motor neuropathies, meningitis, encephalitis, myelopathy, and cerebral angiopathy.

There is no specific treatment. Analgesics provide symptomatic relief. Corticosteroids may reduce the duration and severity of the acute eruption, but not the likelihood that postherpetic neuralgia will occur. The incidence of postherpetic neuralgia may be reduced by oral acyclovir or famciclovir, but this is unsettled. Although postherpetic neuralgia can be very distressing, it sometimes responds to treatment with carbamazepine, up to 1200 mg/d, phenytoin, 300 mg/d, gabapentin, up to 3600 mg/d, or amitriptyline, 10–100 mg at bedtime. Attempts at relieving postherpetic neuralgia by peripheral nerve section are generally unrewarding, but treatment with topically applied local anesthetics is sometimes helpful, as is topically applied capsaicin cream, perhaps because of depletion of pain-mediating peptides from peripheral sensory neurons. A recent trial indicated that intrathecal methylprednisolone may be helpful for intractable pain.

REFERENCES

General

Aminoff MJ: *Electromyography in Clinical Practice,* 3rd ed. Churchill Livingstone, 1998.

Aminoff MJ (editor): *Neurology and General Medicine,* 3rd ed. Churchill Livingstone, 2001.

Dyck PJ et al (editors): *Peripheral Neuropathy,* 3rd ed. Saunders, 1993.

Layzer RB: *Neuromuscular Manifestations of Systemic Disease.* Vol 25 of: *Contemporary Neurology Series.* Davis, 1984.

Mogyros I, Bostock H, Burke D: Mechanisms of paresthesias arising from healthy axons. Muscle Nerve 2000;23:310–320.

Polyneuropathies

Asbury AK, Cornblath DR: Assessment of current diagnostic criteria for Guillain-Barré syndrome. Ann Neurol 1990;27 (Suppl):S21–S24.

Bolton CF, Young GB: *Neurological Complications of Renal Disease.* Butterworths, 1990.

Charness ME, Simon RP, Greenberg DA: Ethanol and the nervous system. N Engl J Med 1989;321:442–454.

Dalakas MC: Intravenous immunoglobulins in the treatment of autoimmune neuromuscular diseases: present status and practical therapeutic guidelines. Muscle Nerve 1999;22:1479–1497.

Dalmau JO, Posner JB: Paraneoplastic syndromes affecting the nervous system. Semin Oncol 1997;24:318–328.

Dyck PJ et al (editors): *Peripheral Neuropathy,* 3rd ed. Saunders, 1993.

Geschwind DH et al: Friedreich's ataxia GAA repeat expansion in patients with recessive or sporadic ataxia. Neurology 1997; 49:1004–1009.

Hahn AF et al: Plasma-exchange therapy in chronic inflammatory demyelinating polyneuropathy: A double-blind, sham-controlled, cross-over study. Brain 1996;119:1055–1066.

Hahn AF: Treatment of chronic inflammatory demyelinating polyneuropathy with intravenous immunoglobulins. Neurology 1998;51(Suppl 5):S16–S21.

Hahn AF: Intravenous immunoglobulins treatment in peripheral nerve disorders—indications, mechanisms of action and side-effects. Curr Opin Neurol 2000;13:575–582.

Harding AE: From the syndrome of Charcot, Marie and Tooth to disorders of peripheral myelin proteins. Brain 1995;118:809–818.

Hartung HP et al: Immunopathogenesis and treatment of the Guillain-Barré syndrome. Muscle Nerve 1995;18:137–153 and 154–164 (two parts).

Hirota N et al: Hereditary neuropathy with liability to pressure palsies: distinguishing clinical and electrophysiological features among patients with multiple entrapment neuropathy. J Neurol Sci 1996;139:187–189.

Kokontis L, Gutmann L: Current treatment of neuromuscular diseases. Arch Neurol 2000;57:939–943.

Lange DJ: Neuromuscular diseases associated with HIV-1 infection. Muscle Nerve 1994;17:16–30.

Latov N: Prognosis of neuropathy with monoclonal gammopathy. Muscle Nerve 2000;23:150–152.

Lewis RA: The challenge of CMTX and connexin 32 mutations. Muscle Nerve 2000;23:147–149.

Manji H: Neuropathy in HIV infection. Curr Opin Neurol 2000; 13:589–592.

Mastaglia FL: Iatrogenic (drug-induced) disorders of the nervous system. Page 593 in: *Neurology and General Medicine,* 3rd ed. Aminoff MJ (editor). Churchill Livingstone, 2001.

Mendell JR et al: Randomized controlled trial of IVIg in untreated chronic inflammatory demyelinating polyradiculoneuropathy. Neurology 2001;56:445–449.

Mishu B et al: Serologic evidence of previous *Campylobacter jejuni* infection in patients with the Guillain-Barré syndrome. Ann Intern Med 1993;118:947–953.

Olney RK: Neuropathies in connective tissue disease. Muscle Nerve 1992;15:531–542.

Pareyson D: Charcot-Marie-Tooth disease and related neuropathies: molecular basis for distinction and diagnosis. Muscle Nerve 1999;22:1498–1509.

Parry GJG: Neurological complications of toxin exposure in the workplace. Pages 645–664 in: *Neurology and General Medicine,* 3rd ed. Aminoff MJ (editor). Churchill Livingstone, 2001.

Parry GJ, Bredesen DE: Sensory neuropathy with low-dose pyridoxine. Neurology 1985;35:1466–1468.

Ponsford S et al: Long-term clinical and neurophysiological follow-up of patients with peripheral neuropathy associated with benign monoclonal gammopathy. Muscle Nerve 2000; 23:164–174.

Priller J et al: Frataxin gene of Friedreich's ataxia is targeted to mitochondria. Ann Neurol 1997;42:265–269.

Quarles RH, Weiss MD: Autoantibodies associated with peripheral neuropathy. Muscle Nerve 1999;22:800–822.

Rees JH et al: *Campylobacter jejuni* infection and Guillain-Barré syndrome. N Engl J Med 1995;333:1374–1379.

Ropper AH: The Guillain-Barré syndrome. N Engl J Med 1992; 326:1130–1136.

Rosenbaum R: Neuromuscular complications of connective tissue disease. Muscle Nerve 2001;24:154–169.

Rudnicki SA, Dalmau J: Paraneoplastic syndromes of the spinal cord, nerve, and muscle. Muscle Nerve 2000;23:1800–1818.

Said G: Vasculitic neuropathy. Curr Opin Neurol 1999;12:627–629.

Saperstein DS et al: Clinical spectrum of chronic acquired demyelinating polyneuropathies. Muscle Nerve 2001;24:311–324.

Schaumburg HH, Berger AR, Thomas PK: *Disorders of Peripheral Nerves,* 2nd ed. Vol 36 of: *Contemporary Neurology Series.* Davis, 1992.

Shannon KM, Goetz CG: Connective tissue diseases and the nervous system. Pages 459–481 in: *Neurology and General Medicine,* 3rd ed. Aminoff MJ (editor). Churchill Livingstone, 2001.

Simpson DM, Olney RK: Peripheral neuropathies associated with human immunodeficiency virus infection. Neurol Clin 1992; 10:685–711.

Smith IS: The natural history of chronic demyelinating neuropathy associated with benign IgM paraproteinaemia: a clinical and neurophysiological study. Brain 1994;117:949–957.

Smith BE, Dyck PJ: Peripheral neuropathy in the eosinophilia-myalgia syndrome associated with L-tryptophan ingestion. Neurology 1990;40:1035–1040.

So YT, Olney RK: Acute lumbosacral polyradiculopathy in acquired immunodeficiency syndrome: experience in 23 patients. Ann Neurol 1994;35:53–58.

Suarez GA, Kelly JJ: Polyneuropathy associated with monoclonal gammopathy of undetermined significance. Neurology 1993; 43:1304–1308.

WHO Expert Committee on Leprosy: World Health Organization Tech Rep Serv 1998;874:1.

Wicklund MP, Kissel JT: Paraproteinemic neuropathy. Curr Treat Options Neurol 2001;3:147–156.

Entrapment Neuropathies

Dawson DM: Entrapment neuropathies of the upper extremities. N Engl J Med 1993;320:2013–2018.

Dawson DM, Hallett M, Wilbourn AJ: *Entrapment Neuropathies,* 3rd ed. Lippincott Williams & Wilkins, 1999.

Spinner RJ, Bachman JW, Amadio PC: The many faces of carpal tunnel syndrome. Mayo Clin Proc 1989;64:829–836.

Stewart JD: *Focal Peripheral Neuropathies,* 3rd ed. Lippincott Williams & Wilkins, 1999.

Root and Plexus Lesions (see also Pain Syndromes)

Ellenberg MR et al: Cervical radiculopathy. Arch Phys Med Rehabil 1994;75:342–352.

Halperin JJ: Spirochetal infections of the nervous system. Pages 683–695 in: *Neurology and General Medicine,* 3rd ed. Aminoff MJ (editor). Churchill Livingstone, 2001.

Hardin JG, Halla JT: Cervical spine and radicular pain syndromes. Curr Opin Rheumatol 1995;7:136–140.

Jaeckle KA, Young DF, Foley KM: The natural history of lumbosacral plexopathy in cancer. Neurology 1985;35:8–15.

Johansson S et al: Brachial plexopathy after postoperative radiotherapy of breast cancer patients—a long-term follow-up. Acta Oncol 2000;39:373–382.

Koes BW et al: Efficacy of non-steroidal antiinflammatory drugs for low back pain: a systematic review of randomized clinical trials. Ann Rheum Dis 1997;56:214–223.

Kori SH, Foley KM, Posner JB: Brachial plexus lesions in patients with cancer: 100 cases. Neurology 1981;31:45–50.

Saal JA: Natural history and nonoperative treatment of lumbar disc herniation. Spine 1996;21(Suppl):2S–9S.

Steere AC: Lyme disease. N Engl J Med 1989;321:586–596.

Thomas JE, Cascino TL, Earle JD: Differential diagnosis between radiation and tumor plexopathy of the pelvis. Neurology 1985;35:1–7.

Myelopathies

Heiss JD et al: Elucidating the pathophysiology of syringomyelia. J Neurosurg 1999;91:553–562.

Hemmer B et al: Subacute combined degeneration: clinical, electrophysiological, and magnetic resonance imaging findings. J Neurol Neurosurg Psychiatry 1998;65:822–827.

Karantanas AH, Markonis A, Bisbiyiannis G: Subacute combined degeneration of the spinal cord with involvement of the anterior columns: a new MRI finding. Neuroradiology 2000; 42:115–117.

Kramer KM, Levin AM: Posttraumatic syringomyelia: a review of 21 cases. Clin Orthop Rel Res 1997;334:190–199.

Sgouros S, Williams B: Management and outcome of posttraumatic syringomyelia. J Neurosurg 1996;85:197–205.

Pain Syndromes

Borenstein DG: Epidemiology, etiology, diagnostic evaluation, and treatment of low back pain. Curr Opin Rheumatol 2001;13: 128–134.

Bovim G et al: Neck pain in the general population. Spine 1994;19:1307–1309.

Choo PW et al: Risk factors for postherpetic neuralgia. Arch Intern Med 1997;157:1217–1224.

Ciricillo SF, Weinstein PR: Lumbar spinal stenosis. West J Med 1993;158:171–177.

Deyo RA: Drug therapy for back pain. Which drugs help which patients? Spine 1996;21:2840–2849.

Fishbain D: Evidence-based data on pain relief with antidepressants. Ann Med 2000;32:305–316.

Frank A: Low back pain. BMJ 1993;306:901–909.

Frymoyer JW: Back pain and sciatica. N Engl J Med 1988;318: 291–300.

Galil K et al: The sequelae of herpes zoster. Arch Intern Med 1997;157:1209–1213.

Hagen KB et al: The Cochrane review of bed rest for acute low back pain and sciatica. Spine 2000;25:2932–2939.

Kost RG, Straus SE: Postherpetic neuralgia. Arch Intern Med 1997;157:1166–1167.

Kotani N et al: Intrathecal methylprednisolone for intractable postherpetic neuralgia. N Engl J Med 2000;343:1514–1519.

Laird MA, Gidal BE: Use of gabapentin in the treatment of neuropathic pain. Ann Pharmacother 2000;34:802–807.

McCleane GJ: Lamotrigine in the management of neuropathic pain: a review of the literature. Clin J Pain 2000;16: 321–326.

Nygaard OP, Kloster R, Solberg T: Duration of leg pain as a predictor of outcome after surgery for lumbar disc herniation: a prospective cohort study with 1-year follow up. J Neurosurg 2000;92(Suppl):131–134.

Paice JA et al: Topical capsaicin in the management of HIV-associated peripheral neuropathy. J Pain Symptom Manage 2000; 19:45–52.

Rowbotham MC: Managing post-herpetic neuralgia with opioids and local anesthetics. Ann Neurol 1994;35:S46–S49.

Stanton-Hicks M, Salamon J: Stimulation of the central and peripheral nervous system for the control of pain. J Clin Neurophysiol 1997;14:46–62.

Straus SE: Shingles: Sorrows, salves, and solutions. JAMA 1993; 269:1836–1839.

Tremont-Lukats IW, Megeff C, Backonja MM: Anticonvulsants for neuropathic pain syndromes: mechanisms of action and place in therapy. Drugs 2000;60:1029–1052.

Tripathi M, Kaushik S: Carbamazepine for pain management in Guillain-Barré syndrome patients in the intensive care unit. Crit Care Med 2000;28:655–658.

Valls I et al: Factors predicting radical treatment after in-hospital conservative management of disk-related sciatica. Bone Joint Surg 2001;68:50–58.

Vroomen PC et al: Conservative treatment for sciatica: a systematic review. J Spinal Disord 2000;13:463–469.

Waxman SG et al: Sodium channels, excitability of primary sensory neurons, and the molecular basis of pain. Muscle Nerve 1999;22:1177-1187.

Movement Disorders

CONTENTS

KEY CONCEPTS

1   *The characterization of abnormal movements is the first step in identifying their cause; age at onset, mode of onset, and clinical course are then diagnostically helpful.*

2   *The relationship of tremor to activity may suggest its cause.*

3   *A variety of medications induce movement disorders. Neuroleptic-induced dyskinesias take many forms; some occur months or years after the start of treatment or after withdrawal of the causal agent, and may be irreversible.*

4   *Pharmacologic treatment of Parkinson's disease should be planned so as to reduce the risk of late management problems related to levodopa therapy.*

Movement disorders (sometimes called **extrapyramidal disorders**) impair the regulation of voluntary motor activity without directly affecting strength, sensation, or cerebellar function. They include hyperkinetic disorders associated with abnormal, involuntary movements and hypokinetic disorders characterized by poverty of movement. Movement disorders result from dysfunction of deep subcortical gray matter structures termed the **basal ganglia.** Although there is no universally accepted anatomic definition of the basal ganglia, for clinical purposes they may be considered to comprise the caudate nucleus, putamen, globus pallidus, subthalamic nucleus, and substantia nigra. The putamen and the globus pallidus are collectively termed the lentiform nucleus; the combination of lentiform nucleus and caudate nucleus is designated the **corpus striatum.**

worsen with stress, diminish during voluntary activity or mental concentration, and disappear during sleep.

Classification

Tics can be classified into four groups depending upon whether they are simple or multiple and transient or chronic.

Transient simple tics are very common in children, usually terminate spontaneously within 1 year (often within a few weeks), and generally require no treatment.

Chronic simple tics can develop at any age but often begin in childhood, and treatment is unnecessary in most cases. The benign nature of the disorder must be explained to the patient.

Persistent simple or multiple tics of childhood or adolescence generally begin before age 15 years. There may be single or multiple motor tics—and often vocal tics—but complete remission occurs by the end of adolescence.

The syndrome of **chronic multiple motor and vocal tics** is generally referred to as **Gilles de la Tourette's syndrome,** after the French physician who was one of the first to describe its clinical features. It is discussed in detail later.

CLINICAL EVALUATION OF PATIENTS

HISTORY

Age at Onset

The age at onset of a movement disorder may suggest the underlying cause. For example, onset in infancy or early childhood suggests birth trauma, kernicterus, cerebral anoxia, or an inherited disorder; abnormal facial movements developing in childhood are more likely to represent tics than involuntary movements of another sort; and tremor presenting in early adult life is more likely to be of the benign essential variety than due to Parkinson's disease.

The age at onset can also influence the prognosis. In **idiopathic torsion dystonia,** for example, progression to severe disability is much more common when symptoms develop in childhood than when they develop in later life. Conversely, **tardive dyskinesia** is more likely to be permanent and irreversible when it develops in the elderly than when it develops in the adolescent years.

Mode of Onset

Abrupt onset of dystonic posturing in a child or young adult should raise the possibility of a drug-induced reaction; a more gradual onset of dystonic movements and postures in an adolescent suggests the possibility of a chronic disorder such as idiopathic torsion dystonia or Wilson's disease. Similarly, the abrupt onset of severe chorea or ballismus suggests a vascular cause, and abrupt onset of severe parkinsonism suggests a neurotoxic cause; more gradual, insidious onset suggests a degenerative process.

Course

The manner in which the disorder progresses from its onset may also be helpful diagnostically. For example, Sydenham's chorea usually resolves within about 6 months after onset and should, therefore, not be confused with other varieties of chorea that occur in childhood.

Medical History

A. DRUG HISTORY

It is important to obtain an accurate account of all drugs that have been taken by the patient over the years, since many of the movement disorders are iatrogenic. The phenothiazine and butyrophenone drugs may lead to the development of abnormal movements either while patients are taking them or after their use has been discontinued, and the dyskinesia may be irreversible. These drugs and the dyskinesias associated with their use are discussed later in this chapter.

Reversible dyskinesia may develop in patients taking certain other drugs, including oral contraceptives, levodopa, and phenytoin. Several drugs, especially lithium, tricyclic antidepressants, valproic acid, and bronchodilators, can cause tremor. Serotonin reuptake inhibitors have been associated with a number of movement disorders including parkinsonism, akathisia, chorea, dystonia, and bruxism.

B. GENERAL MEDICAL BACKGROUND

1. Chorea may be symptomatic of the disease in patients with a history of rheumatic fever, thyroid disease, systemic lupus erythematosus, polycythemia, hypoparathyroidism, or cirrhosis of the liver.

2. Movement disorders, including tremor, chorea, hemiballismus, dystonia, and myoclonus, have been described in patients with acquired immunodeficiency syndrome (AIDS). Opportunistic infections such as cerebral toxoplasmosis appear to be the cause in some cases, but infection with human immunodeficiency virus type 1 (HIV-1) may also have a direct pathogenetic role.

3. A history of birth trauma or perinatal distress may suggest the cause of a movement disorder that develops during childhood.

4. Encephalitis lethargica is no longer encountered clinically; it was epidemic in the 1920s, however, and was often followed by a wide variety of movement disorders, including parkinsonism. It is therefore important to inquire about this disease when elderly patients are being evaluated.

Family History

Some movement disorders have an inherited basis (Table 7–5), and it is essential that a complete family history be obtained, supplemented if possible by personal scrutiny of close relatives. Any possibility of consanguinity should be noted.

EXAMINATION

Clinical examination will indicate the nature of the abnormal movements, the extent of neurologic involvement, and the presence of coexisting disease; these in turn may suggest the diagnosis.

The mental status examination may suggest psychiatric disease, raising the possibility that the abnormal movements are related to the psychiatric disorder or to its treatment with psychoactive drugs—or that the patient has a disorder characterized by both abnormal movements and behavioral disturbances, such as Huntington's disease or Wilson's disease.

Focal motor or sensory deficits raise the possibility of a structural space-occupying lesion, as does papilledema.

Kayser-Fleischer rings suggest Wilson's disease. Signs of vascular, hepatic, or metabolic disease may suggest other causes for a movement disorder, such as acquired hepatocerebral degeneration or vasculitis.

INVESTIGATIVE STUDIES

Several investigations may be of diagnostic help.

Blood & Urine Tests

Serum and urine copper and serum ceruloplasmin levels are important in diagnosing Wilson's disease.

Complete blood count and sedimentation rate are helpful in excluding polycythemia, vasculitis, or systemic lupus erythematosus, any of which can occasionally lead to a movement disorder.

Blood chemistries may reveal hepatic dysfunction related to Wilson's disease or acquired hepatocerebral degeneration; hyperthyroidism or hypocalcemia as a cause of chorea; or a variety of metabolic disorders associated with myoclonus.

Serologic tests are helpful for diagnosing movement disorders caused by systemic lupus erythematosus. Neurosyphilis can be manifested clinically in a variety of ways and should always be excluded by appropriate serologic tests in patients with neurologic disease of uncertain etiology.

Table 7–5. Hereditary movement disorders.

Disorder	Gene	Locus	Protein	Inheritance[1]
Benign hereditary chorea	BCH	Unknown	Unknown	AD
Dentatorubro-pallidoluysian atrophy	DRPLA	12p13	Atrophin-1	AD
Dopa-responsive dystonia	GCH1	14q22.1–q22.2	GTP cyclohydrolase I	AD
Dystonia-parkinsonism	DYT3	Xq13.1	Unknown	XLR
Dystonia-parkinsonism, rapid onset	DYT12	19q13	Unknown	AD
Essential tremor 1	ETM1	3q13	Unknown	AD
Essential tremor 2	ETM2	2p22–p25	Unknown	AD
Familial chorea-acanthocytosis	CHA	Unknown	Unknown	AD, AR
Gilles de la Tourette's syndrome	GTS	18q22.1	Unknown	AD
Huntington's disease	HD	4p16.3	Huntingtin	AD
Myoclonic dystonia	DYT11	7q21	Unknown	AD
Parkinson's disease (familial type 1)	SNCA	4q21–q23	α-Synuclein	AD
Parkinson's disease (juvenile)	PDJ	6q25.2–q27	Parkin	AR
Paroxysmal dystonic choreoathetosis	PNKD	2q33–q35	Unknown	AD
Torsion dystonia[2]	DYT1	9q34	TorsinA	AD
Torsion dystonia, adult onset	DYT6	8p21–q22	Unknown	AD
Torsion dystonia, focal adult onset	DYT7	18p	Unknown	AD
Wilson's disease	ATP7B	13q14.3–q21.1	Copper-transporting ATPase β peptide	AR

[1] AD, autosomal dominant; AR, autosomal recessive; XLR, X-linked recessive.

[2] Other forms with autosomal or X-linked recessive inheritance have been described, but the responsible genes have not been identified.

Electroencephalography

An EEG is sometimes helpful in diagnosing patients with myoclonus; otherwise, it is of limited usefulness.

Imaging

Radiologic studies are occasionally helpful in evaluating patients with movement disorders. In some patients, intracranial calcification may be found by skull x-rays or computed tomography (CT) scans; the significance of this finding, however, is not clear. CT scans or magnetic resonance imaging (MRI) may also reveal a tumor associated with focal dyskinesia or dystonia, caudate atrophy due to Huntington's disease, or basal ganglia abnormalities associated with Wilson's disease.

Genetic Studies

Recombinant DNA technology has been used to generate probes for genes that determine certain inheritable movement disorders. In this manner, the gene responsible for Huntington's disease has been localized to the terminal band of the short arm of chromosome 4, and the gene for Wilson's disease to the long arm of chromosome 13. Genetic markers are therefore of diagnostic value in such disorders. Their use may be limited, however, by the genetic heterogeneity of some diseases, imprecise gene localization by certain probes, ethical concerns about adverse psychological reactions to the presymptomatic diagnosis of fatal disorders, and the potential for misuse of such information by prospective employers, insurance companies, and government agencies.

DISEASES & SYNDROMES MANIFESTED BY ABNORMAL MOVEMENTS

The more common and well-defined diseases or syndromes characterized by abnormal movements are discussed here with the principles of their treatment.

FAMILIAL, OR BENIGN, ESSENTIAL TREMOR

A postural tremor may be prominent in otherwise normal subjects. Although the pathophysiologic basis of this disorder is uncertain, it often has a familial basis with an autosomal dominant mode of inheritance. Two responsible genes have been identified.

Symptoms may develop in the teenage or early adult years but often do not appear until later. The tremor usually involves one or both hands or the head and voice, whereas the legs tend to be spared. Examination usually reveals no other abnormalities. Although the tremor may become more conspicuous with time, it generally leads to little disability other than cosmetic and social embarrassment. In occasional cases, tremor interferes with the ability to perform fine or delicate tasks with the hands; handwriting is sometimes severely impaired. Speech is affected when the laryngeal muscles are involved. Patients commonly report that a small quantity of alcohol provides remarkable but transient relief; the mechanism is not known.

If treatment is warranted, propranolol, 40–120 mg orally twice daily, can be prescribed—but it will need to be taken for an indefinite period. Alternatively, if tremor is particularly disabling under certain predictable circumstances, it can be treated with a single oral dose of 40–120 mg of propranolol taken in anticipation of the precipitating circumstances. Primidone has also been effective, but patients with essential tremor are often very sensitive to this drug, so that it must be introduced more gradually than when it is used to treat epilepsy. Patients are therefore started on 50 mg/d and the daily dose is increased by 50 mg every 2 weeks until benefit occurs or side effects limit further increments. A dose of 100 or 150 mg three times a day is often effective. Occasional patients respond to alprazolam, up to 3 mg/d in divided doses.

Some patients have disabling tremor that is unresponsive to pharmacologic measures. Thalamotomy may be helpful, but a significant morbidity is associated with bilateral procedures. High-frequency thalamic stimulation by an implanted electrode is an effective alternative to thalamotomy and has a low morbidity. It may be particularly useful for treatment of the unoperated side in patients who have already undergone unilateral thalamotomy.

PARKINSONISM

Parkinsonism occurs in all ethnic groups; in the United States and western Europe it has a prevalence of 1–2/1000 population, with an approximately equal sex distribution. The disorder becomes increasingly common with advancing age. It is characterized by tremor, hypokinesia, rigidity, and abnormal gait and posture.

Etiology

A. IDIOPATHIC

A very common variety of parkinsonism occurs without obvious cause; this idiopathic form is called **Parkinson's disease** or **paralysis agitans.**

B. ENCEPHALITIS LETHARGICA

In the first half of the twentieth century, parkinsonism often developed in patients with a history of von Economo's encephalitis. Because this type of infection is not now encountered, cases of **postencephalitic parkinsonism** are becoming increasingly rare.

C. Drug- or Toxin-Induced Parkinsonism

1. Therapeutic drugs—Many drugs, such as phenothiazines, butyrophenones, metoclopramide, reserpine, and tetrabenazine, can cause a reversible parkinsonian syndrome (see p 253).

2. Toxic substances—Environmental toxins such as manganese dust or carbon disulfide can lead to parkinsonism, and the disorder may appear as a sequela of severe carbon monoxide poisoning or exposure to fumes during welding. Experimental studies suggest that pesticide exposure is also associated with the development of parkinsonism.

3. MPTP (1-Methyl-4-phenyl-1,2,5,6-tetrahydropyridine)—A drug-induced form of parkinsonism has been described in individuals who synthesized and self-administered a meperidine analogue, MPTP (Figure 7–2). This compound is metabolized to a toxin that selectively destroys dopaminergic neurons in the substantia nigra and adrenergic neurons in the locus ceruleus and induces a severe form of parkinsonism in humans and in subhuman primates. The ability of this drug to reproduce neurochemical, pathologic, and clinical features of Parkinson's disease suggests that an environmental toxin could be responsible for the idiopathic disorder. MPTP-induced parkinsonism may provide a model that could assist in the development of new drugs for treatment of this disease.

D. Parkinsonism Associated with Other Neurologic Diseases

Parkinsonism that occurs in association with symptoms and signs of other neurologic disorders is considered briefly under *Differential Diagnosis* (p 242).

E. Familial Parkinsonism

Rarely, parkinsonism occurs on a familial basis. In some cases with autosomal dominant inheritance, this results from mutations in the α-synuclein gene (4q21). Mutations in the *parkin* gene (6q25.2–q27) are a major cause of early-onset, autosomal recessive, familial parkinsonism and of sporadic juvenile-onset Parkinson's disease. A number of different rearrangements of exons and different point mutations have been found in such patients.

Pathology

In idiopathic parkinsonism, pathologic examination shows loss of pigmentation and cells in the **substantia nigra** and other brainstem centers, cell loss in the globus pallidus and putamen, and the presence of filamentous eosinophilic intraneural inclusion granules (**Lewy bodies**), containing the protein α-synuclein, in the basal ganglia, brainstem, spinal cord, and sympathetic ganglia. These inclusion bodies are not seen in postencephalitic parkinsonism; instead there may be nonspecific neurofibrillary degeneration in a number of diencephalic structures as well as changes in the substantia nigra.

Pathogenesis

Both dopamine and acetylcholine are present in the corpus striatum, where they act as neurotransmitters (Figure 7–3). In idiopathic parkinsonism, it is generally believed that the normal balance between these two antagonistic neurotransmitters is disturbed because of dopamine depletion in the dopaminergic nigrostriatal system (Figure 7–4). Other neurotransmitters, such as norepinephrine, are also depleted in the brains of patients with parkinsonism, but the clinical relevance of this deficiency is less clear.

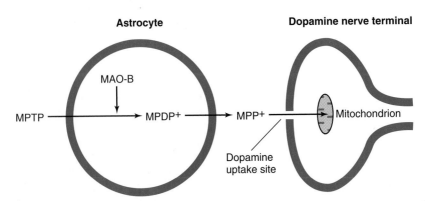

Figure 7–2. Proposed mechanism of MPTP-induced parkinsonism. MPTP enters brain astrocytes and is converted to MPDP$^+$ through the action of monoamine oxidase type B (MAO-B). MPDP$^+$ is then metabolized extracellularly to MPP$^+$, which is taken up through dopamine uptake sites on dopamine nerve terminals and concentrated in mitochondria. The resulting disturbance of mitochondrial function can lead to neuronal death.

Caudate and putamen

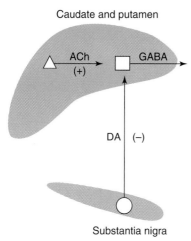

Figure 7–3. Simplified neurochemical anatomy of the basal ganglia. Dopamine (DA) neurons exert a net inhibitory effect and acetylcholine (ACh) neurons a net excitatory effect on the GABAergic output from the striatum.

Disorder of the balance of inhibition and excitation within the basal ganglia and its connections via direct and indirect pathways has been proposed to explain the impaired motor function in Parkinson's disease. These pathways are illustrated in Figure 7–5.

Caudate and putamen

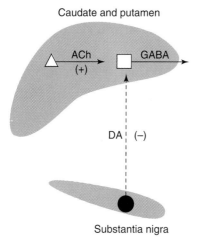

Figure 7–4. Neurochemical pathology of basal ganglia in Parkinson's disease. Dopamine (DA) neurons degenerate (black circle and dashed line), upsetting the normal balance between dopaminergic inhibition and cholinergic (ACh) excitation of striatal output (GABA) neurons. The net effect is to increase GABAergic output from the striatum.

Clinical Findings

A. TREMOR

The 4- to 6-Hz tremor of parkinsonism is characteristically most conspicuous at rest; it increases at times of emotional stress and often improves during voluntary activity. It commonly begins in the hand or foot, where it takes the form of rhythmic flexion-extension of the fingers or of the hand or foot—or of rhythmic pronation-supination of the forearm. It frequently involves the face in the area of the mouth as well. Although it may ultimately be present in all of the limbs, it is not uncommon for the tremor to be confined to one limb—or to the two limbs on one side—for months or years before it becomes more generalized. In some patients tremor never becomes prominent.

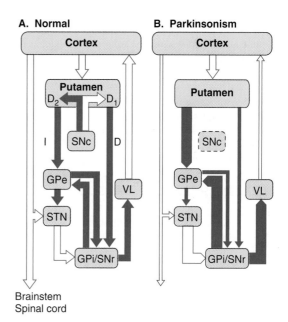

Figure 7–5. A model of the basal ganglia and its connections under normal conditions (**A**) and in the setting of parkinsonism (**B**). I refers to the indirect pathway and D refers to the direct pathway. Blue arrows indicate inhibitory connections; white arrows indicate excitatory connections. The thickness of the arrows indicates the amount of activity in the various projections. GPe, external segment of the globus pallidus; GPi, internal segment of the globus pallidus; SNr, substantia nigra pars reticulata; SNc, substantia nigra pars compacta; STN, subthalamic nucleus; VL, ventrolateral thalamus.
(Reproduced with permission from Wichmann T, Vitej JL, DeLong MR: The Neuroscientist 1995;1:236.)

B. RIGIDITY

Rigidity, or increased tone—ie, increased resistance to passive movement—is a characteristic clinical feature of parkinsonism. The disturbance in tone is responsible for the flexed posture of many patients with parkinsonism. The resistance is typically uniform throughout the range of movement at a particular joint and affects agonist and antagonist muscles alike—in contrast to the findings in spasticity, where the increase in tone is often greatest at the beginning of the passive movement (clasp-knife phenomenon) and more marked in some muscles than in others. In some instances, the rigidity in parkinsonism is described as **cogwheel rigidity** because of ratchet-like interruptions of passive movement that may be due, in part, to the presence of tremor.

C. HYPOKINESIA

The most disabling feature of this disorder is hypokinesia (sometimes called bradykinesia or akinesia)—a slowness of voluntary movement and a reduction in automatic movement, such as swinging the arms while walking. The patient's face is relatively immobile (**masklike facies**), with widened palpebral fissures, infrequent blinking, a certain fixity of facial expression, and a smile that develops and fades slowly. The voice is of low volume (**hypophonia**) and tends to be poorly modulated. Fine or rapidly alternating movements are impaired, but power is not diminished if time is allowed for it to develop. The handwriting is small, tremulous, and hard to read.

D. ABNORMAL GAIT AND POSTURE

The patient generally finds it difficult to get up from bed or an easy chair and tends to adopt a flexed posture on standing (Figure 7–6). It is often difficult to start walking, so that the patient may lean farther and farther forward while walking in place before being able to advance. The gait itself is characterized by small, shuffling steps and absence of the arm swing that normally accompanies locomotion; there is generally some unsteadiness on turning, and there may be difficulty in stopping. In advanced cases, the patient tends to walk with increasing speed to prevent a fall (**festinating gait**) because of the altered center of gravity that results from the abnormal posture.

E. OTHER CLINICAL FEATURES

There is often mild **blepharoclonus** (fluttering of the closed eyelids) and occasionally **blepharospasm** (involuntary closure of the eyelids). The patient may drool, perhaps because of impairment of swallowing. There is typically no alteration in the tendon reflexes, and the plantar responses are flexor. Repetitive tapping (about twice per second) over the bridge of the nose produces a sustained blink response (**Myerson's sign**); the response

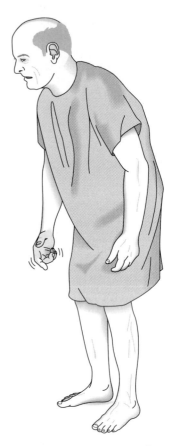

Figure 7–6. Typical flexed posture of a patient with parkinsonism.

is not sustained in normal subjects. Cognitive decline sometimes occurs but is usually mild and late. Depression and visual hallucinations are frequent.

Differential Diagnosis

The diagnosis may be difficult to make in mild cases.

Depression may be accompanied by a somewhat expressionless face, poorly modulated voice, and reduction in voluntary activity; it can thus simulate parkinsonism. Moreover, the two diseases often coexist in the same patient. A trial of antidepressant drug treatment may be helpful if diagnostic uncertainty cannot be resolved by the presence of more widespread neurologic signs indicative of parkinsonism.

Essential (benign, familial) tremor has been considered separately (see earlier). An early age at onset, a family history of tremor, a beneficial effect of alcohol on the tremor, and a lack of other neurologic signs distinguish this disorder from parkinsonism. Furthermore, essential tremor commonly affects the head (causing a nod or head shake); parkinsonism typically affects the face and lips rather than the head.

Diffuse Lewy body disease is a disorder of recently evolving definition. It occurs especially in patients aged between 60 and 80 years and is marked clinically by the combination of a rapidly progressing neurobehavioral syndrome of dementia and hallucinations and extrapyramidal motor features characteristic of Parkinson's disease. Myoclonus may also be seen. There is only an incomplete response to levodopa, but patients are extremely sensitive to parkinsonian complications of neuroleptics as well as to the side effects of antiparkinsonian drugs.

Wilson's disease can also lead to a parkinsonian syndrome, but other varieties of abnormal movements are usually present as well. Moreover, the early age at onset and the presence of Kayser-Fleischer rings should distinguish Wilson's disease from Parkinson's disease, as should the abnormalities in serum and urinary copper and serum ceruloplasmin that occur in Wilson's disease.

Huntington's disease may occasionally be mistaken for parkinsonism when it presents with rigidity and akinesia, but a family history of Huntington's disease or an accompanying dementia, if present, should suggest the correct diagnosis, which can be confirmed by genetic studies.

Shy-Drager syndrome is a degenerative disorder characterized by parkinsonian features, autonomic insufficiency (leading to postural hypotension, anhidrosis, disturbance of sphincter control, impotence, etc), and signs of more widespread neurologic involvement (pyramidal or lower motor neuron signs and often a cerebellar deficit). There is no treatment for the motor deficit, but the postural hypotension may respond to a liberal salt diet; fludrocortisone, 0.1–1 mg/d; midodrine (an α-agonist) 10 mg three times daily; wearing waist-high elastic hosiery; and sleeping with the head up at night.

Striatonigral degeneration is a rare disorder that is associated with neuronal loss in the putamen, the globus pallidus, and caudate nucleus, and presents with bradykinesia and rigidity. Antiparkinsonian drugs are typically ineffective. Striatonigral degeneration may be associated with olivopontocerebellar degeneration (see Chapter 3), in which case the term **multiple system atrophy** or Shy-Drager syndrome is applied.

Progressive supranuclear palsy is a disorder in which there may be bradykinesia and rigidity, but its characteristic features are early postural instability and falls, loss of voluntary control of eye movements (especially vertical gaze), frontotemporal dementia, pseudobulbar palsy, dysarthria, and axial dystonia. The disorder responds poorly, if at all, to antiparkinsonian drugs. It is discussed on p 246.

Cortical basal ganglionic degeneration is charac-terized clinically by both cortical and basal ganglionic dysfunction. Rigidity, bradykinesia, tremor, postural disturbances, and dystonia are accompanied by such additional deficits as cortical sensory loss, apraxia, focal reflex myoclonus, dementia, or aphasia. Symptoms are often strikingly asymmetric. Treatment with antiparkinsonian medication is usually unrewarding, although some patients do respond to Sinemet (p 247).

Creutzfeldt-Jakob disease may be accompanied by parkinsonian features, but dementia is usually present, myoclonic jerking is common, and ataxia is sometimes prominent; there may be pyramidal signs and visual disturbances, and the EEG findings of periodic discharges are usually characteristic.

Normal-pressure hydrocephalus leads to a gait disturbance (often mistakenly attributed to parkinsonism), urinary incontinence, and dementia. CT scanning reveals dilation of the ventricular system of the brain without cortical atrophy. The disorder may follow head injury, intracranial hemorrhage, or meningoencephalitis, but the cause is often obscure. Surgical shunting procedures to bypass any obstruction to the flow of cerebrospinal fluid (CSF) are often beneficial.

Treatment

Early parkinsonism requires no drug treatment, but it is important to discuss with the patient the nature of the disorder and the availability of medical treatment if symptoms become more severe and to encourage activity. Treatment, when indicated, is directed toward restoring the dopaminergic:cholinergic balance in the striatum by blocking the effect of acetylcholine with anticholinergic drugs or by enhancing dopaminergic transmission (Figure 7–7).

A. ANTICHOLINERGIC DRUGS

Muscarinic anticholinergic drugs are more helpful in alleviating tremor and rigidity than hypokinesia but are generally less effective than dopaminergic drugs (see below). A number of preparations are available, and individual patients tend to favor different drugs. Among the most commonly prescribed drugs are trihexyphenidyl and benztropine (Table 7–6). Common side effects include dryness of the mouth, constipation, urinary retention, and defective pupillary accommodation; these are caused by muscarinic receptor blockade in parasympathetic end organs. Confusion, especially in the elderly, is due to antimuscarinic effects in the brain. Treatment is started with a small dose of one of the anticholinergics; the dosage is then gradually increased until benefit occurs or side effects limit further increments. If treatment is not helpful, the drug is withdrawn and another anticholinergic preparation is tried.

Caudate and putamen

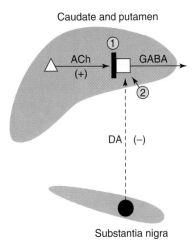

Figure 7–7. Therapeutic approaches in Parkinson's disease. The balance between dopaminergic (DA) and cholinergic (ACh) influences on striatal output (GABA) neurons can be restored by (1) blockade of cholinergic transmission with muscarinic anticholinergic drugs or (2) enhancement of dopaminergic transmission with the dopamine precursor levodopa, dopamine-agonist drugs (eg, bromocriptine), or amantadine (which stimulates the release of dopamine from surviving nerve terminals).

B. AMANTADINE

Amantadine can be given for mild parkinsonism either alone or in combination with an anticholinergic agent. Its precise mode of action is unclear. Its advantages are that it improves all the clinical features of parkinsonism, its side effects (restlessness, confusion, skin rashes, edema, disturbances of cardiac rhythm) are relatively uncommon, its effects are exerted rapidly, and it is given in a standard dose of 100 mg orally twice daily. Unfortunately, however, many patients fail to respond to this drug, or its benefit is short-lived. Amantadine may also be useful in reducing iatrogenic dyskinesias in patients with advanced disease.

C. LEVODOPA

Levodopa, which is converted in the body to dopamine (Figure 7–8), ameliorates all the major clinical features of parkinsonism and, unlike the anticholinergic drugs, is often particularly helpful against hypokinesia. There is controversy about the best time to introduce dopaminergic therapy. Concerns that levodopa loses its effectiveness with time in some patients are probably misplaced, but response fluctuations sometimes occur after it has been used for several years, and these may be particularly disabling and difficult to manage. It may be wise to defer its intro-

Table 7–6. Drugs used in the treatment of Parkinson's disease.

Drug	Total Daily Dose (mg)[1]
Anticholinergics	
Benztropine (Cogentin)	1–6
Trihexyphenidyl (Artane)	6–20
Amantadine (Symmetrel)	100–200
Levodopa (Sinemet)	300–1000[2]
Dopamine agonists	
Ergolides	
Bromocriptine (Parlodel)	15–30
Pergolide (Permax)	2–4
Nonergolides	
Pramipexole (Mirapex)	1.5–4.5
Ropinirole (Requip)	6–24
MAO-B inhibitor	
Selegiline (Eldepryl)	10
COMT inhibitor	
Entacapone (Comtan)	600–1000
Tolcapone (Tasmar)	300–600

[1] Doses are range for total daily maintenance; all drugs are administered in divided doses. Introduction is at a lower dose, which is gradually increased. Drug interactions are common; the addition of one drug may mandate reduction of another. Psychoactive side effects are common with all of these agents.

[2] Refers to the levodopa component of the carbidopa/levodopa combination (eg, 25/250 represents 250 mg of levodopa).

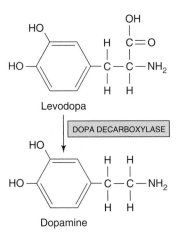

Figure 7–8. Metabolism of levodopa to dopamine.

duction as long as possible and then use dopamine agonists (discussed below) in conjunction with it to keep the levodopa dose as low as possible.

The most common side effects of levodopa are nausea, vomiting, hypotension, abnormal movements (dyskinesias), restlessness, and confusion. Cardiac arrhythmias occur occasionally. The late dyskinesias and behavioral side effects occur as dose-related phenomena, but reduction in dose may diminish any therapeutic benefit. Treatment with clozapine, a dibenzodiazepine derivative that does not block the therapeutic effects of dopaminergic medication, may relieve confusion and psychotic mental disturbances and, in some instances, the dyskinesias. Clozapine requires regular monitoring of the leukocyte count. Olanzepine, quetiapine, and risperidone are alternative agents that may be less effective but do not affect the blood count. Another late complication of levodopa therapy is response fluctuation such as the **wearing-off effect,** in which deterioration occurs shortly before the next dose is to be taken, or the **on-off phenomenon,** in which abrupt but transient fluctuations in the severity of parkinsonism occur at frequent intervals during the day, apparently without any relationship to the last dose of levodopa. This sometimes disabling problem is unaffected by concomitant administration of carbidopa. It can be controlled only partly by varying the dosing intervals, administering levodopa 1 hour before meals, restricting dietary protein intake, or providing treatment with dopamine agonists.

Carbidopa is a drug that inhibits dopa decarboxylase, the enzyme responsible for the breakdown of levodopa to its active metabolite, dopamine (see Figure 7–8), but does not cross the blood-brain barrier. Accordingly, if levodopa is given in combination with carbidopa, the breakdown of levodopa is limited outside the central nervous system. The daily dose of levodopa required for benefit and the incidence of nausea, vomiting, hypotension, and cardiac irregularities can be reduced if levodopa is taken in combination with carbidopa. Carbidopa is generally combined with levodopa in a fixed proportion (1:10 or 1:4) as **Sinemet.** Treatment is started with a small dose, such as Sinemet 10/100 (mg) or Sinemet 25/100 (mg) orally three times daily, and the dose is gradually increased, depending on the response. Most patients ultimately require Sinemet 25/250 (mg) three or four times daily. Carbidopa should total at least 75 mg/d.

Levodopa therapy (either alone or in conjunction with carbidopa) is contraindicated in patients with narrow-angle glaucoma or psychotic illness and should be avoided in patients receiving monoamine oxidase A inhibitors. It should also be used with care in patients with active peptic ulcers or suspected malignant melanomas.

A controlled-release (CR) formulation of Sinemet may reduce response fluctuations and the dosing frequency.

D. DOPAMINE AGONISTS

The older agonists are ergot derivatives. Bromocriptine stimulates dopamine D_2 receptors. It is perhaps slightly less effective than levodopa in relieving the symptoms of parkinsonism but is less likely to cause dyskinesias or the on-off phenomenon. In consequence, it has been recommended that when dopaminergic therapy is to be introduced, the patient be started on Sinemet, 25/100 three times daily, with bromocriptine then added and gradually increased. The starting dose of bromocriptine is 1.25 mg/d for 1 week and 2.5 mg/d for the next week, after which the daily dose is increased by 2.5-mg increments every 2 weeks, depending on the response and the development of side effects. Maintenance doses are usually between 2.5 and 10 mg orally three times daily. Side effects are similar to those associated with levodopa therapy, but psychiatric effects such as delusions or hallucinations are especially common, and bromocriptine is therefore contraindicated in patients with a history of psychotic disorders. Relative contraindications to its use are recent myocardial infarction, severe peripheral vascular disease, and active peptic ulceration. Pericardial, pleural, or retroperitoneal fibrosis are rare, ergot-related side effects.

Pergolide also is an ergot derivative and dopamine receptor agonist; unlike bromocriptine, it activates both D_1 and D_2 receptors. Its indications, side effects, and contraindications are similar to those described above for bromocriptine, and it is unclear whether either compound is clinically superior to the other. The starting dose is 0.05 mg orally daily for 2 days, increased by 0.1–0.15 mg/d every 3 days for 12 days and by 0.25 mg/d every 3 days thereafter. The average maintenance dose is 1 mg orally three times daily.

The new dopamine agonists, pramipexole and ropinirole, are not ergot derivatives. They seem to be as effective as the older agonists but are without their potential ergot-related adverse effects, and may be used in early or advanced Parkinson's disease. Pramipexole is started at 0.125 mg three times daily; the daily dose is doubled after one week and again after another week; it is then increased by 0.75 mg each week according to response and tolerance. A common maintenance dose is between 0.5 and 1.5 mg three times daily. Ropinirole is started at 0.25 mg three times daily and the total daily dose increased at weekly intervals by 0.75 mg until the fourth week and by 1.5 mg thereafter. Most patients need between 2 and 8 mg three times daily for benefit. Adverse effects of these medications include fatigue, somnolence, nausea, peripheral edema, dyskinesias, confusion, hallucinations, and orthostatic hypotension. An irresistable urge to sleep at inappropriate times has also been reported and may lead to injury.

E. Catechol-O-Methyltransferase Inhibitors

These inhibitors may be used to reduce the dose requirements of and any response fluctuations to Sinemet. Their use leads to more sustained plasma levels of levodopa, with improved transport into the blood and across the blood-brain barrier. Side effects include diarrhea, confusion, dyskinesias, and abnormalities of liver function tests. Two of these inhibitors are in widespread use. Tolcapone is taken in a daily dose of 100 or 200 mg three times daily. Acute hepatic necrosis has occurred in rare instances in patients receiving this medication and, accordingly, entacapone (200 mg) taken with Sinemet up to five times daily is generally preferred.

F. Selegiline

Selegiline (also called eldepryl or deprenyl) is a monoamine oxidase type B inhibitor and therefore inhibits the metabolic breakdown of dopamine (Figure 7–9). It thus enhances the antiparkinsonian effect of levodopa and may reduce mild on-off fluctuations in responsiveness. Some clinical studies suggest that selegiline may also delay the progression of Parkinson's disease, although the evidence is incomplete in this regard; when used for neuroprotection, selegiline is best kept for patients with mild disease. The dose is 5 mg orally twice daily, usually given early in the day to avoid insomnia.

G. Surgery

Surgical treatment of parkinsonism by thalamotomy or pallidotomy is often helpful when patients become unresponsive to pharmacologic measures or develop intolerable adverse reactions to antiparkinsonian med-

ication. Lesions of the internal segment of the globus pallidus (GPi), for example, will attenuate its unbalanced inhibitory output (see Figure 7–5). Treatment by surgery is sometimes helpful in relatively young patients with predominantly unilateral tremor and rigidity that have failed to respond to medication; thalamotomy is more helpful for tremor, and pallidotomy for hypokinesia. Diffuse vascular disease or dementia is a contraindication to this approach. The rate of significant complications is less than 5% after unilateral pallidotomy or thalamotomy, but about 20% or more after bilateral procedures, which are therefore best avoided.

Autologous or fetal adrenal medullary tissue or fetal substantia nigra has been transplanted to the putamen or caudate nucleus, in the belief that the transplanted tissue can continue to synthesize and release dopamine. Results from preliminary studies have been contradictory, and this approach is highly controversial. In one recent controlled trial involving intracerebral transplantation of human embryonic mesencephalic tissue containing dopaminergic neurons, benefit occurred in young patients (less than 60 years old) but not in older subjects; among those initially responding favorably, severe uncontrolled dyskinesias and dystonias developed more than 1 year later in some patients despite reduction or discontinuation of antiparkinsonian medication and was attributed to a relative excess of dopamine from continued fiber outgrowth from the transplant. Thus, these approaches remain experimental, are not without hazards, and involve uncertain mechanisms.

H. Deep Brain Stimulation

High-frequency thalamic stimulation is effective for the relief of parkinsonian tremor. Deep brain stimulation of the globus pallidus or subthalamic nucleus may help all the cardinal features of the disease and reduces the time spent in the off-state in patients with response fluctuations. This approach has the advantage of being reversible, of having a lower morbidity than ablative surgical procedures (especially when bilateral procedures are contemplated), and of causing minimal damage to the brain. It is contraindicated in patients with atypical parkinsonism or dementia.

I. Physical Therapy and Aids for Daily Living

Physical therapy and speech therapy are beneficial to many patients with parkinsonism, and the quality of life can often be improved by providing simple aids to daily living. Such aids may include extra rails or banisters placed strategically about the home for additional support, table cutlery with large handles, nonslip rubber table mats, devices to amplify the voice, and chairs that will gently eject the occupant at the push of a button.

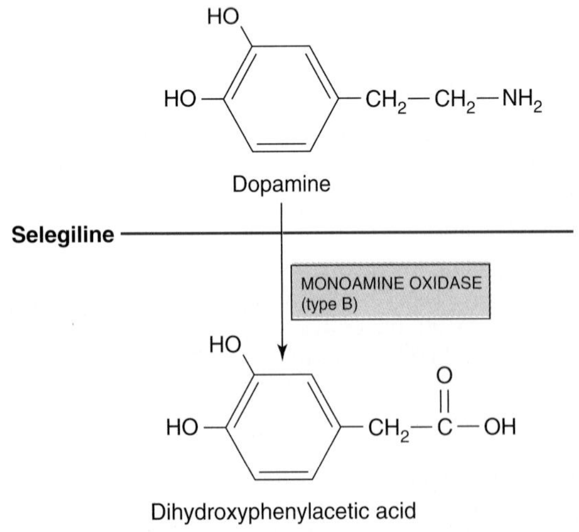

Figure 7–9. Metabolic breakdown of dopamine. Selegiline interferes with the breakdown of dopamine by inhibiting the enzyme monoamine oxidase type B.

PROGRESSIVE SUPRANUCLEAR PALSY

Progressive supranuclear palsy is an idiopathic degenerative disorder that primarily affects subcortical gray matter regions of the brain. The principal neuropathologic finding is neuronal degeneration with the presence of neurofibrillary tangles in the midbrain, pons, basal ganglia, and dentate nuclei of the cerebellum. Associated neurochemical abnormalities include decreased concentrations of dopamine and its metabolite homovanillic acid in the caudate nucleus and putamen. The classic clinical features are gait disturbance with early falls, supranuclear ophthalmoplegia, pseudobulbar palsy, axial dystonia with or without extrapyramidal rigidity of the limbs, and dementia. Men are affected twice as often as women, and the disorder has its onset between ages 45 and 75 years.

Clinical Findings

Supranuclear ophthalmoplegia is characterized by prominent failure of voluntary vertical gaze, with later paralysis of horizontal gaze; oculocephalic and oculovestibular reflexes are preserved. Postural instability and unexplained falls also occur early and may precede vertical gaze palsies. In addition, the neck often assumes an extended posture (**axial dystonia in extension**), with resistance to passive flexion. Rigidity of the limbs and bradykinesia may mimic Parkinson's disease, but tremor is rare. A coexisting **pseudobulbar palsy** produces facial weakness, dysarthria, dysphagia, and often exaggerated jaw jerk and gag reflexes; there may also be exaggerated and inappropriate emotional responses (**pseudobulbar affect**). Hyperreflexia, extensor plantar responses, and cerebellar signs are sometimes seen. The **dementia** of progressive supranuclear palsy is characterized by forgetfulness, slowed thought processes, alterations of mood and personality, and impaired calculation and abstraction. Focal cortical dysfunction is rare.

Differential Diagnosis

Parkinson's disease differs in that voluntary downward and horizontal gaze are not usually lost, axial posture tends to be characterized by flexion rather than extension, tremor is common, the course is less fulminant, and antiparkinsonian medications are more often effective.

Treatment

Dopaminergic preparations are occasionally of benefit for rigidity and bradykinesia. Anticholinergics such as amitriptyline, 50–75 mg orally at bedtime, or benztropine, 6–10 mg/d orally, have been reported to improve speech, gait, and pathologic laughing or crying, and methysergide, 8–12 mg/d orally, may ameliorate dysphagia. There is no treatment for the dementia.

Prognosis

The disorder typically follows a progressive course, with death from aspiration or inanition within 2–12 (usually 4–7) years.

CORTICAL BASAL GANGLIONIC DEGENERATION

Cortical basal ganglionic degeneration is a rare, nonfamilial, degenerative disorder of unknown cause that occurs in middle-aged or elderly persons of either sex. It sometimes simulates Parkinson's disease when bradykinesia and rigidity are conspicuous features. Postural-action tremor may also occur, but the usual cause of profound disability is apraxia and clumsiness rather than extrapyramidal deficits. Other features of the established disorder include speech disturbances (aphasic, apraxic, or dysarthric), cortical sensory deficits (such as neglect syndromes), stimulus-sensitive myoclonus, dysphagia, postural disturbances, dystonic features, and ultimately cognitive decline and behavioral changes. Frontal release signs, brisk tendon reflexes, and extensor plantar responses may also be encountered.

Differential Diagnosis

The disorder is distinguished from Parkinson's disease by the marked apraxia that often leads to a useless limb, difficulty in opening or closing the eyes, or speech disturbances. The presence of pyramidal and cortical deficits in addition to any extrapyramidal dysfunction and the relative preservation of cognitive function, at least until late in the course of the disorder, also help in this regard, but definitive diagnosis can be made only at autopsy.

Treatment

Antiparkinsonian medication is generally unhelpful but is certainly worthy of trial. No specific therapy exists.

Prognosis

The disorder follows a progressive course, leading to increasing disability and dependence. Death typically follows within 10 years, often sooner, from aspiration pneumonia.

HUNTINGTON'S DISEASE

Epidemiology

Huntington's disease is a hereditary disorder of the nervous system characterized by the gradual onset and subsequent progression of chorea and dementia. It occurs throughout the world and in all ethnic groups. Its prevalence rate is about 5 per 100,000 population. Symptoms usually do not appear until adulthood (typically between 30 and 50 years of age), by which time these patients have often started families of their own; thus, the disease continues from one generation to the next.

Genetics

Huntington's disease is an autosomal dominant disorder due to a mutation in the **huntingtin** gene on chromosome 4p16.3. The disease shows complete penetrance, so that offspring of an affected individual have a 50% chance of developing it. Additional features of the inheritance of Huntington's disease include **anticipation,** meaning that there is a trend toward earlier onset in successive generations, and **paternal descent,** which refers to the tendency for anticipation to be most pronounced in individuals who inherit the disease from their father. Both of these phenomena are related to the unstable nature of the mutation responsible for Huntington's disease—expansion of a CAG trinucleotide repeat that codes for a polyglutamine tract. The repeat can expand during gametogenesis, especially in the male germline. This leads to an abnormal protein with longer and longer polyglutamine tracts. Normal subjects have between 11 and 34 CAG repeats whereas nearly all patients with Huntington's disease have more than 40.

Pathology

Postmortem examination of patients with the disease reveals cell loss, particularly in the cerebral cortex and corpus striatum (Figure 7–10). In the latter region, medium-sized spiny neurons that contain γ-aminobutyric acid (GABA) and enkephalin and project to the external segment of the globus pallidus are affected earliest, but other classes of neurons are eventually involved as well. Biochemical studies have shown that the concentrations of the inhibitory neurotransmitter GABA, its biosynthetic enzyme glutamic acid decarboxylase (GAD), and acetylcholine and its biosynthetic enzyme choline acetyltransferase are all reduced in the basal ganglia of patients with Huntington's disease. The concentration of dopamine is normal or slightly increased. Changes in the concentrations of neuropeptides in the basal ganglia have also been found, including decreased substance P, methionine enkephalin, dynorphin, and cholecystokinin and increased somatostatin and neuropeptide Y. Neurons containing NADPH diaphorase activity are spared. Positron emission tomography has shown reduced glucose utilization in an anatomically normal caudate nucleus.

Pathophysiology

How an expanded CAG repeat in huntingtin leads to Huntington's disease is unknown, but at least two factors

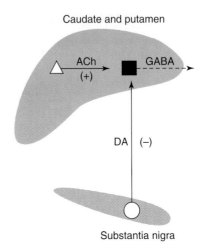

Figure 7–10. Neurochemical pathology of the basal ganglia in Huntington's disease. GABAergic neurons with cell bodies in the striatum degenerate (black square and dashed line), decreasing GABAergic output from the striatum. ACh, acetylcholine; DA, dopamine.

may contribute. First, like other autosomal dominant disorders, Huntington's disease is likely to involve a toxic gain in function of the mutant protein. Mutant huntingtin is cleaved by proteases and conjugated with ubiquitin, then transported in a complex called the proteasome to the cell nucleus, where it may disrupt the gene transcription machinery and thereby promote cell death. However, loss of the normal function of huntingtin, which has not yet been defined but may include an inhibitory effect on programmed cell death, may also contribute to disease pathogenesis.

Clinical Findings

Symptoms usually begin in the fourth or fifth decade, and the disease is progressive, with an average life span after onset of about 15 years.

A. INITIAL SYMPTOMS

Either abnormal movements or intellectual changes may be the initial symptom, but ultimately both are present.

1. Dementia—The earliest mental changes often consist of irritability, moodiness, and antisocial behavior, but a more obvious dementia subsequently develops.

2. Chorea—Movement disturbance may be characterized initially by no more than an apparent fidgetiness or restlessness, but grossly abnormal choreiform movements are eventually seen.

3. Atypical forms—Especially in cases developing during childhood—but occasionally in adult-onset cases as well—the clinical picture is dominated by progressive rigidity and akinesia, with little or no chorea. This is known as the **Westphal variant,** and the correct diagnosis is suggested by the accompanying dementia and positive family history.

Epilepsy and cerebellar ataxia are frequent features of the juvenile form but not of adult cases.

B. FAMILY HISTORY

In cases in which a positive family history cannot be obtained, it must be remembered that the early death of a parent may make the history incomplete and that relatives often conceal the familial nature of the disorder. In addition, a certain degree of eccentric behavior, clumsiness, or restlessness may be regarded as normal by lay people and medical personnel unfamiliar with the disorder. The family history cannot therefore be regarded as negative until all close relatives of the patient have been examined by the physician personally. Nevertheless, apparently sporadic cases are occasionally encountered.

C. GENETIC TESTING

Genetic testing now provides an accurate and definitive means of establishing the diagnosis and also permits the presymptomatic detection of the disease.

D. IMAGING

CT scanning or MRI often demonstrates atrophy of the cerebral cortex and caudate nucleus in established cases.

Differential Diagnosis

Conditions that should be considered in the differential diagnosis of Huntington's disease are listed in Table 7–2. Tardive dyskinesia, which is most common, can usually be identified from the history. Laboratory studies can exclude most medical disorders associated with chorea. Other hereditary disorders in which chorea is a conspicuous feature are described below.

Benign hereditary chorea is a recently recognized disorder that is inherited in either an autosomal dominant or recessive manner and is characterized by choreiform movements that develop in early childhood, do not progress during adult life, and are not associated with dementia.

Familial chorea sometimes occurs in association with circulating acanthocytes (spiny red blood cells), but examination of a wet blood film will clearly distinguish this disorder. Other clinical features of **chorea-acanthocytosis** include orolingual ticlike dyskinesias, vocalizations, mild intellectual decline, seizures, peripheral neuropathy, and muscle atrophy. Parkinsonian features are sometimes present. Unlike certain other disorders associated with circulating acanthocytes, there is no disturbance of β-lipoprotein concentration in the peripheral blood.

Paroxysmal choreoathetosis may occur on a familial basis, but the intermittent nature of the symptoms and their relationship to movement or emotional stress usually distinguish this disorder from Huntington's disease.

The age at onset of symptoms usually distinguishes Huntington's disease from certain rare inherited childhood disorders characterized by choreoathetosis.

Wilson's disease can be distinguished from Huntington's disease by the mode of inheritance, the presence of Kayser-Fleischer rings, and abnormal serum copper and ceruloplasmin levels.

Dentatorubral-pallidoluysian atrophy, another dominantly inherited CAG repeat disorder that is clinically similar to Huntington's disease, is distinguished by genetic testing.

When the early symptoms constitute progressive intellectual failure, it may not be possible to distinguish Huntington's disease from other varieties of dementia unless the family history is characteristic or the movement disorder becomes noticeable.

Treatment & Prognosis

There is no cure for Huntington's disease, which, as a rule, terminates fatally 10–20 years after clinical onset. There is no treatment for the dementia, but the movement disorder may respond to drugs that interfere with dopaminergic inhibition of striatal output neurons. These include dopamine D_2-receptor-blocking drugs such as haloperidol, 0.5–4 mg orally four times daily, or chlorpromazine, 25–50 mg orally three times daily; and drugs that deplete dopamine from nerve terminals, such as reserpine, 0.5–5 mg/d orally, or tetrabenazine (unavailable in the United States), 12.5–50 mg orally three times daily. Drugs that potentiate GABAergic or cholinergic neurotransmission are generally ineffective. Selective serotonin-reuptake inhibitors may help to reduce aggressiveness and agitation. The role of surgical treatment involving the intrastriatal transplantation of fetal striatal neuroblasts is currently being investigated.

Prevention

Patients should be advised of the risk of transmitting the disease, and living offspring should receive genetic counseling. The use of genetic markers for detection of presymptomatic Huntington's disease and the problems associated with this approach are discussed on p 239.

DENTATORUBRAL-PALLIDOLUYSIAN ATROPHY

This disorder, which is inherited in an autosomal dominant manner, is rare except in Japan. It is characterized by dementia, choreoathetosis, ataxia, and myoclonic epilepsy.

The mutant gene is distinct from that in Huntington's disease, despite the similarity of clinical phenotype. The gene maps to 12p13.31, where there is an expanded trinucleotide repeat. The size of the (CAG)n repeat expansion correlates with age on onset and disease severity. Treatment is symptomatic, as for Huntington's disease.

SYDENHAM'S CHOREA

This disorder occurs principally in children and adolescents as a complication of a previous group A hemolytic streptococcal infection. The underlying pathologic feature is probably arteritis. In about 30% of cases, it appears 2 or 3 months after an episode of rheumatic fever or polyarthritis, but in other patients no such history can be obtained. There is usually no recent history of sore throat and no fever. The disorder may have an acute or insidious onset, usually subsiding within the following 4–6 months. It may recur during pregnancy, however, or in patients taking oral contraceptive preparations.

Sydenham's chorea is characterized by abnormal choreiform movements that are sometimes unilateral and, when mild, may be mistaken for restlessness or fidgetiness. There may be accompanying behavioral changes, with the child becoming irritable or disobedient. Obsessive-compulsive symptoms and emotional lability also occur. In 30% of cases there is evidence of cardiac involvement, but the sedimentation rate and antistreptolysin O titer are usually normal.

The traditional treatment is bed rest, sedation, and prophylactic antibiotic therapy even if there are no other signs of acute rheumatism. A course of intramuscular penicillin is generally recommended, and continuous prophylactic oral penicillin daily until about age 20 years is also frequently advised to prevent streptococcal infections.

The prognosis is essentially that of the cardiac complications.

IDIOPATHIC TORSION DYSTONIA

This disorder is characterized by dystonic movements and postures and an absence of other neurologic signs. The birth and developmental histories are normal. Before the diagnosis can be made, other possible causes of dystonia must be excluded on clinical grounds and by laboratory investigations.

Idiopathic torsion dystonia may be inherited as an autosomal dominant (with variable penetrance of 30–40%), autosomal recessive, or X-linked recessive disorder, and the defective genes have been localized in some cases (see Table 7–5). Molecular genetic techniques permit identification of carriers of the responsible trinucleotide (GAG) deletion on the gene for the dominantly inherited disorder, which has been identified, named DYT1, and encodes torsin A, an ATP-binding protein. Other cases seem to occur on a sporadic basis. Changes in the concentrations of norepinephrine, serotonin, and dopamine have been demonstrated in a variety of brain regions, but their role in the pathogenesis of dystonia is uncertain. Onset may be in childhood or later life, and this disorder remains as a lifelong affliction. The diagnosis is made on clinical grounds.

Clinical Findings

A. HISTORY

When onset is in childhood, a family history is usually obtainable. Symptoms generally commence in the legs. Progression is likely, and it leads to severe disability from generalized dystonia.

With onset in adult life, a positive family history is not likely to be obtained. The initial symptoms are usually in the arms or axial structures. Generalized dystonia may ultimately develop in about 20% of patients with adult-onset dystonia, but severe disability does not usually occur.

B. EXAMINATION

The disorder is characterized by abnormal movements and postures that are typically exacerbated by voluntary activity. For example, the neck may be twisted to one side (**torticollis**), the arm held in a hyperpronated position with the wrist flexed and fingers extended, the leg held extended with the foot plantar flexed and inverted, or the trunk held in a flexed or extended position. There is often facial grimacing, and other characteristic facial abnormalities may also be encountered, including **blepharospasm** (spontaneous, involuntary forced closure of the eyelids for a variable period of time) and **oromandibular dystonia.** This consists of spasms of the muscles about the mouth, causing, for example, involuntary opening or closing of the mouth; pouting, pursing, or retraction of the lips; retraction of the platysma muscle; and roving or protruding movements of the tongue.

Differential Diagnosis

It is important to exclude other causes of dystonia (see Table 7–3) before a diagnosis of idiopathic torsion dystonia is made. A normal developmental history prior to the onset of abnormal movements, together with the absence of other neurologic signs and normal results of laboratory investigations, is important in this regard. In patients with primary torsion dystonia that begins before the age of 30 years, genetic testing, especially for DYT1, in conjunction with genetic counseling is helpful by obviating the need for other diagnostic studies and facilitating further advice and management. Testing patients who are older at onset may also be warranted in those with a family history of early-onset disease.

Treatment

The abnormal movements may be helped, at least in part, by drugs. A dramatic response to levodopa suggests a variant of classic torsion dystonia, discussed separately below. Anticholinergic drugs given in the highest doses that can be tolerated (typically, trihexyphenidyl, 40–50 mg/d orally in divided doses) may be very effective. Diazepam is occasionally helpful. Phenothiazines, haloperidol, or tetrabenazine (unavailable in the United States) may be worthwhile; however, at effective doses, these drugs usually lead to a mild parkinsonian syndrome. Other drugs that are sometimes helpful are baclofen and carbamazepine. Stereotactic thalamotomy may help patients with predominantly unilateral dystonia that particularly involves the limbs. Deep brain stimulation of the globus pallidus has shown benefit in a limited number of patients and is currently under study.

Course & Prognosis

If all cases are considered together, about one-third of patients eventually become so severely disabled that they are confined to chair or bed, and another one-third are affected only mildly. In general, severe disability is more likely to occur when the disorder commences in childhood.

DOPA-RESPONSIVE DYSTONIA

Inherited in an autosomal dominant manner, the gene causing this disorder maps to chromosome 14q. Symptom onset is typically in childhood but may occur later. Girls are affected more commonly than boys. Disabling dystonia is accompanied by bradykinesia and rigidity that may lead to a mistaken diagnosis of juvenile Parkinson's disease. Remarkable recovery occurs with low doses of levodopa, to which patients are particularly sensitive.

DYSTONIA-PARKINSONISM

An X-linked recessive form of dystonia-parkinsonism (sometimes called Lubag) has been identified in men from the Philippines, and the responsible gene localized to Xq13. Female heterozygotes are reported to have mild dystonia or chorea. The response to pharmacotherapy is often disappointing.

An autosomal dominant form also occurs, with rapid evolution of symptoms and signs over hours, days, or weeks, but slow progression thereafter. It may first manifest during childhood or adulthood. Levodopa therapy is ineffective. Genetic linkage has been described to markers on chromosome 19q13.

MYOCLONIC DYSTONIA

This is an autosomal dominant disorder with variable expression in which patients exhibit rapid jerks in addition to more sustained abnormal postures. The legs are often spared. The jerks may respond to alcohol. The disorder appears to be distinct from classic idiopathic torsion dystonia. Its onset is usually before the age of 20 years, and it usually has a benign, slowly progressive course over many years.

FOCAL TORSION DYSTONIA

A number of the dystonic features of idiopathic torsion dystonia may also occur as isolated phenomena. They are probably best regarded as focal dystonias that occur as formes frustes of idiopathic torsion dystonia in patients with a positive family history or that represent a focal manifestation of its adult-onset form when there is no family history. In addition, focal adult-onset dystonia may have a familial basis related to a genetic abnormality (DYT7) at 18p31 with autosomal dominant inheritance.

Both **blepharospasm** and **oromandibular dystonia** can occur as isolated focal dystonias.

Spasmodic torticollis usually begins in the fourth or fifth decade and is characterized by a tendency for the neck to twist to one side. This often occurs episodically in early stages, but eventually the neck is held continuously to one side. Although the disorder is usually lifelong once it develops, spontaneous remission does occur occasionally, especially in the first 18 months after onset. Medical treatment is generally unsatisfactory. A trial of the drugs used in treating idiopathic torsion dystonia is worthwhile, as some patients do obtain undoubted benefit. Selective section of the spinal accessory nerve (cranial nerve XI) and the upper cervical nerve roots is sometimes helpful for patients in whom the neck is markedly deviated to the side, but recurrence of the abnormal posture is frequent. Local injection of botulinum toxin into the overactive muscles may also produce benefit for up to several months; it can be repeated as needed. It is the most effective treatment available for this disorder.

Writer's cramp is characterized by dystonic posturing of the hand and forearm when the hand is used for writing and sometimes other tasks such as playing the piano or using a screwdriver or table cutlery. Drug treatment is usually unrewarding, and it is often necessary for patients to learn to use the other hand for these tasks. Injections of botulinum toxin into the involved muscles are sometimes helpful.

WILSON'S DISEASE

Wilson's disease is an autosomal recessive disorder of copper metabolism that produces neurologic and hepatic dysfunction. The gene localizes in the region of chromosome 13q14–21, but the disease is caused by a number of different mutations, two of which are encountered fairly frequently in affected patients. Although the precise nature of the biochemical abnormality in Wilson's disease is unknown, its pathogenesis appears to involve decreased binding of copper to the transport protein **ceruloplasmin**. As a result, large amounts of unbound copper enter the circulation and are subsequently deposited in tissues, including the brain, liver, kidney, and cornea. Studies of mitochondrial function and aconitase activity suggest that free radical formation and oxidative damage, perhaps through mitochondrial copper accumulation, are important in the pathogenesis of the disease.

Clinical Findings

A. MODE OF PRESENTATION

Wilson's disease usually presents in childhood or young adult life. The average age at onset is about 11 years for patients presenting with hepatic dysfunction and 19 years for those with initial neurologic manifestations, but the disease may begin as late as the sixth decade. Hepatic and neurologic presentations are about equally common, and most patients, if untreated, eventually develop both types of involvement. Rare presentations include joint disease, fever, hemolytic anemia, and behavioral disturbances.

B. NONNEUROLOGIC FINDINGS

Ocular and hepatic abnormalities are the most prominent nonneurologic manifestations of Wilson's disease. The most common ocular finding is **Kayser-Fleischer rings** (Figure 7–11): bilateral brown corneal rings that result from copper deposition in Descemet's membrane. The rings are present in virtually all patients with neurologic involvement but may be detectable only by slit lamp examination. Hepatic involvement leads to chronic cirrhosis, which may be complicated by splenomegaly, esophageal varices with hematemesis, or fulminant hepatic failure. Splenomegaly may cause hemolytic anemia and thrombocytopenia.

C. NEUROLOGIC FINDINGS

Neurologic findings in Wilson's disease reflect the disproportionate involvement of the caudate nucleus, putamen, cerebral cortex, and cerebellum. Neurologic signs include resting or postural tremor, choreiform movements of the limbs, facial grimacing, rigidity, hypokinesia, dysarthria, dysphagia, abnormal (flexed) postures, and ataxia. Seizures may also occur. Psychologic disorders in Wilson's disease include dementia, characterized by mental slowness, poor concentration, and memory impairment; disorders of affect, behavior, or personality; and (rarely) psychosis with hallucinations. There is a ten-

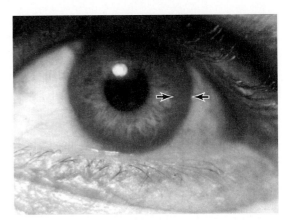

Figure 7–11. Kayser-Fleischer ring in Wilson's disease. This corneal ring **(between arrows)** was golden brown and contrasted clearly against a gray-blue iris. Note that the darkness of the ring increases as the outer border (limbus) of the cornea is approached **(right arrow)**. (Photo courtesy of Hoyt, W.F.)

dency for a dystonic or parkinsonian picture with hyperreflexia and extensor plantar responses to predominate when the disease begins before age 20 years—and for older patients to exhibit wild tremor, chorea, or ballismus. Symptoms may progress rapidly, especially in younger patients, but are more often gradual in development with periods of remission and exacerbation.

Differential Diagnosis

When Wilson's disease presents as a neurologic disorder, other conditions that must be considered in the differential diagnosis include multiple sclerosis and juvenile-onset Huntington's disease.

Investigative Studies

Investigation may reveal abnormal liver function blood tests and aminoaciduria as a result of renal tubular damage. The levels of serum copper and ceruloplasmin (an α_2-globulin to which 90% of the circulating copper is bound) are low, and 24-hour urinary copper excretion is generally increased. Liver biopsy reveals a huge excess of copper; it also usually reveals cirrhosis. No single laboratory feature is reliable in isolation. Brain CT scanning or MRI may show cerebrocortical atrophy and abnormalities in the basal ganglia.

Treatment

The optimal means of removing copper from the brain and other organs is disputed. Most physicians use penicillamine, a copper-chelating agent that promotes extraction of copper from tissue deposition sites, even though instances of penicillamine-induced worsening have been described. Treatment should be started as early as possible and customarily employs 1.5–2 g/d of orally administered penicillamine. The response to treatment may take several months and can be monitored by serial slit lamp examinations and blood chemistries. Side effects of penicillamine include nausea, nephrotic syndrome, myasthenia gravis, arthropathy, pemphigus, diverse blood dyscrasias, and a lupuslike syndrome; moreover, penicillamine may cause an additional worsening of neurologic symptoms. Treatment with tetrathiomolybdate is sometimes helpful. Restriction of dietary copper and administration of zinc sulfate (200 mg/d orally) can decrease copper absorption. Treatment must be continued for the lifetime of the patient, and most patients treated early can expect a complete or nearly complete recovery.

Siblings of affected patients should be screened for presymptomatic Wilson's disease with neurologic and slit lamp examinations and determination of serum ceruloplasmin levels. If no abnormalities are found, serum copper and urinary copper excretion should be assayed and liver biopsy performed if necessary. If these investigations reveal preclinical Wilson's disease, therapy should be instituted as described above for symptomatic disease.

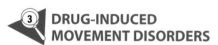

③ DRUG-INDUCED MOVEMENT DISORDERS

Parkinsonism

Parkinsonism frequently complicates treatment with dopamine-depleting agents such as reserpine or antipsychotic dopamine-receptor antagonists such as phenothiazines or butyrophenones. In the case of antipsychotic drugs, the risk of this complication is greatest when agents are used that are potent D_2-receptor antagonists with little anticholinergic effect, such as piperazine phenothiazines, butyrophenones, and thioxanthenes (Table 7–7). In addition, women and elderly patients appear to be at somewhat increased risk. Tremor is relatively uncommon, while hypokinesia tends to be symmetric and the most conspicuous neurologic feature of parkinsonism. These points, together with the history of drug ingestion, often point to the iatrogenic nature of the disorder. Signs usually develop within 3 months after starting the offending drug and disappear over weeks or months following discontinuance.

Depending on the severity of symptoms and the necessity for continuing antipsychotic drug therapy, several strategies are available for treating drug-induced parkinsonism. These include slow tapering and eventual withdrawal of the antipsychotic drug, substituting a less potent dopamine receptor antagonist (see Table 7–7), or adding an anticholinergic drug such as trihexyphenidyl or benztropine (Figure 7–12). Levodopa is of no help if the neuroleptic drugs are continued; it may be helpful if these drugs are discontinued but may aggravate the psychotic disorder for which they were originally prescribed.

Acute Dystonia or Dyskinesia

Acute dystonia or dyskinesia (such as blepharospasm, torticollis, or facial grimacing) is an occasional complication of dopamine receptor antagonist treatment, generally occurring within 1 week after introduction of such medication and often within 48 hours. Men and younger patients show increased susceptibility to this complication. The pathophysiologic basis of the disturbance is unclear, but intravenous treatment with an anticholinergic drug (eg, benztropine, 2 mg, or diphenhydramine, 50 mg) usually alleviates it.

Akathisia

Akathisia is a state of motor restlessness characterized by an inability to sit or stand still, which is relieved by moving about. It is a very common movement disorder induced by chronic treatment with antipsychotic drugs and occurs more often in women than in men. It may be seen as a tardive phenomenon after the discontinuation of neuroleptics. Akathisia is treated in the same manner as drug-induced parkinsonism.

Tardive Dyskinesia

Tardive dyskinesia may develop after long-term treatment with antipsychotic (dopamine-receptor-antagonist) drugs. It is commonly encountered in chronically institutionalized psychiatric patients, and the risk of developing tardive dyskinesia appears to increase with advancing age. The manner in which chronic drug treatment promotes a movement disorder is unknown.

Drug-induced supersensitivity of striatal dopamine receptors has been proposed but is unlikely to be responsible for several reasons. Supersensitivity always accompanies chronic antipsychotic drug treatment, whereas tardive dyskinesia does not. Supersensitivity may occur early in the course of treatment, while tardive dyskinesia does not develop for at least 3 months. In addition, supersensitivity is invariably reversible when drugs are discontinued; tardive dyskinesia is not. The clinical features of tardive dyskinesia, particularly its persistent nature, are more suggestive of an underlying structural abnormality. Such an abnormality may involve GABA neurons, because GABA and its synthesizing enzyme, glutamic acid decarboxylase, are depleted in the basal ganglia following chronic treatment of ani-

Table 7–7. Receptor-blocking properties associated with clinical side effects of antipsychotic drugs.[1,2]

Antipsychotic Drug	Receptor Blocked (Side Effects)			
	Dopamine D$_2$-like (Acute Dystonic Reaction, Akathisia, Parkinsonism)	Muscarinic Cholinergic (Blurred Vision, Dry Mouth, Urinary Retention)	Histamine H$_1$ (Sedation)	α_1-Adrenergic (Hypotension)
Phenothiazine				
Thioridazine (Mellaril)	++	+++	++	+++
Chlorpromazine (Thorazine)	++	+++	+++	+++
Trifluoperazine (Stelazine)	+++	++	++	++
Perphenazine (Trilafon)	+++	+	+++	+++
Fluphenazine (Prolixin)	+++	+	++	+++
Butyrophenone				
Haloperidol (Haldol)	+++	+	+	+++
Thioxanthine				
Thiothixene (Navane)	+++	+	+++	++
Indole compound				
Molindone (Moban)	+	+	+	+
Dibenzoxazepine				
Loxapine (Loxitane)	++	++	+++	++
Dibenzodiazepine				
Clozapine (Clozaril)	+	+++	+++	+++
Benzisoxazole				
Risperidone (Risperdal)	+++	+	++	+++
Thienbenzodiazepine				
Olanzapine (Zyprexa)	++	+++	+++	+++
Dibenzothiazepine				
Quetiapine (Seroquel)	+	++	++	+++

[1] Data from Arnt J, Skarsfeldt T: Do novel antipsychotics have similar pharmacological characteristics? A review of the evidence. Neuropsychopharmacology 1998; 18:63–101 and Black JL, Richelson E: Antipsychotic drugs: Prediction of side-effect profiles based on neuroreceptor data derived from human brain tissue. Mayo Clin Proc 1987;62:369–372.

[2] Antagonists range in potency from most potent (+++) to least potent (+) and produce correspondingly frequent (+++) to infrequent (+) side effects.

mals with antipsychotic drugs and GABA levels in CSF are decreased in patients with tardive dyskinesia. No consistent pathologic features have been found in the brains of patients with tardive dyskinesia, although inferior olive atrophy, degeneration of the substantia nigra, and swelling of large neurons in the caudate nucleus have been described in some cases. The clinical disorder is characterized by abnormal choreoathetoid movements that are often especially conspicuous about the face and mouth in adults and tend to be more obvious in the limbs in children. The onset of dyskinesia is generally not until months—or years—after the start of treatment with the responsible agent. Tardive dyskinesia may be impossible to distinguish from such disorders as Huntington's disease or idiopathic torsion dystonia unless a history of drug exposure is obtained.

Tardive dyskinesia is easier to prevent than to cure. Antipsychotic drugs should be prescribed only on clear indication, and their long-term use should be monitored, with periodic drug holidays to determine whether

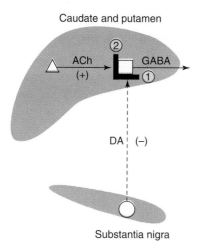

Figure 7–12. Mechanisms and treatment of drug-induced parkinsonism. Symptoms result from pharmacologic blockade of dopamine receptors by antipsychotic drugs (1), which mimics the degeneration of nigrostriatal dopamine (DA) neurons seen in idiopathic parkinsonism. Symptoms may be relieved by the administration of muscarinic anticholinergic drugs (2) or by substituting an antipsychotic drug with anticholinergic properties. These measures restore the normal balance between dopaminergic and cholinergic (ACh) transmission in the striatum.

the need for treatment continues. Drug holidays may also help to unmask incipient dyskinesias—which, curiously, tend to worsen when the drug is withdrawn. Antipsychotic medication should be gradually withdrawn if possible when dyskinesia appears during a drug holiday, as this may allow remission to occur.

Treating the established disorder is generally unsatisfactory, though it sometimes resolves spontaneously, especially in children or young adults. Antidopaminergic agents such as haloperidol or phenothiazines suppress the abnormal movements, but their use for this purpose is not recommended since they may aggravate the underlying disorder. Treatment with reserpine, 0.25 mg gradually increased to 2–4 mg/d orally, or tetrabenazine (not available in the United States), 12.5 mg gradually increased to as much as 200 mg/d orally, may be helpful. Both these drugs deplete monoamine neurotransmitters, including dopamine. A number of other pharmacologic approaches have been suggested and may help in individual cases; these include treatment with carbamazepine, baclofen, lithium, clonazepam, and alprazolam. Anticholinergic drugs should be avoided as they may exacerbate the dyskinesia. In patients requiring continued treatment for psychosis, clozapine, risperidone, olanzapine, or quetiapine should be used in place of the typical antipsychotics.

A variety of other late and often persistent movement disorders may appear during the course of antipsychotic drug treatment. **Tardive dystonia** is usually segmental (affecting two or more contiguous body parts, such as the face and neck or arm and trunk) in nature. It is less often focal; when this is the case, the head and neck are particularly apt to be affected, producing blepharospasm, torticollis, or oromandibular dystonia. Generalized dystonia is least common and tends to occur in younger patients. Treatment is as for tardive dyskinesia, except that anticholinergic drugs may also be helpful; focal dystonias may also respond to local injection of botulinum A toxin. **Tardive akathisia** can also occur; it is treated in the same manner as drug-induced parkinsonism. **Tardive tic,** a drug-induced disorder resembling Gilles de la Tourette's syndrome (see later), is characterized by multifocal motor and vocal tics and can be similarly treated with clonidine (as described later) if symptoms do not remit spontaneously. **Tardive tremor** and **tardive myoclonus** may also occur.

Neuroleptic Malignant Syndrome

This rare complication of treatment with antipsychotic drugs (neuroleptics) is manifested by rigidity, fever, altered mental status, and autonomic dysfunction. Haloperidol is implicated most often, but the syndrome can complicate treatment with any antipsychotic drug; whether concomitant treatment with lithium or anticholinergic drugs increases the risk is uncertain. Symptoms typically develop over 1–3 days and can occur at any time during the course of treatment. The differential diagnosis includes infection, which must be excluded in any febrile patient. Neuroleptic malignant syndrome resembles malignant hyperthermia (see Chapter 5), but the latter disorder develops over minutes to hours rather than days and is associated with the administration of inhalational anesthetics or neuromuscular blocking agents rather than antipsychotics. Treatment of neuroleptic malignant syndrome includes withdrawal of antipsychotic drugs, lithium, and anticholinergics; reduction of body temperature with antipyretics and artificial cooling; and rehydration. Dantrolene (see Chapter 5) may be beneficial, as may bromocriptine, levodopa preparations, or amantadine. The mortality rate is as high as 20%.

Other Drug-Induced Movement Disorders

Levodopa produces a wide variety of abnormal movements as a dose-related phenomenon in patients with parkinsonism. They can be reversed by withdrawing the medication or reducing the dose. Chorea may also develop in patients receiving bromocriptine, anticholinergic drugs, phenytoin, carbamazepine, amphetamines, lithium, and oral contraceptives; it resolves with discontinuance of the responsible drug. Dystonia has resulted from administration of bromocriptine, lithium, serotonin reuptake inhibitors, carbamazepine, and metoclopramide; and postural tremor from administration of theophylline, caffeine, lithium, thyroid hormone, tricyclic antidepressants, valproic acid, and isoproterenol.

GILLES DE LA TOURETTE'S SYNDROME

Gilles de la Tourette's syndrome, characterized by chronic—typically lifelong—multiple motor and verbal tics, is of unknown cause and does not relate to social class, ethnic group, perinatal abnormalities, birth trauma, or birth order. Symptoms begin before 21 years of age, and the course is one of remission and relapse. Most cases are sporadic, although there is occasionally a family history, and partial expression of the trait may occur in siblings or offspring of patients. Inheritance has been attributed to an autosomal dominant gene with variable penetrance. Males are affected more commonly than females. The prevalence in the United States has been estimated to be 0.05%.

The pathophysiology is obscure. Dopaminergic excess in the brains of patients with Gilles de la Tourette's syndrome has been postulated, mainly because of the beneficial effects that dopamine-blocking drugs can have on the tics. The administration of dopamine receptor agonists often fails to produce the exacerbation of symptoms that might be anticipated from this hypothesis, however.

No structural basis for the clinical disorder has been recognized. Only a few cases have come to autopsy, and the findings are conflicting.

Clinical Findings

Symptoms usually commence between ages 2 and 21 years. The first signs consist of motor tics in 80% of cases and vocal tics in 20%; there may be either a single tic or multiple tics. When the initial sign is a motor tic, it most commonly involves the face, taking the form of sniffing, blinking, forced eye closure, etc. It is generally not possible to make the diagnosis at this stage.

All patients ultimately develop a number of different motor tics and involuntary vocal tics, the latter commonly consisting of grunts, barks, hisses, throat-clearing or coughing, and the like, and sometimes taking the form of verbal utterances including **coprolalia** (vulgar or obscene speech). There may also be **echolalia** (parroting the speech of others), **echopraxia** (imitation of others' movements), and **palilalia** (repetition of words or phrases). The tics vary over time in severity, character, and the muscle groups involved. In 40–50% of cases, some of the tics involve self-mutilation with such activities as severe nail-biting or hair-pulling, picking at the nose, or biting the lips or tongue. Sensory tics, consisting of pressure, tickling, and warm or cold sensations, also occur. Behavioral disorders, including obsessive-compulsive disorder and attention deficit hyperactivity disorder, are common in patients with Gilles de la Tourette's syndrome, but their precise relationship to the tic disorder is uncertain.

Physical examination usually reveals no other abnormalities, but there is a higher than expected incidence of left-handedness or ambidexterity. In about 50% of cases, the EEG shows minor nonspecific abnormalities of no diagnostic relevance.

Differential Diagnosis

The differential diagnosis includes the various movement disorders that can present in childhood. Other disorders characterized by tics (see *Tics,* p 236) are distinguished by resolution of the tics by early adulthood or by the restricted number of tics.

Wilson's disease can simulate Gilles de la Tourette's syndrome; it must be excluded because it responds well to medical treatment. In addition to a movement disorder, Wilson's disease produces hepatic involvement, Kayser-Fleischer corneal rings, and abnormalities of serum copper and ceruloplasmin, which are absent in Gilles de la Tourette's syndrome.

Sydenham's chorea can be difficult to recognize if there is no recent history of rheumatic fever or polyarthritis and no clinical evidence of cardiac involvement, but this disorder is a self-limiting one, usually clearing in 3–6 months.

Bobble-head syndrome, which can be difficult to distinguish from Gilles de la Tourette's syndrome, is characterized by rapid, rhythmic bobbing of the head in children with progressive hydrocephalus.

Complications

Gilles de la Tourette's syndrome is often unrecognized for years, the tics being attributed to psychiatric illness or mistaken for some other form of abnormal movement. Indeed, in many cases the correct diagnosis is finally made by the family rather than the physician. In consequence, patients are often subjected to unnecessary and expensive treatment before the true nature of the disorder is recognized. Psychiatric disturbances, sometimes culminating in suicide, may occur because of the cosmetic and social embarrassment produced by the tics.

Drug therapy can lead to a number of side effects, as discussed below.

Treatment

Treatment is symptomatic and, if effective, must be continued indefinitely. Education of the patient, family members, and teachers is important. Extra break periods at school and additional time for test taking are often helpful.

Clonidine has been reported to ameliorate motor or vocal tics in roughly 50% of children so treated. It may act by reducing activity in noradrenergic neurons arising in the locus ceruleus. It is started in a dose of 2–3 µg/kg/d, increasing after 2 weeks to 4 µg/kg/d and then, if necessary, to 5 µg/kg/d. It may cause an initial transient fall in blood pressure. The most frequent side effect is sedation. Other adverse reactions include reduced or excessive salivation and diarrhea.

Haloperidol is often effective. It is started at a low daily dose (0.25 mg), which is gradually increased by 0.25 mg every 4 or 5 days until there is maximum benefit with a minimum of side effects or until side effects limit further increments. A total daily dose of 2–8 mg is usually optimal, but higher doses are sometimes necessary. Side effects include extrapyramidal movement disorders, sedation, dryness of the mouth, blurred vision, and gastrointestinal disturbances. Pimozide, another dopaminergic-receptor antagonist, may be helpful in patients who are either unresponsive to or cannot tolerate haloperidol. Treatment is started with 1 mg/d and the dose is increased by 1 mg every 5 days; most patients require 7–16 mg/d.

Phenothiazines such as fluphenazine are sometimes helpful for the management of tics, as also are dopamine agonists such as pergolide. Recent reports suggest that injection of botulinum toxin A at the site of the most problematic tics may be worthwhile. Treatment of any associated attention deficit disorder may include the use of a clonidine patch, guanfacine, pemoline, methylphenidate, or dextroamphetamine, whereas obsessive-compulsive disorder may require selective serotonin reuptake inhibitors or clomipramine

Patients occasionally respond favorably to clonazepam or carbamazepine, but diazepam, barbiturates, tricyclic antidepressants, phenytoin, and cholinergic agonists (such as deanol) are usually not helpful.

ACQUIRED HEPATOCEREBRAL DEGENERATION

Acquired hepatocerebral degeneration produces a neurologic disorder associated with extrapyramidal, cerebellar, and pyramidal signs as well as dementia. Extrapyramidal signs include rigidity, rest tremor, chorea, athetosis, and dystonia. This condition is discussed in Chapter 1.

RESTLESS LEGS SYNDROME

Restless legs syndrome is characterized by an unpleasant creeping discomfort that is perceived as arising deep within the legs and occasionally in the arms as well. Such symptoms tend to occur when patients are relaxed, especially while lying down or sitting, and lead to a need to move about. They are often particularly troublesome at night and may delay the onset of sleep. A sleep disorder associated with periodic movements during sleep may also occur and can be documented by polysomnographic recording. The cause is unknown, although the disorder seems especially common among pregnant women and is not uncommon among uremic or diabetic patients with neuropathy. Most patients, however, have no obvious predisposing cause. Symptoms sometimes resolve following correction of coexisting iron-deficiency anemia, and they may respond to treatment with drugs such as levodopa, dopamine agonists, diazepam, clonazepam, or opiates. When opiates are required, those with long half-lives or low addictive potential should be used.

REFERENCES

General

Albin RL, Young AB, Penney JB: The functional anatomy of basal ganglia disorders. Trends Neurosci 1989;12:366–375.

Campanella G, Roy M, Barbeau A: Drugs affecting movement disorders. Annu Rev Pharmacol Toxicol 1987;27:113–136.

Gasser T: Advances in the genetics of movement disorders: implications for molecular diagnosis. J Neurol 1997;244:341–348.

Hallett M: Physiology of basal ganglia disorders: an overview. Can J Neurol Sci 1993;20:177–183.

Janavs JL, Aminoff MJ: Involuntary movements in general medical disorders. In Aminoff MJ (editor): *Neurology and General Medicine*, 3rd edition. Churchill Livingstone, 2001.

Martin JB: Molecular basis of the neurodegenerative disorders. N Engl J Med 1999;340:1970–1980.

Nath A, Jankovic J, Pettigrew LC: Movement disorders and AIDS. Neurology 1987;37:37–41.

Special Issue: Basal Ganglia Research. Trends Neurosci 1990;13(7). [Entire issue.]

Watts RL, Koller WC (editors): *Movement Disorders*. McGraw-Hill, 1997.

Familial, or Benign, Essential Tremor

Bain P: A combined clinical and neurophysiological approach to the study of patients with tremor. J Neurol Neurosurg Psychiatry 1993;56:839–844.

Bain PG et al: Assessing tremor severity. J Neurol Neurosurg Psychiatry 1993;56:868–873.

Koller WC, Deuschl G (editors): Essential tremor. Neurology 2000;54(Suppl 4). [Entire issue.]

Koller W et al: High-frequency unilateral thalamic stimulation in the treatment of essential and parkinsonian tremor. Ann Neurol 1997;42:292–299.

Louis ED, Ford B, Barnes LF: Clinical subtypes of essential tremor. Arch Neurol 2000;57:1194–1198.

Parkinsonism

Adler CH et al: Ropinirole for the treatment of early Parkinson's disease. Neurology 1997;49:393–399.

Calne DB et al: Criteria for diagnosing Parkinson's disease. Ann Neurol 1992;32:S125–S127.

Dunnett SB et al: Prospects for new restorative and neuroprotective treatments in Parkinson's disease. Nature 1999;399:A32.

Durif F et al: Low-dose clozapine improves dyskinesias in Parkinson's disease. Neurology 1997;48:658–662.

Freed CR et al:Transplantation of embryonic dopamine neurons for severe Parkinson's disease. N Engl J Med 2001;344: 710–719.

Gottwald MD et al: New pharmacotherapy for Parkinson's disease. Ann Pharmacother 1997;31:1205–1217.

Hallett M, Litvan I: Evaluation of surgery for Parkinson's disease: a report of the Therapeutics and Technology Assessment Subcommittee of the American Academy of Neurology. The task force on surgery for Parkinson's disease. Neurology 1999; 53:1910–1921.

Holm KJ, Spencer CM: Entacapone: a review of its use in Parkinson's disease. Drugs 1999;58:159–177.

Jankovic J: New and emerging therapies for Parkinson disease. Arch Neurol 1999;56:785–790.

Koller WC, Tolos AE: Current and emerging drug therapies for the management of Parkinson's disease. Neurology 1998;50 (Suppl 6). [Entire issue.]

Lang AE: Surgery for Parkinson's disease: a critical evaluation of the state of the art. Arch Neurol 2000;57:1118–1125.

Lang AE, Lozano AM: Parkinson's disease. N Engl J Med 1998; 339:1044–1053; 1130–1143.

Lucking CB et al: Association between early-onset Parkinson's disease and mutations in the *parkin* gene. N Engl J Med 2000; 342:1560–1567.

Metman LV et al: Amantadine as treatment for dyskinesias and motor fluctuations in Parkinson's disease. Neurology 1998; 50:1323–1326.

Obeso JA, Benabid AL, Koller WC (editors): Deep brain stimulation for Parkinson's disease and tremor. Neurology 2000; 55(Suppl 6). [Entire issue.]

Racette BA et al: Welding-related parkinsonism. Neurology 2001; 56:8–13.

Rascol O et al: A five-year study of the incidence of dyskinesia in patients with early Parkinson's disease who were treated with ropinirole or levodopa. N Engl J Med 2000;342:1484–1491.

Riley DE, Lang AE: The spectrum of levodopa-related fluctuations in Parkinson's disease. Neurology 1993;43:1459–1464.

Shannon KM et al: Efficacy of pramipexole, a novel dopamine agonist, as monotherapy in mild to moderate Parkinson's disease. Neurology 1997;49:724–728.

Spillantini MG, Goedert M: The alpha-synucleinopathies: Parkinson's disease, dementia with Lewy bodies, and multiple system atrophy. Ann NY Acad Sci 2000;920:16–27.

Progressive Supranuclear Palsy

Gearing M: Progressive supranuclear palsy: neuropathologic and clinical heterogeneity. Neurology 1994;44:1015–1024.

Litvan I et al: Natural history of progressive supranuclear palsy (Steele-Richardson-Olszewski syndrome) and clinical predictors of survival: a clinicopathological study. J Neurol Neurosurg Psychiatry 1996;60:615–620.

Litvan I et al: Clinical research criteria for the diagnosis of progressive supranuclear palsy (Steele-Richardson-Olszewski syndrome). Neurology 1996;47:1–9.

Santacruz P et al: Progressive supranuclear palsy: a survey of the disease course. Neurology 1998;50:1637–1647.

Cortical-Basal Ganglionic Degeneration

Bergeron C et al: Unusual clinical presentations of cortical-basal ganglionic degeneration. Ann Neurol 1996;40:893–900.

Riley DE et al: Cortical-basal ganglionic degeneration. Neurology 1990;40:1203–1212.

Diffuse Lewy Body Disease

Louis ED et al: Comparison of extrapyramidal features in 31 pathologically confirmed cases of diffuse Lewy body disease and 34 pathologically confirmed cases of Parkinson's disease. Neurology 1997;48:376–380.

McKeith IG: Clinical Lewy body syndromes. Ann NY Acad Sci 2000;920:1–8.

Huntington's Disease

Bachoud-Levi AC et al: Motor and cognitive improvements in patients with Huntington's disease after neural transplantation. Lancet 2000;356:1975–1979.

Bartenstein P et al: Central motor processing in Huntington's disease. A PET study. Brain 1997;120:1553–1567.

Beal MF, Hantraye P: Novel therapies in the search for a cure for Huntington's disease. Proc Natl Acad Sci USA 2001;98: 3–4.

Hersch S et al: The neurogenetics genie: Testing for the Huntington's disease mutation. Neurology 1994;44:1369–1373.

International Huntington Association and World Federation of Neurology Research Group on Huntington's Chorea: guidelines for the molecular genetics predictive test in Huntington's disease. Neurology 1994;44:1533–1536.

Jones AL et al: Huntington disease: Advances in molecular and cell biology. J Inherited Metab Dis 1997;20:125–138.

Mazziotta JC et al: Reduced cerebral glucose metabolism in asymptomatic subjects at risk for Huntington's disease. N Engl J Med 1987;316:357–362.

Quinn N, Schrag A: Huntington's disease and other choreas. J Neurol 1998;245:709–716.

Ross CA et al: Huntington disease and the related disorder, dentatorubral-pallidoluysian atrophy (DRPLA). Medicine 1997; 76:305–338.

Yamada M, Tsuji S, Takahashi H: Pathology of CAG repeat diseases. Neuropathology 2000;20:319–325.

Sydenham's Chorea

Swedo SE et al: Sydenham's chorea: physical and psychological symptoms of St Vitus dance. Pediatrics 1993;91:706–713.

Idiopathic and Focal Torsion Dystonia

Bressman SB: Dystonia update. Clin Neuropharmacol 2000;23: 239–251.

Bressman SB et al: The DYT1 phenotype and guidelines for diagnostic testing. Neurology 2000;54:1746–1752.

Gasser T: Idiopathic, myoclonic and dopa-responsive dystonia. Curr Opin Neurol 1997;10:357–362.

Graeber MB et al: Delineation of the dystonia-parkinsonism syndrome locus in Xq13. Proc Natl Acad Sci USA 1992;89: 8245–8248.

Klein C et al: Genetic testing for early-onset torsion dystonia (DYT1): introduction of a simple screening method, experiences from testing of a large patient cohort, and ethical aspects. Genet Test 1999;3:323–328.

Kramer PL et al: Rapid-onset dystonia-parkinsonism: linkage to chromosome 19q13. Ann Neurol 1999;46:176–182.

Lee LV et al: The phenotype of the X-linked dystonia-parkinsonism syndrome. Medicine 1991;70:179–187.

Leube B et al: Evidence for DYT7 being a common cause of cervical dystonia (torticollis) in central Europe. Am J Med Genet 1997;74:529–532.

Muller U, Steinberger D, Nemeth AH: Clinical and molecular genetics of primary dystonias. Neurogenetics 1998;1:165–177.

Nygaard TG et al: Linkage mapping of dopa-responsive dystonia (DRD) to chromosome 14q. Nat Genet 1993;5:386–391.

Ozelius LJ et al: The early-onset torsion dystonia gene (DYT1) encodes an ATP-binding protein. Nat Genet 1997;17:40–48.

Report of the Therapeutics and Technology Assessment Subcommittee of the American Academy of Neurology: Assessment: the clinical usefulness of botulinum toxin-A in treating neurological disorders. Neurology 1990;40:1332–1336.

Tsui JKC, Calne DB (editors): *Handbook of Dystonia.* Dekker, 1995.

Wilson's Disease

Brewer GJ et al: Treatment of Wilson disease with ammonium tetrathiomolybdate. Arch Neurol 1996;53:1017–1025.

Gow PJ et al: Diagnosis of Wilson's disease: an experience over three decades. Gut 2000;46:415–419.

Gu M et al: Oxidative-phosphorylation defects in liver of patients with Wilson's disease. Lancet 2000;356:469–474.

LeWitt PA: Penicillamine as a controversial treatment for Wilson's disease. Mov Disord 1999;14:555–556.

Thomas GR et al: The Wilson disease gene: spectrum of mutations and their consequences. Nat Genet 1995;9:210–217.

Drug-Induced Movement Disorders

Black JL, Richelson E: Antipsychotic drugs: Prediction of side-effect profiles based on neuroreceptor data derived from human brain tissue. Mayo Clin Proc 1987;62:369–372.

Burke RE: Tardive dyskinesia: Current clinical issues. Neurology 1984;34:1348–1353.

Gerber PE, Lynd LD: Selective serotonin-reuptake inhibitor–induced movement disorders. Ann Pharmacother 1998;32:692–698.

Gratz SS, Simpson GM: Neuroleptic malignant syndrome. CNS Drugs 1994;2:429–439.

Jankovic J: Tardive syndromes and other drug-induced movement disorders. Clin Neuropharmacol 1995;18:197–214.

Kanovsky P et al: Treatment of facial and orolinguomandibular tardive dystonia by botulinum toxin A: evidence of a long-lasting effect. Mov Disord 1999;14:886–888.

Lang AE, Weiner WJ: *Drug-Induced Movement Disorders.* Futura, 1991.

Sachdev P: *Akathisia and Restless Legs.* Cambridge University Press, 1995.

Smego RA Jr, Durack DT: The neuroleptic malignant syndrome. Arch Intern Med 1982;142:1183–1185.

Soares KVS, McGrath JJ: The treatment of tardive dyskinesia—a systemic review and meta-analysis. Schizophr Res 1999;39: 1–16.

Gilles de la Tourette's Syndrome

Chouinard S, Ford B: Adult onset tic disorders. J Neurol Neurosurg Psychiatry 2000;68:738–743.

Evidente VG: Is it a tic or Tourette's? Clues for differentiating simple from more complex tic disorders. Postgrad Med 2000; 108:175–176.

Gilbert DL et al: Tourette's syndrome improvement with pergolide in a randomized, double-blind, cross-over trial. Neurology 2000;54:1310–1315.

Kurlan R: Tourette's syndrome: current concepts. Neurology 1989;39:1625–1630.

Kwak CH, Hanna PA, Jankovic J: Botulinum toxin in the treatment of tics. Arch Neurol 2000;57:1190–1193.

Nee LE et al: Gilles de la Tourette syndrome: clinical and family study of 50 cases. Ann Neurol 1980;7:41–49.

Robertson MM: Tourette syndrome, associated conditions and the complexities of treatment. Brain 2000;123:425–462.

Robertson MM, Stern JS: The Gilles de la Tourette syndrome. Crit Rev Neurobiol 1997;11:1–19.

Sallee FR et al: Relative efficacy of haloperidol and pimozide in children and adolescents with Tourette's disorder. Am J Psychiatry 1997;154:1057–1062.

Singer HS: Current issues in Tourette syndrome. Mov Disord 2000;15:1051–1063.

Van de Wetering BJM, Heutink P: The genetics of the Gilles de la Tourette syndrome: a review. J Lab Clin Med 1993;121: 638–645.

Restless Legs Syndrome

Montplaisir J et al: Restless legs syndrome improved by pramipexole. A double-blind randomized trial. Neurology 1999;52: 938–943.

Sachdev P: *Akathisia and Restless Legs.* Cambridge University Press, 1995.

Silber MH: Restless legs syndrome. Mayo Clin Proc 1997; 72: 261–264.

Seizures & Syncope

8

CONTENTS

KEY CONCEPTS

 1   *Obtaining a thorough history—especially regarding the presence or absence of prodromal symptoms, the patient's position when the episodes occur, and whether episodes are followed by periods of confusion—is critical in evaluating episodic loss of consciousness; therefore, it is important not to neglect the history and proceed too rapidly to the physical examination and laboratory investigation.*

 2   *Prodromal light-headedness before consciousness is lost suggests syncope from brain hypoperfusion, usually due to vasovagal reflex, orthostatic hypotension, or cardiac dysfunction.*

 3   *Syncope that occurs in the recumbent position eliminates orthostatic hypotension and vasovagal reflex as causes, and makes a cardiac disturbance or seizure more likely.*

 4   *Exercise-induced syncope suggests a cardiac cause.*

 5   *Confusion after the spell strongly suggests seizure.*

 6   *Jerking body movements and urinary incontinence are not necessarily indicative of seizure, and can occur during vasovagal and other causes of syncope as well.*

 7   *Prolonged seizures (>30 minutes) may cause brain injury and are thus a medical emergency.*

 8   *When treating seizure disorders, focus on the clinical response—seizure control—rather than on achieving particular blood anticonvulsant levels.*

EPISODIC LOSS OF CONSCIOUSNESS

Consciousness is lost when the function of both cerebral hemispheres or of the brainstem reticular activating system is compromised. Episodic dysfunction of these anatomic regions produces transient, and often recurrent, loss of consciousness. There are two major causes of episodic loss of consciousness.

Seizures

Seizures are disorders characterized by excessive or over-synchronized discharges of cerebral neurons.

Syncope

Syncope is loss of consciousness due to a reduced supply of blood to the cerebral hemispheres or brainstem. It can result from pancerebral hypoperfusion caused by vasovagal reflexes, orthostatic hypotension, or decreased cardiac output or from selective hypoperfusion of the brainstem resulting from vertebrobasilar ischemia. It is important to distinguish seizures from syncope because they have different causes, diagnostic approaches, and treatment.

APPROACH TO DIAGNOSIS

The initial step in evaluating a patient who has suffered a lapse of consciousness is to determine whether the setting in which the event occurred—or associated symptoms or signs—suggests that it was a direct result of a disease requiring prompt attention, such as hypoglycemia, meningitis, head trauma, cardiac arrhythmia, or acute pulmonary embolism. The number of spells and their similarity or dissimilarity should be established. If all spells are identical, then a single pathophysiologic process can be assumed, and the following major differential features should be ascertained.

Phenomena at Onset of Spell

① A detailed inquiry should always be made about prodromal and initial symptoms. The often brief, stereotyped premonitory symptoms (**aura**) at the onset of some seizures may localize the central nervous system abnormality responsible for the seizures.

1. An unambiguous description of a sudden onset of unconsciousness without prodromal features is highly suggestive of seizure.

2. Focal sensory or motor phenomena (eg, involuntary jerking of one hand, hemifacial paresthesias, forced head turning) suggest a seizure originating in the contralateral frontoparietal cortex.

3. A sensation of fear, olfactory or gustatory hallucinations, or visceral or déjà vu sensations are commonly associated with seizures originating in the temporal lobe.

4. Progressive light-headedness, dimming of vision, and faintness, which indicate diffuse central nervous system dysfunction, are associated with decreased cerebral blood flow from any cause (simple faints, cardiac arrhythmias, orthostatic hypotension).

Events During the Spell

1. Generalized tonic-clonic (grand mal, or major motor) seizures are characterized by loss of consciousness, accompanied initially by tonic stiffening and subsequently by clonic (jerking) movements of the extremities.

2. Cerebral hypoperfusion usually produces flaccid unresponsiveness.

3. Cerebral hypoperfusion can also result in stiffening or jerking movements, especially if hypoperfusion is enhanced because the patient is prevented from falling or otherwise assuming a recumbent posture. Such circulatory events are self-limited and do not require anticonvulsant treatment. Loss of consciousness from hypoperfusion rarely lasts more than 15 seconds and is not followed by postictal confusion unless prolonged brain ischemia has occurred.

Posture When Loss of Consciousness Occurs

③ Orthostatic hypotension and simple faints occur in the upright or sitting position. Episodes also (or only) occurring in the lying position suggest seizure or cardiac arrhythmia as a likely cause, although syncope induced by strong emotional stimuli may be responsible (eg, phelobotomy).

Relationship to Physical Exertion

④ Syncope associated with exertion is usually due to cardiac outflow obstruction (eg, aortic stenosis, obstructive hypertrophic cardiomyopathy, atrial myxoma) or arrhythmias.

Phenomena Following the Spell

1. A period of confusion, disorientation, or agitation (**postictal state**) follows a generalized tonic-clonic seizure. The period of confusion is usually brief—lasting only minutes. Although such behavior is often strikingly evident to witnesses, it may not be recalled by the patient.

2. Prolonged alteration of consciousness (**prolonged postictal state**) may follow status epilepticus. It may also occur after a single seizure in patients with diffuse structural cerebral disease (eg, dementia, mental retardation, or encephalitis) or metabolic encephalopathy.

3. Recovery from a simple faint is characterized by a prompt return to consciousness with full lucidity.

SEIZURES

A seizure is a transient disturbance of cerebral function caused by an abnormal neuronal discharge. **Epilepsy,** a group of disorders characterized by recurrent seizures, is a common cause of episodic loss of consciousness; the incidence of epilepsy in the general population is approximately 3%.

An actively convulsing patient or a reported seizure in a known epileptic usually poses no diagnostic difficulty. Because most seizures occur outside the hospital unobserved by medical personnel, the diagnosis must usually be established retrospectively.

5 The two historic features most suggestive of a seizure are the aura associated with seizures of focal onset and the postictal confusional state that follows generalized tonic-clonic seizures (see below).

6 Neither urinary incontinence nor the occurrence of a few tonic or jerking movements is significant in distinguishing seizures from other causes of transient loss of consciousness, since either can also occur with loss of consciousness from cerebral hypoperfusion.

ETIOLOGY

Seizures can result from either primary central nervous system dysfunction or an underlying metabolic derangement or systemic disease. This distinction is critical, since therapy must be directed at the underlying disorder as well as at seizure control. A list of common neurologic and systemic disorders that induce seizures is presented in Table 8–1. The age of the patient may help in establishing the cause of seizures (Figure 8–1).

Table 8–1. Common causes of seizures of new onset.

Primary neurologic disorders
Benign febrile convulsions of childhood
Idiopathic epilepsy
Head trauma
Stroke or vascular malformations
Mass lesions
Meningitis or encephalitis
HIV encephalopathy
Systemic disorders
Hypoglycemia
Hyponatremia
Hyperosmolar states
Hypocalcemia
Uremia
Hepatic encephalopathy
Porphyria
Drug overdose
Drug withdrawal
Global cerebral ischemia
Hypertensive encephalopathy
Eclampsia
Hyperthermia

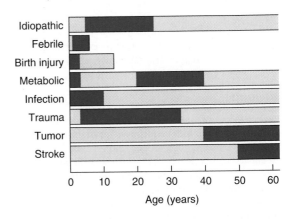

Figure 8–1. Causes of seizures as a function of age at onset. Bars show the range of ages at which seizures from a given cause typically begin; darker shading indicates peak incidence.

Primary Neurologic Disorders

1. Benign febrile convulsions of childhood are seizures that occur in 2–4% of children 3 months to 5 years old, usually during the first day of a febrile illness, and in the absence of central nervous system infection (meningitis or encephalitis). There may be a family history of benign febrile convulsions or other types of seizures. Benign febrile convulsions usually last for less than 15 minutes and lack focal features. About two-thirds of patients experience a single seizure, and fewer than one-tenth have more than three. Seizures occurring during the first hour of fever in children less than 18 months old or in children with a family history of febrile seizures are associated with a significant risk for recurrence; 90% of recurrences occur within 2 years of the initial episode. The differential diagnosis includes meningitis and encephalitis (Chapter 1) and brain abscess (Chapter 10); if present, these should be treated as described elsewhere in this volume. Because benign febrile convulsions are usually self-limited, treatment is often unnecessary; prolonged convulsions (15 minutes) can be treated with diazepam, 0.3 mg/kg orally, intramuscularly, or intravenously or 0.6 mg/kg rectally. Such treatment may decrease the risk of recurrence. The probability of developing a chronic seizure disorder is 2–6% and is highest in patients with persistent neurologic abnormalities; prolonged, focal, or multiple seizures; or a family history of nonfebrile seizures. Long-term administration of phenobarbital to reduce the risk of subsequent afebrile seizures is not indicated, since the efficacy of such prophylactic therapy is disputed, and cognitive impairment is a common side effect of treatment.

2. Idiopathic epilepsy for which no specific cause

can be established accounts for more than 75% of seizure disorders. Idiopathic epilepsy usually begins between the ages of 5 and 25 years, with more than 75% of patients having their first seizure before age 18 years. Less frequently, idiopathic epilepsy begins in later life, although in this age group seizures are also commonly associated with strokes, tumors, trauma, and systemic or metabolic disorders (Figure 8–1). Not all patients with a single idiopathic seizure go on to develop recurrent seizures: recurrence rates vary from about 30% to as high as 70% in different series, and may be higher in patients with electroencephalographic abnormalities such as a generalized spike-and-wave pattern, postictal Todd's paralysis (see below), persistent neurologic abnormalities, status epilepticus, multiple seizures prior to presentation, or a family history of afebrile seizures.

3. Head trauma is a common cause of epilepsy, particularly when it occurs perinatally or is associated with a depressed skull fracture or intracerebral or subdural hematoma. Seizures that occur within the first week after nonpenetrating head injuries are not predictive of a chronic seizure disorder, however. Although patients with serious head injuries are often treated prophylactically with anticonvulsant drugs, this practice has been questioned, since a reduction in the incidence of posttraumatic seizures has not been consistently observed beyond one week of treatment.

4. Stroke affecting the cerebral cortex produces seizures in 5–15% of patients and can occur following thrombotic or embolic infarction or intracerebral hemorrhage (see Chapter 9). As with head trauma, early seizures are not necessarily indicative of chronic epilepsy, and long-term anticonvulsant therapy is not required. Even without rupturing, **vascular malformations** may be associated with seizures, presumably as a result of their irritative effects on adjacent brain tissue.

5. Mass lesions, such as brain tumors (see Chapter 2) or abscesses (see Chapter 10), can present with seizures. Glioblastomas, astrocytomas, and meningiomas are the most common tumors associated with seizures, reflecting their high prevalence among tumors that affect the cerebral hemispheres.

6. Meningitis or **encephalitis** caused by bacterial (eg, *Haemophilus influenzae*), tuberculous, viral (eg, herpes simplex), fungal, or parasitic (eg, cysticercosis) infections can also cause seizures (see Chapter 1). Seizures in patients with AIDS are most often associated with AIDS dementia complex, but also with toxoplasmosis or cryptococcal meningitis.

Systemic Disorders

Metabolic and other systemic disorders, including drug-overdose and drug-withdrawal syndromes, may be associated with seizures that abate with correction of the underlying abnormality. In these cases, the patient is not considered to have epilepsy.

1. Hypoglycemia can produce seizures, especially with serum glucose levels of 20–30 mg/dL, but neurologic manifestations of hypoglycemia are also related to the rate at which serum glucose levels fall. Hypoglycemia is discussed in detail in Chapter 1.

2. Hyponatremia may be associated with seizures at serum sodium levels below 120 meq/L or at higher levels following rapid decline. Hyponatremia is considered further in Chapter 1.

3. Hyperosmolar states, including both hyperosmolar nonketotic hyperglycemia (see Chapter 1) and hypernatremia, may lead to seizures when serum osmolality rises above about 330 mosm/L.

4. Hypocalcemia with serum calcium levels in the range of 4.3–9.2 mg/dL can produce seizures with or without tetany (see Chapter 1).

5. Uremia can cause seizures, especially when it develops rapidly, but this tendency correlates poorly with absolute serum urea nitrogen levels (see Chapter 1).

6. Hepatic encephalopathy is sometimes accompanied by generalized or multifocal seizures (see Chapter 1).

7. Porphyria is a disorder of heme biosynthesis that produces both neuropathy (discussed in Chapter 5) and seizures. The latter may be difficult to treat because most anticonvulsants can exacerbate the disorder. As a result, seizures caused by porphyria have traditionally been treated with bromides, 1–2 g orally three times daily (therapeutic serum levels 10–20 meq/L). Toxicity (manifested by rash, gastrointestinal symptoms, psychiatric disturbances, or impaired consciousness) is common. *In vitro* studies suggest the safety of vigabatrine and gabapentin.

8. Drug overdose can exacerbate epilepsy or cause seizures in nonepileptic patients. Generalized tonic-clonic seizures are most common, but focal or multifocal partial seizures can also occur. The drugs most frequently associated with seizures are antidepressants, antipsychotics, cocaine, insulin, isoniazid, lidocaine, and methylxanthines (Table 8–2).

9. Drug withdrawal, especially withdrawal from ethanol or sedative drugs, may be accompanied by one or more generalized tonic-clonic seizures that usually resolve spontaneously. Alcohol withdrawal seizures occur within 48 hours after cessation or reduction of ethanol intake in 90% of cases, and are characterized by brief flurries of one to six attacks that resolve within 12 hours. Acute abstinence from sedative drugs can also produce seizures in patients habituated to more than 600–800 mg/d of secobarbital or equivalent doses of other short-acting sedatives. Seizures from sedative drug withdrawal typically occur 2–4 days after abstinence but may be delayed for up to 1 week. Focal

Table 8–2. Major categories of drugs reported to cause seizures.

Anticholinesterases (organophosphates, physostigmine)
Antidepressants (tricyclic, monocyclic, heterocyclic)
Antihistamines
Antipsychotics (phenothiazines, butyrophenones, clozapine)
β-Adrenergic receptor blockers (propranolol, oxprenolol)
Chemotherapeutics (etoposide, ifosfamide, cisplatinum)
Cyclosporine, FK 506
Hypoglycemic agents (including insulin)
Hypoosmolar parenteral solutions
Isoniazid
Local anesthetics (bupivacaine, lidocaine, procaine, etidocaine)
Methylxanthines (theophylline, aminophylline)
Narcotic analgesics (fentanyl, meperidine, pentazocine, propoxyphene)
Penicillins
Phencyclidine
Sympathomimetics (amphetamines, cocaine, ephedrine, MDMA[1] "ecstasy," phenylpropanolamine, terbutaline)

[1]Methylenedioxymethamphetamine.

seizures are rarely due to alcohol or sedative drug withdrawal alone; they suggest an additional focal cerebral lesion that requires evaluation.

10. Global cerebral ischemia from cardiac arrest, cardiac arrhythmias, or hypotension may produce, at onset, a few tonic or tonic-clonic movements that resemble seizures, but they probably reflect abnormal brainstem activity instead. Global ischemia may also be associated with spontaneous myoclonus (see Chapter 7) or, after consciousness returns, with myoclonus precipitated by movement (action myoclonus). Partial or generalized tonic-clonic seizures also occur; these may be manifested only by minor movements of the face or eyes and must be treated. Nonetheless, isolated seizures following global cerebral ischemia do not necessarily indicate a poor outcome. Global cerebral ischemia is discussed in more detail in Chapter 9.

11. Hypertensive encephalopathy, which may be accompanied by generalized tonic-clonic or partial seizures, is considered in Chapter 1.

12. Eclampsia refers to the occurrence of seizures or coma in a pregnant woman with hypertension, proteinuria, and edema (**preeclampsia**). As in hypertensive encephalopathy in nonpregnant patients, cerebral edema, ischemia, and hemorrhage may contribute to neurologic complications. Magnesium sulfate has been widely used to treat eclamptic seizures, and may be superior for this purpose to anticonvulsants such as phenytoin.

13. Hyperthermia can result from infection, exposure (heat stroke), hypothalamic lesions, or drugs such as phencyclidine, as well as anticholinergics or neuroleptics (neuroleptic malignant syndrome; see Chapter 7) and inhalational anesthetics or neuromuscular blocking agents (malignant hyperthermia; see Chapter 5). Clinical features of severe hyperthermia (42°C, or 107°F) include seizures, confusional states or coma, shock, and renal failure. Treatment is with antipyretics and artificial cooling to reduce body temperature immediately to 39°C (102°F) and anticonvulsants and more specific therapy (eg, antibiotics for infection, dantrolene for malignant hyperthermia) where indicated. Patients who survive may be left with ataxia as a result of the special vulnerability of cerebellar neurons to hyperthermia.

CLASSIFICATION & CLINICAL FINDINGS

Seizures are classified as follows:
    Generalized seizures
        Tonic-clonic (grand mal)
        Absence (petit mal)
        Other types (tonic, clonic, myoclonic)
    Partial seizures
        Simple partial
        Complex partial (temporal lobe, psychomotor)
        Partial seizures with secondary generalization

Generalized Seizures

A. GENERALIZED TONIC-CLONIC SEIZURES

Generalized tonic-clonic seizures are attacks in which consciousness is lost, usually without aura or other warning. When a warning does occur, it usually consists of nonspecific symptoms.

1. Tonic phase—The initial manifestations are unconsciousness and tonic contractions of limb muscles for 10–30 seconds, producing extension of the extremities and arching of the body in apparent opisthotonos (Figure 8–2). Tonic contraction of the muscles of respiration may produce an expiration-induced vocalization (cry or moan) and cyanosis, and contraction of masticatory muscles may cause tongue trauma. The patient falls to the ground and may be injured.

2. Clonic phase—The tonic phase is followed by a clonic (alternating muscle contraction and relaxation) phase of symmetric limb jerking that persists for an additional 30–60 seconds—or longer. Ventilatory efforts return immediately after cessation of the tonic phase, and cyanosis clears. The mouth may froth with saliva. With time, the jerking becomes less frequent, until finally all movements cease and the muscles are flaccid. Sphincteric relaxation or detrusor muscle contraction may produce urinary incontinence

3. Recovery—As the patient regains consciousness, there is postictal confusion and often headache. Full

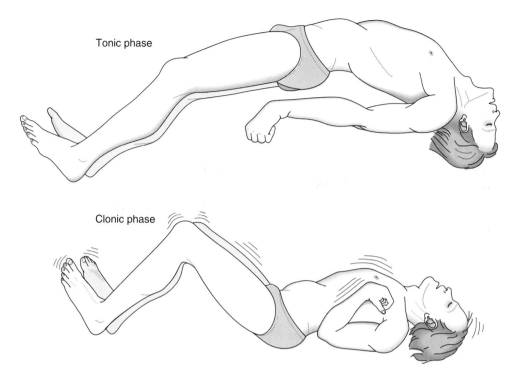

Tonic phase

Clonic phase

Figure 8–2. Generalized tonic-clonic seizure, illustrating the appearance of the patient in the tonic (stiffening) and clonic (shaking) phases.

orientation commonly takes 10–30 minutes—or even longer in patients with status epilepticus (see below) or preexisting structural or metabolic brain disorders. Physical examination during the postictal state is usually otherwise normal in idiopathic epilepsy or seizures of metabolic origin, except that plantar responses may be transiently extensor (Babinski's sign). The pupils always react to light, even when the patient is unconscious. Transient unilateral weakness (hemiparesis) in the postictal period (**Todd's paralysis**) should be sought, because such a finding suggests a focal brain lesion as the cause and calls for further investigation.

4. Status epilepticus—Status epilepticus is defined arbitrarily as seizures that continue for more than 30 minutes without ceasing spontaneously, or which recur so frequently that full consciousness is not restored between successive episodes. Status epilepticus is a medical emergency because it can lead to permanent brain damage—from hyperpyrexia, circulatory collapse, or excitotoxic neuronal damage—if untreated.

B. ABSENCE (PETIT MAL) SEIZURES

Absence (petit mal) seizures are genetically transmitted seizures that always begin in childhood and rarely persist into adolescence. The spells are characterized by brief loss of consciousness (for 5–10 seconds) without loss of postural tone. Subtle motor manifestations, such as eye blinking or a slight head turning, are common. Automatisms are uncommon. Full orientation immediately follows cessation of the seizure. There may be as many as several hundred spells daily, leading to impaired school performance and social interactions, so that children may be mistakenly thought to be mentally retarded before the diagnosis of petit mal epilepsy is made. The spells are characteristically inducible by hyperventilation. The electroencephalogram (EEG) shows a characteristic 3/s spike-and-wave pattern during the seizures (Figure 8–3). In most patients with normal intelligence and normal background activity on EEG, absence spells occur only during childhood; in other cases, however, the attacks continue into adult life, either alone or in association with other types of seizures.

C. OTHER TYPES OF GENERALIZED SEIZURES

These include tonic seizures (not followed by a clonic phase), clonic seizures (not preceded by a tonic phase), and myoclonic seizures.

1. Tonic seizures are characterized by continuing muscle contraction that can lead to fixation of the limbs

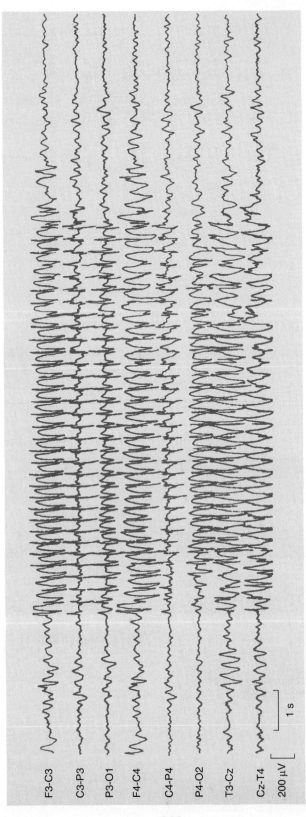

Figure 8–3. EEG of a patient with typical absence (petit mal) seizures, showing a burst of generalized 3-Hz spike-and-wave activity (center of record) that is bilaterally symmetric and bisynchronous. Odd-numbered leads indicate electrode placements over the left side of the head; even numbers, those over the right side.

and axial musculature in flexion or extension and are a cause of drop attacks; the accompanying arrest of ventilatory movements leads to cyanosis. Consciousness is lost, and there is no clonic phase to these seizures.

2. Clonic seizures are characterized by repetitive clonic jerking accompanied by loss of consciousness. There is no initial tonic component.

3. Myoclonic seizures are characterized by sudden, brief, shocklike contractions that may be localized to a few muscles or one or more extremities or that may have a more generalized distribution. Myoclonic seizures may be idiopathic or associated with a variety of rare hereditary neurodegenerative disorders, including Unverricht-Lundborg disease, Lafora body disease, neuronal ceroid lipofuscinosis (late infantile, juvenile, and adult forms), sialidosis, and mitochondrial encephalomyopathy (myoclonus epilepsy with ragged red fibers on skeletal muscle biopsy). Not all myoclonic jerks have an epileptic basis, however, as discussed in Chapter 7.

4. Atonic seizures result from loss of postural tone, sometimes following a myoclonic jerk, leading to a fall or drop attack. They are most common in developmental disorders such as the Lennox-Gastaut syndrome.

Partial Seizures

1. Simple partial seizures begin with motor, sensory, or autonomic phenomena, depending on the cortical region affected. For example, clonic movements of a single muscle group in the face, a limb, or the pharynx may occur and may be self-limited; they may be recurrent or continuous or may spread to involve contiguous regions of the motor cortex (**jacksonian march**).

Autonomic symptoms may consist of pallor, flushing, sweating, piloerection, pupillary dilatation, vomiting, borborygmi, and incontinence. Psychic symptoms include dysphasia, distortions of memory (eg, déjà vu, the sensation that a new experience is being repeated), forced thinking or labored thought processes, cognitive deficits, affective disturbances (eg, fear, depression, an inappropriate sense of pleasure), hallucinations, or illusions. During simple partial seizures, consciousness is preserved unless the seizure discharge spreads to other areas of the brain, producing tonic-clonic seizures (**secondary generalization**). The **aura** is the portion of the seizure that precedes loss of consciousness and of which the patient retains some memory. The aura is sometimes the sole manifestation of the epileptic discharge.

In the postictal state, a focal neurologic deficit such as hemiparesis (**Todd's paralysis**) that resolves over a period of 1/2–36 hours is a manifestation of an underlying focal brain lesion.

2. Complex partial seizures, formerly called temporal lobe or psychomotor seizures, are partial seizures in which consciousness, responsiveness, or memory is impaired. The seizure discharge usually arises from the temporal lobe or medial frontal lobe but can originate elsewhere. The symptoms take many forms but are usually stereotyped for the individual patient. Episodes may begin with an aura. Epigastric sensations are most common, but affective (fear), cognitive (déjà vu), and sensory (olfactory hallucinations) symptoms also occur. Consciousness is then impaired. Seizures generally persist for less than 30 minutes (on the average, 1–3 minutes). The motor manifestations of complex partial seizures are characterized by coordinated involuntary motor activity, termed **automatism**, which takes the form of orobuccolingual movements in about 75% of patients and other facial or neck movements in about 50%. Sitting up or standing, fumbling with objects, and bilateral limb movements are less common. Secondary generalization may occur.

DIAGNOSIS

The diagnosis of seizures is based on clinical recognition of one of the seizure types described above. The EEG can be a helpful confirmatory test in distinguishing seizures from other causes of loss of consciousness (Figure 8–4). However, a normal or nonspecifically abnormal EEG never excludes the diagnosis of seizures. Specific EEG features that suggest epilepsy include abnormal spikes, polyspike discharges, and spike-wave complexes.

A standard diagnostic evaluation of patients with recent onset of seizures is presented in Table 8–3. Metabolic and toxic disorders (see Table 8–1) should be excluded, because they do not require anticonvulsants.

Seizures with a clearly focal onset or those that begin after age 25 years require prompt evaluation to exclude the presence of a structural brain lesion. Magnetic resonance imaging (MRI) is essential for this purpose [computed tomography (CT) is not adequate]. If no cause is found, the decision to begin chronic anticonvulsant therapy should be based on the probability of recurrence. Following a single generalized tonic-clonic seizure, recurrence can be expected within 3–4 years in 30–70% of untreated adult patients.

SELECTION OF THERAPY

Therapy should be directed toward the cause of the seizures, if known. Seizures associated with metabolic and systemic disorders usually respond poorly to anticonvulsants but cease with correction of the underlying abnormality. Acute withdrawal from alcohol and other sedative drugs produces self-limited seizures that, in general, require no anticonvulsant drug therapy. Acute head trauma and other structural brain lesions that result in seizures must be rapidly diagnosed and treated,

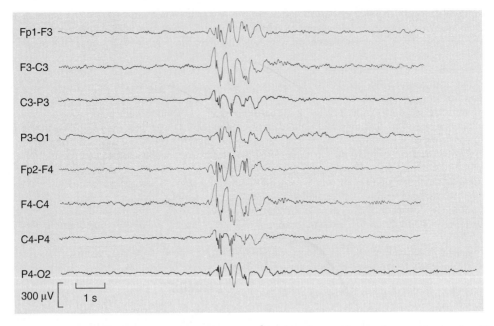

Figure 8–4. EEG of a patient with idiopathic (primary generalized) epilepsy. A burst of generalized epileptiform activity (**center**) is seen on a relatively normal background. These findings, obtained at a time when the patient was not experiencing seizures, support the clinical diagnosis of epilepsy. Odd-numbered leads indicate electrode placements over the left side of the head; even numbers, those over the right side.

and the associated seizures controlled by anticonvulsant drug therapy. Idiopathic epilepsy is treated with anticonvulsant medications.

Anticonvulsant Drug Treatment

Commonly used anticonvulsant drugs and their dosages and methods of administration are listed in Table 8–4. There are four key principles of management:

Establish the diagnosis of epilepsy before starting drug therapy. Therapeutic trials of anticonvulsant drugs intended to establish or reject a diagnosis of epilepsy may yield incorrect diagnoses.

Choose the right drug for the seizure type. Absence seizures, for example, do not respond to most drugs used for complex partial or generalized tonic-clonic seizures.

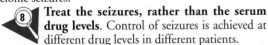 **Treat the seizures, rather than the serum drug levels.** Control of seizures is achieved at different drug levels in different patients.

Evaluate one drug at a time. In most cases, seizures can be controlled with a single drug. Therefore, beginning therapy with multiple drugs may expose patients to increased drug toxicity without added therapeutic benefit.

Most patients with epilepsy fall into one of the following treatment categories.

A. New Seizures

Most epileptologists do not recommend chronic anticonvulsant drug treatment following a single seizure unless an underlying cause is found that is not correctable and is likely to produce recurrent seizures (eg, brain tumor). However, recurrent seizures do require anticonvulsant

Table 8–3. Evaluation of a new seizure disorder in a stable patient.

History (including medications or drug exposure)
General physical examination
Complete neurologic examination
Blood studies
  Fasting glucose
  Serum calcium
  Serum FTA-ABS
  Serum electrolytes
  Complete blood count
  Erythrocyte sedimentation rate
  Renal function studies
  Hepatic function studies
EEG (positive in 20–59% of first EEGs; 59–92% with repeated EEGs)
Brain MRI (especially with abnormal examination, progressive disorder, or onset of seizures after 25 years of age)

Table 8–4. Summary of anticonvulsant drug therapy.

Drug	Usual Preparation	Loading or Initial Dose	Maintenance Dose	Serum Half-Life (Normal Renal and Hepatic Function)	Therapeutic Serum Levels	Indications[1]
Phenytoin (Dilantin)	100-mg capsule. Also 30-mg capsule, 50-mg tablet	Oral loading: 1000 mg in two to four divided doses over 12–24 hours Intravenous loading: 1000–1500 mg (15–18 mg/kg) not exceeding 50 mg/min Fosphenytoin is prodrug form for intramuscular or intravenous use	300–400 mg/d in a single dose or divided doses	Oral: 18–24 hours Intravenous: 12 hours (kinetics are dose dependent and may vary widely)	10–20 µg/mL	P, G
Carbamazepine (Tegretol)	200, 300 mg XR: 100, 200, 400 mg	100 mg twice a day; increase by 200 mg/d to maintenance dose	400–1600 mg/d in three or four doses, or in two doses if XR form	12–18 hours monotherapy	4–12 µg/mL	P, G
Oxcarbazepine (Trileptal)	150, 300, 600 mg	300 mg twice a day	1200–2400 mg/d in two divided doses	8–10 hours	Not established	P
Phenobarbital (Luminal)	15, 30, 60, 100 mg	Oral loading: 180 mg twice a day for 3 days or same as maintance	90–180 mg/d in a single dose	3–5 days	20–40 µg/mL	G
Valproic acid (Depakote, Depakene)	250 mg	Same as maintenance dose	750–3000 mg/d in two or three doses	6–18 hours	50–150 µg/mL	G, M, A, P
Ethosuximide (Zarontin)	250-mg capsules	15 mg/kg/d, then increase by 25 mg/d at weekly intervals to maintenance dose	15–40 mg/kg/d in two or three doses	24–36 hours (children); 60 hours (adult)	40–100 µg/mL	A
Clonazepam (Klonopin)	0.5, 1, 2 mg	Children: 0.01–0.03 mg/kg/d in two or three divided doses Adults: 0.5 mg/d	Children: 0.01–0.02 mg/kg/d Adults: 1.5–2.0 mg/d; in two or three divided doses	20–40 hours	0.02–0.10 µg/mL	A
Gabapentin (Neurontin)	100, 300, 400 mg	300 mg three times a day	900–4800 mg/d in three divided doses	5–7 hours	Not established	P, SG, Adj

continued

Table 8–4. Summary of anticonvulsant drug therapy (continued).

Drug	Usual Preparation	Loading or Initial Dose	Maintenance Dose	Serum Half-Life (Normal Renal and Hepatic Function)	Therapeutic Serum Levels	Indications[1]
Lamotrigine (Lamictal)	50, 100, 200 mg	25 mg twice a day then slow increase[2]	200–500 mg/d 100–700 in two doses[2]	24 hours 12–60 hours[2]	Not established	P, SG, Adj
Levetiracetam (Keppra)	250, 500, 750 mg	250–500 twice a day	1000–3000 mg/d in two divided doses	8–10 hours	Not established	P, Adj
Vigabatrin[3] (Sabril)	500 mg	500 mg twice a day; increase by 500 mg every week	2–4 g/d in two divided doses	5–8 hours	Not established	P, Adj
Topiramate (Topamax)	25, 100, 200 mg	25 mg/d; increase by 25–50 mg every 2 weeks	200–400 mg/d in two divided doses	16–30 hours	Not established	P, Adj
Tiagabine (Gabatril)	4, 12, 16, 20 mg	4 mg/d; increase by 4–8 mg every week	12–56 mg/d in three divided doses	5–13 hours	Not established	P, Adj
Zonisamide (Zonegran)	100 mg	100 mg/d	400–600 mg/d in one to two doses	52–69 hours	Not established	P, Adj

[1] A, absence; Adj, adjunctive; G, generalized tonic-clonic; M, myoclonic; P, partial; S, secondarily generalized tonic-clonic.

[2] Varies depending on interaction with coadministered anticonvulsant drugs; 25 mg every other day for 2 weeks when taking valproic acid; see Table 8–8.

[3] Not approved in the United States.

treatment, and if such therapy is to be administered, the oral loading schedules presented in Table 8–4 can be used. Note that starting a drug at its daily maintenance dose produces stable serum drug levels only after approximately five half-lives have elapsed. Therefore, loading doses should be given whenever possible to achieve therapeutic drug levels promptly in patients with frequent seizures. **Phenytoin, carbamazepine,** or **valproic acid** are the current drugs of first choice for treating generalized tonic-clonic or partial seizures in adults, and **valproic acid** or **carbamazepine** is preferred for children. Phenobarbital is also very effective in treating generalized tonic-clonic seizures in adults, but it is less helpful for treatment of complex partial seizures.

Absence attacks of the petit mal variety are treated with **valproic acid** or **ethosuximide** (Table 8–4). The former has the advantage of also providing protection against tonic-clonic seizures but has caused fatalities from hepatic damage in children under 10 (usually under 2) years of age.

Myoclonic seizures are treated with **valproic acid** or **clonazepam** (see Table 8–4).

B. Recurrent Seizures on Drug Therapy

1. Determining serum levels of drugs—Blood levels of the anticonvulsant drugs the patient has been taking should be measured in samples taken just prior to a scheduled dose. For a single seizure no acute change in medication is mandated even if there has been no interruption of drug therapy and anticonvulsant drug levels are in the therapeutic range, but a slight increase in prescribed dose may be considered. If the history or serum drug levels suggest that treatment has been interrupted, the prescribed drug should be started again as for new seizures.

2. Changing to a second drug—A second anticonvulsant should be introduced only if seizures continue to occur after maximum therapeutic benefit has been achieved with the initial drug. This means not only that blood levels of the drug are in the therapeutic range but also that drug toxicity precludes further dosage increments. An anticonvulsant that has failed to alter seizure frequency should be discontinued gradually once therapeutic levels of the second drug have been achieved. If the first drug has produced partial control of the seizure disorder, however, it is often continued along with the second drug. The newer anticonvulsants **gabapentin**, **lamotrigine**, **topiramate**, **vigabatrin**, **oxcarbazepine**, **levetiracetam**, **zonisamide**, and **tiagabine** may be helpful adjunctive medications for patients who respond suboptimally to conventional anticonvulsant drugs.

3. Treating refractory seizures—In some patients, disabling seizures persist despite trials of all major anticonvulsants, alone and in combination—and at the highest doses the patient can tolerate. When no treatable cause can be found, seizures are not due to a progressive neurodegenerative disease, and medical treatment has been unsuccessful for at least 2 years, evaluation for possible surgical therapy should be considered. Presurgical evaluation begins with a detailed history and neurologic examination to explore the cause of seizures and their site of origin within the brain and to document the adequacy of prior attempts at medical treatment. MRI and electrophysiologic studies are performed to identify the epileptogenic zone within the brain. Several electrophysiologic techniques can be used: **EEG**, in which cerebral electrical activity is recorded noninvasively from the scalp; **stereotactic depth electrode EEG**, in which activity is recorded from electrodes inserted (depth electrodes) into the brain or placed over the brain surface (subdural electrodes); and **electrocorticography**, which involves intraoperative recording from the surface of the brain. When an epileptogenic zone can be identified in this manner and its removal is not expected to produce undue neurologic impairment, surgical excision may be indicated. Patients with complex partial seizures arising from a single temporal lobe are the most frequent surgical candidates; unilateral anterior temporal lobectomy abolishes seizures and auras in about 50% of these patients and significantly reduces their frequency in another 25%. Hemispherectomy and corpus callosum section are also sometimes used to treat intractable epilepsy. Left vagal nerve stimulation has been shown to reduce seizure frequency by as much as 50% in adults and children with refractory epilepsy. The mechanism of action is unknown. Afferent responses from the vagus are received in n. tractus solitarius in the medulla and projected widely.

C. Multiple Seizures or Status Epilepticus

1. Early management
a. Immediate attention should be given to ensuring that the airway is patent and the patient positioned to prevent aspiration of stomach contents.

b. The laboratory studies listed in Table 8–5 should be ordered without delay.

c. Dextrose, 50 mL of 50% solution, should be given intravenously.

d. If fever or meningeal signs are present, immediate lumbar puncture is mandatory, and a gram-stained smear of spinal fluid should be examined to exclude bacterial meningitis. Patients without these signs should also undergo lumbar puncture if the cause of the seizures has not been determined (eg, by their cessation upon administration of dextrose), unless signs of increased intracranial pressure or of focal brain dysfunction are present. It should be noted that **postictal pleocytosis** is detectable in cerebrospinal fluid (CSF) in approximately 2% of patients with single generalized tonic-clonic seizures (and about 15% of those with status epilepticus) in the absence of infection. The white blood cell count may be as high as 80/mm^3, with either polymorphonuclear or mononuclear predominance. Serum protein content may be slightly elevated, but glucose concentration is normal, and Gram's stain is negative. The postictal pleocytosis resolves in 2–5 days.

Table 8–5. Emergency evaluation of serial seizures, or status epilepticus.

Treatment with anticonvulsants should be instituted immediately (Table 8–6), while the following measures are taken.
Vital signs:
  Blood pressure: exclude hypertensive encephalopathy and shock
  Temperature: exclude hyperthermia
  Pulse: exclude life-threatening cardiac arrhythmia
Draw venous blood for serum glucose, calcium, electrolytes, hepatic and renal function blood studies, complete blood count, erythrocyte sedimentation rate, and toxicology
Insert intravenous line
Administer glucose (50 mL of 50% dextrose) intravenously
Obtain any available history
Rapid physical examination, especially for
  Signs of trauma
  Signs of meningeal irritation or systemic infection
  Papilledema
  Focal neurologic signs
  Evidence of metastatic, hepatic, or renal disease
Arterial blood gases
Lumbar puncture, unless the cause of seizures has already been determined or signs of increased intracranial pressure of focal neurologic signs are present
ECG
Calculate serum osmolality: 2 (serum sodium concentration) + serum glucose/20 + serum urea nitrogen/3 (normal range: 270–290)
Urine sample for toxicology, if indicated

2. Drug therapy to control seizures—Every effort must be made to establish a precise etiologic diagnosis so that treatment of the underlying disorder can be started. Because generalized seizure activity per se damages the brain if it persists for more than 30 minutes, drug therapy to terminate seizures should be instituted immediately. An outline for rapid pharmacologic control of acute multiple seizures is presented in Table 8–6.

3. Management of hyperthermia—The metabolic consequences of status epilepticus are related to increased motor activity and high levels of circulating catecholamines; they include hyperthermia [to 42–43°C (108–109°F)], lactic acidosis (to pH <7.00), and peripheral blood leukocytosis (to 60,000 cells/mm³). These derangements typically resolve over a few hours after cessation of the seizures. Only hyperthermia, which is known to increase the risk of brain damage from status epilepticus, requires specific attention.

Severe hyperthermia must be treated with a cooling blanket and, if necessary, the induction of motor paralysis with a neuromuscular blocking agent such as curare. Mild or moderate hyperthermia (101–102°F), not requiring specific intervention, may persist for 24–48 hours. Lactic acidosis resolves spontaneously over 1 hour and should not be treated. Infection should, of course, be excluded.

Discontinuance of Anticonvulsants

Patients (usually children) with epilepsy who are seizure free on medication for 2–5 years may wish to discontinue anticonvulsant drugs. In patients with normal intelligence and a normal neurologic examination, the risk of seizure recurrence may be as low as 25%. Risk factors for recurrence include slowing or spikes (maximum risk with both present) on EEG. When anticonvulsants are to be withdrawn, one drug is eliminated at a time by tapering the dose slowly over 6 weeks. Recurrence of seizures has been reported in approximately

Table 8–6. Drug treatment of status epilepticus in adults.

Drug	Dosage/Route	Advantages/Disadvantages/Complications
Lorazepam or	0.1 mg/kg IV[1] at rate not greater than 2 mg/min	Fast acting. Effective half-life 15 minutes for diazepam and 14 hours for lorazepam. Abrupt respiratory depression or hypotension in 5%, especially when given in combination with other sedatives. Seizure recurrence in 50% of patients; therefore must add maintenance drug (phenytoin or phenobarbital)
diazepam or	10 mg IV over 2 minutes	
diazepam gel	0.2 mg/kg rectally	
	PROCEED IMMEDIATELY TO FOSPHENYTOIN OR PHENYTOIN	
Fosphenytoin or	1000–1500 mg (20 mg/kg) IV at 150 mg/min in saline or dextrose solution	Peak serum concentration 10–20 minutes following IV infusion. Little or not respiratory depression
phenytoin	1000–1500 mg (20 mg/kg) slowly at rate not greater than 50 mg/min (cannot be given in dextrose solution)	Drug levels in the brain are therapeutic at completion of infusion. Effective as maintenance drug. Hypotension and cardiac arrhythmias can occur
	IF SEIZURES PERSIST, ANOTHER 10 mg/kg OF FOSPHENYTOIN OR PHENYTOIN CAN BE ADMINISTERED; IF SEIZURES STILL CONTINUE, PROCEED IMMEDIATELY TO PHENOBARBITAL, PROPOFOL, PENTOBARBITAL, OR MIDAZOLAM	
Phenobarbital	1000–1500 mg (20 mg/kg) IV slowly (50 mg/min)	Peak brain levels within 30 minutes. Effective as maintenance drug. Respiratory depression and hypotension common at higher doses. (Intubation and ventilatory support should be immediately available)
	IF ABOVE IS INEFFECTIVE, PROCEED IMMEDIATELY TO GENERAL ANESTHESIA	
Propofol or	1–2 mg/kg IV bolus and 2–4 mg/kg/h infusion; titrate infusion between 1 and 15 mg/kg/h	Intubation and ventilatory support required. Hypotension is limited factor. Pressors may be required to maintain blood pressure (dopamine up to 10 µg/kg/min)
pentobarbital or	15 mg/kg IV slowly, followed by 0.5–4 mg/kg/h	
midazolam	0.2 mg/kg IV slowly, followed by 0.75–10 µg/kg/min	

[1]IV, intravenous.

20% of children and 40% of adults following medication withdrawal, in which case prior medication should be reinstituted at the previously effective levels.

COMPLICATIONS OF EPILEPSY & ANTICONVULSANT THERAPY

Complications of Epilepsy

When the diagnosis of epilepsy is made, the patient should be warned against working around moving machinery or at heights and reminded of the risks of swimming alone. The issue of driving must also be addressed. Many state governments have notification requirements when a diagnosis of epilepsy is made.

Side Effects of Anticonvulsant Drugs

The side effects of anticonvulsant drug therapy are summarized in Table 8–7. All anticonvulsant drugs may lead to blood dyscrasias, but carbamazepine and valproic acid have been associated with the highest incidence of hema-

Table 8–7. Side effects of anticonvulsant drugs.

Drug	Dose Related	Idiosyncratic
Phenytoin	Diplopia Ataxia Gingival hyperplasia Hirsutism Coarse facial features Polyneuropathy Osteomalacia Megaloblastic anemia	Skin rash Fever Lymphoid hyperplasia Hepatic dysfunction Blood dyscrasia Stevens-Johnson syndrome
Carbamazepine	Diplopia Ataxia Gastrointestinal distress Sedation	Skin rash Blood dyscrasia Hepatic dysfunction Stevens-Johnson syndrome SIADH
Oxcarbazepine	Hyponatremia	Skin rash
Phenobarbital	Sedation Insomnia Behavioral disturbance Diplopia Ataxia	Skin rash Stevens-Johnson
Valproic acid	Gastrointestinal distress Tremor Sedation Weight gain Hair loss Thrombocytopenia	Hepatic dysfunction Peripheral edema
Ethosuximide	Gastrointestinal distress Sedation Ataxia Headache	Skin rash Blood dyscrasia

Drug	Dose Related	Idiosyncratic
Clonazepam	Sedation Diplopia Ataxia Behavioral disturbance Hypersalivation	
Gabapentin	Drowsiness Fatigue	Drugged sensation Loss of libido
Lamotrigine	Dizziness Ataxia	Skin rash in 1–2% (frequency increased by concomitant valproic acid therapy and reduced by gradual build-up of dose) Stevens-Johnson syndrome
Vigabatrin	Sedation Vertigo Psychosis	Peripheral visual constriction (irreversible)
Topiramate	Ataxia Confusion	Renal stones Glaucoma
Tiagabine	Dizziness Sedation Nausea	Rash
Zonisamide	Drowiness Nephrolithiasis	Ataxia Anorexia Headache Skin rash

tologic—and hepatic—toxicity. For this reason, a complete blood count and liver function tests should be obtained before initiating administration of these drugs and at intervals during the course of treatment. *The authors recommend performing these tests at 2 weeks, 1 month, 3 months, 6 months, and every 6 months thereafter.* Carbamazepine should be discontinued if the total neutrophil count falls below 1500/mL or if aplastic anemia is suspected. Valproic acid should be terminated if symptoms of hepatotoxicity, such as nausea, vomiting, anorexia, or jaundice occur. Lamotrigine has a 1:1000 incidence of Stevens-Johnson syndrome in the first 8 weeks.

Most anticonvulsant drugs (especially barbiturates) affect cognitive function to some degree, even in therapeutic doses.

Drug Interactions

A variety of drugs alter the absorption or metabolism of anticonvulsants when given concomitantly. The changes in anticonvulsant levels are summarized in Table 8–8.

Epilepsy & Anticonvulsant Therapy in Pregnancy

The incidence of stillbirth, microcephaly, mental retardation, and seizure disorders is increased in children born to epileptic mothers. Anticonvulsant therapy during pregnancy, however, is also associated with a greater than normal frequency of congenital malformations—especially cleft palate, cleft lip, and cardiac anomalies. Such malformations are about twice as common in the offspring of medicated than of unmedicated epileptic mothers, but because patients with more severe epilepsy are more likely to be treated, it is difficult to know whether epilepsy or its treatment is the more important risk factor. Folic acid supplementation (1 mg/d) should be provided for all women of child-bearing age who take antiepileptic drugs.

Among commonly used anticonvulsants, valproic acid and to some degree carbamazepine are associated with an increased incidence of neural tube defects (2% and 0.5%, respectively). Phenobarbital and phenytoin pose some teratogenic risk, but the extent of the risk is controversial. The fetal risks of the newer anticonvulsants are not known.

When an epileptic patient who has been seizure free for several years is contemplating pregnancy, an attempt should be made to withdraw anticonvulsants prior to conception. The safest anticonvulsant drug for use in pregnancy is controversial; some centers use carbamazepine or oxcarbazepine for generalized tonic-clonic seizures and ethosuximide for absence seizures. In contrast to generalized tonic-clonic seizures, partial and absence seizures present little risk to the fetus, and it may be possible to tolerate imperfect control of these

Table 8–8. Some major anticonvulsant drug interactions.

Drug	Levels Increased by	Levels Decreased by
Phenytoin	Benzodiazepines Chloramphenicol Disulfiram Ethanol Isoniazid Phenylbutazone Sulfonamides Topiramate Trimethoprim Warfarin Zonisamide	Carbamazepine Phenobarbital Pyridoxine Vigabatrin
Carbamazepine	Erythromycin Felbamate[1] Isoniazid Propoxyphene Valproic acid	Phenobarbital Phenytoin Oxcarbazepine Zonisamide
Phenobarbital	Primidone Valproic acid	
Valproic acid		Topiramate Tiagabrin Lamotrigine Phenytoin Carbamazepine
Ethosuximide	Valproic acid	—
Clonazepam	—	—
Gabapentin	—	—
Lamotrigine	Valproic acid	Carbamazepine Phenobarbital Phenytoin
Vigabatrin	—	—
Topiramate	—	Carbamazepine Phenytoin Valproic acid
Tiagabine	—	Carbamazepine Phenytoin Phenobarbital
Zonisamide	Lamotrigine	Carbamazepine Phenytoin

[1] Levels of the parent compound are diminished, but levels of active metabolite increase.

seizures during pregnancy to avoid fetal drug exposure. Every effort should be made to use only a single drug. Status epilepticus is treated as described above for nonpregnant patients.

Plasma levels of anticonvulsant drugs may decrease during pregnancy because of the patient's enhanced drug metabolism, and higher doses may be required to maintain control of seizures. It is therefore important to monitor drug levels closely in this setting.

PROGNOSIS

After a single unprovoked seizure, only one-third to one-half of patients will have a recurrence (develop epilepsy). If a second seizure occurs, however, the recurrence rate approaches 75% and anticonvulsants should therefore be started. With appropriate anticonvulsant drug treatment, seizures can be well controlled, although not always eliminated, in most epileptic patients. At the onset of treatment patients should be seen every few months to monitor seizure frequency and make dose adjustments.

PSEUDOSEIZURES

Attacks that resemble seizures (psychogenic seizures, or pseudoseizures) may be manifestations of a psychiatric disturbance such as conversion disorder, somatization disorder, factitious disorder with physical symptoms, or malingering. In conversion or somatization disorder, the patient is unaware of the psychogenic nature of symptoms and the motivation for their production. In factitious disorder, the patient recognizes that the spells are self-induced, but not the reason for doing so. In malingering, there is conscious awareness of both the production of symptoms and the underlying motivation.

Pseudoseizures can usually be distinguished both clinically and by the EEG findings. In patients with pseudoseizures resembling tonic-clonic attacks, there may be warning and preparation before the attack; there is usually no tonic phase, and the clonic phase consists of wild thrashing movements during which the patient rarely comes to harm or is incontinent. In some instances, there are abnormal movements of all extremities without loss of consciousness; in others, there is shouting or obscene utterances during apparent loss of consciousness or goal-directed behavior. There is no postictal confusion or abnormal clinical signs following the attack. The EEG recorded during the episode does not show organized seizure activity, and postictal slowing does not occur. The differential diagnosis should include **frontal lobe seizures**, which may be marked by unusual midline movements (pelvic thrusting, bicycling) and by very brief postictal states. Ictal EEG abnormalities may escape detection as well.

It is important to appreciate that many patients with pseudoseizures also have genuine epileptic attacks that require anticonvulsant medications, but these should be prescribed at an empirically appropriate dose. Psychiatric referral may be helpful.

SYNCOPE

Syncope is episodic loss of consciousness associated with loss of postural tone. The pathophysiology is distinct from that of seizures and involves global hypoperfusion of the brain or brainstem. The most common causes of syncope are given in Table 8–9.

VASOVAGAL SYNCOPE (SIMPLE FAINTS)

Vasovagal syncope, which is exceedingly common, occurs in all age groups. Precipitating factors include emotional stimulation, pain, the sight of blood, fatigue,

Table 8–9. Common causes of syncope.

Cause	Percentage of Patients
Reflex mediated	
Vasovagal	18
Carotid sinus sensitivity	1
Situational	
Micturition, defecation, cough	5
Orthostatic hypotension	8
Medication induced	3
Psychiatric/hyperventilation	2
Neurologic (seizures, transient ischemic attacks, subclavian steal)	10
Cardiac	
Organic heart disease[1]	4
Arrhythmias[2]	14
Unknown[3]	34

[1] Aortic stenosis, hypertrophic cardiomyopathy, pulmonary embolism, atrial myxoma, myocardial infarction, coronary artery spasm, cardiac tamponade, aortic dissection.

[2] Sinus node disease, second- and third-degree heart block, pacemaker failure, drug-induced bradyarrhythmias, ventricular tachycardia, torsades de pointes, supraventricular tachycardia.

[3] One-half would have neurocardiogenic syncope by tilt-table testing.

Data from Lizner et al. (1997), compiled from studies published 1980–1997 (prior to tilt-table testing).

From Simon RP: Syncope. Pages 2028–2013 in: *Cecil Textbook of Medicine,* 21st ed. Goldman L, Bennett JC (editors). WB Saunders, 2000.

medical instrumentation, blood loss, or prolonged motionless standing. Vagally mediated decreases in arterial blood pressure and heart rate combine to produce central nervous system hypoperfusion and subsequent syncope. Severe cerebral ischemia resulting in tonic-clonic movements can occur if the unconscious patient remains in an upright position during the episode.

Vasovagal episodes generally begin while the patient is in a standing or sitting position and only rarely in a horizontal position (eg, with phlebotomy or IUD insertion). A prodrome lasting 10 seconds to a few minutes usually precedes syncope and can include lassitude, light-headedness, nausea, pallor, diaphoresis, salivation, blurred vision, and tachycardia. The patient, who then loses consciousness and falls to the ground, is pale and diaphoretic and has dilated pupils. Bradycardia replaces tachycardia as consciousness is lost. During unconsciousness, abnormal movements may occur; these are mainly tonic or opisthotonic, but seizurelike tonic-clonic activity is occasionally seen, which can lead to a misdiagnosis of epilepsy. Urinary incontinence may also occur.

The patient recovers consciousness very rapidly (seconds to a few minutes) after assuming the horizontal position, but residual nervousness, dizziness, headache, nausea, pallor, diaphoresis, and an urge to defecate may be noted. A postical confusional state with disorientation and agitation either is very brief (<30 seconds) or does not occur. Syncope may recur, especially if the patient stands up within the next 30 minutes.

Reassurance and a recommendation to avoid precipitating factors are usually the only treatment necessary.

Recurrent vasovagal syncope (often termed **neuro-cardiogenic syncope**) can be documented by head-up tilt-testing. The bradycardia and hypotension can be ameliorated by oral metoprolol, theophylline, or disopyramide; artificial pacing is ineffective.

CARDIOVASCULAR SYNCOPE

A cardiovascular cause is suggested when syncope occurs with the patient in a recumbent position, during or after physical exertion, or in a patient with known heart disease. Loss of consciousness related to cardiac disease is most often due to an abrupt decrease in cardiac output with resultant cerebral hypoperfusion. Such cardiac dysfunction can result from cardiac arrest, rhythm disturbances (either brady- or tachyarrhythmias), cardiac inflow or outflow obstruction, intracardiac right-to-left shunts, leaking or dissecting aortic aneurysms, or acute pulmonary embolus (Table 8–10).

1. Cardiac Arrest

Cardiac arrest (ventricular fibrillation, or asystole) from any cause will result in loss of consciousness in 3–5 sec-

Table 8–10. Causes of syncope from cardiovascular disease.

Cardiac arrest
Cardiac dysrhythmias
  Tachyarrythmias
    Supraventricular
      Paroxysmal atrial tachycardia
      Atrial filter
      Atrial fibrillation
      Accelerated junctional tachycardia
    Ventricular
      Ventricular tachycardia
      Ventricular fibrillation
  Bradyarrhythmias
    Sinus bradycardia
    Sinus arrest
    Second- or third-degree heart block
    Implanted pacemaker failure or malfunction
  Mitral valve prolapse (click-murmur syndrome)
  Prolonged QT-interval syndromes
  Sick-sinus syndrome (tachycardia-bradycardia syndrome)
  Drug toxicity (especially digitalis, quinidine, procainamide, propranolol, phenothiazines, tricyclic antidepressants, potassium)
Cardiac inflow obstruction
  Left atrial myxoma or thrombus
  Tight mitral stenosis
  Constrictive pericarditis or cardiac tamponade
  Restrictive cardiomyopathies
  Tension pneumothorax
Cardiac outflow obstruction
  Aortic stenosis
  Pulmonary stenosis
  Hypertrophic obstructive cardiomyopathy (asymmetric septal hypertrophy, idiopathic hypertrophic subaortic stenosis)
Dissecting aortic aneurysm
Severe pulmonary-vascular disease
  Pulmonary hypertension
  Acute pulmonary embolus

onds if the patient is standing or within 15 seconds if the patient is recumbent. Seizurelike activity and urinary and fecal incontinence may be seen as the duration of cerebral hypoperfusion increases.

2. Tachyarrhythmias

Supraventricular Tachyarrhythmias

Supraventricular tachyarrhythmias (atrial or junctional tachycardia, atrial flutter, or atrial fibrillation) may be paroxysmal or chronic.

Heart rates faster than 160–200/min reduce cardiac output by decreasing the ventricular filling period or inducing myocardial ischemia. Prolonged tachycardia of 180–200 beats or more per minute will produce syncope in 50% of normal persons in the upright posture; in patients with underlying heart disease, a heart rate of 135/min may impair cardiac output enough to induce loss of consciousness. Patients with sinus node dysfunction (**sick-sinus syndrome**) may develop profound bradycardia or even asystole upon termination of their tachyarrhythmias. The diagnosis is established when arrhythmias are demonstrated during a symptomatic episode. Continuous electrocardiogram (ECG) or outpatient portable Holter monitoring may be required; event monitors triggered by the patient at the onset of symptoms may be particularly helpful.

Ventricular Tachyarrhythmias

Ventricular tachyarrhythmias (ventricular tachycardia or multiform, frequent, or paired premature ventricular contractions) are found on prolonged ECG monitoring in some patients with syncope. The syncope associated with ventricular tachycardia is characterized by a very brief prodrome (less than 5 seconds). Frequent or repetitive premature ventricular contractions alone do not often coincide with syncopal symptoms but are predictive of sudden death.

Mitral Valve Prolapse

Mitral valve prolapse (**click-murmur syndrome**) is a common disorder associated with supraventricular and ventricular arrhythmias, and with syncope in a small percentage of patients. Other symptoms include nonexertional chest pain, dyspnea, and fatigue. Serious ventricular arrhythmias and profound bradycardia may occur. The ECG may be normal or show nonspecific ST-T wave changes or frequent premature ventricular contractions. Diagnosis is by echocardiography.

Prolonged QT Syndrome

The congenital prolonged QT-interval syndrome consists of paroxysmal ventricular arrhythmias (often torsade de pointes), syncope, and sudden death and is inherited as an autosomal recessive condition associated with deafness or in an autosomal dominant form without deafness. Sporadic cases also occur. Quinidine, hypocalcemia, and hypokalemia can also produce QT prolongation. Hereditary cases may respond to β-blockers.

3. Bradyarrhythmias

Sinoatrial Node Disease

Sinoatrial node disease may cause syncope with profound sinus bradycardia, prolonged sinus pauses, or sinus arrest with a slow atrial, junctional, or idioventricu-

lar escape rhythm. Patients should be promptly evaluated by a cardiologist, since a permanent pacemaker is necessary in many cases.

Complete Heart Block

Complete heart block (third-degree atrioventricular block) is the most common bradyarrhythmia that produces syncope. Permanent atrioventricular conduction abnormalities are easily noted on a routine ECG, but intermittent conduction abnormalities may not be present on a random tracing. A normal PR interval on an ECG obtained after the episode does not exclude the diagnosis of transient complete heart block.

Patients with syncope and documented or suspected complete heart block should be promptly hospitalized. Patients with acute inferior myocardial infarctions are at high risk for atrioventricular block.

4. Cardiac Inflow Obstruction

Atrial or ventricular **myxomas** and atrial **thrombi** usually present with embolic events, but they may also produce a left ventricular inflow or outflow obstruction that results in a sudden decrease in cardiac output, followed by syncope. A history of syncope occurring with change in position is classic but uncommon. Echocardiography can confirm the diagnosis. Surgical removal of the myxoma is indicated.

With **constrictive pericarditis** or **pericardial tamponade**, any maneuver or drug that decreases heart rate or venous return can result in suddenly inadequate cardiac output and syncope.

5. Cardiac Outflow Obstruction

Aortic Stenosis

Loss of consciousness from congenital or acquired severe aortic stenosis usually occurs following exercise, and is often associated with dyspnea, angina, and diaphoresis. The pathophysiology may involve acute left ventricular failure resulting in coronary hypoperfusion and subsequent ventricular fibrillation, or abrupt increases in left ventricular pressure that stimulate baroreceptors, leading to peripheral vasodilation. Echocardiography can help confirm the diagnosis.

Symptomatic aortic stenosis requires valve replacement; without treatment, the average survival following syncope from aortic stenosis is 18 months to 3 years.

Pulmonary Stenosis

Severe pulmonary stenosis can produce syncope, especially following exertion. A hemodynamic process similar to that occurring in aortic stenosis is responsible.

Obstructive Hypertrophic Cardiomyopathy

Obstructive hypertrophic cardiomyopathy comprises a group of congenital cardiomyopathies inherited as autosomal dominant disorders of variable severity. Symptoms usually begin between the second and fourth decades. Dyspnea is the most common presenting complaint, but syncope occurs in 30% of patients and is the presenting complaint in 10% of patients. Syncope characteristically develops during or following exercise, but orthostatic and posttussive episodes also occur. Syncope may be due to left ventricular outflow obstruction, inflow obstruction, or transient arrhythmias. The diagnosis can be confirmed by echocardiography and propranolol may control symptoms.

6. Dissecting Aortic Aneurysm

Approximately 5–10% of patients with acute aortic dissections present with isolated syncope; other neurologic abnormalities may or may not be present. In 15% of patients, the dissection is painless.

7. Pulmonary Hypertension & Pulmonary Embolus

Syncope, often exertional, may be the presenting symptom of pulmonary hypertension. A history of exertional dyspnea is usual, and blood gas analysis shows hypoxemia, even at rest. Syncope is the presenting symptom in about 20% of patients experiencing a massive pulmonary embolus. Upon recovery, such patients often complain of pleuritic chest pain, dyspnea, and apprehension. Hypotension, tachycardia, tachypnea, and arterial hypoxemia frequently accompany these large emboli.

CEREBROVASCULAR SYNCOPE

Cerebrovascular disease is an often suspected but actually uncommon cause of episodic unconsciousness.

1. Basilar Artery Insufficiency

Basilar artery transient ischemic attacks usually occur after the sixth decade. The symptom complex of diplopia, vertigo, dysphagia, dysarthria, various sensory or motor symptoms, drop attacks, and occipital headaches suggests diffuse brainstem ischemia. Attacks are typically sudden in onset and brief in duration (seconds to minutes), but when consciousness is lost, recovery is frequently prolonged (30–60 minutes or longer). Isolated unconsciousness without other symptoms of brainstem ischemia is rarely due to basilar artery insufficiency. Two-thirds of patients have recurrent attacks,

and strokes eventually occur in about one-fifth of all cases. Treatment is discussed in Chapter 9.

2. Subclavian Steal Syndrome

The subclavian steal syndrome results from subclavian or innominate artery stenosis that causes retrograde blood flow in the vertebral artery, with subsequent brainstem hypoperfusion. The degree of subclavian artery stenosis that will produce symptoms is variable, and minor (about 40%) stenosis may cause the syndrome in some patients. A difference between blood pressures measured in the two arms is nearly always found, the average difference being a 45 mm Hg decrease in systolic pressure in the arm supplied by the stenotic vessel. Stroke is rare. If this diagnosis is suspected, arteriography and surgical correction may be indicated.

3. Migraine

Syncope occurs in 10% of patients with migraine during the headache, often on rapid rising to a standing position, suggesting that loss of consciousness is due to orthostatic hypotension. In some patients, **basilar migraine** produces symptoms similar to those of basilar artery transient ischemic attacks. Antimigraine drug therapy (see Chapter 2) is often effective in preventing attacks.

4. Takayasu's Disease

Takayasu's disease is a panarteritis of the great vessels that is most common in Asian women. Symptoms of cerebral hypoperfusion such as impaired vision, confusion, and syncope are often prominent. Precipitating factors include exercise, standing, or head movement. Examination reveals decreased or absent brachial pulses with low blood pressures in both arms. The erythrocyte sedimentation rate is moderately elevated in the acute stage. Corticosteroid treatment is indicated.

5. Carotid Sinus Syncope

Carotid sinus syncope is uncommon. Men are affected twice as often as women, and most affected individuals are over 60 years of age. Drugs known to predispose to carotid sinus syncope include propranolol, digitalis, and methyldopa. Pressure on the carotid sinus by a tight collar, a neck mass, enlarged cervical lymph nodes, or a tumor causes vagal stimulation, which inhibits the cardiac sinoatrial and atrioventricular nodes and reduces sympathetic vascular tone. The resultant bradycardia or systemic hypotension may then produce syncope; pure cardioinhibitory or vasodepressor syncope also occurs. The bradycardia can be abolished or prevented by administration of atropine.

Carotid sinus syncope may be mistakenly diagnosed

when symptoms result from compression of a normal carotid artery contralateral to an occluded internal carotid artery. Under these circumstances, unilateral compression transiently interrupts the entire anterior cerebral circulation. Performing carotid sinus massage in an attempt to diagnose carotid sinus syncope in patients with carotid atherosclerotic disease entails a risk of distal embolization of atheromatous material.

MISCELLANEOUS CAUSES OF SYNCOPE

1. Orthostatic Hypotension

Orthostatic hypotension occurs more often in men than in women and is most common in the sixth and seventh decades. It may, however, appear even in teenagers. Loss of consciousness usually occurs upon rapidly rising to a standing position, standing motionless for a prolonged period (especially following exercise), and standing after prolonged recumbency (especially in elderly patients).

Numerous conditions can produce orthostatic hypotension (Table 8–11), which generally results from

Table 8–11. Causes of orthostatic hypotension.

Hypovolemia or hemorrhage
Addison's disease
Drug-induced hypotension
Antidepressants
Antihypertensives
Bromocriptine
Diuretics
Levodopa
Monoamine oxidase inhibitors
Nitroglycerin
Phenothiazines
Polyneuropathies
Amyloid neuropathy
Diabetic neuropathy
Guillain-Barré syndrome
Porphyric neuropathy
Vincristine neuropathy
Other neurologic disorders
Idiopathic orthostatic hypotension
Multiple sclerosis
Parkinsonism
Posterior fossa tumor
Shy-Drager syndrome
Spinal cord injury with paraplegia
Surgical sympathectomy
Syringomyelia/syringobulbia
Tabes dorsalis
Wernicke's encephalopathy
Cardiovascular disorders
Prolonged bed rest

either reduced blood volume or autonomic nervous system dysfunction. The latter may be due to sympathetic drugs, autonomic neuropathy, or central nervous system disorders affecting sympathetic pathways in the hypothalamus, brainstem, or spinal cord. Two neurogenic causes of orthostatic hypotension deserve special consideration. **Idiopathic orthostatic hypotension** is associated mainly with the degeneration of postganglionic sympathetic neurons without other neuropathologic changes. In **Shy-Drager syndrome**, orthostatic hypotension appears to be related to degeneration of preganglionic sympathetic neurons; this occurs in combination with parkinsonian, pyramidal, cerebellar, or lower motor neuron signs.

The diagnosis of orthostatic hypotension is established by demonstrating a drop in blood pressure of at least 30 mm Hg systolic or 10 mm Hg diastolic when the patient changes from the lying to the standing position. In equivocal cases, tilt-table testing may be necessary. A detailed general physical and neurologic examination and laboratory studies (hematocrit, stool occult blood, serum glucose and electrolytes, FTA-ABS, nerve conduction studies) should be directed toward establishing the cause of the disorder.

Any medication that might be responsible should be discontinued if possible, and the patient should be instructed to stand up gradually, to elevate the head of the bed on blocks, and to use waist-high elasticized support hosiery. Other therapy is dictated by the specific cause of hypotension. The potent mineralocorticoid fludrocortisone has been effective in idiopathic cases and in diabetic patients in doses beginning with 0.1 mg/d orally and increased gradually, as necessary, up to 1 mg/d orally. Its mode of action is unclear, but its benefit may relate to increased responsiveness to circulating norepinephrine, as well as to an increased plasma volume. Side effects include recumbent hypertension, but to treat this compounds the primary problem of orthostasis.

2. Hyperventilation Syncope

Hyperventilation is a frequent cause of faintness or dizziness but rarely culminates in syncope. Common symptoms include light-headedness, shortness of breath, circumoral numbness and tingling, and muscular twitching. Pathophysiologically, **hypocapnia** produces cerebral vasoconstriction and results in central nervous system hypoperfusion. Patients are usually between 20 and 40 years of age, and women are affected far more frequently than men. The disorder is usually benign, with anxiety a prominent precipitant, but serious cardiopulmonary causes of hyperventilation or subjective dyspnea must be excluded. Symptoms commonly occur in the lying position, which can be diagnostically helpful. Patients often report prolonged unconsciousness, but upon close questioning this rarely proves to be true. Hyperventilation at the examiner's request often reproduces the symptoms.

3. Cough Syncope

Cough syncope occurs chiefly in middle-aged men with chronic obstructive pulmonary disease but has also been reported in children. Coughing need not be prolonged and immediately precedes unconsciousness, which may occur while the patient is supine. Prodromal symptoms are absent, and the duration of unconsciousness is brief—often only a few seconds. Full recovery of consciousness occurs immediately. A history of similar episodes is common, and symptoms may be reproduced by having the patient cough on request. The cause may be a decrease in cerebral blood flow from increased intracranial pressure, which results from transmission of increased intrathoracic pressure to the intracranial compartment via the spinal fluid or venous connections.

The condition is usually benign, and there is no specific treatment except for antitussive drugs such as dextromethorphan.

4. Micturition Syncope

Micturition syncope occurs almost exclusively in men, probably because of the standing position for urination. Episodes can occur immediately before, during, or after micturition. They are more likely to occur at night following the prolonged recumbency of sleep and are due to peripheral pooling of blood plus a vagally induced bradycardia. Urination in a sitting position usually eliminates the symptoms.

5. Glossopharyngeal Neuralgia

Glossopharyngeal neuralgia is a rare syndrome of intermittent, agonizing paroxysmal pain localized to the tonsillar pillar or occasionally to the external auditory meatus. The pain is triggered by contact with or movement of the tonsillar pillars, especially during swallowing or talking. Syncope occurs as a consequence of the activation of a glossopharyngeal-vagal reflex arc, producing a transient bradyarrhythmia with resultant cerebral hypoperfusion.

Carbamazepine, 400–1000 mg/d orally, will prevent pain and bradycardia in most patients.

6. Psychogenic Syncope

Psychogenic syncope is a diagnosis of exclusion and is often made erroneously. Suggestive features are lack of any prodrome, possible secondary gain, bizarre postures and movements, lack of pallor, and a prolonged period of apparent unresponsiveness. Psychogenic spells rarely occur when the patient is alone and they rarely are associated with incontinence or result in injury. Most patients are young or have a well-documented history of conversion disorder. Without such a history, diagnosis after the third decade is suspect.

The EEG during psychogenic unconsciousness is normal, without the slowing that typically occurs with cerebral hypoperfusion and follows unconsciousness from a seizure. Caloric testing (see Chapter 10), which produces nystagmus in conscious patients, and tonic eye deviation in unconscious patients, can distinguish psychogenic unresponsiveness from coma caused by a metabolic or structural lesion.

REFERENCES

SEIZURES

General

Devinsky O: Patients with refractory seizures. N Engl J Med 1999; 340:1565–1570.

Engel J Jr: *Seizures and Epilepsy.* Vol 31 of: *Contemporary Neurology Series.* Davis, 1989.

Hauser WA et al: Risk of recurrent seizures after two unprovoked seizures. N Engl J Med 1998;338:429–434.

Sillanpää M et al: Long-term prognosis of seizures with onset in childhood. N Engl J Med 1998;338:1715–1722.

Etiology

Annegers JF et al: A population-based study of seizures after traumatic brain injuries. N Engl J Med 1998;338:20–24.

Berg AT et al: A prospective study of recurrent febrile seizures. N Engl J Med 1992;327:1122–1127.

Burn J et al: Epileptic seizures after a first stroke: the Oxfordshire Community Stroke Project. BMJ 1997;315:1582–1587.

Delanty N, Vaughan CJ, French JA: Medical causes of seizures. Lancet 1998;352:383–390.

Ettinger AB, Shinnar S: New-onset seizures in an elderly hospitalized population. Neurology 1993;43:489–492.

Fox MW, Harms RW, Davis DH: Selected neurological complications of pregnancy. Mayo Clin Proc 1990;65:1595–1618.

Kurtz Z et al: Epilepsy in young people: 23 year follow up of the British national child development study. BMJ 1998;316: 339–342.

Leppik IE (editor): Status epilepticus in perspective. Neurology 1990;40(Suppl 2):1–51. [Entire issue.]

Lowenstein DH, Alldredge BK: Status epilepticus. N Engl J Med 1998;338:970–976.

Messing RO, Closson RG, Simon RP: Drug-induced seizures: a 10-year experience. Neurology 1984;34:1582–1586.

Messing RO, Simon RP: Seizures as a manifestation of systemic disease. Neurol Clin 1986;4:563–584.

Pomeroy SL et al: Seizures and other neurological sequelae of bacterial meningitis in children. N Engl J Med 1990;323: 1651–1657.

Verity CM et al: Long-term intellectual and behavioral outcomes of children with febrile convulsions. N Engl J Med 1998;338: 1723 –1728.

Treatment

Anonymous: The Brain Trauma Foundation. The American Association of Neurological Surgeons. The Joint Section on Neurotrauma and Critical Care. Role of antiseizure prophylaxis following head injury. J Neurotrauma 2000;17:549–553.

Cascino GD: Intractable partial epilepsy: evaluation and treatment. Mayo Clin Proc 1990;65:1578–1586.

Dalessio DJ: Seizure disorders and pregnancy. N Engl J Med 1985;312:559–563.

Jones KL et al: Pattern of malformations in the children of women treated with carbamazepine during pregnancy. N Engl J Med 1989;320:1661–1666.

Kwan P, Brodie MJ: Early identification of refractory epilepsy. N Engl J Med 2000;342:314–319.

Lucas MJ et al: A comparison of magnesium sulfate with phenytoin for the prevention of eclampsia. N Engl J Med 1995;333:201–205.

Marson AG, Chadwick DW: New drug treatments for epilepsy. J Neurol Neurosurg Psychiatry 2001;70:143–148.

Mattson RH et al: Comparison of carbamazepine, phenytoin, and primidone in partial and secondarily generalized tonic-clonic seizures. N Engl J Med 1985;313:145–151.

Medical Research Council Antiepileptic Drug Withdrawal Study Group: prognostic index for recurrence of seizures after remission of epilepsy. BMJ 1993;306:1374–1378.

Pitt-Miller PL et al: The management of status epilepticus with a continuous propofol infusion. Anesth Analg 1994;78: 1193–1194.

Rosman NP et al: A controlled trial of diazepam administered during febrile illnesses to prevent recurrence of febrile seizures. N Engl J Med 1993;329:79–84.

Sachdeo R: Challenging our past paradigm in the management of epilepsy. Neurology 2000;55(11 Suppl 3):S1–4.

Shinnar S et al: Discontinuing antiepileptic drugs in children with epilepsy: a prospective study. Ann Neurol 1994;35:534–545.

Temkin NR et al: A randomized, double-blind study of phenytoin for the prevention of post-traumatic seizures. N Engl J Med 1990;323:497–502.

Tennison M et al: Discontinuing antiepiletic drugs in children with epilepsy. N Engl J Med 1994;330:1407–1410.

PSEUDOSEIZURES

Lesser RP: Psychogenic seizures. Neurology 1996;46:1499–1507.

SYNCOPE

General

Brenner RP: Electroencephalography in syncope. J Clin Neurophysiol 1997;14:197–209.

Kapoor WN: Syncope. N Engl J Med 2000;343:1856–1862.

Lempert T, Bauer M, Schmidt D: Syncope: a videometric analysis of 56 episodes of transient cerebral hypoxia. Ann Neurol 1994;36:233–237.

Linzer M et al: Diagnosing syncope. Part 1: Value of history, physical examination, and electrocardiography. Clinical Efficacy Assessment Project of the American College of Physicians. Ann Intern Med 1997;126:989–996.

Linzer M et al: Diagnosing syncope. Part 2: Unexplained syncope. Clinical Efficacy Assessment Project of the American College of Physicians. Ann Intern Med 1997;127:76–86.

Mathias CJ, Deguchi K, Schatz I: Observations on recurrent syncope and presyncope in 641 patients. Lancet 2001;357: 348–353.

Vasovagal

Ammirati F et al: Electroencephalographic correlates of vasovagal syncope induced by head-up tilt testing. Stroke 1998;29: 2347–2351.

Barron SA, Rogovski Z, Hemli Y: Vagal cardiovascular reflexes in young persons with syncope. Ann Intern Med 1993;118: 943–946.

Sra JS et al: Comparison of cardiac pacing with drug therapy in the treatment of neurocardiogenic (vasovagal) syncope with bradycardia or asystole. N Engl J Med 1993;328:1085–1090.

Cardiovascular

Calkins H et al: The value of the clinical history in the differentiation of syncope due to ventricular tachycardia, atrioventricular block, and neurocardiogenic syncope. Am J Med 1995; 98:365–373.

Fogel RI et al: Utility and cost of event recorders in the diagnosis of palpitations, presyncope, and syncope. Am J Cardiol 1997; 79:207–208.

Koutkia P, Wachtel TJ: Pulmonary embolism presenting as syncope: case report and review of the literature. Heart Lung 1999;28:342–347.

McIntosh SJ, Lawson J, Kenny RA: Clinical characteristics of vasodepressor, cardioinhibitory, and mixed carotid sinus syndrome in the elderly. Am J Med 1993;95:203–208.

Pacia SV: The prolonged QT syndrome presenting as epilepsy: a report of two cases and literature review. Neurology 1994; 44:1408–1410.

Cerebrovascular

Delaney CP et al: Investigation and management of subclavian steal syndrome. Br J Surg 1994;81:1093–1095.

Tea SH et al: New insights into the pathophysiology of carotid sinus syndrome. Circulation 1996;93:1411–1416.

Miscellaneous Causes

Evans RW: Neurologic aspects of hyperventilation syndrome. Semin Neurol 1995;15:115–125.

Ferrante L et al: Glossopharyngeal neuralgia with cardiac syncope. Neurosurgery 1995;36:58–63.

Mattle HP et al: Transient cerebral circulatory arrest coincides with fainting in cough syncope. Neurology 1995;45:498–501.

Saper CB: "All fall down": the mechanism of orthostatic hypotension in multiple systems atrophy and Parkinson's disease. Ann Neurol 1998;43:149–151.

Stroke

CONTENTS

KEY CONCEPTS

 Stroke is a syndrome characterized by the acute onset of a neurologic deficit that persists for at least 24 hours, reflects focal involvement of the central nervous system, and is the result of a disturbance of the cerebral circulation.

 Stroke results from either of two types of cerebral vascular disturbance: ischemia or hemorrhage.

 Ischemia, the most common cause of stroke, can be caused by either local thrombosis or embolization from a distant site, such as the heart.

 Transient ischemic attack and acute stroke are medical emergencies that require prompt diagnosis, because they may be treatable with antiplatelet drugs, anticoagulants, thrombolytic agents, or surgery.

Stroke is the third most common cause of death in the United States and the most common disabling neurologic disorder. About 750,000 new strokes occur and about 150,000 people die from stroke in the United states each year. The incidence increases with age, with about two-thirds of all strokes occurring in those over age 65 years, and is somewhat higher in men than in women and in African-Americans than in whites. Risk factors for stroke include systolic or diastolic hypertension, hypercholesterolemia, cigarette smoking, heavy alcohol consumption, and oral contraceptive use. The incidence of stroke has decreased in recent decades, largely because of improved treatment of hypertension.

APPROACH TO DIAGNOSIS

Stroke is a syndrome characterized by the acute onset of a neurologic deficit that persists for at least 24 hours, reflects focal involvement of the central nervous system, and is the result of a disturbance of the cerebral circulation. The acute onset and subsequent duration of symptoms are documented by the history. The site of central nervous system involvement is suggested by the nature of the symptoms. It is delineated more precisely by the neurologic examination and confirmed by imaging studies [computed tomography (CT) scans or magnetic resonance imaging

(MRI)]. A vascular etiology may be inferred from the acute onset of symptoms and often from the patient's age, the presence of risk factors for stroke, and the occurrence of symptoms and signs referable to the territory of a particular cerebral blood vessel. When this is confirmed by imaging studies, further investigations can be undertaken to identify a specific cause.

Acute Onset

Strokes begin abruptly. Neurologic deficits may be maximal at onset, as is common in embolic stroke, or may progress over seconds to hours (or occasionally days), which is characteristic of progressive arterial thrombosis or recurrent emboli. A stroke that is actively progressing as a direct consequence of the underlying vascular disorder (but not because of associated cerebral edema) or has done so in recent minutes is termed **stroke in evolution** or **progressing stroke** (Figure 9–1). Focal cerebral deficits that develop slowly (over weeks to months) are unlikely to be due to stroke and are more suggestive of tumor or inflammatory or degenerative disease.

Duration of Deficits

By definition, stroke produces neurologic deficits that persist for at least 24 hours. When symptoms and signs resolve completely after briefer periods (usually within 30 minutes), the term **transient ischemic attack (TIA)** is used (see Figure 9–1). Recurrent TIAs with identical clinical features are usually caused by thrombosis or embolism arising within the cerebral circulation. TIAs that differ in character from event to event suggest recurrent emboli from a cardiac source. Although TIAs do not themselves produce lasting neurologic dysfunction, they are important to recognize because about one-third of patients with TIAs will go on to have a stroke within 5 years—and because this risk may be reduced with treatment.

In some cases, deficits last for longer than 24 hours but resolve completely or almost completely within a few days; the term **reversible ischemic neurological deficit (RIND)** or **minor stroke** is sometimes used to describe these events.

As their names imply, TIAs and RINDs are uniquely associated with cerebral ischemia, as opposed to hemorrhage.

Focal Involvement

Stroke produces focal symptoms and signs that correlate with the area of the brain supplied by the affected blood vessel. In ischemic stroke, occlusion of a blood vessel interrupts the flow of blood to a specific region of the brain, interfering with neurologic functions dependent on that region and producing a more or less stereotyped pattern of deficits. Hemorrhage produces a less pre-

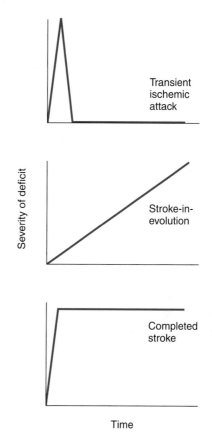

Figure 9–1. Time course of cerebral ischemic events. A transient ischemic attack (TIA) produces neurologic deficits that resolve completely within 24 hours and usually within 30 minutes. Stroke-in-evolution, or progressing stroke, causes deficits that continue to worsen even as the patient is seen. Completed stroke is defined by the presence of residual deficits (which may be stable or improving) at 24 hours; it does not necessarily imply that the entire territory of the involved vessel is affected or that no improvement has occurred since the onset.

dictable pattern of focal involvement because complications such as increased intracranial pressure, cerebral edema, compression of brain tissue and blood vessels, or dispersion of blood through the subarachnoid space or cerebral ventricles can impair brain function at sites remote from the hemorrhage.

Cerebrovascular disorders can also affect the brain in more diffuse fashion and produce global cerebral dysfunction, but the term *stroke* should not be applied in these cases. These disorders include **global cerebral ischemia** (usually from cardiac arrest) and **subarachnoid hemorrhage** (discussed in Chapter 2). In most cases of stroke, the history and neurologic examination provide enough information to localize the lesion to one side of the brain (eg, to the side opposite a hemiparesis or hemisensory deficit or to the left side if aphasia is present) and to the anterior or posterior cerebral circulation.

A. ANTERIOR CIRCULATION

The anterior cerebral circulation, which supplies most of the cerebral cortex and subcortical white matter, basal ganglia, and internal capsule, consists of the internal carotid artery and its branches: the anterior choroidal, anterior cerebral, and middle cerebral arteries. The middle cerebral artery in turn gives rise to deep, penetrating lenticulostriate branches (Figure 9–2). The specific territory of each of these vessels is shown in Table 9–1. Anterior circulation strokes are commonly associated with symptoms and signs that indicate hemispheric dysfunction (Table 9–2), such as aphasia, apraxia, or agnosia. They also produce hemiparesis, hemisensory disturbances, and visual field defects, which can also occur with posterior circulation strokes.

B. POSTERIOR CIRCULATION

The posterior cerebral circulation supplies the brainstem, cerebellum, and thalamus and portions of the occipital and temporal lobes. It consists of the paired vertebral arteries, the basilar artery, and their branches: the posterior inferior cerebellar, anterior inferior cerebellar, superior cerebellar, and posterior cerebral arteries (see Figure 9–2). The posterior cerebral artery also gives off thalamoperforate and thalamogeniculate branches. Areas supplied by these arteries are listed in Table 9–1. Posterior circulation strokes produce symptoms and signs of brainstem dysfunction (see Table 9–2), including coma, drop attacks (sudden collapse without loss of consciousness), vertigo, nausea and vomiting, cranial nerve palsies, ataxia, and crossed sensorimotor deficits that affect the face on one side of the body and the limbs on the other. Hemiparesis, hemisensory disturbances, and visual field deficits also occur, but are not specific to posterior circulation strokes.

Vascular Origin

Although hypoglycemia, other metabolic disturbances, trauma, and seizures can produce focal central neurologic deficits that begin abruptly and last for at least 24 hours, the term *stroke* is used only when such events are caused by cerebrovascular disease.

The underlying pathologic process in stroke can be either ischemia or hemorrhage, usually from an arterial lesion. In recent series, ischemia accounted for about two-thirds and hemorrhage for about one-third of strokes. It may not be pos-

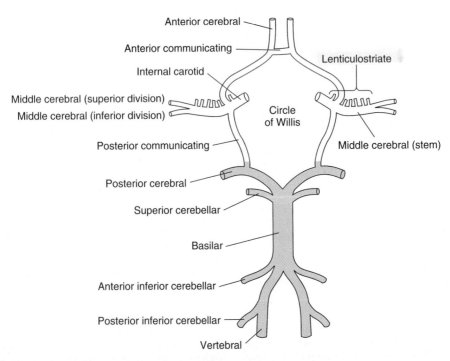

Figure 9–2. Arteries of the anterior (white) and posterior (blue) cerebral circulation in relation to the circle of Willis.

Table 9–1. Territories of the principal cerebral arteries.

Artery	Territory
Anterior circulation	
Internal carotid	
Anterior choroidal	Hippocampus, globus pallidus, lower internal capsule
Anterior cerebral	Medial frontal and parietal cortex and subjacent white matter, anterior corpus callosum
Middle cerebral	Lateral frontal, parietal, occipital, and temporal cortex and subjacent white matter
Lenticulostriate branches	Caudate nucleus, putamen, upper internal capsule
Posterior circulation	
Vertebral	
Posterior inferior cerebellar	Medulla, lower cerebellium
Basilar	
Anterior inferior cerebellar	Lower and midpons, mid cerebellum
Superior cerebellar	Upper pons, lower midbrain, upper cerebellum
Posterior cerebral	Medial occipital and temporal cortex and subjacent white matter, posterior corpus callosum, upper midbrain
Thalamoperforate branches	Thalamus
Thalamogeniculate branches	Thalamus

sible to distinguish between ischemia and hemorrhage from the history and neurologic examination, but CT scan or MRI permits a definitive diagnosis.

A. ISCHEMIA

Interruption of blood flow to the brain deprives neurons and other cells of substrate glucose and oxygen and, unless blood flow is promptly restored, leads ultimately to cell death. The pattern of cell death depends on the

Table 9–2. Symptoms and signs of anterior and posterior circulation ischemia.[1]

Symptom or Sign	Incidence (%)[2]	
	Anterior	Posterior
Headache	25	3
Altered consciousness	5	16
Aphasia[3]	20	0
Visual field defect	14	22
Diplopia[3]	0	7
Vertigo[3]	0	48
Dysarthria	3	11
Drop attacks[3]	0	16
Hemi- or monoparesis	38	12
Hemisensory deficit	33	9

[1] Modified from Hutchinson EC, Acheson EJ: *Strokes: Natural History, Pathology and Surgical Treatment.* Saunders, 1975.

[2] Most patients have multiple symptoms and signs.

[3] Most useful distinguishing features.

severity of ischemia. With mild ischemia, as may occur in cardiac arrest with reperfusion, **selective vulnerability** of certain neuronal populations results in their preferential loss. More severe ischemia produces **selective neuronal necrosis,** in which all neurons die but glia and endothelial cells are preserved. Complete, permanent ischemia causes **pannecrosis,** affecting all cell types, and results in the chronic cavitary brain lesions seen after clinical stroke.

Ischemic neuronal injury is an active biochemical process that evolves over time (Figure 9–3). Lack of glucose and oxygen depletes the cellular energy stores required to maintain membrane potentials and transmembrane ion gradients. Potassium leaks out of cells, causing depolarization-induced calcium entry, and also stimulates the release of glutamate through glial glutamate transporters. Synaptic glutamate activates **excitatory amino acid receptors** coupled to calcium- and sodium-preferring ion channels. The resulting influx of sodium into postsynaptic neuronal cell bodies and dendrites causes depolarization and acute swelling. Calcium influx that exceeds the ability of the cell to extrude, sequester, or buffer calcium activates calcium-dependent enzymes (proteases, lipases, and nucleases). These enzymes and their metabolic products, such as eicosanoids and oxygen free radicals, cause the breakdown of plasma membranes and cytoskeletal elements, leading to cell death. This sequence of events has been termed **excitotoxicity** because of the pivotal role of excitatory amino acids such as glutamate.

Where ischemia is incomplete and therefore permits more prolonged cell survival—as in the **border zone** or **penumbra** surrounding the **core** of an ischemic brain

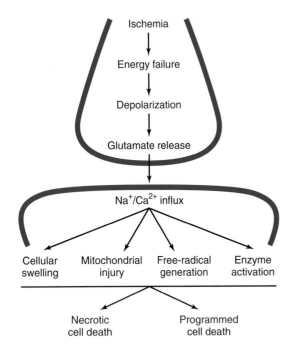

Ischemia
↓
Energy failure
↓
Depolarization
↓
Glutamate release
↓
Na^+/Ca^{2+} influx

Cellular swelling   Mitochondrial injury   Free-radical generation   Enzyme activation

Necrotic cell death   Programmed cell death

Figure 9–3. Pathogenesis of ischemic neuronal death. Ischemia deprives the brain of metabolic substrates, especially oxygen and glucose, making it impossible for cells to carry out energy-dependent functions such as the maintenance of trans-membrane ion gradients. Loss of these gradients depolarizes cell membranes, leading to the influx of calcium through voltage-gated calcium channels and triggering the release of neurotransmitters such as glutamate from presynaptic nerve terminals. Glutamate binds to receptors on the postsynaptic neuronal membrane to activate the influx of sodium and calcium. This sets in motion a cascade of biochemical events that causes cellular swelling, injures mitochondria, generates toxic free radicals, and activates proteases, nucleases, and other enzymes. Depending on the severity and duration of ischemia, neurons may die rapidly, from necrosis, or more gradually, from programmed cell death or apoptosis. Necrotic cell death is characterized by shrinkage of the nucleus (pyknosis), early loss of membrane integrity, structural changes in mitochondria, and eventually cellular lysis. Apoptosis, which depends on the synthesis of new proteins, is associated with margination of nuclear chromatin, relative preservation of cell membrane and mitochondrial integrity, and the formation of membrane-bound extracellular blebs (apoptotic bodies). Necrosis and apoptosis can coexist in different regions of an ischemic lesion.

region—other biochemical processes that regulate cell death may be set into motion. These include the expression of proteins involved in **programmed cell death,** such as Bcl (B-cell lymphoma)-2-family proteins and caspases (proenzymes for cysteine proteases that cleave at aspartate residues). The action of these proteins may lead to **apoptosis,** a form of programmed cell death that is distinct from **necrosis** and is characterized by margination of nuclear chromatin, cleavage of DNA into fragments of defined length (nucleosomes), relative preservation of cell membrane integrity, blebbing of the plasma membrane to form apoptotic bodies, and phagocytosis without inflammation.

If the blood flow to ischemic brain tissue is restored before neurons are irreversibly injured, the clinical symptoms and signs are transient. Prolonged interruption of blood flow, however, leads to irreversible ischemic injury (**infarction**) and persistent neurologic deficits.

Two pathogenetic mechanisms can produce ischemic stroke—thrombosis and embolism. While about two-thirds of ischemic strokes are attributed to thrombosis and about one-third to embolism, the distinction is often difficult or impossible to make on clinical grounds.

1. Thrombosis produces stroke by occluding large cerebral arteries (especially the internal carotid, middle cerebral, or basilar), small penetrating arteries (as in lacunar stroke), cerebral veins, or venous sinuses. Symptoms typically evolve over minutes to hours. Thrombotic strokes are often preceded by TIAs, which tend to produce similar symptoms because they affect the same territory recurrently.

2. Embolism produces stroke when cerebral arteries are occluded by the distal passage of thrombus from the heart, aortic arch, or large cerebral arteries. Emboli in the anterior cerebral circulation most often occlude the middle cerebral artery or its branches, since about 85% of the hemispheric blood flow is carried by this vessel. Emboli in the posterior cerebral circulation usually lodge at the apex of the basilar artery or in the posterior cerebral arteries. Embolic strokes characteristically produce neurologic deficits that are maximal at onset. When TIAs precede embolic strokes, especially those arising from a cardiac source, symptoms typically vary between attacks since different vascular territories are affected.

B. Hemorrhage

Hemorrhage may interfere with cerebral function through a variety of mechanisms, including destruction or compression of brain tissue and compression of vascular structures, leading to secondary ischemia and edema. Intracranial hemorrhage is classified by its location as intracerebral, subarachnoid, subdural, or epidural, all of which—except subdural hemorrhage—are usually caused by arterial bleeding.

1. Intracerebral hemorrhage causes symptoms by compressing adjacent tissue (which can then produce local ischemia) and, to a lesser extent, by destroying tissue. Unlike ischemic stroke, intracerebral hemorrhage tends to cause more severe headache and depression of consciousness as well as neurologic deficits that do not correspond to the distribution of any single blood vessel.

2. Subarachnoid hemorrhage leads to cerebral dysfunction by elevating intracranial pressure as well as by exerting still poorly understood toxic effects of subarachnoid blood on brain tissue. In addition, subarachnoid hemorrhage may be complicated by vasospasm (leading to ischemia), rebleeding, extension of blood into brain tissue (producing an intracerebral hematoma), or hydrocephalus. Subarachnoid hemorrhage typically presents with headache rather than focal neurologic deficits; it is discussed in Chapter 2.

3. Subdural or epidural hemorrhage produces a mass lesion that can compress the underlying brain. These hemorrhages are often traumatic in origin, and usually present with headache or altered consciousness. Because their recognition is most critical in the setting of coma, subdural and epidural hemorrhage are discussed in Chapter 10.

FOCAL CEREBRAL ISCHEMIA

Etiology

A variety of disorders of the blood, blood vessels, and heart can lead to focal cerebral ischemia (Table 9–3).

A. VASCULAR DISORDERS

1. Atherosclerosis—Atherosclerosis of the large extracranial arteries in the neck and at the base of the brain is the underlying cause of focal cerebral ischemia in the great majority of cases. Atherosclerosis affects large and medium-sized elastic and muscular arteries. Within the cerebral circulation, the sites of predilection (Figure 9–4) are the origin of the common carotid artery, the internal carotid artery just above the common carotid bifurcation and within the cavernous sinus, the origin of the middle cerebral artery, the vertebral artery at its origin and just above where it enters the skull, and the basilar artery.

The pathogenesis of atherosclerosis is incompletely understood, but injury to and resulting dysfunction of vascular endothelial cells is thought to be an early step. Endothelial cells may be injured by low-density lipoproteins, free radicals, hypertension, diabetes, homocysteine, or infectious agents. Blood monocytes and T lymphocytes adhere to the sites of endothelial injury and subsequently migrate subendothelially, where monocytes and monocyte-derived macrophages are transformed into lipid-laden foam cells. The resulting lesion is called a

Table 9–3. Conditions associated with focal cerebral ischemia.

Vascular disorders
  Atherosclerosis
  Fibromuscular dysplasia
  Inflammatory disorders
    Giant cell arteritis
    Systemic lupus erythematosus
    Polyarteritis nodosa
    Granulomatous angiitis
    Syphilitic arteritis
    AIDS
  Carotid or vertebral artery dissection
  Lacunar infarction
  Drug abuse
  Migraine
  Multiple progressive intracranial occlusions (moyamoya syndrome)
  Venous or sinus thrombosis
Cardiac disorders
  Mural thrombus
  Rheumatic heart disease
  Arrhythmias
  Endocarditis
  Mitral valve prolapse
  Paradoxic embolus
  Atrial myxoma
  Prosthetic heart valves
Hematologic disorders
  Thrombocytosis
  Polycythemia
  Sickle cell disease
  Leukocytosis
  Hypercoagulable states

fatty streak. The release of growth and chemotactic factors from endothelial cells and macrophages stimulates the proliferation and migration of intimal smooth muscle cells, and leads to formation of a **fibrous plaque.** Platelets adhere to sites of endothelial injury and release growth and chemotactic factors. The resulting atheromatous lesion (Figure 9–5) may enlarge or rupture to occlude the vessel lumen, or it may provide a source of atheromatous or platelet emboli. Ulcerated atheromas may be especially likely sources of emboli.

The most important risk factor for atherosclerosis leading to stroke is systolic or diastolic hypertension. In one study of more than 5000 symptom-free men and women aged from 30 to 60 years followed prospectively for 18 years, the likelihood of hypertensive subjects developing stroke was seven times that of the nonhypertensive subjects. Furthermore, the incidence of all the

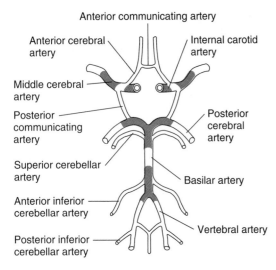

Anterior communicating artery

Anterior cerebral artery

Internal carotid artery

Middle cerebral artery

Posterior communicating artery

Posterior cerebral artery

Superior cerebellar artery

Basilar artery

Anterior inferior cerebellar artery

Vertebral artery

Posterior inferior cerebellar artery

Figure 9–4. Sites of predilection (blue areas) for atherosclerosis in the intracranial arterial circulation.

major cardiac and cerebrovascular sequelae of hypertension increased in direct proportion to the blood pressure even in the nonhypertensive range, without any identifiable critical or safe value. A blood pressure of 160 mm Hg systolic or 95 mm Hg diastolic observed during any clinic visit tripled the risk of stroke, suggesting that such patients should receive antihypertensive treatment.

Atherosclerosis can also occur in the absence of hypertension. In such cases, other factors such as diabetes, elevated serum cholesterol and triglycerides, hyperhomocysteinemia, cigarette smoking, hereditary predisposition, and the use of oral contraceptives may be implicated. Genetic disorders associated with accelerated atherosclerosis include homocystinuria and dyslipoproteinemias.

2. Other inflammatory disorders

a. Giant cell arteritis (see Chapter 2), also called temporal arteritis, produces inflammatory changes that affect branches of the external carotid, cervical internal carotid, posterior ciliary, extracranial vertebral, and intracranial arteries. Inflammatory changes in the arterial wall may stimulate platelet adhesion and aggregation on damaged surfaces, leading to thrombosis or distal embolism. Physical examination may show tender, nodular, or pulseless temporal arteries. Laboratory findings include an increased erythrocyte sedimentation rate and evidence of vascular stenosis or occlusion on angiography or color duplex ultrasonography. Definitive diagnosis is by temporal artery biopsy. Although it is an uncommon cause of cerebral ischemic symptoms, giant cell arteritis should be considered in patients with transient monocu-

lar blindness or transient cerebral ischemic attacks—especially elderly patients—because the disorder is responsive to corticosteroid therapy and its complications (especially permanent blindness) may thus be avoided.

b. Systemic lupus erythematosus is associated with a vasculopathy that involves small cerebral vessels and leads to multiple microinfarctions. Inflammatory changes characteristic of true vasculitis are absent. Libman-Sacks endocarditis may also be a source of cardiogenic emboli.

c. Polyarteritis nodosa is a segmental vasculitis of small and medium-sized arteries that affects multiple organs. Transient symptoms of cerebral ischemia, including typical spells of transient monocular blindness, can occur.

d. Granulomatous angiitis (also called primary angiitis of the central nervous system) is an idiopathic inflammatory disease that affects small arteries and veins in the central nervous system and can cause transient or progressive multifocal lesions. Clinical features include headache, hemiparesis and other focal neurologic abnormalities, and cognitive disturbances. The cerebrospinal fluid (CSF) usually shows pleocytosis and elevated protein, but because the systemic vasculature is spared, the erythrocyte sedimentation rate is typically normal. The diagnosis should be suspected in any patient with multifocal central nervous system dysfunction and CSF pleocytosis. Angiography demonstrates focal and segmental narrowing of small arteries and veins, and a meningeal biopsy is diagnostic. Treatment with corticosteroids, alone or in combination with cyclophosphamide, may be beneficial.

e. Syphilitic arteritis occurs within 5 years after a primary syphilitic infection and reflects the underlying meningeal inflammatory process. It is important to recognize and treat the disorder at this early stage to prevent the development of tertiary parenchymal neurosyphilis (general paresis or tabes dorsalis). Medium-sized penetrating vessels are typically involved (Figure 9–6), producing punctate areas of infarction in the deep white matter of the cerebral hemisphere, that can be seen on CT scan or MRI.

f. AIDS is associated with an increased incidence of TIAs and ischemic stroke. In some cases, ischemic neurologic complications of AIDS are associated with endocarditis or with opportunistic infections of the central nervous system, such as toxoplasmosis or cryptococcal meningitis.

3. Fibromuscular dysplasia—This affects large arteries of children and young adults, producing segmental thinning of the media and fragmentation of the elastic lamina, alternating with rings of fibrous and muscular hyperplasia within the media. Extracranial vessels are involved more often than intracranial ones, and the cervical portion of the internal carotid artery is involved more than

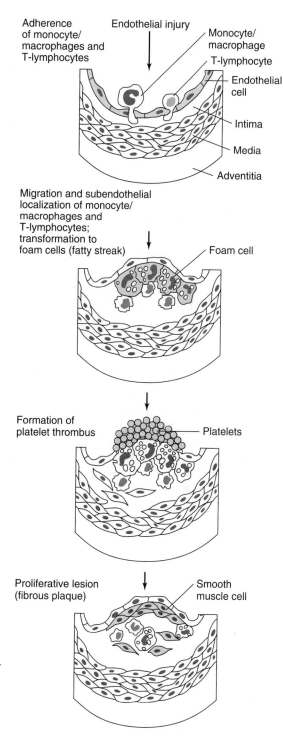

Figure 9–5. Arterial lesion in atherosclerosis. Endothelial injury permits circulating mononuclear cells to adhere to the vessel wall and then migrate beneath the endothelial layer, where they form a fatty streak. The subsequent attachment of platelets and proliferation of smooth muscle cells within this lesion produce a fibrous plaque arising from the intimal surface. This encroaches on the arterial lumen and may occlude the vessel or provide a source of emboli.

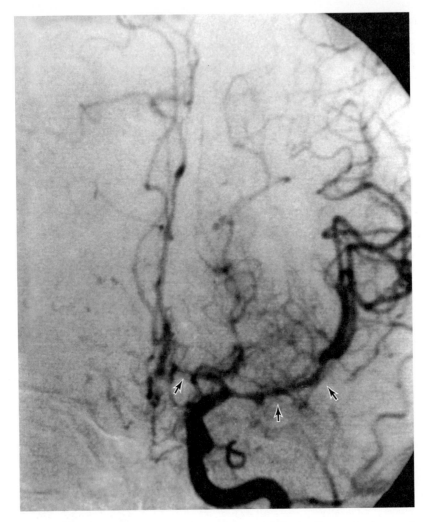

Figure 9–6. Left carotid angiogram (AP projection) in syphilitic arteritis showing marked narrowing of the proximal middle cerebral artery **(arrows at right)** and anterior cerebral artery **(arrow at left)**. (Reproduced, with permission, from Lowenstein DH, Mills C, Simon RP: Acute syphilitic transverse myelitis: unusual presentation of meningovascular syphilis. Genitourin Med 1987;63:333–338.)

the vertebral artery. Lesions are often bilateral. Fibromuscular dysphasia may be inherited as an autosomal dominant disorder and is more common in women than in men. Symptoms may be due to the embolization of vascular thrombi. There is a characteristic "string-of-beads" appearance on angiography. Antiplatelet drugs or intraluminal dilation of affected extracranial vessels may be beneficial in symptomatic cases.

4. Carotid or vertebral artery dissection—Dissection of the carotid or vertebral artery is associated with hemorrhage into the vessel wall, which can occlude the vessel or predispose to thrombus formation and em-

bolization. Posttraumatic carotid dissections present little difficulty in diagnosis. Certain patients, however—usually young men—suffer cerebral infarction after apparently spontaneous carotid artery dissection. Internal carotid artery dissections usually originate near the carotid bifurcation and can extend to the base of the skull. The underlying pathologic process is usually **cystic medial necrosis**. Prodromal transient hemispheric ischemia or monocular blindness sometimes precedes a devastating stroke. Carotid dissection may be accompanied by pain in the jaw or neck, visual abnormalities akin to those that occur in migraine, or Horner's syndrome.

Dissection of the vertebral or basilar artery is less common. The clinical features of this disorder include headache, posterior neck pain, and the sudden onset of signs of brainstem dysfunction.

The treatment of carotid or vertebral artery dissection is controversial. Approaches include no treatment, removal of the intramural hematoma, and measures to prevent embolization from the site of dissection (aspirin, anticoagulants, or occlusion of the vessel distal to the dissection). Recurrent dissection is uncommon and usually occurs within 1 month of the initial event.

5. Lacunar infarction—Lacunar infarction of the brain results from the occlusion of small penetrating branches of the major cerebral arteries, especially those that supply the basal ganglia, thalamus, internal capsule, and pons. Lacunar infarcts are believed to be caused by either atherosclerosis or degenerative changes in arterial walls (including lipohyalinosis and fibrinoid necrosis) that are related to long-standing hypertension. Both hypertension and diabetes appear to predispose to this type of stroke.

6. Drug abuse—Use of **cocaine** hydrochloride, alkaloidal (crack) cocaine, amphetamines, or heroin is a risk factor for stroke in patients younger than 35 years old. Patients who take these agents intravenously may develop infective endocarditis (see below) leading to embolic stroke. Stroke also occurs in drug users without endocarditis, however, including those who take drugs only intranasally or by smoke or vapor inhalation, and often has its onset within hours of drug use. Mechanisms that have been proposed to explain these events include drug-induced vasospasm, vasculitis, and the rupture of preexisting aneurysms or vascular malformations. Cocaine hydrochloride is most often associated with intracerebral hemorrhage but can also cause subarachnoid hemorrhage or ischemic stroke. Stroke from crack cocaine is most commonly ischemic in origin, but intracerebral or subarachnoid hemorrhage also occurs. **Amphetamines** can produce vasculitis, with necrosis of the vessel wall leading to intracerebral hemorrhage; ischemic stroke and subarachnoid hemorrhage are less frequent. Other sympathomimetic amines, including **phenylpropanolamine** and **ephedrine,** are also associated with an increased risk of stroke. **Heroin** is associated primarily with embolic stroke resulting from endocarditis.

7. Multiple progressive intracranial arterial occlusions (moyamoya)—This syndrome has two essential features: bilateral narrowing or occlusion of the distal internal carotid arteries and the adjacent anterior and middle cerebral artery trunks; and the presence of a fine network of collateral channels at the base of the brain. The term *moyamoya* derives from a Japanese word meaning *smoke* or *haze,* which characterizes the angiographic appearance of these fine collaterals (Figure 9–7). Moyamoya is most common in Japanese girls and is sometimes inherited as an autosomal recessive disorder that maps to chromosome 3p26–p24.2, but occurs in all ethnic groups and in patients with atherosclerosis, sickle cell anemia, or a history of basilar meningitis. The term therefore denotes an angiographic pattern of collateral vessels rather than a clinical or pathologic syndrome. Children tend to present with ischemic strokes; adults present with intracerebral, subdural, or subarachnoid hemorrhage. Transient episodes of cerebral ischemia are infrequent.

8. Migraine—Migraine with aura has been proposed as a cause of stroke, but in many cases, other stroke risk factors (eg, oral contraceptive use) may coexist. Stroke in migraineurs may occur during an attack of classic migraine and in the same vascular territory affected by previous migraine attacks. The anterior (especially the middle cerebral artery) and posterior (especially the posterior cerebral artery) cerebral circulations are affected about equally often. Investigative studies show no other cause of stroke (eg, occlusion of large cerebral arteries).

9. Venous or sinus thrombosis—This uncommon cause of stroke is typically associated with a predisposing condition such as otitis or sinusitis, a postpartum state, dehydration, or coagulopathy. Clinical features include headache, papilledema, impaired consciousness, seizures, and focal neurologic deficits. CSF pressure is typically increased, and in cases of septic thrombosis, pleocytosis may occur. A CT scan may demonstrate hemorrhage associated with venous infarction, and in superior sagittal sinus thrombosis a CT scan with contrast sometimes shows a filling defect corresponding to the clot (delta sign). However, MRI with contrast is the diagnostic procedure of choice in most cases. The diagnosis may be confirmed by MR angiography, but conventional intraarterial x-ray angiography is now rarely indicated. In patients presenting with headache and papilledema, venous or sinus thrombosis must be differentiated from intracranial mass lesions and idiopathic pseudotumor cerebri. The radiologic studies mentioned above are useful in this regard. Septic thromboses are treated with antibiotics. Anticoagulation has been used for aseptic thrombosis, but its efficacy has not been proved, and it may precipitate intracranial hemorrhage.

B. Cardiac Disorders

1. Mural thrombus—Mural thrombus complicating myocardial infarction or cardiomyopathy is a recognized source of cerebral embolism. The risk of stroke in the first weeks after myocardial infarction is related to the size of the cardiac lesion. More extensive myocardial damage may increase the tendency for mural thrombi to form; it may exacerbate the generalized hypercoagulable

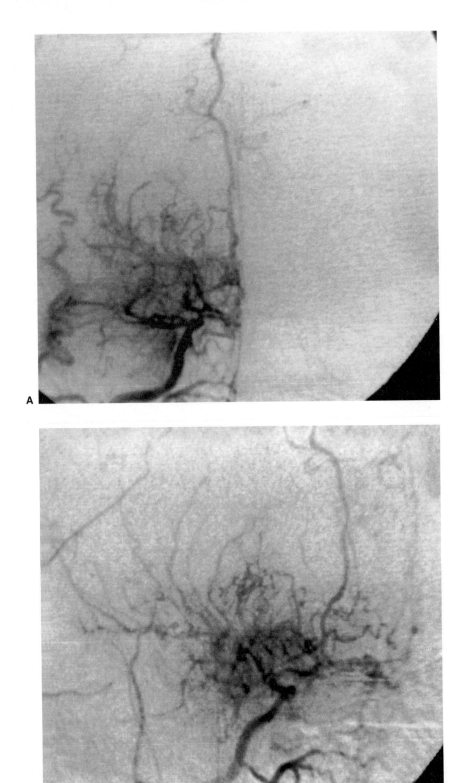

Figure 9–7. Right carotid angiogram in moyamoya. The middle cerebral artery and its branches are replaced by a diffuse capillary pattern that has the appearance of a puff of smoke. **A:** AP view. **B:** lateral view.

state that accompanies the infarct—or it may do both. Accordingly, patients with large transmural myocardial infarcts require anticoagulation therapy to substantially reduce the incidence of early thromboembolic events, including stroke.

2. Rheumatic heart disease—The incidence of focal cerebral ischemia is increased in patients with rheumatic heart disease—particularly those with mitral stenosis and atrial fibrillation—presumably as a result of embolization. In other cases, symptoms are temporally related to exertion, suggesting hypoperfusion as the cause.

3. Arrhythmias—Atrial fibrillation (especially when associated with rheumatic heart disease) and the bradycardia-tachycardia (sick sinus) syndrome are well-recognized causes of embolic stroke. Other cardiac arrhythmias are more likely to produce pancerebral hypoperfusion with diffuse rather than focal symptoms (eg, syncope, dimming of vision, nonspecific lightheadedness, generalized seizures) unless severe carotid artery stenosis is also present.

4. Endocarditis

a. Infective (bacterial or fungal) endocarditis is a cause of transient cerebral ischemia and embolic cerebral infarction during the active phase of infection and during the first few months following antibiotic cure. At autopsy, cerebral emboli are identified in 30% and systemic emboli in 60% of such patients. The middle cerebral artery is the most common site of cerebral embolization. Intracerebral or subarachnoid hemorrhage can also occur as a result of bleeding into an infarct or rupture of a mycotic aneurysm. Infective endocarditis is seen most often in intravenous drug users and patients with valvular heart disease or prosthetic valves. Streptococci and staphylococci are the most common causes, but gram-negative bacilli (eg, *Pseudomonas*) and fungi (especially *Candida* and *Aspergillus*) are also frequent pathogens in intravenous drug users and prosthetic valve recipients.

Signs of infective endocarditis include heart murmurs, petechiae, subungual splinter hemorrhages, retinal Roth's spots (red spots with white centers), Osler's nodes (painful red or purple digital nodules), Janeway's lesions (red macules on the palms or soles), and clubbing of the fingers or toes. The diagnosis is usually made by culturing the responsible organism from the blood. Treatment is with antibiotics; valve replacement is sometimes required. Anticoagulation should be avoided because of the risk of intracranial hemorrhage.

b. Nonbacterial (marantic) endocarditis is most frequent in patients with cancer and is responsible for the vast majority of ischemic strokes in this population. The tumors most often associated with this type of stroke are adenocarcinomas of the lung or gastrointestinal tract. Vegetations are present on the mitral or aortic valves; associated murmurs are rare. Identification of valvular vegetations by two-dimensional echocardiography may be diagnostic, but failure to demonstrate vegetations does not exclude the diagnosis. Anticoagulation with heparin may be useful in patients with treatable tumors or with other treatable causes of marantic endocarditis, such as sepsis.

5. Mitral valve prolapse—Buckling of the mitral valve due to stretching of the mitral annulus (mitral valve prolapse) is common, occurring in 4–8% of young adults, and usually produces no symptoms. In some cases there appears to be an association with cerebral ischemia, but the degree to which the disorder increases the risk of stroke is apparently small, and massive strokes related to mitral valve prolapse are rare.

6. Paradoxic embolus—Congenital cardiac anomalies associated with a pathologic communication between the right and left sides of the heart, such as atrial septal defect or patent foramen ovale, permit the passage of embolic material from the systemic venous circulation to the brain. Under these circumstances, venous thrombi can give rise to embolic stroke.

7. Atrial myxoma—This rare disorder can lead to either embolization (producing stroke) or cardiac outflow obstruction (producing syncope). Embolic events occur in one-fourth to one-half of patients with nonhereditary left atrial myxoma; some cases, however, are familial. Hemorrhagic strokes may occur. Diagnosis is by echocardiography.

8. Prosthetic heart valves—Patients with prosthetic heart valves are at particular risk for cerebral emboli and are generally treated with anticoagulants on a long-term basis.

C. HEMATOLOGICAL DISORDERS

1. Thrombocytosis—Thrombocytosis occurs in myeloproliferative disorders, other neoplastic or infections diseases, and following splenectomy. Thrombocytosis may predispose to focal cerebral ischemia when the platelet count exceeds 1,000,000/μL.

2. Polycythemia—Patients with polycythemia may have focal neurologic symptoms that respond to venesection. Hematocrits above 46% are associated with reduced cerebral blood flow, and the risk of stroke. This risk increases with hematocrits of more than 50%, and rises dramatically above 60%.

3. Sickle cell disease—Sickle cell (hemoglobin S) disease is due to a single amino acid substitution (Glu-6-Val) in the hemoglobin beta locus on chromosome 11 (11p15.5) that results in an abnormal beta hemoglobin chain. Persons of African, especially West African, descent are most frequently affected. The mutation causes the sickle-shaped deformation of erythrocytes when the partial pressure of oxygen in blood is reduced, and produces hemolytic anemia and vascular occlusions, which may be extremely painful (sickle cell crises). Homozygotes are more severely affected than heterozygotes. The most frequent neurologic complication is stroke, which characteristically affects the intracranial internal carotid or proximal middle or anterior cerebral artery. Detection of increased cerebral blood flow velocity by transcranial Doppler studies may help to identify individuals at increased risk for stroke. Therapies in clinical or experimental use include hydration and analgesia for painful crises, blood transfusion, hydroxyurea (which increases levels of fetal hemoglobin), and bone marrow or hematopoietic stem cell transplantation. In patients with sickle cell disease who must undergo angiography, the level of hemoglobin S should be reduced by exchange transfusion to less than 20%, since radiologic contrast media may induce sickling.

4. Leukocytosis—Transient cerebral ischemia has been reported in association with leukocytosis, usually in patients with leukemia and white blood cell counts in excess of 150,000/μL.

5. Hypercoagulable states—Hyperviscosity of the serum from paraproteinemia (especially macroglobulinemia) is an infrequent cause of focal cerebral ischemia. Estrogen therapy, oral contraceptive use, postpartum and postoperative states, and cancer may be accompanied by coagulopathies that lead to cerebral thrombosis or embolism.

Antiphospholipid antibodies, including lupus anticoagulants and anticardiolipin antibodies, may be associated with an increased incidence of ischemic stroke. Stroke has also been reported in patients with hereditary coagulopathies, including heparin cofactor II deficiency, protein C deficiency, defective release of plasminogen activator, and factor XII deficiency.

Pathology

A. Infarction in Major-Cerebral-Artery Distribution

On gross inspection at autopsy, a recent infarct is a swollen, softened area of brain that usually affects both gray and white matter. Microscopy shows acute ischemic changes in neurons (shrinkage, microvacuolization, dark staining), destruction of glial cells, necrosis of small blood vessels, disruption of nerve axons and myelin, and accumulation of interstitial fluid from vasogenic edema. In some cases, perivascular hemorrhages are observed in the infarcted area.

Cerebral infarcts are typically associated with cerebral edema, which is maximal during the first 4 or 5 days after onset. Most deaths that occur within 1 week after massive cerebral infarction are attributable to cerebral edema, with swelling of the affected hemisphere causing herniation of the ipsilateral cingulate gyrus across the midline beneath the free edge of the dural falx, followed by downward displacement of the brain through the tentorial incisure.

B. Lacunar Infarction

In contrast to infarcts associated with major cerebral blood vessels, smaller lacunar infarcts result from lipohyalinosis of small resistance vessels, usually in patients with chronic hypertension. Lacunar infarcts—often multiple—are found in about 10% of brains at autopsy. The pathologic appearance is of small cavities ranging in size from 0.5 to 15 mm in diameter.

Clinicoanatomic Correlation

A rational clinical approach to cerebral ischemia depends on the ability to identify the neuroanatomic basis of clinical deficits.

A. Anterior Cerebral Artery

1. Anatomy—The anterior cerebral artery supplies the parasagittal cerebral cortex (Figures 9–8 and 9–9), which includes portions of motor and sensory cortex related to the contralateral leg and the so-called bladder inhibitory or micturition center.

2. Clinical syndrome of anterior cerebral artery occlusion—Anterior cerebral artery strokes are uncommon, perhaps because emboli from the extracranial vessels or the heart are more apt to enter the larger-caliber middle cerebral artery, which receives the bulk of cerebral blood flow. There is a contralateral paralysis and sensory loss affecting the leg. Voluntary control of micturition may be impaired because of failure to inhibit reflex bladder contractions, resulting in precipitate micturition.

B. Middle Cerebral Artery

1. Anatomy—The middle cerebral artery supplies most of the remainder of the cerebral hemisphere and deep subcortical structures (see Figures 9–8 and 9–9). The cortical branches of the middle cerebral artery include the **superior division,** which supplies the entire motor and sensory cortical representation of the face, hand, and arm; and the **expressive language (Broca's) area** of the dominant hemisphere (Figure 9–10). The **inferior division** supplies the visual radiations, the region of visual cortex related to macular vision, and the **receptive language (Wernicke's) area** of the dominant hemisphere. **Lenticulostriate** branches of the most proximal portion (stem) of the middle cerebral artery supply the basal ganglia as well as motor fibers related to the face, hand, arm, and leg as they descend in the genu and the posterior limb of the internal capsule.

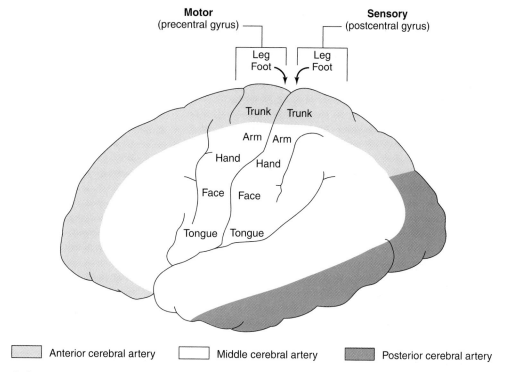

Figure 9–8. Arterial supply of the primary motor and sensory cortex (lateral view).

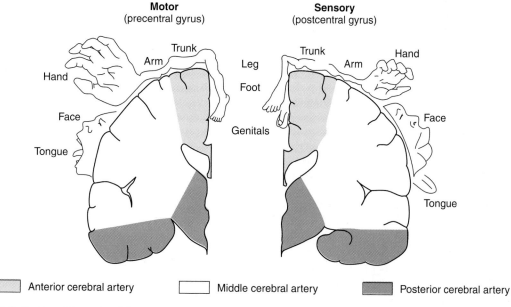

Figure 9–9. Arterial supply of the primary motor and sensory cortex (coronal view).

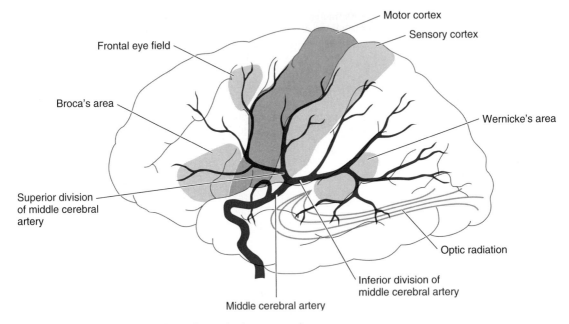

Figure 9–10. Anatomic basis of middle cerebral artery syndromes.

2. Clinical syndrome of middle cerebral artery occlusion—The middle cerebral artery is the vessel most commonly involved in ischemic stroke. Depending on the site of involvement, several clinical syndromes can occur (see Figure 9–10).

a. Superior division stroke results in contralateral hemiparesis that affects the face, hand, and arm but spares the leg; contralateral hemisensory deficit in the same distribution; but no homonymous hemianopia. If the dominant hemisphere is involved, these features are combined with Broca's (expressive) aphasia, which is characterized by impairment of language expression with intact comprehension.

b. Inferior division stroke is less common in isolation and results in contralateral homonymous hemianopia that may be denser inferiorly; marked impairment of cortical sensory functions, such as graphesthesia and stereognosis on the contralateral side of the body; and disorders of spatial thought, including a lack of awareness that a deficit exists (anosognosia), neglect of and failure to recognize the contralateral limbs, neglect of the contralateral side of external space, dressing apraxia, and constructional apraxia. If the dominant hemisphere is involved, Wernicke's (receptive) aphasia occurs and is manifested by impaired comprehension and fluent but often nonsensical speech. With involvement of the nondominant hemisphere, an acute confusional state may occur.

c. Occlusion at the bifurcation or trifurcation of the middle cerebral artery involves a lesion situated at the point where the artery splits into two (superior and inferior) or three (superior, middle, and inferior) major divisions. This severe stroke syndrome combines the features of superior and inferior division stroke. Its clinical features include contralateral hemiparesis and hemisensory deficit involving the face and arm far more than the leg; homonymous hemianopia; and, if the dominant hemisphere is affected, global (combined expressive and receptive) aphasia.

d. Occlusion of the stem of the middle cerebral artery occurs proximal to the origin of the lenticulostriate branches. Because the entire territory of the artery is affected, this is the most devastating of middle cerebral artery strokes. The resulting clinical syndrome is similar to that seen following occlusion at the trifurcation except that, in addition, infarction of motor fibers in the internal capsule causes paralysis of the contralateral leg. The result is a contralateral hemiplegia and sensory loss affecting the face, hand, arm, and leg.

C. INTERNAL CAROTID ARTERY

1. Anatomy—The internal carotid artery arises where the common carotid artery divides into internal and external carotid branches in the neck. In addition to its anterior cerebral and middle cerebral branches discussed above, the internal carotid artery also gives rise to the ophthalmic artery, which supplies the retina. The severity of internal carotid artery strokes is highly variable, depending on the adequacy of collateral circulation, which tends to develop in compensation for a slowly evolving occlusion.

2. Clinical syndrome of internal carotid artery occlusion—Intra- or extracranial internal carotid artery occlusion is responsible for about one-fifth of ischemic strokes. In approximately 15% of cases, progressive atherosclerotic occlusion of the internal carotid artery is preceded by premonitory TIAs or by **transient monocular blindness** caused by ipsilateral retinal artery ischemia.

Carotid artery occlusion may be asymptomatic. Symptomatic occlusion results in a syndrome similar to that of middle cerebral artery stroke (contralateral hemiplegia, hemisensory deficit, and homonymous hemianopia; aphasia is also present with dominant hemisphere involvement).

D. Posterior Cerebral Artery

1. Anatomy—The paired posterior cerebral arteries arise from the tip of the basilar artery (Figure 9–11) and supply the occipital cerebral cortex, medial temporal lobes, thalamus, and rostral midbrain. Emboli carried up the basilar artery tend to lodge at its apex, where they can occlude one or both posterior cerebral arteries. These emboli can subsequently break up and produce signs of asymmetric or patchy posterior cerebral artery infarction.

2. Clinical syndrome of posterior cerebral artery occlusion—Occlusion of a posterior cerebral artery produces homonymous hemianopia affecting the contralateral visual field. Macular vision may be spared, however, because of the dual (middle and posterior cerebral artery) blood supply to the portion of the visual cortex representing the macula (see Chapter 4). In contrast to visual field defects from infarction in the middle cerebral artery territory, those caused by posterior cerebral artery occlusion may be denser superiorly. With occlusions near the origin of the posterior cerebral artery at the level of the midbrain, ocular abnormalities can include vertical gaze palsy, oculomotor (III) nerve palsy, internuclear ophthalmoplegia, and vertical skew deviation of the eyes. When posterior cerebral artery occlusion affects the occipital lobe of the dominant (usually left) hemisphere, patients may exhibit anomic aphasia (difficulty in naming objects), alexia without agraphia (inability to read, with no impairment of writing), or visual agnosia. The last is a failure to identify objects presented in the left side of the visual field, caused by a lesion of the corpus callosum that disconnects the right visual cortex from language areas of the left hemisphere. Bilateral posterior cerebral artery infarction may result in **cortical blindness,** memory impairment (from temporal lobe involvement), or the inability to recognize familiar faces (**prosopagnosia**), as well as a variety of exotic visual and behavioral syndromes.

E. Basilar Artery

1. Anatomy—The basilar artery usually arises from the junction of the paired vertebral arteries (Figure 9–11), though in some cases only a single vertebral artery is present. The basilar artery courses over the ventral surface of the brainstem to terminate at the level of the midbrain, where it bifurcates to form the posterior cerebral arteries (see above). Branches of the basilar artery supply the occipital and medial temporal lobes, the medial thalamus, the posterior limb of the internal capsule, and the entire brainstem and cerebellum.

2. Clinical syndromes of basilar artery occlusion—

a. Thrombosis—Thrombotic occlusion of the basilar artery (Figure 9–11A)—a serious event that is often

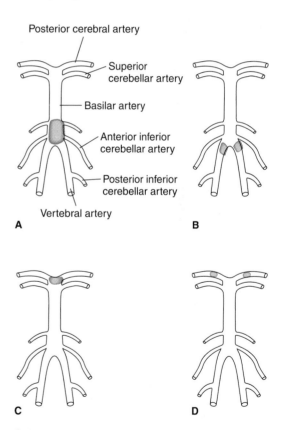

Figure 9–11. Sites of thrombotic and embolic occlusions in the vertebrobasilar circulation. **A:** Thrombotic occlusion of the basilar artery. **B:** Thrombotic occlusion of both vertebral arteries. **C:** Embolic occlusion at the apex of the basilar artery. **D:** Embolic occlusion of both posterior cerebral arteries.

incompatible with survival—produces bilateral neurologic signs referable to involvement of multiple branch arteries (Figure 9–12). Occlusion of both vertebral arteries (Figure 9–11B) or of a lone unpaired vertebral artery produces a similar syndrome. Temporary occlusion of one or both vertebral arteries can also occur in relation to rotation of the head in patients with cervical spondylosis, leading to transient symptoms and signs of brainstem dysfunction.

Major stenosis or occlusion of the subclavian artery before it has given rise to the vertebral artery can lead to the **subclavian steal syndrome,** in which blood passes from the vertebral artery into the distal subclavian artery with physical activity of the ipsilateral arm. The syndrome is a manifestation of generalized atherosclerosis and is not predictive of stroke in the vertebrobasilar system. Patients are usually asymptomatic, and stroke, when it occurs, is typically due to coexisting carotid lesions.

Basilar thrombosis usually affects the proximal portion of the basilar artery (Figure 9–11A), which supplies the pons. Involvement of the dorsal portion (tegmentum) of the pons produces unilateral or bilateral abducens (VI) nerve palsy; horizontal eye movements are impaired, but vertical nystagmus and ocular bobbing may be present. The pupils are constricted as a result of the involvement of descending sympathetic pupillodilator fibers in the pons, but they may remain reactive. Hemiplegia or quadriplegia is usually present, and coma is common. Although the syndrome of basilar occlusion in unconscious patients may be confused with pontine hemorrhage, a CT or MRI brain scan will differentiate the two.

In some patients with basilar occlusion, the ventral portion of the pons (basis pontis) is infarcted and the tegmentum is spared. Such patients remain conscious but quadriplegic. The term **locked-in syndrome** has been applied to this state. Locked-in patients may be able to signify that they are conscious by opening their eyes or moving their eyes vertically on command. In other cases, a conventional electroencephalogram (EEG) with stimulation may be needed to distinguish the locked-in state (in which the EEG is normal) from coma (see Chapter 10).

b. Embolism—Emboli small enough to pass through the vertebral arteries into the larger basilar artery are usually arrested at the top of the basilar artery, where it bifurcates into the posterior cerebral arteries (Figure 9–11C). The resulting reduction in blood flow to the ascending reticular formation of the midbrain and thalamus produces immediate loss or impairment of consciousness. Unilateral or bilateral oculomotor (III) nerve palsies are characteristic. Hemiplegia or quadriplegia with decerebrate or decorticate posturing occurs because of the involvement of the cerebral peduncles in the midbrain. Thus, the **top of the basilar syndrome** may be confused with midbrain failure

caused by transtentorial uncal herniation. Less commonly, an embolus may lodge more proximally in an atheromatous narrowed portion of the basilar artery, producing a syndrome indistinguishable from basilar thrombosis.

Smaller emboli may occlude the rostral basilar artery transiently before fragmenting and passing into one or both posterior cerebral arteries (Figure 9–11D). In such cases, portions of the midbrain, thalamus, and temporal and occipital lobes can be infarcted. If conscious, these patients display a variety of visual (homonymous hemianopia, cortical blindness), visuomotor (impaired convergence, paralysis of upward or downward gaze, diplopia), and behavioral (especially confusion) abnormalities without prominent motor dysfunction. Sluggish pupillary responses are a helpful sign of midbrain involvement.

**F. Long Circumferential
Vertebrobasilar Branches**

1. Anatomy—The long circumferential branches arising from the vertebral and basilar arteries are the posterior inferior cerebellar, the anterior inferior cerebellar, and the superior cerebellar arteries (Figure 9–12). These vessels supply the dorsolateral brainstem, including dorsolaterally situated cranial nerve nuclei (V, VII, VIII) and pathways entering and leaving the cerebellum in the cerebellar peduncles.

2. Clinical syndrome of long circumferential artery occlusion—Occlusion of one of the circumferential branches produces infarction in the dorsolateral area of the medulla or pons.

a. Posterior inferior cerebellar artery occlusion results in the **lateral medullary (Wallenberg's) syndrome** (see Chapter 3). This syndrome varies in its presentation with the extent of infarction, but it can include ipsilateral cerebellar ataxia, Horner's syndrome, and facial sensory deficit; contralateral impaired pain and temperature sensation; and nystagmus, vertigo, nausea, vomiting, dysphagia, dysarthria, and hiccup. The motor system is characteristically spared because of its ventral location in the brainstem.

b. Anterior inferior cerebellar artery occlusion leads to infarction of the lateral portion of the caudal pons and produces a syndrome with many of the same features. Horner's syndrome, dysphagia, dysarthria, and hiccup do not occur, however, but ipsilateral facial weakness, gaze palsy, deafness, and tinnitus are common findings.

c. The syndrome of lateral rostral pontine infarction from **superior cerebellar artery occlusion** resembles that associated with anterior inferior cerebellar artery lesions, but impaired optokinetic nystagmus or skew deviation of the eyes may occur. Auditory function is unaffected, and the contralateral sensory disturbance

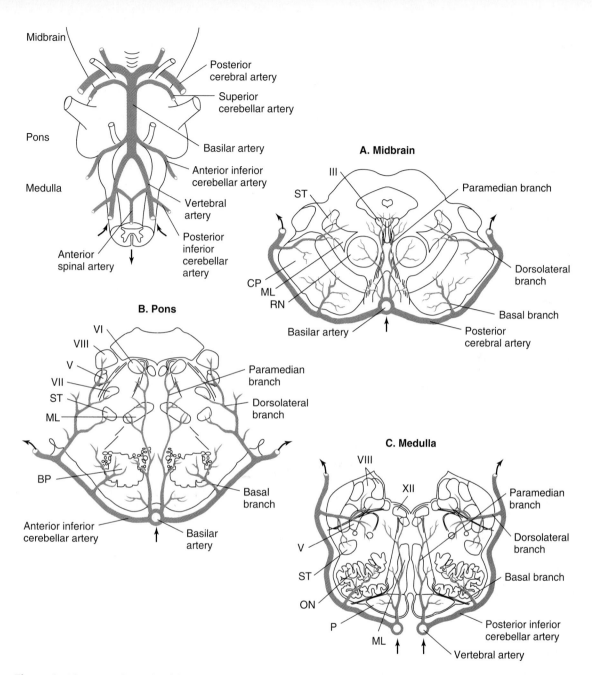

Figure 9–12. Arterial supply of the brainstem. **A:** Midbrain. The basilar artery gives off paramedian branches that supply the oculomotor (III) nerve nucleus and the red nucleus (RN). A larger branch, the posterior cerebral artery, courses laterally around the midbrain, giving off a basal branch that supplies the cerebral peduncle (CP) and a dorsolateral branch supplying the spinothalamic tract (ST) and medial lemniscus (ML). The posterior cerebral artery continues **(upper arrows)** to supply the thalamus, occipital lobe, and medial temporal lobe. **B:** Pons. Paramedian branches of the basilar artery supply the abducens (VI) nucleus and the medial lemniscus (ML). The anterior inferior cerebellar artery gives off a basal branch to the descending motor pathways in the basis pontis (BP) and a dorsolateral branch to the trigeminal (V) nucleus, the vestibular (VIII) nucleus, and the spinothalamic tract (ST), before passing to the cerebellum **(upper arrows)**. **C:** Medulla. Paramedian branches of the vertebral arteries supply descending motor pathways in the pyramid (P), the medial lemniscus (ML), and the hypoglossal (XII) nucleus. Another vertebral branch, the posterior inferior cerebellar artery, gives off a basal branch to the olivary nuclei (ON) and a dorsolateral branch that supplies the trigeminal (V) nucleus, the vestibular (VIII) nucleus, and the spinothalamic tract (ST), on its way to the cerebellum **(upper arrows)**.

may involve touch, vibration, and position sense as well as pain and temperature sense.

G. Long Penetrating Paramedian Vertebrobasilar Branches

1. Anatomy—Long penetrating paramedian arteries supply the medial brainstem from its ventral surface to the floor of the fourth ventricle. Structures located in this region include the medial portion of the cerebral peduncle, sensory pathways, the red nucleus, the reticular formation, and the midline cranial nerve nuclei (III, IV, VI, XII).

2. Clinical syndrome of long penetrating paramedian artery occlusion—Occlusion of a long penetrating artery causes paramedian infarction of the brainstem and results in contralateral hemiparesis if the cerebral peduncle is affected. Associated cranial nerve involvement depends on the level of the brainstem at which occlusion occurs. Occlusion in the **midbrain** results in ipsilateral third nerve palsy, which may be associated with contralateral tremor or ataxia from involvement of pathways connecting the red nucleus and cerebellum. Ipsilateral 6th and 7th nerve palsies are seen in the **pons,** and 12th nerve involvement can occur in the **medulla.**

If the lesion appears patchy or involves both sides of the brainstem (as manifested by coma or quadriparesis), the differential diagnosis includes occlusion of a main trunk vessel (both vertebral arteries or the basilar artery); intramedullary lesions such as hemorrhage, pontine glioma, or multiple sclerosis; and compression of the brainstem by a cerebellar mass (hemorrhage, infarct, or tumor).

H. Short Basal Vertebrobasilar Branches

1. Anatomy—Short branches arising from the long circumferential arteries (discussed above) penetrate the ventral brainstem to supply the brainstem motor pathways.

2. Clinical syndrome of basal brainstem infarction—The most striking finding is contralateral hemiparesis caused by corticospinal tract involvement in the cerebral peduncle or basis pontis. Cranial nerves (eg, III, VI, VII) that emerge from the ventral surface of the brainstem may be affected as well, giving rise to ipsilateral cranial nerve palsies.

I. Lacunar Infarction

Small penetrating arteries located deep in the brain may become occluded as a result of changes in the vessel wall induced by chronic hypertension. The resulting lacunar infarcts are most common in deep nuclei of the brain (putamen, 37%; thalamus, 14%; caudate nucleus, 10%), the pons (16%), and the posterior limb of the internal capsule (10%) (Figure 9–13). They occur in

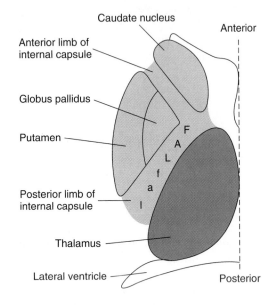

Figure 9–13. Arterial supply of deep cerebral structures frequently involved in lacunar infarction. Descending motor fibers to the face (F), arm (A), and leg (L) and ascending sensory fibers from face (f), arm (a), and leg (l) are shown in the posterior limb of the internal capsule.

lesser numbers in the deep cerebral white matter, the anterior limb of the internal capsule, and the cerebellum. Because of their small size and their frequent location in relatively silent areas of the brain, many lacunar infarctions are not recognized clinically. In as many as three-fourths of autopsy-proved cases, there is no history of stroke or clear evidence of neurologic deficit on antemortem examinations.

In many cases, the isolated nature of the neurologic deficit makes the clinical picture of lacunar infarction distinctive. The onset of lacunar stroke may be gradual, developing over several hours or days. Headache is absent or minor, and the level of consciousness is unchanged.

Recognition of lacunar stroke syndromes is important because the prognosis for complete or nearly complete recovery is good. In addition, the likelihood of future lacunar strokes can be reduced by treating the hypertension that is usually associated with and causally related to them. Because the arteries involved are small, angiography is normal (for that reason, it is not required). The CSF is also normal, and it is possible that a CT brain scan or MRI will not disclose the lesion. CT scanning or MRI should be performed to exclude other causes of stroke, however. Anticoagulation is not indicated since there is no evidence that it confers any benefit in this context. Aspirin is also of uncertain benefit, but it is often given because of the low risk of serious complications. Although a wide variety of deficits can be produced, there are four classic and distinctive lacunar syndromes.

1. Pure motor hemiparesis—This consists of hemiparesis affecting the face, arm, and leg to a roughly equal extent, without an associated disturbance of sensation, vision, or language. When lacunar in origin, it is usually due to a lesion in the contralateral internal capsule or pons. Pure motor hemiparesis may also be caused by internal carotid or middle cerebral artery occlusion, subdural hematoma, or intracerebral mass lesions.

2. Pure sensory stroke—This is characterized by hemisensory loss, which may be associated with paresthesia, and results from lacunar infarction in the contralateral thalamus. It may be mimicked by occlusion of the posterior cerebral artery or by a small hemorrhage in the thalamus or midbrain.

3. Ataxic hemiparesis—In this syndrome, sometimes called **ipsilateral ataxia and crural (leg) paresis,** pure motor hemiparesis is combined with ataxia of the hemiparetic side and usually predominantly affects the leg. Symptoms result from a lesion in the contralateral pons, internal capsule, or subcortical white matter.

4. Dysarthria-clumsy hand syndrome—This consists of dysarthria, facial weakness, dysphagia, and mild weakness and clumsiness of the hand on the side of facial involvement. When the syndrome is caused by a lacunar infarct, the lesion is in the contralateral pons or internal capsule. Infarcts or small intracerebral hemorrhages at a variety of locations can produce a similar syndrome, however. In contrast to the lacunar syndromes described above, premonitory TIAs are unusual.

Clinical Findings

A. HISTORY

1. Predisposing factors—In patients with cerebrovascular disorders, possible risk factors such as TIAs, hypertension, and diabetes should be sought. In women, the use of oral contraceptives has been associated with cerebral arterial and venous occlusive disease, especially in the presence of hypertension and cigarette smoking. The presence of such medical conditions as ischemic or valvular heart disease or cardiac arrhythmias must also be ascertained. A variety of systemic disorders involving the blood or blood vessels (see Table 9–3) also increase the risk of stroke. Antihypertensive drugs can precipitate cerebrovascular symptoms if the blood pressure is lowered excessively in patients with nearly total cerebrovascular occlusion and poor collateral circulation.

2. Onset and course—The history must address whether the clinical picture is that of TIA, stroke in evolution, or completed stroke. In some cases, it may also be possible to evaluate whether a stroke is likely to be thrombotic or embolic in origin from the clinical history.

a. Features suggesting thrombotic stroke—Patients with thrombotic vascular occlusion often present with stepwise incremental neurologic deficits; the occlusion may be preceded by a series of TIAs. TIAs, for example, precede infarction in 25–50% of patients with occlusive atherosclerotic disease of the extracranial internal carotid arteries. In approximately one-third of such patients, however, the onset of infarction is abrupt, suggesting that embolization from the distal extracranial artery to the intracranial artery may be the cause of stroke.

b. Features suggesting embolic stroke—Cerebral embolism typically causes neurologic deficits that occur abruptly with no warning and are maximal at onset. In many patients, a cardiac origin of emboli is suggested by signs of multifocal cerebral infarction, cardiac valvular disease, cardiomegaly, arrhythmias, or endocarditis.

3. Associated symptoms

a. Seizures accompany the onset of stroke in a small number of cases; in other instances, they follow the stroke by weeks to years. The presence of seizures does not definitively distinguish embolic from thrombotic strokes, but seizure at the onset of stroke may be more common with embolus. If patients with vertebrobasilar stroke or an additional condition predisposing to seizures are not considered, the incidence of epilepsy after stroke is about 10%. The risk of epilepsy increases to about 25% with cortical strokes and to 50% when cortical strokes are associated with a persistent motor deficit.

b. Headache occurs in about 25% of patients with ischemic stroke, possibly because of the acute dilation of collateral vessels.

B. PHYSICAL EXAMINATION

1. General physical examination—The general physical examination of a patient with a cerebrovascular disorder should focus on searching for an underlying systemic cause, especially a treatable one.

a. The blood pressure should be measured to ascertain whether hypertension—a known risk factor for stroke—is present.

b. Comparison of blood pressure and pulse on the two sides can reveal differences related to atherosclerotic disease of the aortic arch or coarctation of the aorta.

c. Ophthalmoscopic examination of the retina can provide evidence of embolization in the anterior circulation in the form of visible embolic material in retinal blood vessels.

d. Examination of the neck may reveal the absence of carotid pulses or the presence of carotid bruits. Reduced carotid artery pulsation in the neck is a poor indicator of internal carotid artery disease, however. Although carotid bruits have been associated with cerebrovascular disease, significant carotid stenosis can occur without an audible bruit; conversely, a loud bruit can occur without stenosis.

e. A careful cardiac examination is essential in order to detect arrhythmias or murmurs related to valvular disease, either of which may predispose to embolization from heart to brain.

f. Palpation of the temporal arteries is useful in the diagnosis of giant cell arteritis, in which these vessels may be tender, nodular, or pulseless.

2. Neurologic examination—Patients with cerebrovascular disorders may or may not have abnormal neurologic findings on examination. A normal examination is expected, for example, after a TIA has resolved. Where deficits are found, the goal of the neurologic examination is to define the anatomic site of the lesion, which may suggest the cause or optimal management of the stroke. Thus, clear evidence that the anterior circulation is involved may lead to angiographic evaluation in contemplation of possible surgical correction of an internal carotid lesion. Establishing that the symptoms are referable to the vertebrobasilar circulation or to a lacunar infarction is likely to dictate a different course of action.

a. Cognitive deficits that indicate cortical lesions in the anterior circulation should be sought. For example, if aphasia is present, the underlying disorder cannot be in the posterior circulation and is unlikely to represent lacunar infarction. The same is true for nondominant hemisphere lesions producing parietal lobe syndromes such as unilateral neglect or constructional apraxia (see discussion of inferior division middle cerebral artery stroke, above).

b. The presence of visual field abnormalities similarly excludes lacunar infarction. Hemianopia may occur, however, with involvement of either the anterior or posterior cerebral arteries. Isolated hemianopia suggests posterior cerebral artery infarction.

c. Ocular palsies, nystagmus, or internuclear ophthalmoplegia assign the underlying lesion to the brainstem and thus to the posterior circulation.

d. Hemiparesis can be due to lesions in cerebral cortical regions supplied by the anterior circulation, descending motor pathways in the brainstem supplied by the vertebrobasilar system, or lacunae at subcortical (corona radiata, internal capsule) or brainstem sites. However, hemiparesis affecting the face, hand, and arm more than the leg is characteristic of lesions within the distribution of the middle cerebral artery. Hemiparesis that is nonselective with respect to the face, arm, and leg is consistent with occlusion of the internal carotid artery or the stem of the middle cerebral artery, lacunar infarction in the internal capsule or basal ganglia, or brainstem disease. A crossed hemiparesis—ie, one that involves the face on one side and the rest of the body on the other—means that the abnormality must lie between the level of the facial nerve nucleus in the pons and the decussation of the pyramids in the medulla.

e. Cortical sensory deficits such as astereognosis and agraphesthesia with preserved primary sensory modalities imply a cerebral cortical deficit within the territory of the middle cerebral artery. Isolated hemisensory deficits without associated motor involvement are usually lacunar in origin. Crossed sensory deficits result from brainstem lesions in the medulla, as seen in the lateral medullary syndrome (Wallenberg's syndrome).

f. Hemiataxia usually points to a lesion in the ipsilateral brainstem or cerebellum but can also be produced by lacunae in the internal capsule.

Investigative Studies

A. BLOOD TESTS

These should be obtained routinely to detect treatable causes of stroke and to exclude conditions that can mimic stroke. The recommended studies are listed below.

1. Complete blood count to investigate such possible causes of stroke as thrombocytosis, thrombocytopenia, polycythemia, anemia (including sickle cell disease), and leukocytosis (eg, leukemia).

2. Erythrocyte sedimentation rate to detect elevations indicative of giant cell arteritis or other vasculitides.

3. Serologic assay for syphilis—treponemal assay in blood, such as the FTA-ABS or MHA-TP, or the CSF VDRL test.

4. Serum glucose to document hypoglycemia or hyperosmolar nonketotic hyperglycemia, which can present with focal neurologic signs and thereby masquerade as stroke.

5. Serum cholesterol and lipids to detect elevations that can represent risk factors for stroke.

B. ELECTROCARDIOGRAM (ECG)

An ECG should be obtained routinely to detect unrecognized myocardial infarction or cardiac arrythmias, such as atrial fibrillation, which predispose to embolic stroke.

C. CT Scan or MRI

A CT scan or MRI (Figure 9–14) should be obtained routinely to distinguish between infarction and hemorrhage as the cause of stroke, to exclude other lesions (eg, tumor, abscess) that can mimic stroke, and to localize the lesion. CT is usually preferred for initial diagnosis because it is widely available and rapid and can readily make the critical distinction between ischemia and hemorrhage. MRI may be superior to CT scan for demonstrating early ischemic infarcts, showing ischemic strokes in the brainstem or cerebellum, and detecting thrombotic occlusion of venous sinuses.

D. Lumbar Puncture

This should be performed in selected cases to exclude subarachnoid hemorrhage (manifested by xanthochromia and red blood cells) or to document meningovascular syphilis (reactive VDRL) as the cause of stroke.

E. Cerebral Angiography

Intaarterial angiography is used to identify operable extracranial carotid lesions in patients with anterior circulation TIAs who are good surgical candidates. It is also useful in the diagnosis of certain vascular disorders associated with stroke, including vasculitis, fibromuscular dysplasia, and carotid or vertebral artery dissection. Transfemoral arch aortography with selective catheterization of the carotid (and, if indicated, vertebral) arteries is the procedure of choice. **Magnetic resonance angiography** may detect stenosis of large cerebral arteries, aneurysms, and other vascular lesions, but its sensitivity is generally inferior to that of conventional angiography.

F. Ultrasonography

Doppler ultrasonography can detect stenosis or occlusion of the internal carotid artery, but it lacks the sensitivity of angiography. In cases in which the likelihood of finding operable symptomatic carotid stenosis is insufficient to justify the risk of angiography or in which the risk is especially high because of coexisting illness or the lack of angiographic expertise, the finding of normal carotid blood flow or complete occlusion by Doppler studies can obviate the need for angiography. **Transcranial doppler ultrasonography** is sometimes used in the evaluation of suspected stenosis of the intracranial internal carotid artery, middle cerebral artery, or basilar artery and for detecting and following the course of cerebral vasospasm after aneurysmal subarachnoid hemorrhage.

G. Echocardiography

Echocardiography may be useful for demonstrating the cardiac lesions responsible for embolic stroke in patients with clinically evident cardiac disease, such as atrial fibrillation.

H. Electroencephalogram (EEG)

The EEG is rarely useful in evaluating stroke. It may, however, help differentiate between a seizure disorder and TIAs or between lacunar and cortical infarcts in the occasional patient in whom these possibilities cannot otherwise be distinguished.

Differential Diagnosis

In patients presenting with focal central nervous system dysfunction of sudden onset, ischemic stroke must be distinguished from structural and metabolic processes that can mimic it. An underlying process other than focal cerebral ischemia should be suspected when the resulting neurologic deficit does not conform to the distribution of any single cerebral artery. In addition, strokes do not typically impair consciousness in the absence of profound focal deficits, whereas other cerebral disorders may do so.

Vascular disorders mistaken for ischemic stroke include intracerebral hemorrhage, subdural or epidural hematoma, and subarachnoid hemorrhage from rupture of an aneurysm or vascular malformation. These conditions can often be distinguished by a history of trauma or of excruciating headache at onset, by a more marked depression of consciousness, or by the presence of neck stiffness on examination. They can be excluded by CT scan or MRI.

Other structural brain lesions such as tumor or abscess can also produce focal cerebral symptoms of acute onset. Brain abscess is suggested by concurrent fever, and both abscess and tumor can usually be diagnosed by CT scan or MRI. Metabolic disturbances, particularly hypoglycemia and hyperosmolar nonketotic hyperglycemia, may present in strokelike fashion. The serum glucose level should therefore be determined in all patients with apparent stroke.

Treatment

The treatment options commonly available for cerebrovascular disease are summarized in Table 9–4.

A. Asymptomatic Carotid Bruit or Stenosis

Carotid bruits are commonly detected during routine examinations of asymptomatic patients, with a frequency that reaches 7% above age 65. Carotid artery stenosis is also common, and can be demonstrated by ultrasonography in as many as 30% of men over age 75. Because the natural history of carotid artery stenosis is variable, the relationship of asymptomatic bruit or stenosis to an individual's risk for stroke is difficult to assess. In large studies, severe stenosis is associated with increased stroke risk (2.5% per year for ipsilateral stroke with 75% stenosis), but the risk of contralateral

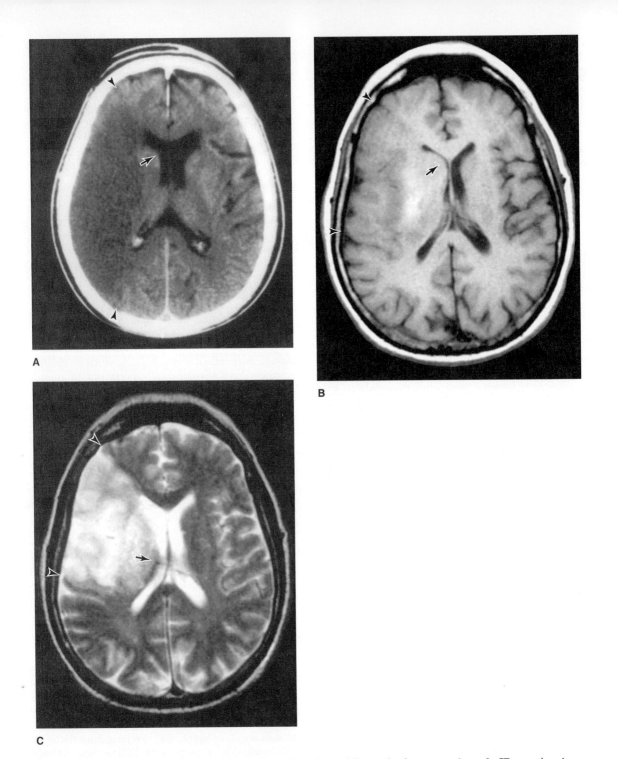

Figure 9–14. Imaging studies in ischemic stroke in the right middle cerebral artery territory. **A:** CT scan showing low density and effacement of cortical sulci **(between arrowheads)** and compression of the anterior horn of the lateral ventricle **(arrow). B:** T$_1$-weighted MRI scan showing loss of sulcal markings **(between arrowheads)** and compression of the anterior horn of the lateral ventricle **(arrow). C:** T$_2$-weighted MRI scan showing increased signal intensity **(between arrowheads)** and ventricular compression **(arrow).**

Table 9–4. Recommended treatment of cerebrovascular disease.[1]

Condition	Antiplatelet Agents[2]	Anticoagulants[2]	Thrombolytics[4]	Endarterectomy[5]
Asymptomatic carotid bruit or stenosis	+	−	−	±
Transient ischemic attack				
Cardiac source	±	+	−	−
Extracranial carotid source	+	±	−	+
Intracranial or vertebrobasilar source	+	±	−	−
Stroke-in-evolution	−	±		
Completed stroke[6]				
Cardiac source	±	+	−	−
Extracranial carotid source	+	±	+	+
Intracranial or vertebrobasilar source	+	±	+	−

[1] +, probably effective; ±, less evidence for efficacy or similarly effective but associated with greater risk; −, ineffective or efficacy untested.

[2] Aspirin, 80–1300 mg orally daily (optimal dose uncertain); aspirin/extended release dipyridamole, 25 mg/200 mg orally twice daily; ticlopidine, 250 mg orally twice daily; or clopidogrel, 75 mg orally daily.

[3] Heparin, given by continuous intravenous infusion to achieve an activated partial thromboplastin time (aPTT) = 1.5–2.5 times control, followed by warfarin, given orally daily to achieve an international normalized ratio (INR) = 3.0–4.0.

[4] Recombinant tissue plasminogen activator (rt-PA), 0.9 mg/kg intravenously over 1 hour, begun within 3 hours of the onset of symptoms (contraindicated in hemorrhagic stroke).

[5] For 50–99% stenosis, assuming a low (<2%) risk of perioperative death or disabling stroke.

[6] For prophylaxis against subsequent events in another vascular territory, or in the same territory in the case of completed stroke involving less than the entire area supplied by the affected vessel (partial stroke), or for dissolution of the existing thrombus (thrombolytics).

stroke is increased as well, and the risk of myocardial ischemia in these patients is even higher. Moreover, carotid endarterectomy—which has been advocated in this setting—carries significant perioperative risk of stroke or death, and this risk varies widely across institutions. Although asymptomatic patients with high-grade carotid stenosis have appeared to benefit from endarterectomy in some studies, this effect was dependent on an extremely low surgical morbidity and mortality rate. For these reasons, antiplatelet therapy with aspirin (see below) is probably the approach of choice for asymptomatic carotid bruit or stenosis at present.

B. TRANSIENT ISCHEMIC ATTACK

(4) Because TIAs can indicate an impending stroke and because it may be possible to prevent such an event by appropriate treatment, TIAs must be accurately and promptly diagnosed and treatment instituted (Table 9–4).

1. Antiplatelet therapy—Of the various medical treatments proposed for stroke prophylaxis in patients with noncardiogenic TIAs, antiplatelet agents appear to have the best benefit-to-risk ratio. The rationale for this approach is that embolism from platelet-fibrin thrombi on arterial surfaces may be responsible for many cases of TIA and stroke. Antiplatelet agents interfere with platelet function by irreversibly inhibiting the enzyme cyclooxygenase-1, which catalyzes the synthesis of thromboxane A_2, an eicosanoid with procoagulant and platelet-aggregating properties.

Aspirin, when administered to patients with TIAs or minor stroke (defined as little or no neurologic deficit after 1 week), has been shown to reduce the incidence of subsequent TIAs, stroke, or death in several studies. Although most studies have focused on noncardiogenic TIA or stroke, aspirin is also beneficial for preventing recurrent cerebral ischemia caused by cardiac emboli. In some cases (eg, patients with artificial heart valves), the combination of aspirin and anticoagulation may be more effective than anticoagulation alone. Doses of aspirin between 80 and 1300 mg orally daily (one baby aspirin to four adult aspirin tablets) appear to be effective, and daily oral administration of 325 mg of aspirin is probably used most often in North America. A sex-related difference in benefit favoring men has been observed, but only inconsistently. Administration of low-dose aspirin (325 mg orally every other day) to men age 40 and older *without* a history of TIA or stroke does not reduce the risk of stroke, although it decreases the incidence of myocardial infarction. Adverse effects of aspirin include dyspepsia, nausea, abdominal pain, diarrhea, skin rash, peptic ulcer, gastritis, and gastrointestinal bleeding.

Ticlopidine (250 mg orally twice daily), another antiplatelet agent, may be somewhat more effective than aspirin in preventing stroke and reducing mortality in patients with TIAs or mild stroke. However, ticlopidine is more expensive than aspirin and appears to be associated with such side effects as diarrhea, skin rash, and occasional cases of severe but reversible neutropenia.

Clopidogrel (75 mg orally daily), which inhibits platelet aggregation by binding irreversibly to adenosine diphosphate (ADP) receptors on the platelet surface, has also been shown to reduce the incidence of ischemic stroke, myocardial infarction, or death from other vascular causes in patients with recent ischemic stroke, myocardial infarction, or symptomatic peripheral arterial disease. Diarrhea and skin rash were more common than with aspirin, but neutropenia and thrombocytopenia occurred at the same rate. Thrombotic thrombocytopenic purpura (see Chapter 1) has complicated clopidogrel treatment in some patients.

Other antiplatelet drugs such as **sulfinpyrazone** and **dipyridamole** are commonly used to treat thrombotic vascular disease. Some experts recommend the use of a combination of aspirin (25 mg) and extended-release dipyridamole (200 mg), taken twice daily to prevent stroke in patients with prior TIA or stroke. **Glycoprotein IIb/IIIa antagonists** are also under investigation as platelet aggregation inhibitors.

2. Anticoagulation—Anticoagulation is indicated for patients with TIAs caused by cardiac embolus and is typically continued indefinitely or for as long as the cause of embolization (eg, atrial fibrillation or prosthetic heart valve) persists. The value of anticoagulation for TIAs from arterial thrombosis is uncertain.

Heparin is the drug of choice for acute anticoagulation, whereas warfarin is used for long-term therapy. Heparin is usually administered by continuous intravenous infusion at 1000–2000 units/h. The activated partial thromboplastin time (aPTT) is measured at least daily, and the dose of heparin is adjusted to maintain the aPTT at about 1.5 to 2.5 times the pretreatment value.

Warfarin (the usual maintenance dose is 5–15 mg/d orally) can be started simultaneously with heparin therapy. About 2 days after the prothrombin time (PT) reaches roughly one and one-half times the pretreatment value (typically about 5 days), heparin can be discontinued. The PT or international normalized ratio (INR) should be measured at least every 2 weeks and the dose of warfarin adjusted to maintain PT = 1.5 times control or INR = 3.0–4.0.

Enthusiasm for the use of anticoagulant therapy should be tempered by an appreciation of its potential hazards. The risk of intracranial hemorrhage is greatest in hypertensive patients and those over 65 years of age.

3. Carotid endarterectomy—Carotid endarterectomy involves the surgical removal of thrombus from a stenotic common or internal carotid artery in the neck. In patients with anterior-circulation TIAs and moderate (50–70%) or high-grade (70–99%) carotid stenosis on the side appropriate to account for the symptoms, the combination of endarterectomy and aspirin is superior to aspirin alone in preventing stroke. Endarterectomy has no place in the treatment of vertebrobasilar TIAs or those related to intracranial arterial disease or complete carotid occlusion. The value of carotid endarterectomy for minimally stenotic but ulcerated carotid lesions is uncertain. The operative mortality rate for carotid endarterectomy has ranged from 1 to 5% or more.

4. Angioplasty and intralumenal stents—Transluminal angioplasty of the carotid and vertebral arteries and surgical placement of tubular metal stents to maintain lumen patency in stenotic cerebral arteries are under investigation. The Carotid and Vertebral Artery Transluminal Angioplasty Study (CAVATAS), in which patients with carotid stenosis were randomized to receive carotid endarterectomy or percutaneous transluminal angioplasty, provided preliminary evidence for the greater safety of angioplasty, but also a higher rate of restenosis. A second phase of the study, the International Carotid Stenting Study (ICSS), is underway to evaluate the efficacy of stenting for symptomatic carotid stenosis.

5. Extracranial-intracranial bypass—Many patients with TIAs referable to the carotid circulation have stenoses in intracranial portions of the artery not accessible through the neck, or they exhibit tandem lesions in both the extracranial and intracranial cerebral circulations. Because carotid endarterectomy does not correct these problems, an alternative approach has been explored involving anastomosis of the extracranial (temporal artery) and intracranial (middle cerebral artery) circulations distal to the stenosis. The bulk of current evidence suggests that this bypass procedure is ineffective.

6. Conclusions—In experienced hands, carotid endarterectomy can be a safe procedure that reduces the risk of subsequent TIAs or stroke in patients with carotid TIAs. Angiography should be used with these patients to define surgically accessible moderate to high-grade (50–99%) stenotic lesions.

Medical treatment with aspirin should be instituted with both nonsurgical and postoperative patients. For patients who continue to have TIAs despite aspirin treatment, increasing the dose of aspirin, substituting ticlopidine or clopidogrel, or adding sulfinpyrazone or dipyridamole should be considered. Alternatively, a 3-month course of warfarin should be substituted unless there are contraindications such as active peptic ulcer disease or severe hypertension. The prothrombin time should be maintained at one and one-half times the control value (INR = 3.0–4.0). In addition to the above measures, such contributory risk factors as hypertension and cardiac disease should be treated and cigarette smoking discontinued.

C. STROKE IN EVOLUTION

The optimal treatment for stroke in evolution is uncertain. The onset of aspirin's antiplatelet effect is delayed after oral administration, and endarterectomy also involves considerable delay in treatment.

The most widely used treatment is **anticoagulation** with heparin and subsequent administration of warfarin at the doses described above, although the efficacy of this approach has not been proved.

Thrombolytic agents such as tissue plasminogen activator might also be of value for stroke in evolution, but require further study in this context.

D. COMPLETED STROKE

1. Intravenous thrombolytic therapy—Tissue plasminogen activator (t-PA) is a serine protease that maps to chromosome 8 (8p12) in humans and catalyzes the conversion of plasminogen to plasmin. This accounts for its ability to lyse fibrin-containing clots such as those found in cerebrovascular thrombotic lesions. Some but not all controlled clinical data suggest that the intravenous administration of recombinant t-PA (rt-PA) within 3 hours of the onset of symptoms reduces disability and mortality from ischemic stroke (technically, from TIA, since stroke is defined by a deficit that persists for at least 24 hours). The drug is administered at a dose of 0.9 mg/kg, up to a maximum total dose of 90 mg; 10% of the dose is given as an intravenous bolus and the remainder as a continuous intravenous infusion over 60 minutes. The efficacy of rt-PA given more than 3 hours after symptoms begin, of other thrombolytic agents such as urokinase, or of intraarterial administration of these agents has not been demonstrated in stroke.

The major complication of rt-PA treatment is hemorrhage, which may affect the brain or other tissues. The lack of proven benefit when rt-PA is given after 3 hours, the risk of bleeding complications, and the importance of a correct diagnosis when treatment is potentially dangerous dictate that rt-PA not be given in certain settings. It is important that the time of onset of symptoms can be established with confidence. The CT scan should not already show evidence of a large ischemic stroke or of

hemorrhage. Patients whose coagulation function has been compromised by the administration of warfarin or heparin or by thrombocytopenia (platelet count <100,000/mm³) should not receive rt-PA, nor should those who are at increased risk of hemorrhage because of seizures at the onset of symptoms, prior intracranial hemorrhage, another intracranial disorder (including stroke or trauma) within 3 months, a major surgical procedure within 14 days, bleeding from the gastrointestinal or urinary tract within 21 days, or marked hypertension (systolic blood pressure >185 mm Hg or diastolic blood pressure >110 mm Hg). To avoid treating TIAs that are already resolving or other conditions unlikely to respond to rt-PA, or for which the risk exceeds likely benefit, patients whose deficits are improving rapidly and spontaneously, patients with mild and isolated deficits, and those with blood glucose concentrations consistent with a hypo- or hyperglycemic origin of symptoms (<50 mg/dl or >400 mg/dl) should be excluded.

Patients receiving rt-PA for stroke should be managed in facilities in which the capacity exists to diagnose stroke with a high degree of certainty and to manage bleeding complications. Within the first 24 hours after administration of rt-PA, anticoagulants and antiplatelet agents should not be given, blood pressure should be carefully monitored, and arterial puncture and placement of central venous lines, bladder catheters, and nasogastric tubes should be avoided.

2. Intraarterial thrombolytic therapy—Intraarterial administration of urokinase, prourokinase, or rt-TPA has also been investigated for the acute treatment of stroke. Early results with this approach suggest that prourokinase, and perhaps the other thrombolytic agents, given together with low-dose intravenous heparin, may be beneficial for patients with middle cerebral artery distribution stroke who can be treated within 3–6 hours of the onset of symptoms. Less is known about the benefit of intraarterial thrombolytic therapy for vertebrobasilar stroke, and about the comparative efficacy of intravenous and intrarterial thrombolysis.

3. Antiplatelet agents—As noted above in discussing the treatment of TIAs, some but not all studies have shown a decrease in the incidence of subsequent stroke when aspirin is administered chronically following a stroke. The regimen is as described in the section on treatment of TIA.

4. Anticoagulation—Anticoagulation has not been shown to be useful in most cases of completed stroke. An exception is where a persistent source of cardiac embolus is present; anticoagulation is then indicated to prevent subsequent embolic strokes, although it does not affect the course of the stroke that has already occurred. Recent evidence indicates that although immediate anticoagulation of such patients may result in

hemorrhage into the infarct, this rarely affects the ultimate outcome adversely unless the infarct is massive. The risk of hemorrhage is more than offset by the particularly high risk of recurrent embolization soon after an embolic stroke, and anticoagulation should not be delayed in this setting. Heparin and warfarin are administered as described in the section on treatment of TIA.

5. Surgery—The indications for surgical treatment of completed stroke are extremely limited. When patients deteriorate as a consequence of brainstem compression following cerebellar infarction, however, posterior fossa decompression with evacuation of infarcted cerebellar tissue can be lifesaving.

6. Antihypertensive agents—Although hypertension contributes to the pathogenesis of stroke and many patients with acute stroke have elevated blood pressures, attempts to reduce the blood pressure in stroke patients can have disastrous results, since the blood supply to ischemic but as yet uninfarcted brain tissue may be further compromised. Therefore, such attempts should not be made. In the usual course of events, the blood pressure declines spontaneously over a period of hours to a few days.

7. Antiedema agents—Antiedema agents such as mannitol and corticosteroids have not been shown to be of benefit for cytotoxic edema (cellular swelling) associated with cerebral infarction.

8. Neuroprotective agents—A variety of drugs with diverse pharmacologic actions have been proposed as neuroprotective agents that might reduce ischemic brain injury by decreasing cerebral metabolism or interfering with the cytotoxic mechanisms triggered by ischemia. These include barbiturates, the opioid antagonist naloxone, voltage-gated calcium channel antagonists, and excitatory amino acid receptor antagonists. Thus far, however clinical trials with these agents have yielded disappointing results.

Prognosis

Outcome following stroke is influenced by a number of factors, the most important being the nature and severity of the resulting neurologic deficit. The patient's age, the cause of stroke, and coexisting medical disorders also affect prognosis. Overall, somewhat less than 80% of patients with stroke survive for at least 1 month, and 10-year survival rates in the neighborhood of 35% have been cited. The latter figure is not surprising, considering the advanced age at which stroke commonly occurs. Of patients who survive the acute period, about one-half to two-thirds regain independent function, while approximately 15% require institutional care.

INTRACEREBRAL HEMORRHAGE

Hypertensive Hemorrhage

Hypertension is the most common underlying cause of nontraumatic intracerebral hemorrhage.

A. PATHOPHYSIOLOGY

1. Cerebral autoregulation—Autoregulation of cerebral blood flow (Figure 9–15), which is achieved by changes in the caliber of small resistance cerebral arteries, maintains constant cerebral blood flow as systemic blood pressure rises and falls. The range of autoregulated blood pressures is variable.

In normotensive individuals, the lowest mean blood pressure at which autoregulation is effective is approximately 60 mm Hg. Below this level, changes in the caliber of cerebral arteries cannot compensate for decreased perfusion pressure; cerebral blood flow therefore declines, producing symptoms of hypoxia, such as lightheadedness, confusion, and dimming of vision. These symptoms are followed by somnolence and loss of consciousness if the mean blood pressure falls below 35–40 mm Hg. In contrast, at blood pressures above the upper limit of the range of autoregulation (150–200 mm Hg), cerebral blood flow is increased, which can produce hypertensive encephalopathy.

In chronically hypertensive individuals, the lower limit of the autoregulatory range is higher (Figure 9–15), which may be due to damage to small arterial walls. As a result, cerebral blood flow declines when the mean arterial blood pressure falls below about 120 mm Hg. The clinical relevance of this observation is that blood pressure should be reduced rarely, if ever—and never to hypotensive levels—in patients with stroke.

2. Chronic hypertension—Chronic hypertension appears to promote structural changes in the walls of penetrating arteries, predisposing them to intracerebral hemorrhage. In 1888, Charcot and Bouchard found minute aneurysms on the small intraparenchymal arteries of hypertensive patients and postulated that aneurysmal rupture led to intracerebral hemorrhage. Subsequently, Ross Russell showed microaneurysms of small resistance arteries in cerebral sites at which hypertensive hemorrhages occur most commonly. Some aneurysms were surrounded by small areas of hemorrhage, and the aneurysmal walls often showed changes of lipohyalinosis or fibrinoid necrosis. These processes are characterized by destruction of the vessel wall with deposition of fibrinoid material, focal aneurysmal expansion of the involved vessel, thrombotic occlusion, and extravasation of red cells. There is now general agreement that massive cerebral hemorrhage often follows the rupture of either a microaneurysmal or lipohyalinotic segment of a small resistance artery and that the underlying lesion is caused by chronic hypertension.

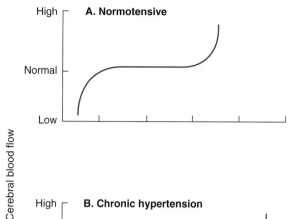

Figure 9–15. Cerebrovascular autoregulation. **A:** Cerebral blood flow is maintained in the normal range over a wide range of blood pressures. At very low pressures, cerebral hypoperfusion occurs, producing syncope. Pressures that rise beyond the autoregulatory range can cause hypertensive encephalopathy. **B:** Structural changes in cerebral arteries shift the autoregulatory range to higher blood pressures. Hypoperfusion and syncope can occur at normal pressures, and pressures associated with hypertensive encephalopathy are increased.

3. Acute hypertension—In addition to structural changes in the cerebral arterial wall produced by chronic hypertension, acute elevation of blood pressure appears to play a role in the pathogenesis of intracerebral hemorrhage. Although most patients with intracerebral hemorrhage are hypertensive following the event, many have no history of hypertension and lack such signs of hypertensive end-organ disease as left ventricular hypertrophy, retinopathy, or nephropathy. It has therefore been suggested that a sudden increase in blood pressure may itself be sufficient to cause intracerebral hemorrhage, as with amphetamine or cocaine abuse. Acute elevation of blood pressure may also be the immediate precipitating cause of intracerebral hemorrhage in chronically hypertensive patients with Charcot-Bouchard aneurysms.

B. PATHOLOGY

Most hypertensive hemorrhages originate in certain areas of predilection, corresponding to long, narrow, penetrating arterial branches along which Charcot-Bouchard aneurysms are found at autopsy (Figure 9–16). These include the caudate and putaminal branches of the middle cerebral arteries (42%); branches of the basilar artery supplying the pons (16%); thalamic branches of the posterior cerebral arteries (15%); branches of the superior cerebellar arteries supplying the dentate nuclei and the deep white matter of the cerebel-

lum (12%); and some white matter branches of the cerebral arteries (10%), especially in the parietooccipital and temporal lobes.

C. CLINICAL FINDINGS

Hypertensive hemorrhage occurs without warning, most commonly while the patient is awake. Headache is present in 50% of patients and may be severe; vomiting is common. Blood pressure is elevated after the hemorrhage has occurred. Thus, normal or low blood pressure in a patient with stroke makes the diagnosis of hypertensive hemorrhage unlikely, as does onset before 50 years of age.

Following the hemorrhage, edema surrounding the area of hemorrhage produces clinical worsening over a period of minutes to days. The duration of active bleeding, however, is brief. Once the deficit stabilizes, improvement occurs slowly. Because the deficit is caused principally by hemorrhage and edema, which compress rather than destroy brain tissue, considerable return of neurologic function can occur.

Massive hypertensive hemorrhages may rupture through brain tissue into the ventricles, producing bloody CSF; direct rupture through the cortical mantle is unusual. A fatal outcome is most often due to herniation caused by the combined mass effect of the hematoma and the surrounding edema.

Clinical features vary with the site of hemorrhage (Table 9–5).

A. Cerebral hemispheres

Anterior

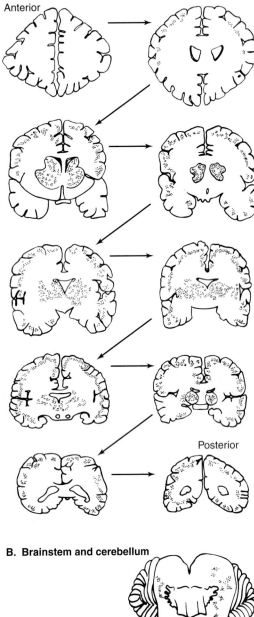

Posterior

B. Brainstem and cerebellum

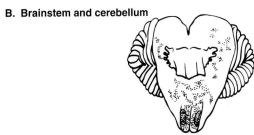

Figure 9–16. Distribution of Charcot-Bouchard aneurysms (stippling) underlying hypertensive intracerebral hemorrhage.

1. Deep cerebral hemorrhage—The two most common sites of hypertensive hemorrhage are the **putamen** and the **thalamus,** which are separated by the posterior limb of the internal capsule. This segment of the internal capsule is traversed by descending motor fibers and ascending sensory fibers, including the optic radiations (Figure 9–17). Pressure on these fibers from an expanding lateral (putaminal) or medial (thalamic) hematoma produces a contralateral sensorimotor deficit. In general, putaminal hemorrhage leads to a more severe motor deficit and thalamic hemorrhage to a more marked sensory disturbance. Homonymous hemianopia may occur as a transient phenomenon after thalamic hemorrhage and is often a persistent finding in putaminal hemorrhage. In large thalamic hemorrhages, the eyes may deviate downward, as in staring at the tip of the nose, because of impingement on the midbrain center for upward gaze. Aphasia may occur if hemorrhage at either site exerts pressure on the cortical language areas. A separate aphasic syndrome has been described with localized hemorrhage into the thalamus; it carries an excellent prognosis for full recovery.

2. Lobar hemorrhage—Hypertensive hemorrhages also occur in subcortical white matter underlying the frontal, parietal, temporal, and occipital lobes. Symptoms and signs vary according to the location; they can include headache, vomiting, hemiparesis, hemisensory deficits, aphasia, and visual field abnormalities. Seizures are more frequent than with hemorrhages in other locations, while coma is less so.

3. Pontine hemorrhage—With bleeding into the pons, coma occurs within seconds to minutes and usually leads to death within 48 hours. Ocular findings typically include pinpoint pupils. Horizontal eye movements are absent or impaired, but vertical eye movements may be preserved. In some patients, there may be ocular bobbing, a bilateral downbeating excursion of the eyes at about 5-second intervals. Patients are commonly quadriparetic and exhibit decerebrate posturing. Hyperthermia is sometimes present. The hemorrhage usually ruptures into the fourth ventricle, and rostral extension of the hemorrhage into the midbrain with resultant midposition fixed pupils is common. In contrast to the classic presentation of pontine hemorrhage described above, small hemorrhages that spare the reticular activating system—and that are associated with less severe deficits and excellent recovery—also occur.

4. Cerebellar hemorrhage—The distinctive symptoms of cerebellar hemorrhage (headache, dizziness, vomiting, and the inability to stand or walk) begin suddenly, within minutes after onset of bleeding. Although patients may initially be alert or only mildly confused, large hemorrhages lead to coma within 12 hours in 75% of patients and within 24 hours in 90%. When

Table 9–5. Clinical features of hypertensive intracerebral hemorrhage.

Location	Coma	Pupils	Eye Movements	Sensorimotor Disturbance	Hemianopia	Seizures
Putamen	Common	Normal	Ipsilateral deviation	Hemiparesis	Common	Uncommon
Thalamus	Common	Small, sluggish	Downward and medial deviation may occur	Hemisensory deficit	May occur transiently	Uncommon
Lobar	Uncommon	Normal	Normal or ipsilateral deviation	Hemiparesis or hemisensory deficit	Common	Common
Pons	Early	Pinpoint	Absent horizontal	Quadriparesis	None	None
Cerebellum	Delayed	Small, reactive	Impaired late	Gait ataxia	None	None

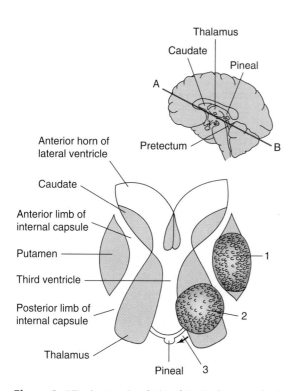

Figure 9–17. Anatomic relationships in deep cerebral hemorrhage. **Top:** Plane of section. **Bottom:** Putaminal (1) and thalamic (2) hemorrhages can compress or transect the adjacent posterior limb of the internal capsule. Thalamic hemorrhages can also extend into the ventricles or compress the hypothalamus or midbrain upgaze center (3).

coma is present at the onset, the clinical picture is indistinguishable from that of pontine hemorrhage.

Common ocular findings include impairment of gaze to the side of the lesion or forced deviation away from the lesion caused by pressure on the pontine lateral gaze center. Skew deviation may also occur, in which case the eye ipsilateral to the lesion is depressed. The pupils are small and reactive. Ipsilateral facial weakness of lower motor neuron type occurs in about 50% of cases, but strength in the limbs is normal. Limb ataxia is usually slight or absent. Plantar responses are flexor early in the course but become extensor as the brainstem becomes compromised and the patient deteriorates. Impairment of voluntary or reflex upward gaze indicates upward transtentorial herniation of the cerebellar vermis and midbrain, leading to compression of the pretectum. It implies a poor prognosis.

D. DIFFERENTIAL DIAGNOSIS

Putaminal, thalamic, and lobar hypertensive hemorrhages may be difficult to distinguish from cerebral infarctions. To some extent, the presence of severe headache, nausea and vomiting, and impairment of consciousness are useful clues that a hemorrhage may have occurred; the CT scan (Figure 9–18) identifies the underlying disorder definitively.

Brainstem stroke or cerebellar infarction can mimic cerebellar hemorrhage. When cerebellar hemorrhage is a possibility, CT scan or MRI is the most useful diagnostic procedure, since hematomas can be quickly and accurately localized. If neither CT nor MRI is available, vertebral angiography should be performed. The angiogram shows a cerebellar mass effect in about 85% of cases, but the procedure is time consuming. Bloody CSF will confirm the diagnosis of hemorrhage, but a clear tap does not exclude the possibility of an intracere-

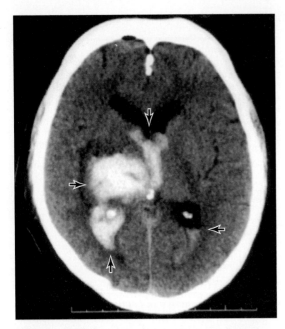

Figure 9–18. CT scan in hypertensive intracerebral hemorrhage. Blood is seen as a high-density signal at the site of hemorrhage in the thalamus **(left arrow)** and extends into the third ventricle **(top arrow)** and the occipital horns of the ipsilateral **(bottom arrow)** and contralateral **(right arrow)** lateral ventricles.

bellar hematoma—and lumbar puncture may hasten the process of herniation. Lumbar puncture is therefore not advocated if a cerebellar hemorrhage is suspected.

Like cerebellar hemorrhage, acute peripheral vestibulopathy also produces nausea, vomiting, and gait ataxia. Severe headache, impaired consciousness, elevated blood pressure, or later age at onset, however, strongly favors cerebellar hemorrhage.

E. TREATMENT

1. Surgical measures

a. Cerebellar decompression—The most important therapeutic intervention in hypertensive hemorrhage is surgical decompression for cerebellar hematomas. Unless this step is taken promptly, there may be a fatal outcome or unexpected deterioration. Note that this procedure may also reverse the neurologic deficit. Because surgical results are much better for responsive than unresponsive patients, surgery should be performed early in the course when the patient is still conscious.

b. Cerebral decompression—Surgery can be useful when a superficial hemorrhage in the cerebral white matter is large enough to cause a mass effect with shift of midline structures and incipient herniation. The

prognosis is directly related to the level of consciousness before the operation, and surgery is usually fruitless in an already comatose patient.

c. Contraindications to surgery—Surgery is not indicated for pontine or deep cerebral hypertensive hemorrhages, because in most cases spontaneous decompression occurs with rupture into the ventricles—and the areas in question are accessible only at the expense of normal overlying brain.

2. Medical measures—The use of antihypertensive agents in acute intracerebral hemorrhage is controversial. Attempts to lower systemic blood pressure may compromise cerebral blood flow and lead to infarction, but continued hypertension may exacerbate cerebral edema. On this basis, it seems reasonable to lower blood pressure to diastolic levels of approximately 100 mm Hg following intracerebral hemorrhage, but this must be done with great care because the cerebral vasculature may be unusually sensitive to antihypertensive agents. The use of nitroglycerin paste (½–1 in. topically) has an advantage—if the blood pressure declines excessively, the drug can be wiped off the skin and its effect rapidly terminated. If volume overload is considered to contribute to the hypertension, the judicious use of a diuretic such as furosemide (from 10 mg intravenously in patients unused to the drug to 40 mg intravenously in patients accustomed to receiving it) can be helpful.

There is no other effective medical treatment for intracerebral hemorrhage. Rebleeding at the site of a hypertensive intracerebral hemorrhage is uncommon, and antifibrinolytic agents are not indicated. Corticosteroids are commonly prescribed to reduce vasogenic edema in patients with intracerebral hemorrhage, but the evidence of their benefit is poor. Antiedema agents provide only temporary benefit.

Other Causes of Intracerebral Hemorrhage

A. TRAUMA

Intracerebral hemorrhage is a frequent consequence of closed-head trauma. Such hemorrhages may occur under the skull at the site of impact or directly opposite the site of impact (contrecoup injury). The most common locations are the frontal and temporal poles. The appearance of traumatic hemorrhages on CT scans may be delayed for as much as 24 hours after injury; MRI permits earlier detection.

B. VASCULAR MALFORMATIONS

Bleeding from cerebral angiomas and aneurysms can lead to both intracerebral and subarachnoid hemorrhage. Angiomas may come to medical attention because of seizures, in which case anticonvulsants are the treatment of choice, or because of bleeding. In the latter instance, surgical removal is indicated to prevent rebleeding—provided the malformation is surgically accessible. Aneurysms usually present with intracranial hemorrhage but occasionally with compressive focal deficits such as third-nerve palsy. Their treatment is considered in Chapter 2.

C. HEMORRHAGE INTO CEREBRAL INFARCTS

Some cases of cerebral infarction, especially when embolic in origin, are accompanied by hemorrhage into the infarct.

D. AMPHETAMINE OR COCAINE ABUSE

Intravenous, intranasal, and oral amphetamine or cocaine use can result in intracerebral hemorrhage, which typically occurs within minutes to hours after the drug is administered. Most such hemorrhages are located in subcortical white matter and may be related to either acute elevation of blood pressure, leading to spontaneous hemorrhage or rupture of a vascular anomaly, or drug-induced arteritis.

E. CEREBRAL AMYLOID ANGIOPATHY

Cerebral amyloid (congophilic) angiopathy is a rare cause of intracerebral hemorrhage. Amyloid deposits are present in the walls of small cortical blood vessels and in the meninges. The disorder is most common in elderly patients (a mean age of 70 years) and typically produces lobar hemorrhages at multiple sites. Some cases are familial.

F. ACUTE HEMORRHAGIC LEUKOENCEPHALITIS

This is a demyelinating and hemorrhagic disorder that characteristically follows a respiratory infection and has a fulminant course resulting in death within several days. Multiple small hemorrhages are found in the brain, and red blood cells may be present in the CSF.

G. HEMORRHAGE INTO TUMORS

Bleeding into primary or metastatic brain tumors is an occasional cause of intracerebral hemorrhage. Tumors associated with hemorrhage include glioblastoma multiforme, melanoma, choriocarcinoma, renal cell carcinoma, and bronchogenic carcinoma. Bleeding into a tumor should be considered when a patient with known cancer experiences acute neurologic deterioration; it may also be the presenting manifestation of cancer.

H. COAGULOPATHIES

Intracerebral hemorrhage is a complication of disorders of both clotting factors and platelets, such as hemophilia (factor VIII deficiency) and idiopathic thrombocytopenic purpura. Acute myelogenous leukemia with white blood cell counts greater than 150,000/μL may also predispose to intracerebral hemorrhage.

I. ANTICOAGULATION

Patients receiving heparin or warfarin are at increased risk for developing spontaneous or traumatic intracerebral hemorrhage.

GLOBAL CEREBRAL ISCHEMIA

Etiology

Global cerebral ischemia occurs when the blood flow is inadequate to meet the metabolic requirements of the brain, as in cardiac arrest. The result is a spectrum of neurologic disorders. The greater severity of neurologic involvement in ischemia than in pure anoxia may be due to the fact that in the former condition, the delivery of glucose and removal of potentially toxic metabolites are also impaired.

Pathology

Neuropathologic changes depend on the degree and duration of cerebral ischemia.

A. DISTRIBUTION

Complete interruption of cerebral blood flow followed by reperfusion, such as occurs in cardiac arrest with resuscitation, produces damage that selectively affects metabolically vulnerable neurons of the cerebral cortex, basal ganglia, and cerebellum.

With less profound hypotension for prolonged periods, the damage is concentrated in the anatomically vulnerable border zones between the territories supplied by the major arteries of cerebral cortex, cerebellum, basal ganglia, and spinal cord. It is most severe in the watershed region between the territories supplied by the anterior, middle, and posterior cerebral arteries (Figure 9–19).

B. MODIFYING FACTORS

Reducing cerebral energy requirements, such as with deep anesthesia or hypothermia, can minimize or prevent brain damage from ischemic insults. Hyperglycemia or hypermetabolic states such as status epilepticus, on the other hand, can increase ischemic damage. Superimposed occlusive atherosclerotic disease of the craniocervical arteries may lead to asymmetries in the distribution of cerebral damage from panhypoperfusion.

Clinical Findings

A. BRIEF ISCHEMIC EPISODES

Reversible encephalopathies are common following brief episodes of systemic circulatory arrest. In such cases, coma persists for less than 12 hours. Transient confusion or amnesia may occur on awakening, but

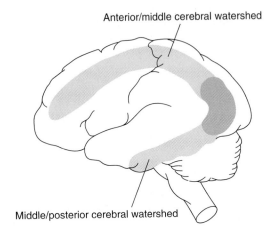

Anterior/middle cerebral watershed

Middle/posterior cerebral watershed

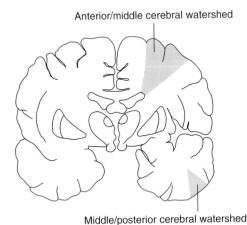

Anterior/middle cerebral watershed

Middle/posterior cerebral watershed

Figure 9–19. Distribution of watershed cerebral infarctions (blue areas).

recovery is rapid and complete. Some patients show a severe anterograde and variable retrograde amnesia and a bland, unconcerned affect with or without confabulation. Recovery often occurs within 7–10 days but may be delayed by 1 month or longer. This syndrome may reflect reversible bilateral damage to the thalamus or hippocampus.

B. PROLONGED ISCHEMIC EPISODES

1. Focal cerebral dysfunction—Patients are usually comatose for at least 12 hours and may have lasting focal or multifocal motor, sensory, and cognitive deficits if they awaken. Full recovery may not occur or may require weeks to months. Some patients are eventually capable of leading an independent existence, whereas those who are more severely disabled may require institutional care.

Focal neurologic signs after cardiac arrest include partial or complete cortical blindness, weakness of both arms (bibrachial paresis), and quadriparesis. Cortical blindness is usually transient but can rarely be permanent. It probably results from disproportionate ischemia of the occipital poles because of their location in the border zone between the middle and posterior cerebral arteries (see Figure 9–19). Bibrachial paresis (**man-in-a-barrel syndrome**) results from bilateral infarction of the motor cortex in the border zone between the anterior and middle cerebral arteries (see Figure 9–19).

2. Persistent vegetative state—Some patients who are initially comatose following cardiac arrest survive and awaken but remain functionally decorticate and unaware of their surroundings. They typically regain spontaneous eye-opening, sleep-wake cycles, and roving eye movements and brainstem and spinal cord reflexes. The persistent vegetative state is thus distinct from coma and appears to be associated with destruction of the neocortex. A persistent vegetative state associated with an isoelectric (flat) EEG is termed **neocortical death.** Persistent vegetative states must be distinguished from brain death (see Chapter 10), in which both cerebral and brainstem function are absent.

3. Spinal cord syndromes—The spinal cord seems to be more resistant to transient ischemia than the brain, so that cord damage from hypoperfusion is usually accompanied by profound cerebral involvement. Hypoperfusion does occasionally lead to isolated spinal cord infarction, however. In such cases, the anterior and central structures of the spinal cord are more involved because of their location in the critical border zones between territories supplied by the anterior and posterior spinal arteries (see Chapter 5). These watersheds, especially in the upper and lower levels of the thoracic cord, are vulnerable to profound drops in perfusion pressure. In the acute period, spinal stroke from hypotension produces a flaccid paraplegia and urinary retention. The sensory level in the thoracic region is characterized more by marked impairment of pain and temperature sensation than of light touch. With time, flaccid paralysis is replaced by spastic paraplegia with brisk tendon reflexes in the legs and extensor plantar responses.

Treatment

A. ESTABLISHED MEASURES

The clinical management of patients in coma caused by global cerebral ischemia involves immediate restoration of adequate cerebral circulation, elimination of cardiac dysrhythmias, maintenance of effective systemic blood pressure, and correction of acid-base or electrolyte abnormalities. Ventilatory assistance may be necessary if either medullary depression or injury to the chest wall prevents adequate ventilation, and supplemental oxygen can also be administered.

Beyond these measures, there are no other uniformly satisfactory methods of treatment. Attempts to prevent cerebral edema in this setting have not been successful, and treatment with corticosteroids, dehydrating agents, calcium channel antagonists, hypothermia, and hyperventilation have not improved the prognosis.

B. Experimental Measures

Although barbiturates have a protective effect in some experimental models of global cerebral ischemia, a similar benefit does not appear to occur in patients.

Excitatory amino acid receptor antagonists may find application in the treatment of cerebral anoxic ischemia but are at present experimental. The rationale for considering the use of these drugs lies in existing evidence that ischemia or hypoxia may trigger the release of excitatory amino acid neurotransmitters, which may in turn interact with vulnerable neurons to promote cell death.

REFERENCES

General

Barnett HJM et al: *Stroke: Pathophysiology, Diagnosis and Management*, 3rd ed. WB Saunders, 1998.

Epidemiology

Berger K et al: Light-to-moderate alcohol consumption and the risk of stroke among US male physicians. N Engl J Med 1999; 341:1557–1564.

Bousser MG, Kittner SJ: Oral contraceptives and stroke. Cephalalgia 2000;20:183–189.

Elkind MS, Sacco RL: Stroke risk factors and stroke prevention. Semin Neurol 1998;18:429–440.

Gillum RF: Stroke mortality in blacks: disturbing trends. Stroke 1999;30:1711–1715.

Kittner SJ et al: Pregnancy and the risk of stroke. N Engl J Med 1996;335:768–774.

Sagie A, Larson MG, Levy D: The natural history of borderline isolated systolic hypertension. N Engl J Med 1993;329:1912–1917.

White HD et al: Pravastatin therapy and the risk of stroke. N Engl J Med 2000;343:317–326.

Focal Cerebral Ischemia

Dirnagl U, Iadecola C, Moskowitz MA: Pathobiology of ischaemic stroke: an integrated view. Trends Neurosci 1999;22:391–397.

Graham SH, Chen J: Programmed cell death in cerebral ischemia. J Cereb Blood Flow Metab 2001;21:99–109.

Sharp FR et al: Multiple molecular penumbras after focal cerebral ischemia. J Cereb Blood Flow Metab 2000;20:1011–1032.

Tatu L et al: Arterial territories of human brain: brainstem and cerebellum. Neurology 1996;47:1125–1135.

Atherosclerosis

Lusis AJ: Atherosclerosis. Nature 2000;407:233–241.

Russell, R: Atherosclerosis—an inflammatory disease. N Engl J Med 1999;340:115–126.

Other Vascular Causes

Ferro JM: Vasculitis of the central nervous system. J Neurol 1998; 245:766–776.

Haller CA, Benowitz NL: Adverse cardiovascular and central nervous system events associated with dietary supplements containing ephedra alkaloids. N Engl J Med 2000;343:1833–1838.

Ikeda H et al: Mapping of a familial moyamoya disease gene to chromosome 3p24.2–p26. Am J Hum Genet 1999;64:533–537.

Kernan WN et al: Phenylpropanolamine and the risk of hemorrhagic stroke. N Engl J Med 2000;343:1826–1832.

Neiman J, Haapaniemi HM, Hillbom M: Neurological complications of drug abuse: pathophysiological mechanisms. Eur J Neurol 2000;7:595–606.

Pantoni L, Garcia JH: Pathogenesis of leukoaraiosis: a review. Stroke 1997;28:652–659.

Schievink WI: Spontaneous dissection of the carotid and vertebral arteries. N Engl J Med 2001;344:898–906.

Tzourio C et al: Migraine and stroke in young women. Cephalalgia. 2000;20:190–199.

Welch GN, Loscalzo J: Homocysteine and atherothrombosis. N Engl J Med 1998;338:1042–1050.

Cardiac Causes

Babikian VL, Caplan LR: Brain embolism is a dynamic process with variable characteristics. Neurology 2000;54:797–801.

Falk R H: Atrial fibrillation. N Engl J Med 2001;344:1067–1078.

Gilon D et al: Lack of evidence of an association between mitral-valve prolapse and stroke in young patients. N Engl J Med 1999;341:8–13.

Maggioni AP et al: The risk of stroke in patients with acute myocardial infarction after thrombolytic and antithrombotic treatment. N Engl J Med 1992;327:1–6.

Hematologic Causes

Adams RJ et al: Prevention of a first stroke by transfusions in children with sickle cell anemia and abnormal results on transcranial doppler ultrasonography. N Engl J Med 1998;339: 5–11.

Medical Treatment

Albers GW et al: Antithrombotic and thrombolytic therapy for ishemic stroke. Chest 2001;119:300S–320S.

Bath PMW, Iddenden R, Bath FJ: Low-molecular-weight heparins and heparinoids in acute ischemic stroke: a meta-analysis of randomized controlled trials. Stroke 2000;31:1770–1778.

Bednar MM, Gross CE: Antiplatelet therapy in acute cerebral ischemia. Stroke 1999;30:887–893.

Brott T, Bogousslavsky J: Treatment of acute ischemic stroke. N Engl J Med 2000;343:710–722.

CAPRIE Steering Committee: A randomised, blinded, trial of clopidogrel versus aspirin in patients at risk of ischaemic events (CAPRIE). Lancet 1996;348:1329–1339.

International Stroke Trial Collaborative Group: The International Stroke Trial (IST): a randomised trial of aspirin, subcutaneous heparin, both, or neither among 19435 patients with acute ischaemic stroke. Lancet 1997;349:1569–1581.

Kwiatkowski TG et al: Effects of tissue plasminogen activator for acute ischemic stroke at one year. N Engl J Med 1999;340:1781–1787.

Lyden PD et al: Intravenous thrombolysis for acute stroke. Neurology 1997;49:14–20.

National Institute of Neurological Disorders and Stroke rt-PA Stroke Study Group: Tissue plasminogen activator for acute ischemic stroke. N Engl J Med 1995;333:1581–1587.

Powers WJ: Acute hypertension after stroke: the scientific basis for treatment decisions. Neurology 1993;43:461–467.

Report of the Quality Standards Subcommittee of the American Academy of Neurology: Practice advisory: Thrombolytic therapy for acute ischemic stroke—summary statement. Neurology 1996;47:835 –839.

Ridker PM et al: Inflammation, aspirin, and the risk of cardiovascular disease in apparently healthy men. N Engl J Med 1997;336:973–979.

Surgical Treatment

Barnett HJM et al: Benefit of carotid endarterectomy in patients with symptomatic moderate or severe stenosis. N Engl J Med 1998;339:1415–1425.

European Carotid Surgery Trialists' Collaborative Group: Randomised trial of endarterectomy for recently symptomatic carotid stenosis: final results of the MRC European Carotid Surgery Trial (ECST). Lancet 1998;351:1379–1387.

Wong JH et al: Regional performance of carotid endarterectomy: Appropriateness, outcomes, and risk factors for complications. Stroke 1997;28:891–898.

Prognosis

Sacco RL: Risk factors and outcomes for ischemic stroke. Neurology 1995;45:S10–14.

Intracerebral Hemorrhage

Brilstra EH et al: Treatment of intracranial aneurysms by embolization with coils: a systematic review. Stroke 1999;30:470–476.

Fernandes HM et al: Surgery in intracerebral hemorrhage: the uncertainty continues. Stroke 2000;31:2511–2516.

Qureshi AI et al: Spontaneous intracerebral hemorrhage. N Engl J Med 2001;344:1450–1460.

Global Cerebral Ischemia

Hossmann KA: Reperfusion of the brain after global ischemia: hemodynamic disturbances. Shock 1997;8:95–101.

White BC et al: Global brain ischemia and reperfusion. Ann Emerg Med 1996;27:588–594.

Coma

CONTENTS

KEY CONCEPTS

 Coma is produced by disorders that affect both cerebral hemispheres or the brainstem reticular activating system.

 The possible causes of coma are limited: mass lesion, metabolic encephalopathy, infection of the brain (encephalitis) or its coverings (meningitis), and subarachnoid hemorrhage.

 The examination of a comatose patient should be focused and brief: assess whether the pupils constrict in response to light, whether eye movements

can be elicited by rotating the head (doll's-head maneuver) or by irrigating the tympanic membrane with cold water (caloric stimulation), the nature (especially bilateral symmetry or asymmetry) of the motor response to a painful stimulus, and the presence or absence of signs of meningeal irritation.

 Immediately exclude hypoglycemia.

 Patients who can open their eyes are not in coma.

Coma is a sleeplike state in which the patient makes no purposeful response to the environment and from which he or she cannot be aroused. The eyes are closed and do not open spontaneously. The patient does not speak, and there is no purposeful movement of the face or limbs. Verbal stimulation produces no response. Mechanical (eg, painful) stimulation may produce no response or may elicit nonpurposeful reflex movements mediated through spinal cord or brainstem pathways.

 Coma results from a disturbance in the function of either the brainstem reticular activating system above the midpons or both cerebral

hemispheres (Figure 10–1), since these are the brain regions that maintain consciousness.

APPROACH TO DIAGNOSIS

The approach to diagnosis of the comatose patient consists first of emergency measures to stabilize the patient and treat presumptively certain life-threatening disorders, followed by efforts to establish an etiologic diagnosis.

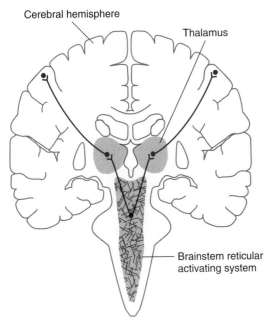

Figure 10–1. Anatomic basis of coma. Consciousness is maintained by the normal functioning of the brainstem reticular activating system above the mid pons and its bilateral projections to the thalamus and cerebral hemispheres. Coma results from lesions that affect either the reticular activating system or both hemispheres.

EMERGENCY MANAGEMENT

As summarized in Table 10–1, emergency management of the comatose patient includes the following steps:

1. Ensure patency of the airway and adequacy of ventilation and circulation. This is accomplished by rapid visual inspection and by measuring the vital signs. If the **airway** is obstructed, the obstruction should be cleared and the patient intubated. If there is evidence of trauma that may have affected the cervical spine, however, the neck should not be moved until this possibility has been excluded by x-rays of the cervical spine. In this case, if intubation is required, it should be performed by tracheostomy. Adequacy of **ventilation** can be established by the absence of cyanosis, a respiratory rate greater than 8/min, the presence of breath sounds on auscultation of the chest, and the results of arterial blood gas and pH studies (see below). If any of these suggest inadequate ventilation, the patient should be ventilated mechanically. Measurement of the pulse and blood pressure provides a rapid assessment of the status of the **circulation**. Circulatory embarrassment should be treated with intravenous fluid replacement, pressors, and antiarrhythmic drugs, as indicated.

2. Insert an intravenous catheter and withdraw blood for laboratory studies. These studies should include measurement of serum glucose and electrolytes, hepatic and renal function tests, prothrombin time, partial thromboplastin time, and a complete blood count. Extra tubes of blood should also be obtained for additional studies that may be useful in certain cases, such as drug screens, and for tests that become necessary as diagnostic evaluation proceeds.

Table 10–1. Emergency management of the comatose patient.[1]

Immediately	Next	Later
Ensure adequacy of airway, ventilation, and circulation	If signs of meningeal irritation are present (Figure 2–3) perform LP to rule out meningitis Obtain a history if possible	ECG
Draw blood for serum glucose, electrolytes, liver and renal function tests, PT, PTT, and CBC	Perform detailed general physical and neurologic examination	Correct hyper- or hypothermia
Start IV and administer 25 g of dextrose, 100 mg of thiamine, and 0.4–1.2 mg of naloxone IV	Order CT scan of head if history or findings suggest structural lesion or subarachnoid hemorrhage	Correct severe acid-base and electrolyte abnormalities
Draw blood for arterial blood gas determinations		Chest x-ray
Treat seizures (see Chapter 8)		Blood and urine toxicology studies; EEG

[1] CBC, complete blood count; IV, intravenous; LP, lumbar puncture; PT, prothrombin time; PTT, partial thromboplastin time.

3. Begin an intravenous infusion and administer dextrose, thiamine, and naloxone. Every comatose patient should be given 25 g of **dextrose** intravenously, typically as 50 mL of a 50% dextrose solution, to treat possible hypoglycemic coma. Since administration of dextrose alone may precipitate or worsen Wernicke's encephalopathy in thiamine-deficient patients, all comatose patients should also receive 100 mg of **thiamine** by the intravenous route. To treat possible opiate overdose, the opiate antagonist **naloxone**, 0.4–1.2 mg intravenously, should also be administered routinely to comatose patients. The benzodiazepine antagonist **flumazenil** should not be used in coma of unknown cause (see p 332).

4. Withdraw arterial blood for blood gas and pH determinations. In addition to assisting in the assessment of ventilatory status, these studies can provide clues to metabolic causes of coma (Table 10–2).

5. Institute treatment for seizures, if present. Persistent or recurrent seizures in a comatose patient should be considered to represent status epilepticus and treated accordingly, as described in Chapter 8 (see particularly Table 8–6).

After these measures have been taken, the history (if available) is obtained and general physical and neurologic examinations are performed.

HISTORY & EXAMINATION

History

The most crucial aspect of the history is the time over which coma develops. In the absence of precise details about the mode of onset, information about when the patient was last seen in an apparently normal state may assist in establishing the time course of the disease process.

Table 10–2. Metabolic coma: Differential diagnosis by acid-base abnormalities.[1]

Respiratory acidosis	Metabolic acidosis
Sedative drug intoxication	Diabetic ketoacidosis
Pulmonary encephalopathy	Uremic encephalopathy
Respiratory alkalosis	Lactic acidosis
Hepatic encephalopathy	Paraldehyde intoxication
Salicylate intoxication	Methanol intoxication
Sepsis	Ethylene glycol intoxication
	Isoniazid intoxication
	Salicylate intoxication
	Sepsis (terminal)
	Metabolic alkalosis
	Coma unusual

[1] Adapted from Plum, F, Posner JB: *The Diagnosis of Stupor and Coma,* 3rd ed. Vol 19 of: *Contemporary Neurology Series.* Davis, 1980.

 1. A sudden onset of coma suggests a vascular origin, especially a brainstem stroke or subarachnoid hemorrhage.

 2. Rapid progression from hemispheric signs, such as hemiparesis, hemisensory deficit, or aphasia, to coma within minutes to hours is characteristic of intracerebral hemorrhage.

 3. A more protracted course leading to coma (days to a week or more) is seen with tumor, abscess, or chronic subdural hematoma.

 4. Coma preceded by a confusional state or agitated delirium, without lateralizing signs or symptoms, is probably due to a metabolic derangement.

General Physical Examination

A. SIGNS OF TRAUMA

1. Inspection of the head may reveal signs of **basilar skull fracture**, including the following:

a. Raccoon eyes—Periorbital ecchymoses.

b. Battle's sign—Swelling and discoloration overlying the mastoid bone behind the ear.

c. Hemotympanum—Blood behind the tympanic membrane.

d. Cerebrospinal fluid (CSF) rhinorrhea or otorrhea—Leakage of CSF from the nose or ear. CSF rhinorrhea must be distinguished from other causes of rhinorrhea, such as allergic rhinitis. It has been suggested that CSF can be distinguished from nasal mucus by the higher glucose content of CSF, but this is not always the case. The chloride level may be more useful, since CSF chloride concentrations are 15–20 meq/L higher than those in mucus.

2. Palpation of the head may demonstrate a **depressed skull fracture** or **swelling of soft tissues** at the site of trauma.

B. BLOOD PRESSURE

Elevation of blood pressure in a comatose patient may reflect long-standing hypertension, which predisposes to intracerebral hemorrhage or stroke. In the rare condition of hypertensive encephalopathy, the blood pressure is above 250/150 mm Hg in chronically hypertensive patients; it may be lower following acute elevation of blood pressure in previously normotensive patients (eg, in acute renal failure). Elevation of blood pressure may also be a consequence of the process causing the coma, as in intracerebral or subarachnoid hemorrhage or, rarely, brainstem stroke.

C. TEMPERATURE

Hypothermia can occur in coma caused by ethanol or sedative drug intoxication, hypoglycemia, Wernicke's encephalopathy, hepatic encephalopathy, and myxedema.

Coma with hyperthermia is seen in heat stroke, status epilepticus, malignant hyperthermia related to inhalational anesthetics, anticholinergic drug intoxication, pontine hemorrhage, and certain hypothalamic lesions.

D. SIGNS OF MENINGEAL IRRITATION

Signs of meningeal irritation [eg, nuchal rigidity or the Brudzinski sign (see Figure 2–3)] are of great importance in leading to the prompt diagnosis of meningitis or subarachnoid hemorrhage, but they are lost in deep coma.

E. OPTIC FUNDI

Examination of the optic fundi may reveal papilledema or retinal hemorrhages compatible with chronic or acute hypertension or an elevation in intracranial pressure. Subhyaloid (superficial retinal) hemorrhages in an adult strongly suggest subarachnoid hemorrhage (Figure 2–5).

Neurologic Examination

The neurologic examination is the key to etiologic diagnosis in the comatose patient. Pupillary size and reactivity, oculocephalic and oculovestibular reflexes, and the motor response to pain should be evaluated in detail (Figure 10–2).

A. PUPILS

1. Normal pupils—Normal pupils are 3–4 mm in diameter and equal bilaterally; they constrict briskly and symmetrically in response to light. Normal pupils, however, are larger in children and smaller in the old.

2. Thalamic pupils—Slightly smaller reactive pupils are present in the early stages of thalamic compression from mass lesions, perhaps because of the interruption of the descending sympathetic pathways.

3. Fixed dilated pupils—Pupils greater than 7 mm in diameter and fixed (nonreactive to light) usually result from compression of the oculomotor (III) cranial nerve anywhere along its course from the midbrain to the orbit but may also be seen in anticholinergic or sympathomimetic drug intoxication. The most common cause of a fixed dilated pupil in a comatose patient is transtentorial herniation of the medial temporal lobe from a supratentorial mass.

4. Fixed midsized pupils—Pupils fixed at about 5 mm in diameter are the result of brainstem damage at the midbrain level.

5. Pinpoint pupils—Pinpoint pupils (1–1.5 mm in diameter) in a comatose patient usually indicate opioid overdose or focal damage at the pontine level. Under these conditions, the pupils may appear unreactive to light except, perhaps, with a magnifying glass. Pinpoint pupils are also caused by organophosphate poisoning, miotic eye drops, or neurosyphilis.

6. Asymmetric pupils—Asymmetry of pupillary size (anisocoria) with a difference of 1 mm or less in diameter is a normal finding in 20% of the population; the pupils constrict to a similar extent in response to light, and extraocular movements are not impaired. In contrast, a pupil that constricts less rapidly or to a lesser extent than its fellow usually implies a structural lesion affecting the midbrain or oculomotor nerve.

B. EXTRAOCULAR MOVEMENTS

1. Pathways tested—The neuronal pathways to be tested begin at the pontomedullary junction [vestibular (VIII) nerve and nucleus], synapse in the caudal pons [horizontal gaze center and abducens (VI) nerve nucleus], ascend through the central core of the brainstem reticular activating system (medial longitudinal fasciculus), and arrive at the midbrain level [oculomotor (III) nucleus and nerve; Figure 10–3].

2. Methods of testing—In the comatose patient, eye movements are tested by stimulating the vestibular system (semicircular canals of the middle ear) by means of passive head rotation (the **oculocephalic reflex**, or **doll's-head maneuver**) or by the stronger stimulus of ice-water irrigation against the tympanic membrane (**oculovestibular reflex**, or **cold-water calorics** testing) (see Chapter 3 and Figures 3–1 and 10–3).

3. Normal movements—A comatose patient without brainstem disease will often demonstrate full conjugate horizontal eye movements during the doll's-head maneuver and always exhibits tonic conjugate movement of both eyes to the side of the ice-water irrigation during caloric testing. The presence of full reflex eye movements in the comatose patient attests to the integrity of the brainstem from the pontine to the midbrain level and excludes a mass lesion in the brainstem.

4. Abnormal movements—

a. With lesions of the oculomotor nerve or nucleus (such as in the rostral-caudal herniation syndrome; Figure 10–2), oculovestibular testing will reveal failure of ocular adduction with unimpaired contralateral abduction.

b. Complete absence of response on oculovestibular testing in a comatose patient implies either a structural lesion of the brainstem at the level of the pons or a metabolic disorder with a particular predilection for brainstem involvement; this is usually caused by sedative drug intoxication.

c. Downward deviation of one or both eyes in response to unilateral cold-water irrigation is most suggestive of sedative drug intoxication.

C. MOTOR RESPONSE TO PAIN

The motor response to pain is tested by applying strong pressure on the supraorbital ridge, sternum, or nail beds.

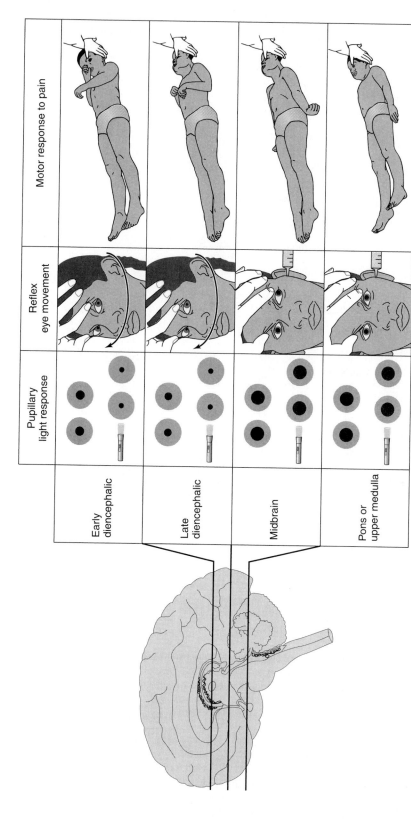

Figure 10–2. Neurologic signs in coma with downward transtentorial herniation. In the **early diencephalic** phase, the pupils are small (about 2 mm in diameter) and reactive, reflex eye movements are intact, and the motor response to pain is purposeful or semipurposeful (localizing) and often asymmetric. The **late diencephalic** phase is associated with similar findings, except that painful stimulation results in decorticate (flexor) posturing, which may also be asymmetric. With **midbrain** involvement, the pupils are fixed and midsized (about 5 mm in diameter), reflex adduction of the eyes is impaired, and pain elicits decerebrate (extensor) posturing. Progression to involve the **pons or medulla** also produces fixed, midsized pupils, but these are accompanied by loss of reflex abduction as well as adduction of the eyes and by no motor response or only leg flexion upon painful stimulation. Note that although a lesion restricted to the pons produces pinpoint pupils as a result of the destruction of descending sympathetic (pupillodilator) pathways, downward herniation to the pontine level is associated with midsized pupils. This happens because herniation also interrupts parasympathetic (pupilloconstrictor) fibers in the oculomotor (III) nerve.

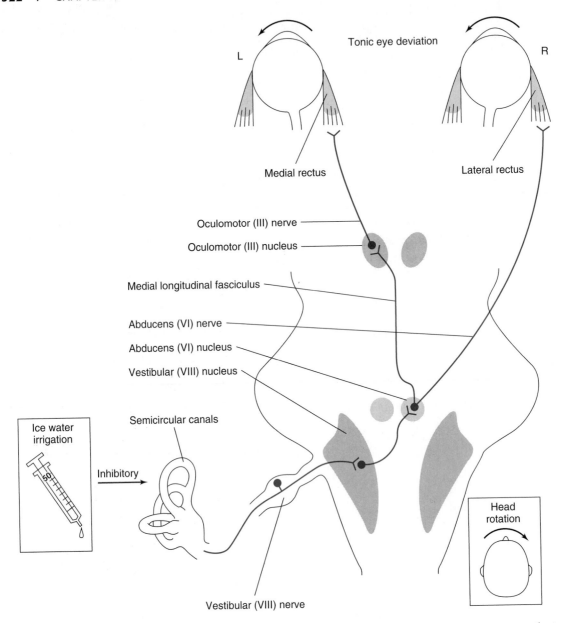

Tonic eye deviation

L

R

Medial rectus

Lateral rectus

Oculomotor (III) nerve

Oculomotor (III) nucleus

Medial longitudinal fasciculus

Abducens (VI) nerve

Abducens (VI) nucleus

Vestibular (VIII) nucleus

Ice water irrigation

Semicircular canals

Inhibitory

Head rotation

Vestibular (VIII) nerve

Figure 10–3. Brainstem pathways mediating reflex conjugate horizontal eye movements. In a comatose patient with intact brainstem function, irrigation of the tympanic membrane with ice water inhibits the vestibuloocular pathways shown, resulting in tonic deviation of both eyes toward the irrigated side; head rotation causes eye deviation away from the direction of rotation.

The response to such stimuli may be helpful in localizing the level of cerebral dysfunction in comatose patients or providing a guide to the depth of coma.

1. With cerebral dysfunction of only moderate severity, patients may localize the offending stimulus by reaching toward the site of stimulation. Although semipurposeful localizing responses to pain can sometimes be difficult to distinguish from the reflex responses described below, movements that involve limb abduction are virtually never reflexive in nature.

2. A **decorticate** response to pain (flexion of the arm at the elbow, adduction at the shoulder, and extension of the leg and ankle) is classically associated with lesions that involve the thalamus directly or large hemispheric masses that compress it from above.

3. A **decerebrate** response (extension at the elbow, internal rotation at the shoulder and forearm, and leg extension) tends to occur when midbrain function is compromised. Decerebrate posturing generally implies more severe brain dysfunction than decorticate posturing, but neither response localizes the site of disease precisely.

4. Bilateral symmetric posturing may be seen in both structural and metabolic disorders.

5. Unilateral or asymmetric posturing suggests structural disease in the contralateral cerebral hemisphere or brainstem.

6. In patients with pontine and medullary lesions, there is usually no response to pain, but occasionally some flexion at the knee is noted (a spinal reflex).

PATHOPHYSIOLOGIC ASSESSMENT

The most important step in evaluating the comatose patient is to decide whether unconsciousness is the result of a structural brain lesion (for which emergency neurosurgical intervention may be critical) or is secondary to a diffuse encephalopathy caused by metabolic disturbance, meningitis, or seizures (for which surgical procedures are unnecessary and medical treatment may be required). The most common diagnostic dilemma is to try to differentiate between a supratentorial (hemispheric) mass lesion and metabolic encephalopathy.

Supratentorial Structural Lesions

When coma is the result of a supratentorial mass lesion, the history and physical findings early in the course usually point to a hemispheric disorder. Hemiparesis with hemisensory loss is typical. Aphasia occurs with dominant (usually left) hemispheric lesions, and agnosia (indifference to or denial of the deficit) with injury to the nondominant hemisphere. As the mass expands (commonly from associated edema), somnolence supervenes because of the compression of the contralateral hemisphere or downward pressure on the diencephalon. Stupor progresses to coma, but the findings often remain asymmetric. As rostral-caudal compression progresses, the thalamus, midbrain, pons, and medulla become sequentially involved, and the neurologic examination reveals dysfunction at successively lower anatomical levels (see Figure 10–2). Such segmental involvement strongly supports the diagnosis of a supratentorial mass with downward transtentorial herniation (Figure 10–4) and dictates the need for neurosurgical

intervention. Once the pontine level is reached, a fatal outcome is inevitable. Even at the fully developed midbrain level, chances of survival without severe neurologic impairment decrease rapidly, especially in adults.

When supratentorial mass lesions produce herniation of the medial portion of the temporal lobe (the uncus) across the cerebellar tentorium (see Figure 10–4), thus exerting direct pressure on the rostral brainstem, signs of oculomotor nerve and midbrain compression such as ipsilateral pupillary dilatation and impaired adduction of the eye (**uncal syndrome**) may precede loss of consciousness. As consciousness is lost with progressive uncal herniation, the fully developed midbrain stage rapidly appears, with marked ipsilateral pupillary dilation and loss of reactivity to light. Neurosurgical treatment must be given early in the course of third-nerve involvement if useful recovery is to be achieved.

Subtentorial Structural Lesions

Coma of sudden onset with focal brainstem signs strongly supports a diagnosis of a subtentorial structural lesion. Pupillary function and extraocular movements are the most helpful features of the neurologic examination, especially if the abnormalities are asymmetric. With focal midbrain lesions, pupillary function is lost: the pupils are midsized (about 5 mm in diameter) and nonreactive to light. Pinpoint pupils are found in pontine hemorrhage

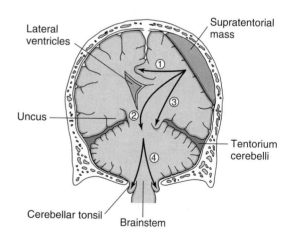

Figure 10–4. Anatomic basis of herniation syndromes. An expanding supratentorial mass lesion may cause brain tissue to be displaced into an adjacent intracranial compartment, resulting in (1) cingulate herniation under the falx, (2) downward transtentorial (central) herniation, (3) uncal herniation over the edge of the tentorium, or (4) cerebellar tonsillar herniation into the foramen magnum. Coma and ultimately death result when (2), (3), or (4) produces brainstem compression.

and less often in pontine infarction or pontine compression caused by cerebellar hemorrhage or infarction. Conjugate gaze deviation away from the side of the lesion and toward the hemiparesis—or disconjugate eye movements, such as internuclear ophthalmoplegia (selective impairment of eye adduction)—strongly suggests a subtentorial lesion. Motor responses are generally not helpful in separating subtentorial from supratentorial lesions. Ventilatory patterns associated with subtentorial lesions are abnormal but variable and may be ataxic or gasping (Figure 10–5). Because the fully developed syndrome of transtentorial herniation from a supratentorial mass is characterized by extensive brainstem dysfunction, its differentiation from a primary subtentorial process may be impossible except by history.

Diffuse Encephalopathies

Diffuse encephalopathies that result in coma (sometimes termed **metabolic coma**) include not only metabolic disorders such as hypoglycemia and drug intoxication but other processes that affect the brain diffusely, such as meningitis, subarachnoid hemorrhage, and seizures.

The clinical presentation is distinct from that of a mass lesion. There are usually no focal signs, such as

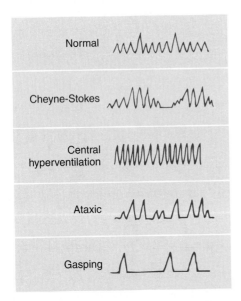

Figure 10–5. Ventilatory patterns in coma. Cheyne-Stokes respiration and central hyperventilation are seen with metabolic disturbances and with structural lesions at a variety of sites in the brain. They are therefore not useful for anatomic localization of disorders producing coma. Ataxic and gasping ventilatory patterns are most commonly seen with pontomedullary lesions.

hemiparesis, hemisensory loss, or aphasia, and—except in some cases of subarachnoid hemorrhage—no sudden loss of consciousness. Instead, the history reveals a period of progressive somnolence or toxic delirium followed by gradual descent into a stuporous and finally comatose state.

A symmetric neurologic examination supports a metabolic cause of coma. Hepatic encephalopathy, hypoglycemia, and hyperosmolar nonketotic hyperglycemia may uncommonly be accompanied by focal signs—especially hemiparesis, which may alternate from side to side. Asterixis, myoclonus, and tremor preceding coma are important clues that suggest metabolic disease. Symmetric decorticate or decerebrate posturing can be seen with hepatic, uremic, anoxic, hypoglycemic, or sedative-drug-induced coma.

The finding of reactive pupils in the presence of otherwise impaired brainstem function is the hallmark of metabolic encephalopathy. Although coma with intact pupillary reactivity is also seen in the early stages of transtentorial herniation (see Figure 10–2), this latter syndrome is associated with asymmetric neurologic findings (hemiparesis). The few metabolic causes of coma that also impair pupillary reflexes include glutethimide overdose, massive barbiturate overdose with apnea and hypotension, acute anoxia, marked hypothermia, and anticholinergic poisoning (large pupils); and opioid overdose (pinpoint pupils). Even in these conditions, however, completely nonreactive pupils are uncommon.

The respiratory patterns in metabolic coma vary widely, and measurement of arterial blood gases and pH may provide a further basis for establishing an etiologic diagnosis. Arterial blood gas abnormalities in coma are outlined in Table 10–2.

Summary

The relationship between neurologic signs and the pathophysiologic basis of coma is summarized in Table 10–3. Examining pupillary size and reactivity and testing reflex eye movements and the motor response to pain help determine whether brain function is disrupted at a discrete anatomic level (**structural lesion**) or in a diffuse manner (**metabolic coma**).

Supratentorial structural lesions compromise the brain in an orderly way, producing dysfunction at progressively lower anatomic levels. In patients with metabolic coma, such localization is not possible, and scattered, anatomically inconsistent findings are noted on examination. An impressive example of the anatomically discordant findings characteristic of metabolic encephalopathy is the retention of pupillary reactivity in the face of otherwise depressed brainstem functions: paralysis of eye movements, respiratory depression, flac-

Table 10–3. Pathophysiologic assessment of the comatose patient.

	Supratentorial Structural Lesion	Subtentorial Structural Lesion	Diffuse Encephalopathy/Meningitis
Pupil size and light reaction	Usually normal size (3–4 mm) and reactive; large (>7 mm) and unreactive after transtentorial herniation	Midsized (about 5 mm) and unreactive with midbrain lesions; pinpoint (1–1.5 mm) and unreactive with pontine lesion	Usually normal size (3–4 mm) and reactive; pinpoint (1–1.5 mm) and sometimes unreactive with opiates; large (>7mm) and unreactive with anticholinergics
Reflex eye movements	Normal	Impaired adduction with midbrain lesion; impaired adduction and abduction with pontine lesion	Usually normal; impaired by sedative drugs or Wernicke's encephalopathy
Motor responses	Usually asymmetric; may be symmetric after transtentorial herniation	Asymmetric (unilateral lesion) or symmetric (bilateral lesion)	Usually symmetric; may be asymmetric with hypoglycemia, hyperosmolar nonketotic hyperglycemia, or hepatic encephalopathy

cid muscle tone, and unresponsiveness to painful stimuli such as is typical with sedative drug overdose. The same degree of low brainstem dysfunction produced by a supratentorial mass lesion would have to first compromise the more rostrally situated midbrain structures that mediate pupillary reactivity before affecting the lower brainstem centers.

ETIOLOGY

SUPRATENTORIAL STRUCTURAL LESIONS

1. Subdural Hematoma

Subdural hematoma is a correctable supratentorial mass lesion and must be considered in any comatose patient. It is more common in older patients, since cerebral atrophy makes bridging cortical veins more subject to laceration from shearing injury or to apparently spontaneous rupture.

Trauma is the most common cause, and in the acute stage following head injury, focal neurologic deficits are often conspicuous. The severity of injury needed to produce a subdural hematoma becomes less with advancing age, so that in perhaps 25% of cases a history of trauma is not present.

The most common clinical findings are headache and altered consciousness, but symptoms and signs may be absent, nonspecific, or nonlocalizing, especially with chronic subdural hematomas that appear months or years after injury (Table 10–4). The classic history of

Table 10–4. Clinical features of subdural hematoma.[1]

	Acute[2] (82 Cases) (%)	Subacute[3] (91 Cases) (%)	Chronic[4] (216 Cases) (%)
Symptoms			
Depression of consciousness	100	88	47
Vomiting	24	31	30
Weakness	20	19	22
Confusion	12	41	37
Headache	11	44	81
Speech disturbance	6	8	6
Seizures	6	3	9
Vertigo	0	4	5
Visual disturbance	0	0	12
Signs			
Depression of consciousness	100	88	59
Pupillary inequality	57	27	20
Motor asymmetry	44	37	41
Confusion and memory loss	17	21	27
Aphasia	6	12	11
Papilledema	1	15	22
Hemianopia	0	4	3
Facial weakness	0	3	3

[1] Data from McKissock W: Lancet 1960;1:1365–1370.
[2] Within 3 days of trauma.
[3] 4–20 days after trauma.
[4] More than 20 days after trauma.

waxing and waning signs and symptoms is too infrequent to be relied on for diagnosis. Hemiparesis, when present, is contralateral to the lesion in about 70% of cases. Pupillary dilation, when present, is ipsilateral in approximately 90% of cases. The frequency of bilateral hematomas makes localization of the lesion even more difficult, as may coexisting cerebral contusion.

Diagnosis is made by computed tomography (CT) scan or magnetic resonance imaging (MRI) (Figure 10–6). Lumbar puncture will not be diagnostic and is therefore not indicated.

Treatment of symptomatic subdural hematoma is by surgical evacuation.

2. Epidural Hematoma

Epidural hematoma typically results from head trauma associated with a lateral skull fracture and tearing of the middle meningeal artery and vein. Patients may or may not lose consciousness initially. There is often a lucid interval of several hours before the onset of coma during which headache, vomiting, obtundation, seizures, and focal neurologic signs may occur. The diagnosis is made by CT scan or MRI (Figure 10–6), which classically shows a radiodense biconvex lens-shaped mass com-

pressing the cerebral hemisphere. Lumbar puncture is contraindicated. Prompt surgical evacuation of the hematoma is essential to prevent a fatal outcome.

3. Cerebral Contusion

Cerebral contusion caused by head trauma is associated with initial unconsciousness from which the patient recovers. Edema surrounding the contusion may cause the level of consciousness to fluctuate, and seizures and focal neurologic signs may develop. Patients must be carefully monitored for neurologic deterioration related to progressive edema and herniation.

Lumbar puncture is unnecessary and potentially dangerous. CT scan or MRI is the diagnostic procedure of choice. In contrast to subdural and epidural hematomas, cerebral contusions are rarely operated upon.

4. Intracerebral Hemorrhage

Etiology

The most common cause of nontraumatic intracerebral hemorrhage is chronic hypertension. This and other causes are discussed in more detail in Chapter 9.

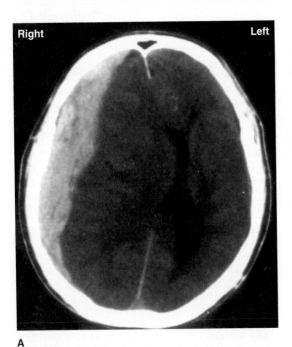
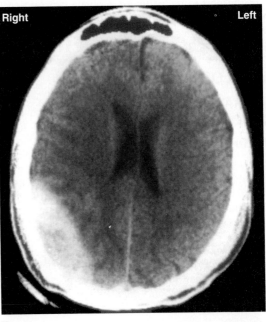

A   B

Figure 10–6. **A:** Subdural hematoma. Unenhanced CT scan showing a large, high-density crescentic mass over the right cerebral hemisphere, with shift of the lateral ventricles across the midline. **B:** Epidural hematoma. Unenhanced CT scan showing a large, high-density lens-shaped mass in the right parietooccipital region. Fracture of the occipital bone was seen on bone windows.

Clinical Findings

A. SYMPTOMS

Hemorrhage usually occurs when the patient is awake and is not preceded by prodromal symptoms such as the transient ischemic attacks often associated with cerebral infarction. Headache occurs in many cases and can be moderate to severe. If present, headache may overlie the site of hemorrhage or be generalized. Nausea and vomiting are common. Hemiparesis is a frequent early symptom because of the proximity of common hemorrhage sites, such as the basal ganglia and thalamus, to the internal capsule. Seizures occur in about 10% of cases and are often focal. Altered consciousness is common and may progress steadily to stupor or coma over minutes to hours. Neurologic deficits do not fluctuate spontaneously.

B. PHYSICAL EXAMINATION

Patients are nearly always hypertensive (blood pressure 170/90 mm Hg or higher) even in the late stages of transtentorial herniation. The funduscopic examination usually shows vascular changes associated with chronic hypertension. Nuchal rigidity is common, as is conjugate deviation of the eyes toward the side of hemorrhage in the cerebral hemisphere—and thus away from the hemiparetic side.

C. INVESTIGATIVE STUDIES

CT brain scan without contrast or MRI confirms the diagnosis, showing the presence of intraparenchymal blood. Lumbar puncture is generally unnecessary and can be dangerous if intracranial pressure is markedly increased. The spinal fluid is bloody in 90% of cases.

Treatment

Treatment for intracerebral hemorrhage is limited, in particular because the hemorrhage usually occurs over a brief period and then stops. Bleeding generally does not recur, but the patient's condition worsens because of cerebral edema.

A. ACUTE MANAGEMENT OF BLOOD PRESSURE

Acute reduction of systemic blood pressure is usually ineffective in decreasing edema. In addition, it may result in dangerous hypoperfusion of the brain although autoregulation is preserved. Once the acute phase is over, the blood pressure should be controlled pharmacologically.

B. SURGICAL TREATMENT

Surgical evacuation of the clot would seem appropriate, but because the hematoma is usually deep within the brain, surgical results are disappointing. Operation may be useful, however, in the cases (approximately 10%) in which the hemorrhage is located superficially in the cerebral hemisphere and produces a mass effect.

C. TREATMENT OF CEREBRAL EDEMA

Cerebral edema may be treated with steroids, mannitol, glycerol, or intravenous urea (Table 10–5), but such measures rarely alter the eventual outcome.

Table 10–5. Drug therapy for cerebral edema.

Drug	Dose	Route	Indications and Comments
Glucocorticoids			
Dexamethasone	10–100 mg, then 4 mg four times daily	Intravenous or orally	Dexamethasone preferred for lowest mineralocorticoid effect. Antacid treatment indicated. Effective for edema associated with brain tumor or abscess, perhaps also intracerebral hemorrhage, but not infarction
Prednisone	60 mg, then 25 mg four times daily	Orally	
Methylprednisone	60 mg, then 25 mg four times daily	Intravenous or orally	
Hydrocortisone	300 mg, then 130 mg four times daily	Intravenous or orally	
Osmotic diuretic agents			
Mannitol	1.5–2 g/kg over 30 minutes to 1 hour	20% Intravenous solution	Effective acutely. Major dehydrating effect on normal tissue; osmotic effect short-lived, and more than two intravenous doses rarely effective. Side effects include osmotic diuresis, electrolyte imbalance, and (with glycerol) nausea and vomiting
Urea	1–5 g/kg	Intravenously	
Glycerol	1.5–4 g/kg/d	Orally	

Prognosis

Many patients experience a rapid downhill course leading to death. Those who do survive may be left with a surprisingly mild deficit as the clot resolves over a period of weeks to months.

5. Brain Abscess

Brain abscess is an uncommon disorder, accounting for only 2% of intracranial masses.

Etiology

The common conditions predisposing to brain abscess, in approximate order of frequency, are blood-borne metastasis from distant systemic (especially pulmonary) infection; direct extension from parameningeal sites (otitis, cranial osteomyelitis, sinusitis); an unknown source; infection associated with recent or remote head trauma or craniotomy; and infection associated with cyanotic congenital heart disease.

The most common pathogenic agents are aerobic, anaerobic, and microaerophilic streptococci, and gram-negative anaerobes such as bacteroides, fusobacterium, and prevotella. *Staphylococcus aureus, Proteus,* and other gram-negative bacilli are less common. *Actinomyces, Nocardia,* and *Candida* are also found. Multiple organisms are present in many cases.

Clinical Findings

The course is that of an expanding mass lesion, and its usual presentation is with headache and focal signs in a conscious patient. Coma may develop over days but rarely over hours. Common presenting signs and symptoms are shown in Table 10–6. Of importance is the fact that the common correlates of infection may be absent: The temperature is within normal limits in 40% of patients, and the peripheral white blood cell count is below 10,000/mm^3 in 20% of patients.

Investigative Studies

The diagnosis is strongly supported by the finding of an avascular mass on angiography or a lesion with a contrast-enhanced rim on CT scan or MRI. Examination of the CSF reveals an opening pressure greater than 200 mm water in 75% of patients; pleocytosis of 25–500 or more white cells/mm^3, depending on the proximity of the abscess to the ventricular surface and its degree of encapsulation; and elevation of protein (45–500 mg/dL) in about 60% of patients. CSF cultures are usually negative. Marked clinical deterioration may follow lumbar puncture in patients with brain abscess, however, so lumbar puncture should not be performed if brain abscess is suspected.

Table 10–6. Brain abscess: Presenting features in 43 cases.[1]

Headache	72%
Lethargy	71%
Fever	60%
Nuchal rigidity	49%
Nausea, vomiting	35%
Seizures	35%
Ocular palsy	27%
Confusion	26%
Visual disturbance	21%
Weakness	21%
Dysarthria	12%
Stupor	12%
Papilledema	10%
Aphasia	9%
Hemiparesis	9%
Dizziness	7%

[1] Data from Chun CH et al: Medicine 1986;65:415–431.

Treatment

Treatment of pyogenic brain abscess can be with antibiotics alone or combined with surgical drainage. Surgical therapy should be strongly considered when there is a significant mass effect or the abscess is near the ventricular surface, because catastrophic rupture into the ventricular system may occur. Medical treatment alone is indicated for surgically inaccessible, multiple, or early abscesses. If the causal organism is unknown, broad coverage with antibiotics is indicated. A suggested regimen includes penicillin G, 3–4 million units intravenously every 4 hours, and metronidazole, 7.5 mg/kg intravenously or orally every 6 hours. If staphylococcal infection is suspected, oxacillin or nafcillin should be added at a dose of 3 g intravenously every 6 hours. To cover staphylococci and aerobic gram-negative bacilli (trauma patients), nafcillin plus cefotaxime or ceftriaxone is recommended. Glucocorticoids (see Table 10–5) may attenuate edema surrounding the abscess. Response to medical treatment is assessed by the clinical examination and by frequent CT scans or MRIs. When medically treated patients do not improve, needle aspiration of the abscess is indicated to identify the organisms present.

6. Cerebral Infarction (Stroke)

Embolic or thrombotic occlusion of one carotid artery does not cause coma directly, because bihemispheric dysfunction is required for coma to occur. Cerebral edema following massive hemispheric infarction, however, can produce contralateral hemispheric compression or transtentorial herniation that will result in coma.

Such cerebral swelling becomes maximal within 48–72 hours after the infarct. Thus, the history is of the stroke-like onset of a focal neurologic deficit, with progression over hours or days to stupor and coma. A cerebral hemorrhage is excluded by CT scan or MRI.

The use of corticosteroids and dehydrating agents to treat associated cerebral edema has produced no clear benefit. Cerebral infarction is discussed in more detail in Chapter 9.

7. Brain Tumor

Clinical Findings

Primary or metastatic tumors of the central nervous system (see Chapter 2) rarely present with coma, although they can do so when hemorrhage into the tumor or tumor-induced seizures occur. More often, coma occurs late in the clinical course of brain tumor, and there is a history of headache, focal neurologic deficits, and altered consciousness. Papilledema is a presenting sign in 25% of cases.

Investigative Studies

If brain tumor is suspected, a CT scan or MRI should be obtained. It may or may not be possible to determine the nature of the tumor by its radiographic appearance alone; biopsy may be required. Chest x-ray is useful, because lung carcinoma is the most common source of intracranial metastasis and because other tumors that metastasize to the brain commonly involve the lungs first.

Treatment

In contrast to its lack of therapeutic effect in cerebral infarction, corticosteroid treatment (see Table 10–5) is often remarkably effective in reducing tumor-associated vasogenic brain edema (leaking capillaries) and improving related neurologic deficits. Specific approaches to the treatment of tumors include excision, radiotherapy, and chemotherapy, depending on the site and nature of the lesion.

SUBTENTORIAL STRUCTURAL LESIONS

1. Basilar Artery Thrombosis or Embolic Occlusion

Clinical Findings

These relatively common vascular syndromes (discussed in more detail in Chapter 9) produce coma by impairing blood flow to the brainstem reticular activating system. Patients are typically middle-aged to elderly and often have a history of hypertension, atherosclerotic vascular disease, or transient ischemic attacks (TIAs). Thrombosis usually affects the midportion, and embolic occlu-sion the top, of the basilar artery. Virtually all patients present with some alteration of consciousness, and 50% of patients are comatose at presentation. Focal signs are present from the outset.

Pupillary abnormalities vary with the site of the lesion and include midsized fixed pupils with midbrain involvement and pinpoint pupils with pontine lesions. Vertically skewed deviation of the eyes is common, and horizontal eye movements may be absent or asymmetric during doll's-head or caloric testing. Conjugate eye deviation, if present, is directed away from the side of the lesion and toward the hemiparesis. Vertical eye movements may be impaired or intact.

Symmetric or asymmetric long-tract signs, such as hemiparesis, hyperreflexia, and Babinski responses, may be present. There is no blood in the CSF.

Treatment & Prognosis

Current practice supports anticoagulation for progressive subtotal basilar artery thrombosis, despite the absence of clear evidence of efficacy. Anticoagulation will reduce the frequency of recurrent cardiac emboli. The prognosis depends directly upon the degree of brainstem injury.

2. Pontine Hemorrhage

Pontine hemorrhage is essentially restricted to hypertensive patients and is the least common of the hypertensive intracerebral hemorrhages (6% of cases). The apoplectic onset of coma is the hallmark of this syndrome. Physical examination reveals many of the findings noted in basilar artery infarction, but transient ischemic episodes are not encountered. Features especially suggestive of pontine involvement include ocular bobbing (spontaneous brisk, periodic, mainly conjugate downward movements of the eyes, with slower return to the primary position), pinpoint pupils, and loss of lateral eye movements. Hyperthermia [with temperature elevations to 39.5°C (103 °F) or greater] occurs in most patients surviving for more than several hours. The diagnosis is made by CT scan or MRI. CSF is grossly bloody and under increased pressure, but lumbar puncture is not indicated. There is no effective treatment. Pontine hemorrhage is considered in greater detail in Chapter 9.

3. Cerebellar Hemorrhage or Infarction

The clinical presentation of cerebellar hemorrhage or infarction ranges from sudden onset of coma, with rapid evolution to death, to a progressive syndrome developing over hours or even several days. Acute deterioration may occur without warning; this emphasizes the need for careful observation and early treatment of all patients. CT scan or MRI is helpful in confirming the diagnosis.

Surgical decompression may produce dramatic reduction of symptoms, and with proper surgical treatment, lethargic or even stuporous patients may survive with minimal or no residual deficits and intact intellect. If the patient is deeply comatose, however, the likelihood of useful survival is small. Additional discussion of these disorders can be found in Chapter 9.

4. Posterior Fossa Subdural & Epidural Hematomas

These very uncommon lesions have similar clinical pictures and are important to recognize because they are treatable. The history is frequently of occipital trauma that precedes the onset of brainstem involvement by hours to many weeks. Physical findings are those of extraaxial (extrinsic) compression of the brainstem: ataxia, nystagmus, vertigo, vomiting, and progressive obtundation. Nuchal rigidity may be present, as may papilledema in more chronic cases. CT scans of the skull often reveal a fracture line crossing the transverse and sigmoid sinuses. The source of the hematoma is the traumatic tearing of these vessels. Examination of the CSF is not helpful.

Treatment is by surgical decompression.

DIFFUSE ENCEPHALOPATHIES

1. Meningeal Irritation

Meningitis & Encephalitis

Meningitis and encephalitis may be manifested by an acute confusional state or coma, which is characteristically associated with fever and headache. In meningitis, signs of meningeal irritation are also typically present and should be sought meticulously so that lumbar puncture, diagnosis, and treatment are not delayed. These signs include resistance of the neck to full forward flexion, knee flexion during passive neck flexion, and flexion of the neck or contralateral knee during passive elevation of the extended straight leg (see Figure 2–3). Meningeal signs may be absent in encephalitis without meningeal involvement and in meningitis occurring at the extremes of age—or in patients who are deeply comatose or immunosuppressed. The findings on examination are usually symmetric, but focal features may be seen in certain infections, such as herpes simplex encephalitis or bacterial meningitis complicated by vasculitis. CSF findings and treatment are considered in Chapter 1. If signs of meningeal irritation are present, CSF examination should not be delayed in order to obtain a CT scan.

Subarachnoid Hemorrhage

In subarachnoid hemorrhage, discussed in detail in Chapter 2, symptoms are sudden in onset and almost always include headache that is typically, but not invariably, severe. Consciousness is frequently lost, either transiently or permanently, at onset. Decerebrate posturing or, rarely, seizures may occur at this time. Because bleeding is confined mainly to the subarachnoid space about the surface of the brain, prominent focal neurologic signs other than oculomotor (III) or abducens (VI) nerve palsies are uncommon, although bilateral extensor plantar responses occur frequently. Subarachnoid blood also causes irritation and meningeal signs. Examination of the optic fundi may show acute hemorrhages secondary to suddenly increased intracranial pressure or the more classic superficial subhyaloid hemorrhages (see Figure 2–5). In coma-producing subarachnoid hemorrhage, the CSF is bloody and the CT brain scan shows blood in the subarachnoid space (see Figure 2–6).

2. Hypoglycemia

Etiology

In most cases, the cause of hypoglycemic encephalopathy is insulin overdose. Other causes include alcoholism, severe liver disease, oral hypoglycemic agents, insulin-secreting neoplasms (insulinoma), and large retroperitoneal tumors.

Clinical Findings

As the blood glucose level falls, signs of sympathetic nervous system hyperactivity (tachycardia, sweating, and anxiety) may warn patients of impending hypoglycemia. These prodromal symptoms may be absent, however, in patients with diabetic autonomic neuropathy. Neurologic findings in hypoglycemia include seizures, focal signs that may alternate sides, delirium, stupor, and coma. Progressive hypothermia is common during coma.

Investigative Studies

There is no precise correlation between blood levels of glucose and symptoms, so that levels of 30 mg/dL can result in coma in one patient, delirium in a second, and hemiparesis with preserved consciousness in a third. Coma, stupor, and confusion have been reported with blood glucose concentrations of 2–28, 8 –59, and 9–60 mg/dL, respectively.

Treatment

 Permanent brain damage can be avoided if glucose is rapidly administered, intravenously, orally, or by nasogastric tube. Because this condition is so easily treated and because a delay in instituting therapy may have tragic consequences, every patient presenting with a syndrome of altered consciousness (psychosis, acute confusional state, or coma) should have blood drawn for subsequent glucose determination and immediately receive 50 mL of 50% dextrose intravenously. This allows blood to be analyzed without delaying therapy.

Prognosis

The duration of hypoglycemia that will result in permanent damage to the brain is variable. Hypoglycemic coma may be tolerated for 60–90 minutes, but once the stage of flaccidity with hyporeflexia has been reached, glucose must be administered within 15 minutes if recovery is to be expected. If the brain has not been irreparably damaged, full recovery should occur within seconds after intravenous administration of glucose and within 10–30 minutes after nasogastric administration. Rapid and complete recovery is the rule, but gradual improvement to full normality may take place over hours to several days. Any lingering signs or symptoms suggest irreversible brain damage from hypoglycemia or the presence of an additional neuropathologic process.

3. Global Cerebral Ischemia

Global cerebral ischemia produces encephalopathy that culminates in coma; it most often occurs following cardiac arrest. The pupils dilate rapidly, and there may be tonic, often opisthotonic, posturing with a few seizurelike tonic-clonic movements. Fecal incontinence is common. With prompt reestablishment of cerebral perfusion, recovery begins at the brainstem level with the return of reflex eye movements and pupillary function. Reflex motor activity (extensor or flexor posturing) then gives way to purposive movements, and consciousness is regained. The persistence of impaired brainstem function (fixed pupils) in adults following the return of cardiac function makes the outlook virtually hopeless. Incomplete recovery may occur, leading to the return of brainstem function and wakefulness (ie, eye opening with sleep-wake cycles) without higher-level intellectual functions. The condition of such patients—**awake but not aware**—has been termed **persistent vegetative state** (see below). Although such an outcome is possible following other major brain insults such as trauma, bihemispheric stroke, or subarachnoid hemorrhage, global ischemia is the most common cause.

The prognosis in anoxic-ischemic encephalopathy is related to the rapidity with which central nervous system function returns. Patients without pupillary reactivity within 1 day—or those who fail to regain consciousness within 4 days—have a poor prognosis for functional recovery (Table 10–7).

Table 10–7. Prognostic signs in coma from global cerebral ischemia. Comparison of the findings in two studies.[1,2,3]

Sign	Probability of Recovering Independent Function (%) Time Since Onset of Coma (Days)			
	0	1	3	7
Data from Levy et al[2]				
No verbal response	13	8	5	6
No eye opening	11	6	4	0
Unreactive pupils	0	0	0	0
No spontaneous eye movements	6	5	2	0
No caloric responses	5	6	6	0
Extensor posturing	18	0	0	0
Flexor posturing	14	3	0	0
Absent motor responses	4	3	0	0
Data from Edgren et al[3]				
No eye opening to pain	31	8	0	0
Absent or reflex motor responses	25	9	0	0
Unreactive pupils	17	7	0	0

[1] It can be seen that there is some variation in the prognostic utility of individual signs in the early phase of acute hypoxic encephalopathy.

[2] Data from Levy DE et al: Predicting outcome from hypoxic-ischemic coma. JAMA 1985;253:1420–1426 (N = 210).

[3] Data from Edgren E et al: Assessment of neurological prognosis in comatose survivors of cardiac arrest. Lancet 1994;343:1055–1059 (N = 131).

4. Drug Intoxication

Sedative-Hypnotic Drugs

Sedative-hypnotic drug overdose is the most common cause of coma in many series; barbiturates and benzodiazepines are the prototypical drugs. Coma is preceded by a period of intoxication marked by prominent nystagmus in all directions of gaze, dysarthria, and ataxia. Shortly after consciousness is lost, the neurologic examination may briefly suggest an upper motor neuron lesion as hyperreflexia, ankle clonus, extensor plantar responses, and (rarely) decerebrate or decorticate posturing appear. With the single exception of glutethimide, which regularly produces midsized pupils nonreactive to light, the characteristic feature of sedative-hypnotic overdose is the absence of extraocular movements on oculocephalic testing, with preservation of the pupillary light reflex. Rarely, concentrations of barbiturates or other sedative drugs sufficient to produce severe hypotension and respiratory depression requiring pressors and ventilatory support can compromise pupillary reactivity, resulting in pupils 2–3 mm in diameter that are nonreactive to light. The electroencephalogram (EEG) may be flat—and in overdose with long-acting barbiturates may remain isoelectric for at least 24 hours—yet full recovery will occur with support of cardiopulmonary function. Bullous skin eruptions and hypothermia are also characteristic of barbiturate-induced coma.

Treatment should be supportive, centered upon maintaining adequate ventilation and circulation. Barbiturates are dialyzable; however, with the shorter-acting barbiturates, morbidity and mortality rates are clearly lower in more conservatively managed patients. The use of benzodiazepine-receptor antagonists such as **flumazenil** (0.2–0.3 mg intravenously, repeated once, then 0.1-mg intravenous dosing to maximum of 1 mg) can be used to reverse sedative-hypnotic drug intoxication in settings such as conscious sedation. It should not be included as standard treatment of coma of unknown cause, since in patients with some combined drug overdoses with, eg, cocaine or a tricyclic agent in addition to a benzodiazepine, flumazenil treatment can precipitate status epilepticus.

Ethanol

Ethanol overdose produces a similar syndrome, although nystagmus during wakefulness, early impairment of lateral eye movements, and progression to coma are not as common. Peripheral vasodilation is prominent, producing tachycardia, hypotension, and hypothermia. Stupor is typically associated with blood ethanol levels of 250–300 mg/dL and coma with levels of 300–400 mg/dL, but alcoholic patients who have developed tolerance to the drug may remain awake and even apparently sober with considerably higher levels.

Opioids

Opioid overdose is characterized by pupillary constriction that is mimicked by miotic eye drops, pontine hemorrhage, Argyll Robertson pupils, and organophosphate poisoning. The diagnosis of opioid intoxication is confirmed by rapid pupillary dilation and awakening after intravenous administration of 0.4–1.2 mg of the narcotic antagonist naloxone. The duration of action of naloxone is typically 1–4 hours. Repeated doses may therefore be necessary, especially following intoxication with long-acting narcotics such as methadone.

5. Hepatic Encephalopathy

Clinical Findings

Hepatic encephalopathy (also discussed in Chapter 1) leading to coma can occur in patients with severe liver disease, especially those with portacaval shunting. Jaundice need not be present. Coma may be precipitated by an acute insult, especially gastrointestinal hemorrhage, and the production of ammonia by colonic bacteria may contribute to pathogenesis. Neuronal depression may result from an increase in inhibitory γ-aminobutyric acid (GABA)-mediated neurotransmission, perhaps from elevated levels of endogenous benzodiazepine receptor agonists in the brain. As in other metabolic encephalopathies, the patient presents with somnolence or delirium. Asterixis may be especially prominent. Muscle tone is often increased, hyperreflexia is common, and alternating hemiparesis and decorticate or decerebrate posturing have been described. Generalized and focal seizures occur but are infrequent.

Investigative Studies

A helpful diagnostic clue is the nearly invariable presence of hyperventilation with resultant respiratory alkalosis; serum bicarbonate levels are rarely depressed below 16 meq/L, however. The CSF is usually normal but may appear yellow (xanthochromic) in patients with serum bilirubin levels greater than 4–6 mg/dL. The diagnosis is confirmed by an elevated CSF glutamine concentration. Coma is usually associated with concentrations above 50 mg/dL but may occur with values as low as 35 mg/dL. Hepatic encephalopathy is treated by controlling gastrointestinal bleeding or systemic infection, decreasing protein intake to less than 20 g/d, and decreasing intracolonic pH with lactulose (30 mg orally two to three times per day or titrated to produce two to four bowel movements daily). Abdominal cramping may occur during the first 48 hours of lactulose treatment. Production of ammonia by colonic bacteria may be reduced with neomycin, 6 g/d orally in three or four divided doses.

6. Hyperosmolar States

Coma with focal seizures is a common presentation of the hyperosmolar state, which is most often associated with nonketotic hyperglycemia. Hyperosmolar nonketotic hyperglycemia is discussed in Chapter 1.

7. Hyponatremia

Hyponatremia can cause neurologic symptoms if serum sodium levels fall below 120 meq/L, especially when the serum sodium level falls rapidly. Delirium and seizures are common presenting features.

Hyponatremia is considered in detail in Chapter 1.

8. Hypothermia

All patients with temperatures below 26°C (79°F) are comatose, whereas mild hypothermia [temperatures

>32.2°C (90°F)] does not cause coma. Causes of coma associated with hypothermia include hypoglycemia, sedative drug intoxication, Wernicke's encephalopathy, and myxedema. Exposure can also produce hypothermia, such as may occur when a structural brain lesion causes acute coma out of doors or in another unheated area; therefore, such a lesion should not be excluded from consideration in the differential diagnosis of coma with hypothermia.

On physical examination, the patient is obviously cold to the touch but may not be shivering [it ceases at temperatures below 32.5°C (90.5°F)]. Standard thermometers do not record values below 35°C (95°F). Neurologic examination shows the patient to be unresponsive to pain, with diffusely increased muscle tone. Pupillary reactions may be sluggish or even absent.

The electrocardiogram (ECG) may show prolonged PR, QRS, and QT intervals; bradycardia; and characteristic J point elevation (Osborn waves). Serum creatine phosphokinase (CPK) may be elevated in the absence of myocardial infarction, and high levels of serum amylase are common. Arterial blood gas values and pH must be corrected for temperature; otherwise, falsely high P_{O_2} and P_{CO_2} and falsely low pH values will be reported.

Treatment is aimed at the underlying disease and at restoration of normal body temperature. The optimal method and speed of rewarming are controversial, but passive rewarming with blankets in a warm room is an effective and simple treatment. Ventricular fibrillation may occur during rewarming. Because warming produces vasodilation and can lead to hypotension, intravenous fluids may be required.

Most patients who recover from hypothermia do so without neurologic sequelae; except in myxedema, however, there is no direct correlation between recorded temperature and survival. Death, when it occurs, is caused by the underlying disease process responsible for hypothermia or by ventricular fibrillation, to which the human myocardium becomes especially susceptible at temperatures below 30°C (86°F); myocardial sensitivity is maximal below 21–24°C (70–75°F).

9. Hyperthermia

At body temperatures over 42–43°C (107.6–109.4°F), the metabolic activity of the central nervous system is unable to provide for increased energy demands, and coma ensues. The cause of hyperthermia in most cases is exposure to elevated environmental temperatures—what is commonly known as heat stroke. Additional causes include status epilepticus, idiosyncratic reactions to halogenated inhalational anesthetics (malignant hyperthermia), anticholinergic drugs, hypothalamic damage, and delirium tremens. Patients surviving pontine hemorrhage for more than a few hours have centrally mediated temperature elevations ranging from 38.5 to 42.8°C (101.3–109°F). The neurological examination in hyperthermia reveals reactive pupils and a diffuse increase in muscle tone as well as coma.

Treatment is immediate reduction of body temperature to 39°C (102.2°F) by sponging the patient with ice water and alcohol and using an electric fan or cooling blanket. Care must be taken to prevent overhydration, since cooling results in vasoconstriction that may produce pulmonary edema in volume-expanded patients.

10. Other Causes

Rare causes of coma include disseminated intravascular coagulopathy, sepsis, pancreatitis, vasculitis, thrombotic thrombocytopenic purpura, fat emboli, hypertensive encephalopathy, and diffuse micrometastases.

SEIZURE OR PROLONGED POSTICTAL STATE

Status epilepticus should always be considered in the differential diagnosis of coma. Motor activity may be restricted to repetitive movements of part of a single limb or one side of the face. Although these signs of seizure activity can be subtle, they must not escape notice: status epilepticus requires urgent treatment (see Chapter 8).

Coma may also be due to a prolonged postictal state, which is also discussed in Chapter 8.

DIFFERENTIAL DIAGNOSIS

Coma can be confused with a variety of psychiatric and neurologic disorders.

PSYCHOGENIC UNRESPONSIVENESS

Psychogenic unresponsiveness is a diagnosis of exclusion that should be made only on the basis of compelling evidence. It may be a manifestation of schizophrenia (catatonic type), somatoform disorders (conversion disorder or somatization disorder), or malingering. The general physical examination reveals no abnormalities; neurologic examination generally reveals symmetrically decreased muscle tone, normal reflexes, and a normal (flexor) response to plantar stimulation. The pupils are 2–3 mm in diameter or occasionally larger and respond briskly to light. Lateral eye movements on oculocephalic (doll's-head) testing may or may not be present, since visual fixation can suppress this reflex. The slow conjugate roving eye movements of metabolic coma cannot be imitated, however, and, if present, are incompatible with a diagnosis of psychogenic unresponsiveness. Likewise, the slow, often asymmetric and incomplete eye closure commonly seen after the eyes of a comatose patient are passively opened cannot be voluntarily reproduced. The patient with psychogenic unresponsiveness usually exhibits some voluntary muscle tone in the eyelids during passive eye opening. A helpful diagnostic test is irrigation of the tympanic membrane with cold water. Brisk nystagmus is the characteristic response in conscious patients, whereas no nystagmus occurs in coma. The EEG in psychogenic unresponsiveness is that of a normal awake person.

PERSISTENT VEGETATIVE STATE

Some patients who are comatose because of cerebral hypoxia or ischemia—or structural brain lesions (Figure 10–7)—regain wakefulness but not awareness. After 1 month, this condition is termed **persistent vegetative state**. Such patients exhibit spontaneous eye opening and sleep-wake cycles, which distinguish them from patients in coma, and demonstrate intact brainstem and autonomic function. However, they neither comprehend nor produce language, and they make no purposeful motor responses. This condition may persist for years. Recovery of consciousness from nontraumatic causes is rare after 3 months, and from traumatic causes is rare after 12 months.

LOCKED-IN SYNDROME

Because the portion of the reticular formation responsible for consciousness lies above the level of the midpons, functional transection of the brainstem below this level—by pontine infarct (Figure 10–8), hemorrhage, central pontine myelinolysis, tumor, or encephalitis—can interrupt descending neural pathways to produce an akinetic and mute state, with preserved consciousness. Such patients appear comatose but are awake and alert although mute and quadriplegic. Decerebrate posturing or flexor spasms may be seen. The diagnosis is made by noting that voluntary eye opening, vertical eye movements, ocular convergence, or some combination of these midbrain-mediated movements is preserved. During the examination of any apparently comatose patient, the patient should be told to "open your eyes," "look up," "look down," and "look at the tip of your nose" to elicit such movements. The EEG is normal. Outcome is variable and related to the underlying cause and the extent of the brainstem lesion. Mortality, usually from pneumonia, is approximately 70% when the cause is a vascular disturbance and about 40% in nonvascular cases. Survivors may recover partially or completely over a period of weeks to months.

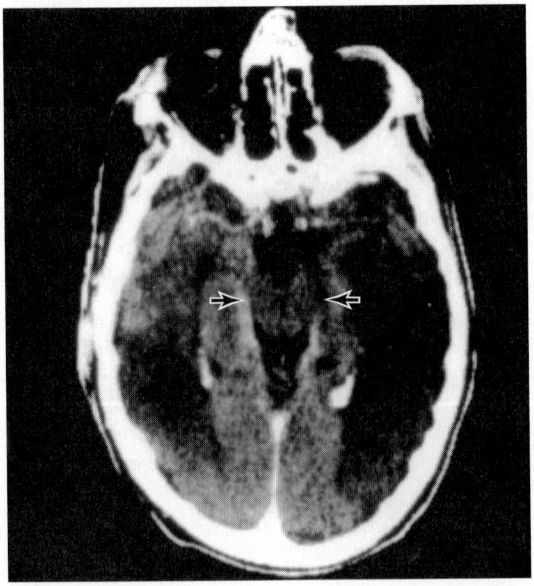

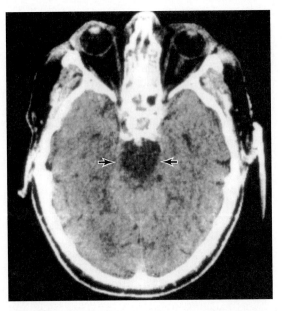

Figure 10–7. CT brain scan (contrast-enhanced) of a patient with bilateral middle cerebral artery infarcts, who is in a persistent vegetative state. The reticular activating system in the intact midbrain **(arrows)** allows wakefulness, but the bihemispheric lesions preclude awareness.

Figure 10–8. CT brain scan (contrast-enhanced) of a man with basilar artery occlusion who exhibits the "locked-in" syndrome. The pontine infarction **(arrows)** is below the level of the reticular activating system, allowing wakefulness, but the bilateral descending motor tracts have been effectively transected.

BRAIN DEATH

Current standards for the determination of brain death, developed by the President's Commission for the Study of Ethical Problems in Medicine and Biomedical and Behavioral Research (1981), are summarized below. Irreversible cessation of all brain function is required for a diagnosis of brain death. The diagnosis of brain death in children under 5 years of age must be made with caution.

Cessation of Brain Function

A. UNRESPONSIVENESS

The patient must be unresponsive to sensory input, including pain and speech.

B. ABSENT BRAINSTEM REFLEXES

Pupillary, corneal, and oropharyngeal responses are absent, and attempts to elicit eye movements with the oculocephalic and vestibuloocular maneuvers are unsuccessful. Respiratory responses are also absent, with no ventilatory effort after the patient's PCO_2 is permitted to rise to 60 mm Hg, while oxygenation is maintained by giving 100% oxygen by a cannula inserted into the endotracheal tube (apnea test).

Irreversibility of Brain Dysfunction

The cause of coma must be known; it must be adequate to explain the clinical picture; and it must be irreversible.

Sedative drug intoxication, hypothermia [32.2°C (90°F)], neuromuscular blockade, and shock must be ruled out, since these conditions can produce a clinical picture that resembles brain death but in which neurologic recovery may still be possible.

Persistence of Brain Dysfunction

The criteria for brain death described above must persist for an appropriate length of time, as follows:

1. Six hours with a confirmatory isoelectric (flat) EEG, performed according to the technical standards of the American Electroencephalographic Society.
2. Twelve hours without a confirmatory isoelectric EEG.
3. Twenty-four hours for anoxic brain injury without a confirmatory isoelectric EEG.

REFERENCES

General

Buettner UW, Zee DS: Vestibular testing in comatose patients. Arch Neurol 1989;46:561–563.

Fisher CM: The neurological examination of the comatose patient. Acta Neurol Scand 1969;45(Suppl 36):1–56.

Fisher CM: Brain herniation: a revision of classical concepts. Can J Neurol Sci 1995;22:83–91.

Plum F, Posner JB: *The Diagnosis of Stupor and Coma*, 3rd ed. Vol 19 of: *Contemporary Neurology Series.* Davis, 1980.

Simon RP: Coma. Pages 1–51 in: *Clinical Neurology.* Joynt RJ, Griggs RC (editors). Lippincott Raven, 1997.

Young GB et al (editors): *Coma and Impaired Consciousness: A Clinical Perspective.* McGraw-Hill, 1998.

Structural Lesions

Dunne JW, Chakera T, Kermode S: Cerebellar hemorrhage—Diagnosis and treatment: a study of 75 consecutive cases. Q J Med 1987; New Series 64:739–754.

Ferbert A, Bruckmann H, Drummen R: Clinical features of proven basilar artery occlusion. Stroke 1990;21:1135–1142.

Macdonnell RAL, Kalnins RM, Donnan GA: Cerebellar infarction: natural history, prognosis, and pathology. Stroke 1987;18: 849–855.

Poungvarin N et al: Effects of dexamethasone in primary supratentorial intracerebral hemorrhage. N Engl J Med 1987;316: 1229–1233.

Seelig JM et al: Traumatic acute subdural hematoma: major mortality reduction in comatose patients treated within four hours. N Engl J Med 1981;304:1511–1518.

Wijdicks EF, St Louis E: Clinical profiles predictive of outcome in pontine hemorrhage. Neurology 1997;49:1342–1346.

Wintzen AR: The clinical course of subdural hematoma: a retrospective study of etiological, chronological and pathological features in 212 patients and a proposed classification. Brain 1980;103:855–867.

Yang SY, Zhao CS: Review of 140 patients with brain abscess. Surg Neurol 1993;39:290–296.

Zhu XL et al: Spontaneous intracranial hemorrhage: which patients need diagnostic cerebral angiography? A prospective study of 206 cases and review of the literature. Stroke 1997;28: 1406–1409.

Diffuse Encephalopathies

Brust JCM: Other agents: phencyclidine, marijuana, hallucinogens, inhalants, and anticholinergics. Neurol Clin 1993;11: 555–562.

Denborough M: Malignant hyperthermia. Lancet 1998;352: 1131–1136.

Edgren E et al: Assessment of neurological prognosis in comatose survivors of cardiac arrest. Lancet 1994;343:1055–1059.

Fischbeck KH, Simon RP: Neurological manifestations of accidental hypothermia. Ann Neurol 1981;10:384–387.

Foley KM: Opioids. Neurol Clin 1993;11:503–522.

Greenberg DA: Ethanol and sedatives. Neurol Clin 1993;11: 523–534.

Levy DE et al: Predicting outcome from hypoxic-ischemic coma. JAMA 1985;253:1420–1426.

Lowenstein DH, Simon RP: Acute drug intoxication. Pages 302–336 in: *Principles of Drug Therapy in Neurology.* Johnston MV, Macdonald RL, Young AB (editors). Vol 37 of: *Contemporary Neurology Series.* Davis, 1992.

Malouf R, Brust JC: Hypoglycemia: causes, neurological manifestations, and outcome. Ann Neurol 1985;17:421–430.

Sanchez-Ramos JR: Psychostimulants. Neurol Clin 1993;11: 535–554.

Simon H: Hyperthermia. Curr Concepts 1993;329:483–487.

Weinbroum A et al: Use of flumazenil in the treatment of drug overdose: a double-blind and open clinical study in 110 patients. Crit Care Med 1996;24:199–206.

Persistent Vegetative State

Adams JH, Graham DI, Jennett B: The neuropathology of the vegetative state after an acute brain insult. Brain 2000;123: 1327–1338.

Zeman A: Persistent vegetative state. Lancet 1997;350:795–799.

Locked-In Syndrome

Katz RT et al: Long-term survival, prognosis, and life-care planning for 29 patients with chronic locked-in syndrome. Arch Phys Rehabil 1992;73:403–408.

Patterson JR, Grabois M: Locked-in syndrome: a review of 139 cases. Stroke 1986;17:758–764.

Brain Death

de Tourtchaninoff M et al: Brain death diagnosis in misleading conditions. Q J Med 1999;92:407–414.

Halevy A, Brody B: Brain death: reconciling definitions, criteria, and tests. Ann Intern Med 1993;119:519–525.

Wijdicks EFM: The diagnosis of brain death. N Engl J Med 2001; 344:1215–1221.

Neurologic Investigations

CONTENTS

KEY CONCEPTS

1. *The investigations that are performed in a particular case depend on the clinical context and the likely diagnosis.*

2. *Investigations are performed not only to suggest or confirm the diagnosis but also to exclude other diagnostic possibilities, aid prognostication, provide a guide to further management, and follow disease progression.*

3. *Physiologic studies evaluate function and are complementary to imaging studies, which evaluate structure.*

4. *The results of investigations need to be interpreted in the context in which they were obtained.*

LUMBAR PUNCTURE

Indications

Lumbar puncture is indicated for the following purposes:

1. Diagnosis of meningitis and other infective or inflammatory disorders, subarachnoid hemorrhage, hepatic encephalopathy, meningeal malignancies, paraneoplastic disorders, or suspected abnormalities of intracranial pressure.

2. Assessment of the response to therapy in meningitis and other infective or inflammatory disorders.

3. Administration of intrathecal medications or radiologic contrast media.

4. Rarely, to reduce cerebrospinal fluid (CSF) pressure.

Contraindications

1. Suspected intracranial mass lesion. In this situation, performing a lumbar puncture can hasten incipient transtentorial herniation.

2. Local infection overlying the site of puncture. Under this circumstance, cervical or cisternal puncture should be performed instead.

3. Coagulopathy. Clotting-factor deficiencies and thrombocytopenia (below 20,000/mm³ or rapidly falling platelet counts) should be corrected before lumbar puncture is undertaken, to reduce the risk of hemorrhage.

4. Suspected spinal cord mass lesion. Lumbar puncture in this case should be performed only in association with myelography, which is used to determine the presence and level of structural spinal pathology.

Preparation

A. PERSONNEL

With a cooperative patient, lumbar puncture can generally be performed by one person. An assistant can be helpful in positioning the patient and handling CSF samples, of course, especially if the patient is uncooperative or frightened.

B. EQUIPMENT AND SUPPLIES

The following items, which are usually included in preassembled lumbar puncture trays, are required. All must be sterile.

1. Gloves.
2. Iodine-containing solution for sterilizing the skin.
3. Sponges.
4. Drapes.
5. Lidocaine (1%).
6. Syringe (5 mL).
7. Needles (22- and 25-gauge).
8. Spinal needles (preferably 22-gauge) with stylets.
9. Three-way stopcock.
10. Manometer.
11. Collection tubes.
12. Adhesive bandage.

C. POSITIONING

Lumbar puncture is usually performed with the patient in the lateral decubitus position (Figure 11–1), lying at the edge of the bed and facing away from the person performing the procedure. The patient's lumbar spine should be maximally flexed to open the intervertebral spaces. The spine should be parallel to the surface of the bed and the hips and shoulders should be aligned in the vertical plane.

Occasionally, it is desirable to perform lumbar puncture with the patient seated. In this case, the patient is seated on the side of the bed, bent over a pillow that rests on a bedside table, while the physician reaches over the bed from the opposite side to perform the procedure.

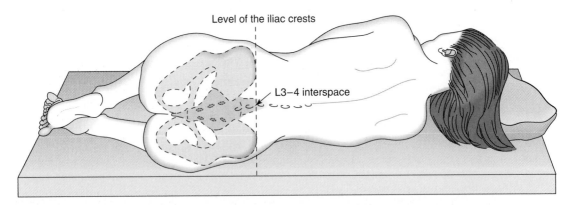

Level of the iliac crests

L3–4 interspace

Figure 11–1. Lateral decubitus position for lumbar puncture.

D. Site of Puncture

The usual practice is to enter the L3–4 or L4–5 interspace, since the spinal cord (conus medullaris) terminates at about the L1–2 level in adults. Thus, the procedure is performed without danger of puncturing the cord. The L3–4 interspace is located at the level of the posterior iliac crests.

Procedure

1. If a comparison between blood and CSF glucose levels is planned, venous blood is drawn for glucose determination. Ideally, blood and CSF glucose levels should be measured in samples obtained simultaneously after the patient has fasted for at least 4 hours.

2. The necessary equipment and supplies are placed within easy reach.

3. Sterile gloves are worn by the person performing the procedure.

4. A wide area surrounding the interspace to be entered is sterilized, using iodine-containing solution applied to sponges; the solution is then wiped off with clean sponges.

5. The area surrounding the sterile field may be draped.

6. The skin overlying the puncture site is anesthetized using lidocaine, a 5-mL syringe, and a 25-gauge needle. A 22-gauge needle is then substituted to anesthetize the underlying tissues.

7. With the stylet in place, the spinal needle is inserted at the midpoint of the chosen interspace. The needle should be parallel to the surface of the bed and angled slightly cephalad, or toward the umbilicus. The bevel of the needle should face upward, toward the face of the person performing the procedure.

8. The needle is advanced slowly until a pop, from penetration of the ligamentum flavum, is felt. The stylet is withdrawn to determine whether the CSF space has been entered, which is indicated by flow of CSF through the needle. If no CSF appears, the stylet is replaced and the needle advanced a short distance; this is continued until CSF is obtained. If at some point the needle cannot be advanced, it is likely that bone has been encountered. The needle is withdrawn partway, maintained parallel to the surface of the bed, and advanced again at a slightly different angle.

9. When CSF is obtained, the stylet is reinserted. The patient is asked to straighten his or her legs, and the stopcock and manometer are attached to the needle. The stopcock is turned to allow CSF to enter the manometer to measure the opening pressure. The pressure should fluctuate with the phases of respiration.

10. The stopcock is turned to allow the CSF to be collected, and the appearance (clarity and color) of the fluid is noted. The amount obtained and the number of tubes required varies, depending on the tests to be performed. Typically, 1–2 mL is collected in each of five tubes for cell count, glucose and protein determination, VDRL, Gram's stain, and cultures. Additional specimens may be collected for other tests, such as oligoclonal bands and glutamine, and for cytologic study. If the CSF appears to contain blood, additional fluid should be obtained so that the cell count can be repeated on the specimen in the last tube collected. Cytologic studies, if desired, require at least 10 mL of CSF.

11. The stopcock and manometer are replaced to record a closing pressure.

12. The needle is withdrawn and an adhesive bandage is applied over the puncture site.

13. It has been customary to have the patient lie prone or supine for 1 or 2 hours after the procedure to reduce the risk of post-lumbar-puncture headache. Current evidence suggests this is unnecessary.

Complications

A. Unsuccessful Tap

A variety of conditions, including marked obesity, degenerative disease of the spine, previous spinal surgery, recent lumbar puncture, and dehydration, can make it difficult to perform lumbar puncture in the conventional manner. When puncture in the lateral decubitus position is impossible, the procedure should be attempted with the patient in a sitting position. If the tap is again unsuccessful, alternative methods include lumbar puncture by an oblique approach or guided by fluoroscopy; lateral cervical puncture; or cisternal puncture. These procedures should be undertaken by a neurologist, neurosurgeon, or neuroradiologist experienced in performing them.

B. Arterial or Venous Puncture

If the needle enters a blood vessel rather than the spinal subarachnoid space, it should be withdrawn and a new needle used to attempt the tap at a different level. Patients who have coagulopathy or are receiving aspirin or anticoagulants should be observed with particular care for signs of spinal cord compression (see Chapter 5) from spinal subdural or epidural hematoma.

C. Post-Lumbar-Puncture Headache

A mild headache, worse in the upright position but relieved by recumbency, is not uncommon following lumbar puncture and will resolve spontaneously over a period of hours to days. Frequency is directly related to the size of the spinal needle. Vigorous hydration or keeping the patient in bed for 1 or 2 hours after the procedure apparently does not reduce the likelihood of such headache. The headache usually responds to nonsteroidal antiinflammatory drugs or caffeine (see

Chapter 2). Severe and protracted headache can be treated by an autologous blood clot patch, which should be applied by experienced personnel.

Analysis of Results

A. Appearance

The clarity and color of the CSF should be observed as it leaves the spinal needle, and any changes in the appearance of fluid during the course of the procedure should be noted. CSF is normally clear and colorless. It may appear cloudy or turbid with white blood cell counts that exceed about 200/μL, but counts as low as about 50/μL can be detected by holding the tube up to direct sunlight and observing the light-scattering (Tyndall) effect of suspended cells. Color can be imparted to the CSF by hemoglobin (pink), bilirubin (yellow), or, rarely, melanin (black).

B. Pressure

With the patient in the lateral decubitus position, CSF pressure in the lumbar region does not normally exceed 180–200 mm water. When lumbar puncture is performed with patients in the sitting position, patients should assume a lateral decubitus posture before CSF pressure is measured. Increased CSF pressure may result from obesity, agitation, or increased intraabdominal pressure related to position; the latter factor may be eliminated by having the patient extend the legs and back once the CSF space has been entered and before the opening pressure is recorded. Pathologic conditions associated with increased CSF pressure include intracranial mass lesions, meningoencephalitis, subarachnoid hemorrhage, and pseudotumor cerebri.

C. Microscopic Examination

This may be performed either by the person who performed the lumbar puncture or by a technician at the clinical laboratory; it always includes a cell count and differential. Gram's stain for bacteria, acid-fast stain for mycobacteria, an India ink preparation for *Cryptococcus,* and cytologic examination for tumor cells may also be indicated. The CSF normally contains up to five mononuclear leukocytes (lymphocytes or monocytes) per microliter, no polymorphonuclear cells, and no erythrocytes. Erythrocytes may be present, however, if the lumbar puncture is traumatic (see below). Normal CSF is sterile, so that in the absence of central nervous system infection, no organisms should be observed with the various stains listed above.

D. Bloody CSF

If the lumbar puncture yields bloody CSF, it is crucial to distinguish between central nervous system hemorrhage and a traumatic tap. The fluid should be watched as it leaves the spinal needle to determine whether the blood clears, which suggests a traumatic tap. This can be established with greater accuracy by comparing cell counts in the first and last tubes of CSF obtained; a marked decrease in the number of red cells supports a traumatic cause. The specimen should be centrifuged promptly and the supernatant examined. With a traumatic lumbar puncture, the supernatant is colorless. In contrast, following central nervous system hemorrhage, enzymatic degradation of hemoglobin to bilirubin in situ renders the supernatant yellow (xanthochromic). The time course of changes in CSF color following subarachnoid hemorrhage is outlined in Table 11–1. Blood in the CSF following a traumatic lumbar puncture usually clears within 24 hours; blood is usually present after subarachnoid hemorrhage for at least 6 days. In addition, blood related to traumatic puncture does not clot, whereas clotting may occur with subarachnoid hemorrhage. Crenation (shriveling) of red blood cells, however, is of no diagnostic value.

In addition to breakdown of hemoglobin from red blood cells, other causes of CSF xanthochromia include jaundice with serum bilirubin levels above 4–6 mg/dL, CSF protein concentrations greater than 150 mg/dL, and, rarely, the presence of carotene pigments.

White blood cells seen in the CSF early after subarachnoid hemorrhage or with traumatic lumbar puncture result from leakage of circulating whole blood. If the hematocrit and peripheral white blood cell count are within normal limits, there is approximately one white blood cell for each 1000 red cells. If the peripheral white cell count is elevated, a proportionate increase in this ratio should be expected. In addition, every 1000 red cells present in CSF will increase the CSF protein concentration by about 1 mg/dL.

Procedure Notes

Whenever a lumbar puncture is performed, notes describing the procedure should be recorded in the patient's chart. These notes should provide the following information:

Table 11–1. Pigmentation of the CSF following subarachnoid hemorrhage.

	Appearance	Maximum	Disappearance
Oxyhemoglobin (pink)	0.5–4 hours	24–35 hours	7–10 days
Bilirubin (yellow)	8–12 hours	2–4 days	2–3 weeks

1. Date and time performed.
2. Name of person or persons performing the procedure.
3. Indication.
4. Position of patient.
5. Anesthetic used.
6. Interspace entered.
7. Opening pressure.
8. Appearance of CSF, including changes in appearance during the course of the procedure.
9. Amount of fluid removed.
10. Closing pressure.
11. Tests ordered, eg:

    Tube #1 (1 mL), cell count.

    Tube #2 (1 mL), glucose and protein levels.

    Tube #3 (1 mL), microbiologic stains.

    Tube #4 (1 mL), bacterial, fungal, and mycobacterial cultures.
12. Results of any studies, such as microbiologic stains, performed by the operator.
13. Complications, if any.

ELECTROPHYSIOLOGIC STUDIES

ELECTROENCEPHALOGRAPHY

The electrical activity of the brain can be recorded noninvasively from electrodes placed on the scalp. Electroencephalography (EEG) is easy to perform, is relatively inexpensive, and is helpful in several different clinical contexts.

Evaluation of Suspected Epilepsy

EEG is useful in evaluating patients with suspected epilepsy. The presence of electrographic seizure activity (abnormal, rhythmic electrocerebral activity of abrupt onset and termination) during a behavioral disturbance that could represent a seizure, but about which there is clinical uncertainty, establishes the diagnosis beyond doubt. Because seizures occur unpredictably, it is often not possible to obtain an EEG during a seizure. Despite that, the EEG findings may be abnormal interictally (at times when the patient is not experiencing clinical attacks) and are therefore still useful for diagnostic purposes. The interictal presence of epileptiform activity (abnormal paroxysmal activity containing some spike discharges) is of particular help in this regard. Such activity is occasionally encountered in patients who have never had a seizure, but its prevalence is greater in patients with epilepsy than in normal subjects. Epileptiform activity in the EEG of a patient with an episodic behavioral disturbance that could on clinical grounds be a manifestation of seizures markedly increases the likelihood that the attacks are indeed epileptic, thus providing support for the clinical diagnosis.

Classification of Seizure Disorders

In known epileptics, the EEG findings may help in classifying the seizure disorder and thus in selecting appropriate anticonvulsant medication. For example, in patients with the typical absences of petit mal epilepsy (see Chapter 8) the EEG is characterized both ictally and interictally by episodic generalized spike-and-wave activity (Figure 8–3). In contrast, in patients with episodes of impaired external awareness caused by complex partial seizures, the EEG may be normal or show focal epileptiform discharges interictally. During the seizures there may be abnormal rhythmic activity of variable frequency with a localized or generalized distribution, or, in some instances, there may be no electrographic correlates. The presence of a focal or lateralized epileptogenic source is of particular importance if surgical treatment is under consideration.

Assessment & Prognosis of Seizures

The EEG findings may provide a guide to prognosis and have been used to follow the course of seizure disorders. A normal EEG implies a more favorable prognosis for seizure control, whereas an abnormal background or profuse epileptiform activity implies a poor prognosis. The EEG findings do not, however, provide a reliable guide to the subsequent development of seizures in patients with head injuries, stroke, or brain tumors. Some physicians have used the electrophysiologic findings to determine whether anticonvulsant medication can be discontinued in patients who have been free of seizures for several years. Although patients are more likely to be weaned successfully if the EEG is normal, the findings provide only a general guide, and patients can certainly have further seizures, despite a normal EEG, after withdrawal of anticonvulsant medication. Conversely, they may have no further seizures despite a continuing EEG disturbance.

Management of Status Epilepticus

The EEG is of little help in managing tonic-clonic status epilepticus unless patients have received neuromuscular blocking agents and are in a pentobarbital-induced coma. In this case, the electrophysiologic findings are useful in indicating the level of anesthesia and determining whether the seizures are continuing. The status itself is characterized by repeated electrographic seizures or continuous epileptiform (spike-and-wave) activity. In patients with nonconvulsive status epilepticus, the EEG findings provide the only means of making the diagnosis with confidence and in distinguishing the two main types. In absence status epilepticus, continuous spike-and-wave activity is seen, whereas repetitive electrographic seizures are found in complex partial status.

Detection of Structural Brain Lesions

Electroencephalography has been used as a noninvasive means of detecting focal structural abnormalities, such as brain tumors. There may be a focal slow-wave disturbance, a localized loss of electrocerebral activity, or a more generalized EEG disturbance that probably relates in part to an altered level of arousal. Noninvasive imaging procedures such as computed tomography (CT) and magnetic resonance imaging (MRI) have supplanted the use of EEG in this context.

Diagnosis of Neurologic Disorders

Certain neurologic disorders produce characteristic but nonspecific abnormalities in the EEG. Their presence is helpful in suggesting, establishing, or supporting the diagnosis. In patients presenting with an acute disturbance of cerebral function, for example, the presence of repetitive slow-wave complexes over one or both temporal lobes suggests a diagnosis of herpes simplex encephalitis. Similarly, the presence of periodic complexes in a patient with an acute dementing disorder suggests a diagnosis of Creutzfeldt-Jakob disease or subacute sclerosing panencephalitis.

Evaluation of Altered Consciousness

The EEG tends to become slower as consciousness is depressed, but the findings depend at least in part upon the etiology of the clinical disorder. The findings, such as the presence of electrographic seizure activity, can suggest diagnostic possibilities that might otherwise be overlooked. Serial records permit the prognosis and course of the disorder to be followed. The EEG response to external stimulation is an important diagnostic and prognostic guide: electrocerebral responsiveness implies a lighter level of coma. Electrocerebral silence in a technically adequate record implies neocortical death, in the absence of hypothermia or drug overdose. In some patients who appear to be comatose, consciousness is, in fact, preserved. Although there is quadriplegia and a supranuclear paralysis of the facial and bulbar muscles, the EEG is usually normal in such patients with locked-in syndrome (see Chapter 10) and helps in indicating the correct diagnosis.

EVOKED POTENTIALS

The spinal or cerebral potentials evoked by noninvasive stimulation of specific afferent pathways are an important means of monitoring the functional integrity of these pathways. They do not, however, indicate the nature of any lesion that may involve these pathways. The responses are very small compared with the background EEG activity (noise), which has no relationship to the time of stimulation. The responses to a number of stimuli are therefore recorded and averaged (with a computer) to eliminate the random noise.

Types of Evoked Potentials

A. VISUAL

Monocular visual stimulation with a checkerboard pattern is used to elicit visual evoked potentials, which are recorded from the midoccipital region of the scalp. The most clinically relevant component is the P100 response, a positive peak with a latency of approximately 100 ms. The presence and latency of the response are noted. Although its amplitude can also be measured, alterations in amplitude are far less helpful in recognizing pathology.

B. AUDITORY

Monaural stimulation with repetitive clicks is used to elicit brainstem auditory evoked potentials, which are recorded at the vertex of the scalp. A series of potentials are evoked in the first 10 ms after the auditory stimulus; these represent the sequential activation of various structures in the subcortical auditory pathway. For clinical purposes, attention is directed at the presence, latency, and interpeak intervals of the first five positive potentials recorded at the vertex.

C. SOMATOSENSORY

Electrical stimulation of a peripheral nerve is used to elicit the somatosensory evoked potentials, which are recorded over the scalp and spine. The configuration and latency of the responses depend on the nerve that is stimulated.

Indications for Use

Evoked potential studies are useful in several clinical contexts.

A. DETECTION OF LESIONS IN MULTIPLE SCLEROSIS

Evoked potentials have been used to detect and localize lesions in the central nervous system. This is particularly important in multiple sclerosis, where the diagnosis depends upon detecting lesions in several regions of the central nervous system. When patients present with clinical evidence of a lesion at only one site, electrophysiologic recognition of abnormalities in other locations helps to establish the diagnosis. When patients with suspected multiple sclerosis present with ill-defined complaints, electrophysiologic abnormalities in the appropriate afferent pathways are helpful in indicating the organic basis of the symptoms. Although noninvasive imaging studies such as MRI are also useful for detecting lesions, they should be used to complement evoked potential studies rather than as a replacement. Evoked potential studies monitor the functional status rather than anatomic integrity of the afferent pathways and can sometimes reveal abnormalities that are not detected by MRI (and the reverse also holds true). Their cost is also considerably lower than MRI. In patients with established multiple sclerosis, the evoked potential findings are sometimes used to follow the course of the disorder or monitor the response to novel forms of treatment, but their value in this regard is unclear.

B. DETECTION OF LESIONS IN OTHER CENTRAL NERVOUS SYSTEM DISORDERS

Evoked potential abnormalities are encountered in disorders other than multiple sclerosis; multimodal evoked potential abnormalities may be encountered in certain spinocerebellar degenerations, familial spastic paraplegia, Lyme disease, acquired immunodeficiency syndrome (AIDS), neurosyphilis, and vitamin E or B_{12} deficiency. The diagnostic value of electrophysiologic abnormalities therefore depends upon the context in which they are found. Although the findings may permit lesions to be localized within broad areas of the central nervous system, precise localization may not be possible because the generators of many of the recorded components are unknown.

C. ASSESSMENT AND PROGNOSIS FOLLOWING CENTRAL NERVOUS SYSTEM TRAUMA OR HYPOXIA

Evoked potentials studies can provide information of prognostic relevance. In posttraumatic or postanoxic coma, for example, the bilateral absence of cortically generated components of the somatosensory evoked potential implies that cognition will not be recovered; the prognosis is more optimistic when cortical responses are present on one or both sides. Such studies may be particularly useful in patients with suspected brain death. Somatosensory evoked potentials have also been used to determine the completeness of a traumatic cord lesion; the presence or early return of a response following stimulation of a nerve below the level of the cord injury indicates that the lesion is incomplete and thus suggests a better prognosis.

D. INTRAOPERATIVE MONITORING

Evoked potentials are also used to monitor the functional integrity of certain neural structures during operative procedures, in an attempt to permit the early recognition of any dysfunction and thereby minimize damage. When the dysfunction relates to a surgical maneuver, it may be possible to prevent or diminish any prominent neurologic deficit by reversing the maneuver.

E. EVALUATION OF VISUAL OR AUDITORY ACUITY

Visual and auditory acuity may be evaluated through evoked potential studies in patients who are unable to cooperate with behavioral testing because of age or abnormal mental state.

ELECTROMYOGRAPHY & NERVE CONDUCTION STUDIES

Electromyography

The electrical activity within a discrete region of an accessible muscle can be recorded by inserting a needle electrode into it. The pattern of electrical activity in muscle (**electromyogram**) both at rest and during activity has been characterized, and abnormalities have been correlated with disorders at different levels of the motor unit.

A. ACTIVITY AT REST

Relaxed muscle normally shows no spontaneous electrical activity except in the end-plate region where neuromuscular junctions are located, but various types of abnormal activity occur spontaneously in diseased muscle. **Fibrillation potentials** and **positive sharp waves** (which reflect muscle fiber irritability) are typically found in denervated muscle; they are not invariably present, however. They are sometimes also found in myopathic disorders, especially inflammatory disorders such as polymyositis. Although **fasciculation potentials**—which reflect the spontaneous activation of individual motor units—are occasionally encountered in normal muscle, they are characteristic of neuropathic disorders, especially those with primary involvement of anterior horn cells (eg, amyotrophic lateral sclerosis). Myotonic discharges (high-frequency discharges of potentials from muscle fibers that wax and wane in amplitude and frequency) are found most commonly in disorders such as myotonic dystrophy or myotonia congenita and occasionally in polymyositis or other, rarer disorders. Other types of abnormal spontaneous activity also occur.

B. ACTIVITY DURING VOLUNTARY MUSCLE CONTRACTION

A slight voluntary contraction of a muscle activates a small number of motor units. The potentials generated by the muscle fibers of individual units within the detection range of the needle electrode can be recorded. Normal motor-unit potentials have clearly defined limits of duration, amplitude, configuration, and firing rates. These limits depend, in part, on the muscle under study, and the number of units activated for a specified degree of voluntary activity is known within broad limits. In many myopathic disorders, there is an increased incidence of small, short-duration, polyphasic motor units in affected muscles, and an excessive number of units may be activated for a specified degree of voluntary activity. There is a loss of motor units in neuropathic disorders, so that the number of units activated during a maximal contraction will be reduced, and units will fire at a faster rate than normal. In addition, the configuration and dimensions of the potentials may be abnormal, depending on the acuteness of the neuropathic process and on whether reinnervation is occurring. Variations in the configuration and size of individual motor-unit potentials are characteristic of disorders of neuromuscular transmission.

C. CLINICAL UTILITY

Lesions can involve the neural or muscle component of the motor unit, or the neuromuscular junction. When the neural component is affected, the pathologic process can be either at the level of the anterior horn cells or at some point along the length of the axon as it traverses a nerve root, limb plexus, and peripheral nerve before branching into its terminal arborizations. Electromyography can detect disorders of the motor units and can indicate the site of the underlying lesion. The technique also permits neuromuscular disorders to be recognized when clinical examination is unrewarding because the disease is still at a mild stage—or because poor cooperation on the part of the patient or the presence of other symptoms such as pain makes clinical evaluation difficult. Note that the electromyographic findings do not, of themselves, permit an etiologic diagnosis to be reached, and the electrophysiologic findings must be correlated with the clinical findings and the results of other laboratory studies.

The electromyographic findings may provide a guide to prognosis. For example, in patients with an acute disorder of a peripheral or cranial nerve (eg, a pressure palsy of the radial nerve or a Bell's palsy) electromyographic evidence of denervation implies a poorer prognosis for recovery than when denervation has not occurred.

In contrast to needle electromyography, the clinical utility of surface-recorded electromyography is not established.

Nerve Conduction Studies

A. MOTOR NERVE CONDUCTION STUDIES

These studies are performed by recording the electrical response of a muscle to stimulation of its motor nerve at two or more points along its course. This permits conduction velocity to be determined in the fastest-conducting motor fibers between the points of stimulation.

B. SENSORY NERVE CONDUCTION STUDIES

These are performed by analogous means, by determining the conduction velocity and amplitude of action potentials in sensory fibers when these fibers are stimulated at one point and their responses are recorded at another point along the course of the nerve.

C. INDICATIONS FOR USE

Nerve conduction studies provide a means of confirming the presence and extent of peripheral nerve damage. Such studies are particularly helpful when clinical examination is difficult (eg, in children). Nerve conduction studies are particularly helpful in the following contexts.

1. Determining whether sensory symptoms are caused by a lesion proximal or distal to the dorsal root ganglia (in the latter case, sensory conduction studies of the involved fibers will be abnormal) and whether neuromuscular dysfunction relates to peripheral nerve disease.

2. Detecting subclinical involvement of other peripheral nerves in patients who present with a mononeuropathy.

3. Determining the site of a focal lesion and providing a guide to prognosis in patients with a mononeuropathy.

4. Distinguishing between a polyneuropathy and a mononeuropathy multiplex. This distinction may not be possible clinically, but it is important because the causes of these conditions differ.

5. Clarifying the extent to which the disabilities experienced by patients with polyneuropathy relate to superimposed compressive focal neuropathies—which are common complications.

6. Following the progression of peripheral nerve disorders and their response to treatment.

7. Indicating the predominant pathologic change in peripheral nerve disorders. In demyelinating neuropathies, conduction velocity is often markedly slowed and conduction block may occur; in axonal neuropathies, conduction velocity is usually normal or slowed only mildly, sensory nerve action potentials are small or absent, and electromyography shows evidence of denervation in affected muscles.

8. Detecting hereditary disorders of the peripheral nerves at a subclinical stage in genetic and epidemiologic studies.

F-RESPONSE STUDIES

When a stimulus is applied to a motor nerve, impulses travel **antidromically** (toward the spinal cord) as well as **orthodromically** (toward the nerve terminals) and lead to the discharge of a few anterior horn cells. This produces a small motor response that occurs considerably later than the direct muscle response elicited by nerve stimulation. The F wave so elicited is sometimes abnormal in patients with lesions of the proximal portions of the peripheral nervous system, such as the nerve roots. These studies may be helpful in detecting abnormalities when conventional nerve conduction studies are normal.

REPETITIVE NERVE STIMULATION

Description

The size of the electrical response of a muscle to supramaximal electrical stimulation of its motor nerve depends on a number of factors but correlates with the number of activated muscle fibers. Neuromuscular transmission can be tested by recording (with surface electrodes) the response of a muscle to supramaximal stimulation of its motor nerve either repetitively or by single shocks or trains of shocks at selected intervals after a maximal voluntary contraction.

Normal Response

In normal subjects, there is little or no change in the size of the compound muscle action potential following repetitive stimulation of a motor nerve at 10 Hz or less, or with a single stimulus or a train of stimuli delivered at intervals after a voluntary muscle contraction of about 10 seconds. This lack of change is the case even though preceding activity in the junctional region influences the amount of acetylcholine released and thus the size of the end-plate potentials elicited by the stimuli. Although the amount of acetylcholine released is increased briefly after maximal voluntary activity and is then reduced, more acetylcholine is normally released than is required to bring the motor end-plate potentials to the threshold for generating muscle-fiber action potentials.

Response in Disorders of Neuromuscular Transmission

A. MYASTHENIA GRAVIS

In myasthenia gravis, depletion of postsynaptic acetylcholine receptors at the neuromuscular junction makes it impossible to compensate for the reduced release of acetylcholine that follows repetitive firing of the motor neuron. Accordingly, repetitive stimulation, particularly between 2 and 5 Hz, may lead to a depression of neuromuscular transmission, with a decrement in the size of the compound muscle action potential recorded from an affected muscle. Similarly, an electrical stimulus of the motor nerve immediately after a 10-second period of maximal voluntary activity may elicit a muscle response that is slightly larger than before, indicating that more muscle fibers are responding. This postactivation facilitation of neuromuscular transmission is followed by a longer-lasting period of depression that is maximal from 2–4 minutes after the conditioning period and lasts up to 10 minutes or so. During this period, the compound muscle action potential is reduced in size.

Decrementing responses to repetitive stimulation at 2–5 Hz can also occur in congenital myasthenic syndromes.

B. MYASTHENIC SYNDROME AND BOTULISM

In Lambert-Eaton myasthenic syndrome, in which there is a defective release of acetylcholine at the neuromuscular junction, the compound muscle action potential elicited by a single stimulus is generally very small. With repetitive stimulation at rates of up to 10 Hz, the first few responses may decline in size, but subsequent responses increase and their amplitude is eventually several times larger than the initial response. Patients with botulism exhibit a similar response to repetitive stimulation, but the findings are somewhat more variable and not all muscles are affected. Incremental responses in Lambert-Eaton syndrome and botulism are more conspicuous with high rates of stimulation and may result from the facilitation of acetylcholine release by the progressive accumulation of calcium in the motor nerve terminal.

CRANIAL IMAGING STUDIES

PLAIN X-RAYS

Abnormalities of bone may be visualized by plain x-rays of the skull. Such abnormalities include metastatic deposits, fractures, and the changes associated with Paget's disease or fibrous dysplasia. In addition, plain films can show areas of abnormal intracranial calcification, alterations in size of the sella turcica, and inflammatory disease of the paranasal sinuses. The advent of computed tomographic scanning (which permits visualization of cerebral tissue as well as bone) has led to a marked decline in the use of plain films.

COMPUTED TOMOGRAPHY

Description

Computed tomographic (CT) scanning is a noninvasive computer-assisted radiologic means of examining anatomic structures (Figure 11–2). It permits the detection of structural intracranial abnormalities with precision, speed, and facility. It is thus of particular use in evaluating patients with progressive neurologic disorders or focal neurologic deficits in whom a structural lesion is suspected as well as patients with dementia or increased intracranial pressure. Intravenous administration of an iodinated contrast agent improves the ability of CT to detect and define lesions, such as tumors and abscesses, associated with a disturbance of the blood-brain barrier. Because the contrast agents may have an adverse effect on the kidneys, they should be used with discrimination. Other adverse effects of the contrast agents in common use are pain, nausea, thermal sensations, and anaphylactoid reactions that include bronchospasm and death. Contrast-enhanced scans may provide more information than that obtained by unenhanced scans in patients with known or suspected primary or secondary brain tumors, arteriovenous malformations (AVMs), multiple sclerosis, chronic isodense subdural hematomas, or hydrocephalus.

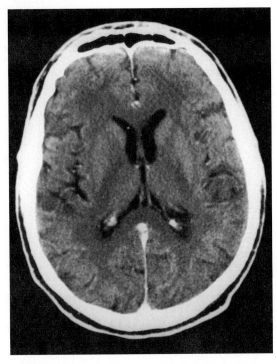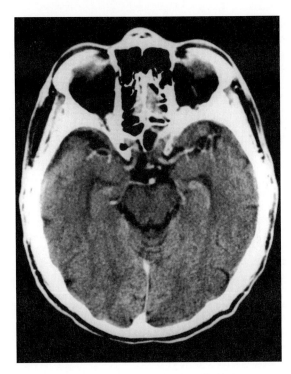

Figure 11–2. Contrast-enhanced CT brain scans from a 62-year-old man, showing the normal anatomy. Images at the level of the mid-brain and lateral ventricles are illustrated (same patient as Figure 11–3).

Indications for Use

A. STROKE

CT is particularly helpful in evaluating strokes because it can distinguish infarction from intracranial hemorrhage; it is particularly sensitive in detecting intracerebral hematomas, and the location of such lesions may provide a guide to their cause. Moreover, the CT scan occasionally demonstrates a nonvascular cause of the patient's clinical deficit, such as a tumor or abscess.

B. TUMOR

CT scans can indicate the site of a brain tumor, the extent of any surrounding edema, whether the lesion is cystic or solid, and whether it has displaced midline or other normal anatomic structures.

C. TRAUMA

The CT scan is an important means of evaluating patients following head injury—in particular for detecting traumatic subarachnoid or intracerebral hemorrhage and bony injuries. It also provides a more precise delineation of associated fractures than do plain x-rays.

D. DEMENTIA

In patients with dementia, CT scan may indicate the presence of a tumor or of hydrocephalus (enlarged ventricles), with or without accompanying cerebral atrophy. The occurrence of hydrocephalus without cerebral atrophy in demented patients suggests normal pressure or communicating hydrocephalus. Cerebral atrophy can occur in demented or normal elderly subjects.

E. SUBARACHNOID HEMORRHAGE

In patients with subarachnoid hemorrhage, the CT scan generally indicates the presence of blood in the subarachnoid space and may even suggest the source of the bleeding. If the CT findings are normal despite clinical findings suggestive of subarachnoid hemorrhage, the CSF should be examined to exclude hemorrhage or meningitis.

MAGNETIC RESONANCE IMAGING

Description

Magnetic resonance imaging (MRI) is an imaging procedure that involves no radiation. The patient lies within a large magnet that aligns some of the protons in the body along the magnet's axis. The protons resonate when stimulated with radio-frequency energy, producing a tiny echo that is strong enough to be detected. The position and intensity of these radio-frequency emissions are recorded and mapped by a computer. The signal intensity depends upon the concentration of mobile hydrogen nuclei (or nuclear-spin density) of the tissues. Spin-lattice (T1) and spin-spin (T2) relaxation times are mainly responsible for the relative differences in signal intensity of the various soft tissues; these parameters are sensitive to the state of water in biologic tissues. Pulse sequences with varying dependence on T1 and T2 selectively alter the contrast between soft tissues (Figure 11–3).

The soft-tissue contrast available with MRI makes it more sensitive than CT scanning in detecting certain structural lesions. MRI provides better contrast than does CT between the gray and white matter of the brain; it is superior for visualizing abnormalities in the posterior fossa and spinal cord and for detecting lesions associated with multiple sclerosis or those that cause seizures. In addition to its greater sensitivity, it is also free of bony artifact and permits multiplane (axial, sagittal, and coronal) imaging with no need to manipulate the position of the patient. Because there are no known hazardous effects, MRI studies can be repeated in a serial manner if necessary. Occasional patients cannot tolerate the procedure because of claustrophobia, but sedation usually alleviates this problem.

Gadopentetate dimeglumine is stable, well-tolerated intravenously, and an effective enhancing MRI agent that is useful in identifying small tumors that, because of their similar relaxation times to normal cerebral tissue, may be missed on unenhanced MRI. It also helps to separate tumor from surrounding edema, identify leptomeningeal disease, and provide information about the blood-brain barrier.

Indications for Use & Comparison with CT

A. STROKE

Within a few hours of vascular occlusion, it may be possible to detect and localize cerebral infarcts by MRI. Breakdown in the blood-brain barrier (which occurs several hours after onset of cerebral ischemia) permits the intravascular content to be extravasated into the extracellular space. This can be detected by T2-weighted imaging and fluid-attenuated inversion-recovery (FLAIR) sequences. Diffusion-weighted MRI also has an important role in the early assessment of stroke, as is discussed in a later section. CT scans, on the other hand, may be unrevealing for up to 48 hours. After that period, there is less advantage to MRI over CT scanning except for the former's ability to detect smaller lesions and its superior imaging of the posterior fossa. Nevertheless, CT scanning without contrast is usually the preferred initial

study in patients with acute stroke, in order to determine whether hemorrhage has occurred. Intracranial hemorrhage is not easily detected by MRI within the first 36 hours, and CT scan is more reliable for this purpose. Hematomas of more than 2–3 days' duration, however, are better visualized by MRI. Although MRI is very effective in detecting and localizing vascular malformations, angiography is still necessary to define their anatomic features and plan effective treatment. In cases of unexplained hematoma, a follow-up MRI obtained 3 months later may reveal the underlying cause, which is sometimes unmasked as the hematoma resolves.

B. TUMOR

Both CT scans and MRI are very useful in detecting brain tumors, but the absence of bone artifacts makes MRI superior for visualizing tumors at the vertex or in the posterior fossa and for detecting acoustic neuromas. Secondary effects of tumors, such as cerebral herniation, can be seen with either MRI or CT scan, but MRI provides more anatomic information. Neither technique, however, permits the nature of the underlying tumor to be determined with any certainty. Pituitary tumors are often visualized more easily by MRI than CT because of the absence of bone or dental metal artifacts.

C. TRAUMA

In the acute phase following head injury, CT scan is preferable to MRI because it requires less time, is superior for detecting intracranial hemorrhage, and may reveal bony injuries. Similarly, spinal MRI should not be used in the initial evaluation of patients with spinal injuries because nondisplaced fractures are often not visualized. For follow-up purposes, however, MRI is helpful for detecting parenchymal pathology of the brain or spinal cord.

D. DEMENTIA

In patients with dementia, either CT or MRI can help in demonstrating treatable structural causes, but MRI appears to be more sensitive.

E. MULTIPLE SCLEROSIS

In patients with multiple sclerosis, it is often possible to detect lesions in the cerebral white matter or the cervical cord by MRI, even though such lesions may not be visualized on CT scans. The demyelinating lesions detected by MRI may have signal characteristics resembling those of ischemic changes, however, and clinical correlation is therefore always necessary. Gadolinium-enhanced MRI permits lesions of different ages to be distinguished. This ability facilitates the diagnosis of multiple sclerosis: the presence of lesions of different ages suggests a multiphasic disease, whereas lesions of similar age suggest a monophasic disorder, such as acute disseminated encephalomyelitis.

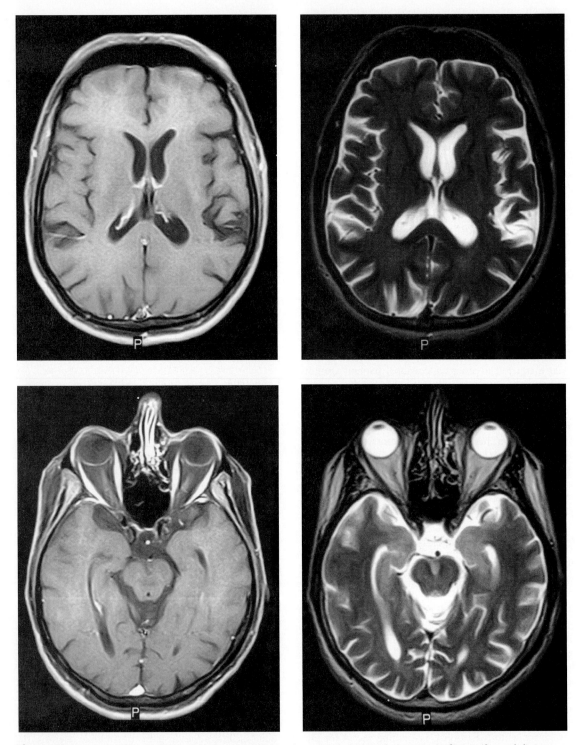

Figure 11–3. Brain MR images from a 62-year-old man, showing the normal anatomy. **Left panels:** gadolinium-enhanced T1-weighted (CSF dark) images; **right panels:** T2-weighted (CSF white) images. Images are at the level of the lateral ventricles **(top panels)** and midbrain **(lower panels).** Midsagittal T1-weighted image on facing page. Brain images from same patient as Figure 11–2.

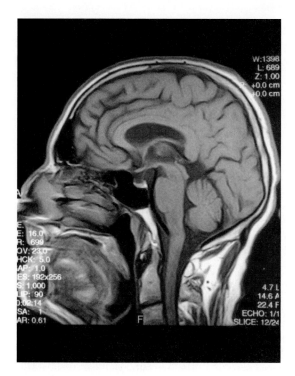

Figure 11–3. (continued)

F. INFECTIONS

MRI is very sensitive in detecting white-matter edema and probably permits earlier recognition of focal areas of cerebritis and abscess formation than is possible with CT.

Contraindications

Contraindications to MRI include the presence of intracranial clips, metallic foreign bodies in the eye or elsewhere, pacemakers, cochlear implants, and conditions requiring close monitoring of patients. Furthermore, it can be difficult to image patients with claustrophobia, gross obesity, uncontrolled movement disorders, or respiratory disorders that require assisted ventilation or carry any risk of apnea. Advances in MRI-compatible mechanical ventilators and monitoring equipment now allow even critically ill patients to be scanned safely.

DIFFUSION-WEIGHTED MAGNETIC RESONANCE IMAGING

This technique, in which contrast within the image is based on the microscopic motion of water protons in tissue, provides information that is not available on standard MRI. It is particularly important in the assessment of stroke because it can discriminate cytotoxic edema (which occurs in strokes) from vasogenic edema (found with other types of cerebral lesion) and thus reveals cerebral ischemia early and with high specificity. It is rapidly and widely being adopted into clinical practice.

Diffusion-weighted MRI permits reliable identification of acute cerebral ischemia during the first few hours after onset, before it is detectable on standard MRI. This is important because it reveals infarcts early enough for treatment with thrombolytic agents. When more than one infarct is found on routine MRI, diffusion-weighted imaging permits the discrimination of acute from older infarcts by the relative hyperdensity of the former. It also permits the identification of intracranial hemorrhage at an early stage.

PERFUSION-WEIGHTED MAGNETIC RESONANCE IMAGING

Perfusion-weighted imaging measures relative blood flow through the brain by either an injected contrast medium (e.g., gadolinium) or an endogenous technique (in which the patient's own blood provides the contrast). It allows cerebral blood-flow abnormalities to be recognized and can confirm the early reperfusion of tissues after treatment. Cerebral ischemia may be detected very soon after clinical onset. Comparison of the findings from diffusion-weighted and perfusion-weighted MRI may have a prognostic role and is currently under study. The distinction of reversible from irreversible ischemic damage is important in this regard.

POSITRON EMISSION TOMOGRAPHY

Positron emission tomography (PET) is an imaging technique that uses positron-emitting radiopharmaceuticals, such as ^{18}F-fluoro-2-deoxy-D-glucose or ^{18}F-L-dopa, to map brain biochemistry and physiology. PET thus complements other imaging methods that provide primarily anatomic information, such as CT and MRI, and may demonstrate functional brain abnormalities before structural abnormalities are detectable. Although its availability is currently limited, PET has proved useful in several clinical settings. When patients with medically refractory epilepsy are being considered for surgical treatment, PET can help identify focal areas of hypometabolism in the temporal lobe as likely sites of the origin of seizures. PET can also be useful in the differential diagnosis of dementia, since common dementing disorders such as Alzheimer's disease and multiinfarct dementia exhibit different patterns of abnormal cerebral metabolism. PET can help distinguish between clinically similar movement disorders, such as Parkinson's disease and progressive supranuclear palsy, and can provide confirmatory evidence of early Huntington's disease. PET may also be of value in grading gliomas, selecting tumor biopsy sites, and distinguishing recurrent tumors from radiation-induced brain necrosis. PET has also been an important tool with which to investigate the functional involvement of different cerebral areas in behavioral and cognitive tasks.

The major problems associated with PET are its expense, the requirement that radioactive isotopes are produced near the site of imaging, and the exposure of subjects to radiation.

SINGLE-PHOTON EMISSION COMPUTED TOMOGRAPHY

Single-photon emission computed tomography (SPECT) involves the administration intravenously or by inhalation of chemicals containing isotopes that emit single photons in order to image the brain. SPECT has been used, in particular, for perfusion studies, the investigation of receptor distribution, and the detection of areas of increased metabolism such as occurs with seizures. At present the technique is more of academic interest than of clinical relevance, but it is considerably cheaper than PET and the isotopes in use do not have to be produced near the site of imaging.

FUNCTIONAL MAGNETIC RESONANCE IMAGING

Functional MRI (fMRI) involves the intravenous administration of contrast material that lowers signal intensity on MRI in relation to blood flow as the material passes through the cerebral vasculature. Studies are performed with the subject at rest and then after an activation procedure, so that the change in signal intensity reflects the effect of the activation procedure on local cerebral blood flow (Figure 11–4). An alternative approach involves pulse sequences that show changes in signal intensity from regional changes in the oxygen concentration of venous blood—focal cerebral activity leads to regional increases in the concentration of oxygenated blood. These techniques permit changes in signal to be related to underlying activity and thus allow functional processes to be localized within the brain. At present, fMRI is an important investigative tool, but its role in the clinical evaluation of patients remains to be established.

MAGNETIC RESONANCE SPECTROSCOPY

Magnetic resonance spectroscopy is an investigational tool available in some centers; it provides information about the chemical composition of tissue. Proton magnetic resonance spectroscopy (¹H-MRS) may be used to determine levels of *N*-acetylaspartate exclusive to neurons

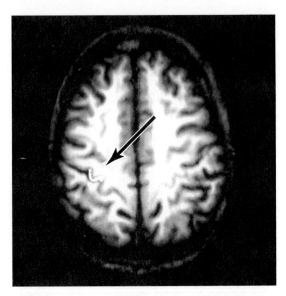

Figure 11–4. A functional MR brain image obtained from a patient during rapid finger tapping of the left hand. An increase in relative blood flow in the region of the right motorstrip is imaged **(arrow)** and superimposed upon a T1-weighted MR scan. (From Waxman SG: *Correlative Neuroanatomy,* 23rd ed., 1996.)

or choline creatinine and lactate (glia and neurons). Measurements of brain concentration may be useful in detecting specific tissue loss in diseases such as Alzheimer's disease or hypoxic-ischemic encephalopathy, or to classify brain tumors or lateralize temporal lobe epilepsy. Phosphorus magnetic resonance (³¹P-MRS) may be useful in the evaluation of metabolic muscle diseases.

ARTERIOGRAPHY

Description

The intracranial circulation is visualized most satisfactorily by arteriography, a technique in which the major vessels to the head are opacified and radiographed. A catheter is introduced into the femoral or brachial artery and passed into one of the major cervical vessels. A radiopaque contrast material is then injected through the catheter, allowing the vessel (or its origin) to be visualized. The technique, generally performed after noninvasive imaging by CT scanning or MRI, has a definite (approximately 1%) morbidity and mortality associated with it and involves considerable exposure to radiation. It is contraindicated in patients with a stroke in evolution (progressing stroke) and in patients who are allergic to the contrast medium. Stroke may result as a complication of arteriography. Moreover, at the conclusion of the procedure, bleeding may occur at the puncture site and occlusion of the catheterized artery (usually the femoral artery) may lead to distal ischemic complications. The puncture site and the distal circulation must therefore be monitored with these complications in mind.

Indications for Use

The major indications for arteriography include the following:

1. Diagnosis of **intracranial aneurysms, arteriovenous malformations,** or **fistulas.** Although these lesions can be visualized by CT scan or MRI, their detailed anatomy and the vessels that feed, drain, or are otherwise implicated in them cannot reliably be defined by these other means. Moreover, arteriography is still required for interventional procedures such as embolization, the injection of occlusive polymers, or the placement of detachable balloons to treat certain vascular anomalies.

2. Detection and definition of the underlying lesion in patients with **subarachnoid hemorrhage** who are considered good operative candidates (see Table 2–2).

3. Localization of vascular lesions in patients with **transient cerebral ischemic attacks** if surgical treatment is being considered.

4. Evaluation of small vessels, such as when a vasculitis is under consideration.

5. Diagnosis of **cerebral venous sinus thrombosis.**

6. Evaluation of **space-occupying intracranial lesions,** particularly when CT scanning or MRI is unavailable. There may be displacement of the normal vasculature, and in some tumors neovasculature may produce a blush or stain on the angiogram. Meningiomas can be recognized by their blood supply from the external carotid circulation.

MAGNETIC RESONANCE ANGIOGRAPHY

Several imaging techniques that have been used to visualize blood vessels by MRI depend upon certain physical properties of blood to generate contrast. These properties include the rate at which blood is supplied to the imaged area, its velocity and relaxation time, and the absence of turbulent flow. MR angiography is a noninvasive technique that has a reduced cost and reduced risks compared with conventional angiography. It has been most useful in visualizing the carotid arteries and proximal portions of the intracranial circulation, where flow is relatively fast. The images are used to screen for stenosis or occlusion of vessels and for large atheromatous lesions. It has particular utility in screening for venous sinus occlusion. Resolution is inferior to that of conventional angiography and, in vessels with slow flow, it may be difficult to recognize occlusive disease. Moreover, intracra-

nial MR angiograms may be marred by irregular or discontinuous signal intensity in vessels close to the skull base. Although current techniques allow visualization of arteriovenous malformations and aneurysms greater than 3 mm in diameter, conventional angiography remains the "gold standard" in this context. Finally, MR angiography may reveal dissection of major vessels: narrowing is produced by the dissection and cross-sectional images reveal the false lumen as a crescent of abnormal signal intensity next to the vascular flow void.

COMPUTED TOMOGRAPHIC ANGIOGRAPHY

Spiral CT angiography is a minimally invasive procedure that requires the CT scanner to be capable of rapidly acquiring numerous thin, overlapping sections after intravenous injection of a bolus of contrast material. It can be performed within minutes, and is less likely to be affected by patient movement than MR angiography. A wide range of vessels can be imaged with the technique.

CT angiography of the carotid bifurcation is being used increasingly, but it cannot reliably distinguish between moderate (50–69%) and severe (70–99%) stenosis, which is an important limitation. It can also be used for intracranial imaging and can detect stenotic or aneurysmal lesions. However, sensitivity is reduced for aneurysms less than 5 mm, and the method cannot adequately define aneurysmal morphology in the preoperative evaluation of patients. It is sensitive in visualizing the anatomy in the circle of Willis, the vasculature of the anterior and posterior circulations, and intracranial vasoocclusive lesions, but it may not reveal plaque ulceration. It is a reliable alternative to MR angiography, but both techniques are less sensitive than conventional angiography in this regard.

In patients with acute stroke, CT angiography provides important information complementary to conventional CT studies, revealing the site and length of vascular occlusion and the contrast-enhanced arteries distal to the occlusion as a reflection of collateral blood flow.

SPINAL IMAGING STUDIES
PLAIN X-RAYS

Plain x-rays of the spine can reveal congenital, traumatic, degenerative or neoplastic bony abnormalities, or narrowing (stenosis) of the spinal canal. Degenerative changes become increasingly common with advancing age, and their clinical relevance depends on the context in which they are found. In patients presenting with neck or low back pain, a plain film is usually the first radiologic investigation undertaken.

MYELOGRAPHY

Injecting radiopaque contrast medium into the subarachnoid space permits visualization of part or all of the spinal subarachnoid system. The cord and nerve roots, which are silhouetted by the contrast material in the subarachnoid space, are visualized indirectly. The procedure is invasive and carries the risks of headache, low back pain, confusion, arachnoiditis, inadvertent intravenous injection of contrast material, and vasovagal reactions. Rarely, traumatic herniated intervertebral disks have occurred because of poor technique, as has damage to nerve roots.

Water-soluble agents (such as iohexol) have now replaced oil-based formulations (pantopaque) as the preferred contrast medium. The dye is absorbed from the CSF and excreted by the kidneys, with approximately 75% eliminated over the first 24 hours. Unlike pantopaque, iohexol does not produce significant arachnoiditis, but tonic-clonic seizures have been reported in some instances when contrast entered the intracranial cavity. Other complications include headaches and nausea and vomiting. Contrast myelography may be followed by a CT scan of the spine while the medium is still in place. This shows the soft tissue structures in or about the spinal cord and provides information complementary to that obtained by the myelogram (see below).

Myelography is indicated in the investigation of patients with suspected spinal cord or nerve root compression or structural anomalies in the foramen magnum region. It is helpful in detecting both extradural and intradural lesions and in providing evidence of an intramedullary abnormality. Although it remains a powerful diagnostic tool, noninvasive CT scanning and MRI have reduced the need for its use.

COMPUTED TOMOGRAPHY

CT scanning after myelography may be helpful when the myelogram either fails to reveal any abnormality or provides poor visualization of the area of interest. The myelogram may be normal, for example, when there is a laterally placed disk protrusion; in such circumstances, a contrast-enhanced CT scan may reveal the lesion. It is also useful in visualizing more fully the area above or below an almost complete block in the subarachnoid space and in providing further information in patients with cord tumors.

An unenhanced CT scan may be helpful in defining the bony anatomy of the spine. CT scanning may show osteophytic narrowing of neural foramina or the spinal canal in patients with cervical spondylosis and may show spinal stenosis or disk protrusions in patients with neurogenic claudication. In patients with neurologic deficits, however, MRI is generally preferred as it provides more useful information.

MAGNETIC RESONANCE IMAGING

In many instances, the information obtained by myelography can now be obtained more simply by MRI of the spine. Imaging of the spinal canal by MRI is direct and noninvasive, and it permits differentiation of solid from cystic intramedullary lesions. MRI is therefore being used increasingly in place of myelography. In syringomyelia, for example, MRI is the preferred imaging method for visualizing cord cavitation and detecting any associated abnormalities at the craniocervical junction. Congenital abnormalities associated with spinal dysraphism are also easily visualized by MRI. In patients with degenerative disk disease, MRI is probably more accurate than myelography for detecting cord or root compression (Figure 11–5). However, abnormal MRI findings in the lumbar spine are common in asymptomatic subjects, especially in middle or later life, and care must therefore be exercised in attributing symptoms such as back pain to anatomic abnormalities that may be coincidental. When a spinal AVM is suspected the myelogram is the most sensitive screening technique.

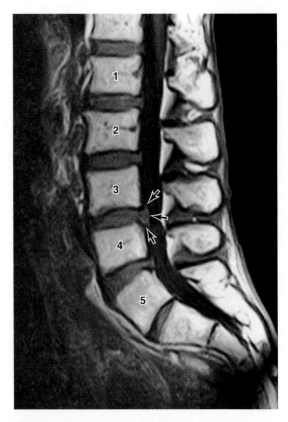

Figure 11–5. Disk herniation at the L3–L4 level **(arrows).**

ULTRASONOGRAPHY

In B-mode ultrasonography, echoes reflected from anatomic structures are plotted on an oscilloscope screen in two dimensions. The resulting brightness at each point reflects the density of the imaged structure. The technique has been used to image the carotid artery and its bifurcation in the neck, permitting evaluation of the extent of extracranial vascular disease. Blood flowing within an artery does not reflect sound, and the lumen of the vessels therefore appears black. The arterial wall can be seen, however, and atherosclerotic lesions can be detected. Note that with severe stenosis or complete occlusion of the internal carotid artery, it may not be possible to visualize the carotid artery bifurcation.

The velocity of blood flow through an artery can be measured by Doppler ultrasonography. Sound waves within a certain frequency range are reflected off red blood cells, and the frequency of the echo provides a guide to the velocity of the flow. Any shift in frequency is proportional to the velocity of the red cells and the angle of the beam of sound waves. When the arterial lumen is narrowed, the velocity of flow increases; increased frequencies are therefore recorded by Doppler ultrasonography. Spectral analysis of Doppler frequencies is also used to evaluate the anatomic status of the carotid artery. Transcranial Doppler studies are now used routinely in many centers to detect intracranial arterial lesions or vasospasm (eg, after subarachnoid hemorrhage) and to assess the hemodynamic consequences of extracranial disease of the carotid arteries.

Duplex instruments, which are now widely used for vascular ultrasound, perform a combination of both B-mode imaging and Doppler ultrasonography, thereby providing information at the same time about both structure and the hemodynamics of the circulation in a color-coded format. The technique is being increasingly used to evaluate patients with suspected atheromatous lesions of the carotid artery in the neck. Such sonographic screening has been helpful in identifying patients who require arteriography, thereby increasing the yield of the latter and reducing the number of unnecessary arteriograms. When sonography shows significant disease that may require operative treatment, angiography is required to provide an overview of the vasculature and aid in the planning of treatment.

■ BIOPSIES

BRAIN BIOPSY

Biopsy of brain tissue can be useful in certain cases when less invasive methods, such as imaging studies, fail to provide a diagnosis. Brain lesions most amenable to biopsy are those that can be localized by imaging studies; are situated in superficial, surgically accessible sites; and do not involve critical brain regions, such as the brainstem or the areas of cerebral cortex involved in language or motor function. Cerebral disorders that can be diagnosed by biopsy include primary and metastatic brain tumors, infectious disorders such as herpes simplex encephalitis or brain abscess, and certain degenerative diseases such as Creutzfeldt-Jakob disease.

MUSCLE BIOPSY

Histopathologic examination of a biopsy specimen of a weak muscle can indicate whether the underlying weakness is neurogenic or myopathic in origin. In neurogenic disorders, atrophied fibers occur in groups, with adjacent groups of larger uninvolved fibers. In myopathies, atrophy occurs in a random pattern; the nuclei of muscle cells may be centrally situated, rather than in their normal peripheral location; and fibrosis or fatty infiltration may also be found. Examination of a muscle biopsy specimen may also permit certain inflammatory diseases of muscle, such as polymyositis, to be recognized and treated.

In some patients with a suspected myopathy, although the electromyographic findings are normal, examination of a muscle biopsy specimen reveals the nature of the underlying disorder. Conversely, electromyographic abnormalities suggestive of a myopathy are sometimes found in patients in whom the histologic or histochemical studies fail to establish a diagnosis of myopathy. The two approaches are therefore complementary.

NERVE BIOPSY

It is not necessary to undertake nerve biopsy to establish a diagnosis of peripheral neuropathy. The nature of any neuropathologic abnormalities can be important, however, in suggesting the underlying disorder of peripheral nerves. In particular, evidence may be found of metabolic storage disease (eg, Fabry's disease, Tangier disease), infection (eg, leprosy), inflammatory change, vasculitis, or neoplastic involvement. The findings are not always of diagnostic relevance, however, and nerve biopsy itself can be performed only on accessible nerves. It is rarely undertaken on more than a single occasion.

ARTERY BIOPSY

In patients with suspected giant cell arteritis, temporal artery biopsy may help to confirm the diagnosis, but the pathologic abnormalities are usually patchy in distribution. Therefore, a normal study should not exclude the diagnosis or lead to withdrawal of treatment.

REFERENCES

Lumbar Puncture

Broadley SA, Fuller GN: Lumbar puncture needn't be a headache. BMJ 1997;315:1324–1325.

Evans RW et al: Prevention of post-lumbar puncture headaches: report of the Therapeutics and Technology Assessment Subcommittee of the American Academy of Neurology. Neurology 2000;55:909–914.

Fishman RA: *Cerebrospinal Fluid in Diseases of the Nervous System,* 2nd ed. Saunders, 1992.

Hayward RA, Shapiro MF, Oye RK: Laboratory testing on cerebrospinal fluid: a reappraisal. Lancet 1987;1:1–4.

Howard SC et al: Safety of lumbar puncture for children with acute lymphoblastic leukemia and thrombocytopenia. JAMA 2000;284:2222–2224.

Electrophysiologic Studies

Aminoff MJ: *Electromyography in Clinical Practice,* 3rd ed. Churchill Livingstone, 1998.

Aminoff MJ (editor): *Electrodiagnosis in Clinical Neurology,* 4th ed. Churchill Livingstone, 1999.

Aminoff MJ: Evoked potential studies in neurological diagnosis and management. Ann Neurol 1990;28:706–710.

Burke D, Hicks RG: Surgical monitoring of motor pathways. J Clin Neurophysiol 1998;15:94–205.

Deuschl G, Eisen A (editors): *Recommendations for the Practice of Clinical Neurophysiology.* Elsevier, 1999.

Gronseth GS, Ashman EJ: Practice parameter: the usefulness of evoked potentials in identifying clinically silent lesions in patients with suspected multiple sclerosis (an evidence-based review): report of the Quality Standards Subcommittee of the American Academy of Neurology. Neurology 2000;55:7–15.

Nuwer M: Spinal cord monitoring. Muscle Nerve 1999;22: 1620–1630.

Pullman SL et al: Clinical utility of surface EMG: report of the Therapeutics and Technology Assessment Subcommittee of the American Academy of Neurology. Neurology 2000;55: 171–177.

Cranial & Spinal Imaging and Arteriographic Studies

Anderson GB et al: CT angiography for the detection and characterization of carotid artery bifurcation disease. Stroke 2000; 31:2168–2174.

Atlas SW: MR angiography in neurologic disease. Radiology 1994; 193:1–16.

Gilman S: Imaging the brain. N Engl J Med 1998;338:812–820, 889–896.

Jensen MC et al: Magnetic resonance imaging of the lumbar spine in people without back pain. N Engl J Med 1994;331:69–73.

Katz DA et al: Circle of Willis: evaluation with spiral CT angiography, MR angiography, and conventional angiography. Radiology 1995;195:445–449.

Knauth M et al: Potential of CT angiography in acute ischemic stroke. AJNR Am J Neuroradiol 1997;18:1001–1010.

Laughlin S, Montanera W: Central nervous system imaging. When is CT more appropriate than MRI? Postgrad Med 1998;104: 73–76, 81–84, 87–88.

Neumann-Haefelin T, Moseley ME, Albers GW: New magnetic resonance imaging methods for cerebrovascular disease: emerging clinical applications. Ann Neurol 2000;47:559– 570.

Oliver TB et al: Atherosclerotic plaque at the carotid bifurcation: CT angiographic appearance with histopathologic correlation. AJNR Am J Neuroradiol 1999;20:897–901.

Provenzale JM, Sorensen AG: Diffusion-weighted MR imaging in acute stroke: theoretical considerations and clinical applications. AJR 1999;173:1459–1467.

Skutta B et al: Intracranial stenoocclusive disease: double-detector helical CT angiography versus digital subtraction angiography. AJNR Am J Neuroradiol 1999;20:791–799.

Tong DC, Albers GW: Diffusion and perfusion magnetic resonance imaging for the evaluation of acute stroke: potential use in guiding thrombolytic therapy. Curr Opin Neurol 2000;13:45–50.

Ueda T, Yuh WTC, Taoka T: Clinical application of perfusion and diffusion MR imaging in acute ischemic stroke. J Magn Reson Imaging 1999;10:305–309.

Positron Emission Tomography

Brooks DJ: Positron emission tomography studies in movement disorders. Neurosurg Clin North Am 1998;9:263–282.

Mohan KK, Chugani DC, Chugani HT: Positron emission tomography in pediatric neurology. Semin Pediatr Neurol 1999; 6:111–119.

Magnetic Resonance Spectroscopy

Argov Z, Lofberg M, Arnold DL: Insights into muscle diseases gained by phosphorus magnetic resonance spectroscopy. Muscle Nerve 2000;23:1316–1334.

Laxer KD: Clinical applications of magnetic resonance spectroscopy. Epilepsia 1997;38(Suppl 4):S13–S17.

Poptani H et al: Diagnostic assessment of brain tumours and non-neoplastic brain disorders in vivo using protein nuclear magnetic resonance spectroscopy and artificial neural networks. J Cancer Res Clin Oncol 1999;125:343–349.

Ultrasonography

Back MR et al: Magnetic resonance angiography is an accurate imaging adjunct to duplex ultrasound scan in patient selection for carotid endarterectomy. J Vasc Surg 2000;32:429–438.

Lewis BD, James EM, Welch TJ: Current applications of duplex and color Doppler ultrasound imaging: carotid and peripheral vascular system. Mayo Clin Proc 1989;64:1147–1157.

Tegeler CH, Babikian VL, Gomez CR (editors): *Neurosonology.* Mosby, 1996.

Wechsler LR, Babikian VL: Transcranial Doppler sonography. Arch Neurol 1994;51:1054–1056.

Nerve Biopsy

Said G: Indications and value of nerve biopsy. Muscle Nerve 1999;22:1617–1619.

Appendices

APPENDIX A: THE NEUROLOGIC EXAMINATION

Despite recent advances in neuroscience and the continuing development of sensitive diagnostic procedures, the essential skill required for diagnosis of neurologic disorders remains the clinical neurologic examination.

DIFFUSE CORTICAL FUNCTION: MENTAL STATUS (CHAPTER 1)

1. Level of Consciousness

The level of consciousness is the first state evaluated in the neurologic examination. Consciousness may be assessed as **normal** (patient awake and alert, attentive to surroundings and to the examiner), **depressed** (patient sleepy, lethargic, stuporous—arousing only briefly in response to pain stimulation; or comatose—not arousable by pain stimulation); or **hyperalert** (patient distractible, jittery, "jumpy").

2. Cognitive Functioning

Assessment of cognitive functioning aims not to determine "how smart the patient is" but how the patient's cognitive capacity has changed from a recent baseline. The examiner must have some way (recent work history, observations of family, other physicians, etc) of assessing the patient's cognitive status before onset of the present illness. Assessment should include (at a minimum) informal evaluation of the following.

Cognitive Functioning Checklist

A. ORIENTATION

Orientation is to person, place, and time.

B. FUND OF COMMON KNOWLEDGE

This is judged by the response to such questions as "Who is the president?" or "How many nickels are there in a dollar?"

C. MEMORY

Short-term—Repeat the names of three common objects, then name them again after 5 minutes; long-term—recount verifiable events from the past.

D. INSIGHT AND JUDGMENT

"Why have you come to see me?"

E. CONCENTRATION

This can often be tested along with calculations (see below) or by instructing the patient (for example) to repeat a series of four to seven digits, arrange the letters in "world" in alphabetical order, or spell "world" backward.

F. CALCULATIONS

The conventional test is serial sevens, but informal "real-life" problems may yield a more objective result:

    1. Serial sevens—Count backward from 100, taking away 7 each time.

    2. Real-life problem—For example, "If an apple costs 29 cents, how many can you buy for $1.50?" Then, "How much change do you have left over?"

G. ABSTRACT THOUGHT

Examples are proverb interpretation or "compare-and-contrast" tasks such as "How is an apple different from an orange?"

H. VERBAL FLUENCY

This can be judged by listening to the patient talk or by asking such questions as "How many words can you say that start with the letter B?" (Time for 30 seconds.)

I. OTHER

The examiner should now be able to form an impression of the patient's mood, content of thought, and appropriateness of behavior.

FUNCTION OF SPECIFIC HEMISPHERES

1. Dominant Hemisphere

The most important function of the dominant hemisphere is **language.** Language skills include comprehension, repetition, naming, reading, and writing. Language mastery can be lost as a consequence of diffuse transient (eg, metabolic derangements) or degenerative (eg, dementia) diseases, but language impairment with otherwise normal cognitive function almost always suggests a focal lesion.

Aphasias

Impairments of the expression or understanding of language are traditionally divided into categories depending on the pattern of the language deficit and the site of the damage. Table A–1 lists the three most frequently seen syndromes of clinical significance: Broca's aphasia, Wernicke's aphasia, and conduction aphasia. The three syndromes are tested for as follows.

A. FLUENCY

Listen to spontaneous speech. Assess speech for fluency, errors of grammar or vocabulary, neologisms (meaningless words), or word substitutions (paraphasias). Determine whether the patient's speech makes sense in the current context. Alternatively, give the patient paper and pencil and say, "Write your name." "Write, The boy and the girl are happy about the dog." "Please write down your reason for being here."

B. COMPREHENSION

Using only words (no gestures), instruct the patient to follow commands of increasing complexity: "Close your eyes." "Show me your left hand." "With your left hand, put a finger in your right ear." Alternatively, present a written command ("Go to the door, knock three times, and come back.") and assess whether the task is performed properly. If the patient does not comply, assess cooperation and physical capacity by repeating the commands with demonstration and miming.

C. REPETITION

Ask the patient to repeat three common nouns ("bread, coffee, pencil") or "No ifs, ands, or buts."

D. WRITING

With rare exceptions, every patient aphasic in speech is also aphasic in writing (agraphic). A patient who cannot speak but can write is mute, and the lesion is not in Broca's area. Muteness occurs in a wide variety of disorders, including severe rigidity, vocal cord paralysis, bilateral corticobulbar lesions, and psychiatric disease.

E. NAMING

Difficulty in naming familiar objects (anomia) may occur in expressive aphasia or other aphasic syndromes but by itself is not diagnostic of any specific entity. It is more likely a consequence of diffuse cerebral dysfunction of structural or metabolic origin. Ask patients to name, or mute patients to point to, a wrist watch, a typewriter keyboard, etc.

2. The Nondominant Hemisphere

Tests for lesions of the nondominant hemisphere are chiefly concerned with the interpretation of incoming stimuli (other than language), visuospatial orientation, and perception of the contralateral body in space. (Lesions of the dominant hemisphere can also produce abnormalities in these areas, but they are usually masked by aphasia.)

Assessment of Sensory Interpretation

Defects of sensory interpretation can be evaluated in a number of ways, though all require reasonably intact primary sensation.

A. GRAPHESTHESIA

Ask the patient to identify a letter or number written on the palm.

B. OBJECT IDENTIFICATION (STEREOGNOSIS)

Have the patient name a common object placed in the hand (key, paper clip, coin, etc).

C. NEGLECT

Misperception of one side of space results in a number of abnormalities collectively called neglect. The patient may not heed information incoming from the side contralateral to the lesion (right brain affecting left side of body). For example, the patient may hunt eagerly for the exam-

Table A–1. Common aphasia syndromes.

Type	Synonym	Characteristic	Associated	Location
Broca's	Anterior, nonfluent, expressive, motor	Paucity of speech, loss of grammar, telegraphic	Hemiparesis	Frontal
Wernicke's	Posterior, fluent, receptive, sensory	Intact grammar, neologisms, paraphasias, "word salad," no comprehension	Visual field cut	Posterior temporal
Conduction		Repetition lost, with spared comprehension and expression		Arcuate fasciculus

iner's face on the right when the voice is calling from the left—or may eat only the food on the right side of a plate. Patients may deny that the left side of the body exists (even a dense hemiparesis may be cheerfully "overlooked"), fail to acknowledge as one's own the left arm held up in plain view by the examiner, or, most dramatically, fail to properly clothe or groom the left side of the body. Clumsiness or "disuse" out of proportion to actual weakness—or a pronounced lag in initiating movement on the involved side—suggests motor **apraxia** as a manifestation of neglect. There are several classic tests, as follows.

Spatial Orientation

Approach the patient quietly on the weak side (particularly when the head and gaze are turned away), speak a greeting and observe whether the patient's head turns ("orients") to the source of the voice or searches only on the wrong side. Then move over to the "good" side and repeat the exercise.

Double Simultaneous Stimulation

Touch the patient gently first on one hand and then the other while identifying the side. Then randomly vary the stimulus, asking the patient to say, with both eyes closed, "left," "right," or "both." Mute patients should be asked to raise the touched hand. If the patient correctly identifies each side in isolation but "extinguishes" the touch on the involved side when both are touched, neglect is present.

Clockface Exercise

Draw (or have the patient draw) a large circle and ask the patient to write in the numbers of the hours of the day. Note if the patient writes all 12 numbers into the hemicircle opposite the neglected side. If the numbers are placed correctly, the patient should then be asked to draw in the hands to indicate a specified time such as "a quarter to four."

Reading, Writing

Ask the patient to read from a book or write on a sheet of paper. The patient may read only the right side of the page or squeeze the sentence into the right half. Give the patient a sheet of lined notebook paper and say, "Cross out all the lines." Note whether lines on the left side of the page are ignored.

Ideomotor Apraxia

Ask the patient to manipulate some familiar object (dial a phone number, hold a pencil in the position of writing) or to raise one arm in the air.

CRANIAL NERVES

1. Olfactory (I)

Ask the patient to identify common scents such as coffee, vanilla, etc, with eyes closed. Do not use irritants. In testing olfactory nerve function, it is less important to determine whether the patient can correctly identify a particular odor than whether the presence or absence of the stimulus is perceived.

2. Optic (II) (Chapter 4)

Visual Acuity

A pocket card or wall chart—or any reading matter—may be used to observe the focal distance (normally, small newspaper print can be read at 32 inches). Patients with refractive errors may wear spectacle lenses or be given a pinhole.

Visual Fields

Visual fields are a measure of the integrity of the optic nerves and the postthalamic optic radiations through the hemispheres. They are tested as follows.

A. CONFRONTATION TESTING

Patient and examiner stand at eye level at about arm's length. Have the patient cover the left eye. The examiner's right arm is extended and then brought forward from the side; the patient says how many fingers are shown. The patient and examiner should see the fingers at the same time. Then repeat with the left hand over the patient's right eye. Test all four quadrants in each eye in this way (see Figure 4–9).

B. THREAT TESTING

Flick an extended finger obliquely toward the patient's pupil from each temporal field and observe for blinking. This crude test is occasionally useful when the patient is less than fully alert or is uncooperative.

Fundus (Ophthalmoscopic) Examination

Look for blurring of the disk margins, loss of venous pulsations, retinal lesions, abnormalities of the vessels, and color of the optic nerve head.

3. Pupillary Reflexes (II, III) (Chapter 4)

A normal pupil will constrict (1) in response to direct light, (2) as a consensual response to light in the opposite eye, and (3) to accommodation (convergence to focus on a close object). A pupil that reacts to accommodation but not to light is an **Argyll-Robertson pupil,** signifying a lesion in the tectum of the midbrain. A **Marcus-Gunn**

pupil is one with impaired constriction to direct light with preservation of the consensual response; in this case, an afferent light stimulus does not reach the lateral geniculate nucleus and a lesion should be sought in the optic tract, preoptic chiasm, optic nerve, or retina.

Constriction to Accommodation

The patient is instructed to gaze at the wall over the examiner's shoulder and then quickly focus on the examiner's forefinger held just in front of the patient's nose. Look for subtle constriction when the patient changes from far vision to very near.

Consensual Constriction (Swinging Flashlight Test)

After shining a flashlight into one eye to constrict the pupil, switch to the other eye and observe if that pupil constricts further (normal response) or dilates (abnormal response).

4. Control of Extraocular Muscle Movements (Chapter 4)

Extraocular muscle movements are controlled by the oculomotor (III), trochlear (IV), and abducens (V) nerves—innervating the lateral, medial, superior, and inferior rectus muscles (LR, MR, SR, IR) and the superior (SO) and inferior oblique (IO), respectively.

Movements are checked in all six directions of gaze: LR (VI) for lateral gaze, MR (III) for medial gaze, IR and SR (III) for down gaze and up gaze with the eye laterally deviated, and SO (IV) and IO (III) for down gaze and up gaze with the eye medially deviated. Ask about **diplopia,** as the patient's perception is more sensitive than the examination results.

Abnormalities of eye movements can result from lesions other than those involving the cranial nerves—anything from muscular or neuromuscular disease to central lesions in the cortex or brainstem. For example, if the patient has had a stroke, horizontal movements may remain **conjugate** (with eyes moving smoothly yoked together) but gaze at rest may be directed to one side—toward the lesion if the lesion is cortical, away from the site of damage if the lesion is in the brainstem.

If the patient is unresponsive or otherwise unable to perform voluntary eye movements, the doll's eye (doll's head) maneuver (oculocephalic reflex) should be performed (see below).

Nystagmus is rhythmic oscillation of the eyes; it can be either conjugate or asymmetric. It can be a normal phenomenon (eg, at the extremes of lateral gaze) or may relate to weakness of an eye muscle or to lesions in the brainstem, cerebellum, or anywhere in the peripheral or central vestibular systems; each type has its characteristic pattern. Nystagmus is most easily observed—as are all disorders of smooth coordinated eye movements—while the patient is following the examiner's finger.

Tests for control of extraocular muscle movements include the following.

Primary Gaze (Straight Ahead)

Look for symmetry of position of the light reflection off the two corneas.

Volitional Eye Movements

Face the patient and put a hand on the patient's forehead and say, "Follow my finger, just with your eyes." Then move the index finger of the other hand horizontally, then up and down on either side, tracing the letter H.

Doll's Head (Oculocephalic) Maneuver

The patient's head is held firmly and rotated from side to side, then up and down. (It may be necessary to hold the eyelids open as well.) If the brainstem is intact, the eyes will move conjugately away from the direction of turning (as if still looking at the examiner rather than fixed straight ahead).

5. Trigeminal Nerve (V)
Facial Sensation

Simultaneously touch both sides of the forehead (V_1), then the cheek (V_2), and then the jaw (V_3) and ask if they feel the same. Check for temperature perception in the same sequence, using the cool surface of a tuning fork or other appropriate stimulus. The stimulus will be perceived as warmer on the side of impaired sensation.

Corneal Reflex

Sweep a wisp of cotton lightly across the lateral surface of the eye (out of the direct visual field) from sclera to cornea. As soon as the stimulus reaches the sensitive cornea, the patient will wince and blink vigorously if nerves V and VII are both intact. Compare the sides for symmetry.

Motor V Testing

Observe the symmetry of opening and closing of the mouth; the jaw will fall faster and farther on the side of the lesion, so that the face looks askew. For more subtle weakness, ask the patient to clench the teeth and then attempt to force jaw opening or lateral jaw displacement. Normal strength cannot be overcome.

6. *Facial Strength (VII)*

A central "supranuclear" lesion, such as a hemispheric stroke, will preserve forehead wrinkling and cause only mild weakness of eye closure, while the lower face is more severely involved. If there is a peripheral lesion of the cranial nerve (or nucleus), the entire hemiface will be flaccid and the eyelids will gape open.

Some cranial neuropathies or neuromuscular diseases cause bilateral facial weakness, and in such cases the usual criterion of facial asymmetry as a marker of weakness will not apply.

Facial Symmetry

Observe the patient's face for symmetry of the palpebral fissures and nasolabial folds at rest. Ask the patient to wrinkle the forehead, then to squeeze the eyes tightly shut (looking for asymmetry in the extent to which the eyelashes protrude), then to smile or snarl, saying, "Show me your teeth."

Bilateral Facial Weakness

Ask the patient to squeeze the eyes tightly shut, then press the lips tightly together, then puff air into the cheeks. If strength is normal, one should not be able to pry the eyelids open, force the lips apart, or forcibly expel air from the mouth (by compressing the cheeks).

7. *Auditory (VIII)*

Auditory acuity can be tested crudely by rubbing thumb and forefinger together about 2 inches from each ear. If there are complaints of deafness or if the patient cannot hear the finger rub, proceed to the following tests.

Rinne Test

Hold the base of a lightly vibrating high-pitched (512-Hz) tuning fork on the mastoid process until the sound is no longer perceived, then bring the still vibrating fork up close to (not touching) the ear. Normally—or if the hearing loss is sensorineural—air conduction is greater than bone conduction and the patient will again hear the tone. If there is significant conductive loss, the patient will not be able to hear the air-conducted tone longer than the bone-conducted tone.

Weber Test

If hearing is impaired in one ear, lightly strike a high-pitched (512-Hz) tuning fork and place the handle on the midline of the forehead. If there is conductive loss, the tone will sound louder in the affected ear; if the loss is sensorineural, the tone will be louder in the unaffected ear.

Vestibular Function

Vestibular function needs to be tested only if there are complaints of dizziness or vertigo or evidence of nystagmus. The Nylen-Bárány (Dix-Hallpike) maneuver tests for positional vertigo and positional nystagmus. In this disorder, as in other types of vertigo of peripheral origin, nystagmus will come on after at least 3–5 seconds, will decrease with time, and will become less prominent with repetition of the test.

Nylen-Bárány (Dix-Hallpike) Maneuver

The patient sits with legs extended on a table while the examiner supports the head and shoulders. Rapidly lower the patient to the supine position with neck hyperextended (head hanging off the table) and rotated to one side; repeat with the head turned to the other side. Look for nystagmus and ask the patient to report vertigo. The patient may need encouragement to keep the eyes open (see Figure 3–6).

8. *Glossopharyngeal (IX) & Vagus (X)*

Some useful tests for detection of deficiencies in motor function of the palate, pharynx, and larynx are described below. Sensory function needs to be checked if one suspects cranial neuropathy or a brainstem lesion.

Palatal Elevation

Ask the patient to say "ah." Look for full and symmetric palatal elevation (not deviation of the uvula). If one side is weak, it will fail to elevate and will be pulled toward the strong side.

Gag Reflex (Afferent IX, Efferent X)

Gently touch each side of the posterior pharyngeal wall with a cotton swab and compare the vigor of the gag.

Sensory Function

Lightly touch each side of the soft palate with the tip of a cotton swab.

Voice Quality

Listen for hoarseness or "breathiness," suggesting laryngeal weakness.

9. *Accessory (XI)*
Sternocleidomastoid

Press a hand against the patient's jaw and have the patient rotate the head against resistance. Pressing against the right jaw tests the left sternocleidomastoid and vice versa.

Trapezius

Have the patient shrug shoulders against resistance and assess weakness.

10. Hypoglossal (XII)

Dysarthria is a defect in the mechanical production of speech sounds. Testing for dysarthria provides a quick functional assessment of the lower cranial nerves, cerebellum, and basal ganglia. Facial weakness (see VII above) can be assessed by asking for labial sounds ("mee-mee-mee"). Pharyngeal weakness (see IX and X above) results in a nasal voice as assessed by asking for guttural sounds ("kay-kay-kay"). Laryngeal dysfunction (see IX and X above) presents as hoarseness or "breathy" speech. Maximal difficulty is found with a high-pitched sound, as this requires vocal cord adduction. Tongue weakness (XII) is manifested by pronounced slurring, particularly of lingual sounds ("la-la-la"). Bilateral corticobulbar tract lesions are manifested by strangled, spastic, labored speech or, if severe enough, no speech at all (along with inability to open the mouth or protrude the tongue and a hyperactive gag reflex).

Tests for hypoglossal nerve function include the following.

Atrophy or Fasciculations

With the patient's tongue resting in the floor of the mouth, first inspect for atrophy or fasciculations (worm-like quivers and twitches). Then ask the patient to protrude the tongue, and observe for deviation to the weak side. Be sure the deviation is real and not just apparent because of facial weakness. Mark the midline of the nose and chin with thumb and forefinger. Then ask the patient to move the tongue rapidly from side to side.

Subtle Weakness

If subtle weakness is suspected, have the patient push the tongue into each cheek against external resistance. Strength of protrusion to one side is a measure of the power of the opposite hypoglossal muscle.

Subtle Dysarthria

Ask the patient to repeat difficult phrases such as "methodist episcopal" or "administrative assistant."

MOTOR COORDINATION (CHAPTER 3)

The **cerebellar hemispheres** are responsible for coordinating and fine-tuning movements already set in motion and for correcting speed, accuracy of direction, and intensity of force to meet the intended purpose. The cerebellar hemispheres control the ipsilateral appendages, particularly the arms.

The following are some tests for cerebellar hemispheric function.

Finger-to-Nose

Ask the patient to alternately touch his or her nose and then the examiner's extended forefinger, held far enough away to require reaching. Look for overshoot or for an oscillatory "hunting" tremor that increases in amplitude as the target is neared. Abnormalities are referred to as **dysmetria.**

Finger-Tapping, Toe-Tapping

Demonstrate and then ask the patient to tap as evenly and rhythmically as possible. Look and listen for irregularities of rhythm or force.

Rapid Alternating Movements

Have the patient strike the thighs rhythmically and rapidly, alternating between the palms and the backs of the hands; rapidly touch the thumb to each finger in succession; or rapidly wiggle the protruded tongue from side to side. **Dysdiadochokinesia** is the technical term for dysrhythmias in performing any of these tasks.

Rebound

The patient flexes an arm as strongly as possible or holds the arm extended against resistance. The examiner then suddenly lets go. If the arm flies upward or toward the face, this signifies that the patient is unable to check the abrupt imbalance between flexors and extensors.

Heel-Knee-Shin

The supine or seated patient is instructed to place one heel against the opposite knee, tap the knee with the heel, then run the heel smoothly down the tibia to the ankle.

Cerebellar Vermis

The cerebellar vermis is concerned with postural stability and axial function—particularly stance and gait. In patients with lesions in this area, the gait will be wide-based and ataxic (staggering) and it may be difficult to sit upright without support. There may be irregular back-and-forth rocking or shaking of the head (**titubation**), and speech may be "scanning," ie, irregular in force and pitch, with words distinctly broken into "syl-luh-bles." Integrity of the vermis can be tested by asking the patient to stand "naturally" while observing how far apart the feet are positioned for a stable base. The examiner then extends the arms (for reassurance and to prevent falls) and asks the patient to bring the feet together until they touch.

Basal Ganglia

Disorders of the basal ganglia (extrapyramidal system) may result in inability either to initiate motor activity (bradykinesia, loss of associated movements such as arm swinging), correct for postural imbalance, or control movements such as tremor or chorea. Tremor or other abnormal movements should be observed with the patient at rest, during arm extension, and during performance of a goal-directed action such as drinking from an imaginary cup.

Other Tests of Motor Coordination

A. TURNING AROUND

How many steps does the patient need to "about face"? A normal turn is made with a one- or two-step pivot. A patient with parkinsonism may require up to 20 small steps ("en bloc turn") or may freeze altogether.

B. DRAWING SPIRALS

The patient is asked to draw a copy of an expanding (Archimedes) spiral. In parkinsonism, there is difficulty enlarging the figure's successive loops.

C. RETROPULSION

The examiner stands behind the patient, announces what is about to happen, then vigorously pulls the patient backward by the shoulders. Normally, the subject will regain the center of gravity with a step or two backward and truncal flexion. The patient with parkinsonism cannot do so and may stagger rigidly backward or fall into the examiner's arms.

MOTOR FUNCTION (CHAPTER 5)

The motor examination includes evaluation of muscle tone, bulk, and strength.

1. Muscle Tone

Tone is defined as resistance of muscle to passive movement at a joint. Tone can be decreased, normal, or increased (Table A–2).

The hardest part of evaluating tone is getting the patient to relax. Diversionary tactics may be required. Once the patient is seen to be relaxed, the following maneuvers can be used.

Arm Muscle Tone

Support the patient's bent arm with one hand cupping the elbow, then smoothly flex and extend the forearm, then pronate and supinate. Grasp the forearm and flop the wrist back and forth, briskly raise the arms as if tossing them into the air, and then abruptly let go and watch how fast and symmetrically they drop.

Table A–2. Classification of muscle tone.

Tone	Type	Description	Anatomic Basis
Decreased		Floppy, flaccid, hypotonic	Motor neuron, cerebellum, acute stroke or cord lesion (spinal shock)
Normal			
Increased	Spastic	"One-way" resistance to extension (arm) or flexion (leg), maximum at the beginning of the extension or with faster stretch	Upper motor neuron (pyramidal)
	Rigid	Resistance equal throughout the range of motion in all directions and at all speeds, like a "lead pipe"; can have a ratchety "cogwheeling" quality that may be from a superimposed tremor	Basal ganglia (extrapyramidal)
	Paratonic ("gegenhalten")	Limb stiffens in response to any contact, and the degree of resistance increases with the force exerted by the examiner; motor perseveration may also occur	Frontal lobes or diffuse

Leg Muscle Tone

With the patient lying prone and relaxed, place a hand under the knee, then abruptly pull vigorously upward. With normal or reduced tone, the heel lifts only momentarily off the bed or remains in contact with the surface as it slides up toward the buttocks. The hypertonic leg lifts entirely off the bed. With the patient seated, grasp the knee and bounce the foot up and down off the floor.

Axial Rotation

Passively rotate the patient's head and observe if the shoulders also move, or gently but firmly flex and extend the neck and assess resistance.

2. Muscle Bulk

Some loss of muscle bulk may be seen with disuse, but significant **atrophy** ("wasting") is characteristic of denervation from lower motor neuron lesions. Atrophy may also be associated with **fasciculations,** or rapid twitching. These spontaneous contractions of a muscle fascicle may resemble worm-like writhing under the skin, or occasionally may be coarse enough to move a joint. Asymmetric atrophy can best be assessed by comparing sides or by careful measurement. If atrophy is diffuse, one can compare the patient's muscle to a "normal" muscle by palpating one's own corresponding muscle mass.

3. Muscle Strength

Strength is measured by the ability to contract the muscle against force or gravity. The classic grading system scores as follows: 5, full strength; 4, movement against gravity and resistance; 3, movement against gravity only; 2, movement only if gravity is eliminated (eg, horizontally along the surface of the bed); 1, palpable contraction but little visible movement ("flicker"); 0, no contraction.

Exactly which muscles are tested—and how carefully—will depend on the patient's complaints and the examiner's suspicions. Tests of strength should be conducted with the following in mind:

1. "Normal" means "to be expected of this patient." A frail elderly man is expected to be less strong than a young weight lifter.

2. The examiner should be on equal footing with the patient. If testing shoulder abduction, the examiner should stand facing the patient and use only the upper arms to oppose the patient rather than standing above a seated patient and pressing down with full body weight. When testing finger extension, only the equivalent finger should be used, not the whole arm and shoulder strength.

3. The patient is a more sensitive observer than the examiner and may have more subtle weakness than is detectable through formal testing. This is particularly true in the legs. If indicated, follow formal testing with "functional" tests such as squatting and rising, walking on the heels, and rising from a low stool with arms crossed.

A pattern frequently seen after a stroke is **pyramidal weakness,** in which abductors and extensors of the arm and flexors of the leg are preferentially affected, so that the arm has a tendency to be held in adducted flexion and the leg in adducted extension.

Tests of strength are as follows.

General Strength

Isolate the specific agonist muscle action and then apply an equal and opposite force in gradually increasing intensity. For example, support the patient's elbow with one hand underneath and attempt to extend the arm by pressing down on the forearm, telling the patient to "bend your elbow up as tightly as you can—don't let me pull it down."

Pyramidal Weakness

Check for weakness of finger or forearm extension by attempting to push down the extended fingers or flex the half-extended elbow. In contrast, the strength of the biceps or hand grip is an insensitive index of pyramidal weakness.

Pronator Drift

Ask the patient to hold the arms straight out with palms up and then to close the eyelids. A weak arm will begin to drift downward and the hand will begin to pronate.

SENSORY FUNCTION (CHAPTER 6)

A basic screening examination should assess both large-fiber and small-fiber modalities in the fingers and toes.

1. Large-Fiber & Dorsal Column Functions

Lesions of large fiber nerves and of the dorsal column of the spinal cord are investigated by tests of **vibration** and **joint position** sense. Normal joint position sense is exquisitely sensitive, and the patient should detect any movement no matter how fine. If joint position sense is diminished distally, test more proximal limb joints. Functional tests for joint position sense include **Romberg's test** and the **finger-to-finger test.**

Vibration Sense

Strike a low-pitched (128-Hz) tuning fork gently and place the base firmly on a bony prominence, with one finger of the other hand supporting the digit and serving as a control. Ask if the patient "feels the buzz," and determine when it can no longer be perceived. Compare sides, and if sensation is decreased at the toe, repeat at the ankle, knee, or hip to determine the extent of impairment. Compare leg and arm sensation as well. Abnormalities in the distal legs but not the arms are found in patients with polyneuropathies or lesions of the thoracolumbar spinal cord.

Joint Position Sense

Grasp the sides of the distal phalanx of a finger or toe and faintly displace the tip up or down. Rehearse first with the patient watching, then test with the patient's eyes closed to determine the threshold for correctly perceiving the direction of movement.

Romberg's Test

Instruct the patient to stand with the feet as close together as possible. (If the patient cannot stand with the feet together, a cerebellar lesion is present and Romberg's test is not applicable.) The patient is then observed with eyes closed. An abnormal result consists of swaying or other evidence of instability.

Finger-to-Finger Test

Instruct the patient to bring the extended forefingers together with eyes closed through two or three feet of space, or have the patient touch the tip of the nose with a finger. As in the Romberg test, the patient is demonstrating "pseudoataxia," a disorder of sensory input, if finger placement is clumsy with the eyes closed but not with the eyes open.

2. Small-Fiber & Spinothalamic Function

Temperature Sensation

Using the cold flat disk of a tuning fork or other cold object, first establish the patient's ability to detect its temperature in a presumably normal area. Then have the patient compare the relative temperature of the stimulus from the dorsum of the feet upward, or from side to side, or between dermatomes.

Superficial Pain Sensation

Use a disposable instrument, such as a safety pin, for each patient. Prick the skin with enough force to be unpleasant but not harmful, and ask if the prick feels sharp or "hurts like a pin." As always, work from side to side, distal to proximal, or dermatome to dermatome—and from area of deficit toward normal regions.

Light Touch Sensation

The sensation of light touch is served by both the large-fiber–posterior column system and the small-fiber–spinothalamic system. Testing is done with a very light stimulus such as a wisp of cotton, the teased-out tip of a cotton swab, or a brush motion with the examiner's fingertips. Ask the patient to indicate with closed eyes where the stimulus is perceived.

REFLEXES

1. Deep Tendon Reflexes

A deep tendon reflex is the reaction of a muscle to being passively stretched by percussion on the tendon. These reflexes are a measure of the integrity both of the afferent and efferent peripheral nerves and of their central inhibitory controls. Tendon reflexes are graded on a scale according to the force of the contraction or the minimum force needed to elicit the response: 4, very brisk, often with clonus (record the number of beats); 3, brisk but normal; 2, normal; 1, minimal; 0, absent.

In some cases, deep tendon reflexes are difficult to elicit without such reinforcement as having the patient clench the opposite fist or interlock the fingers and attempt to pull them apart. Hypoactivity or hyperactivity is generally of less significance than asymmetry; however, absent reflexes may be a clue to an unsuspected neuropathy, and hyperactivity may be associated with spasticity.

The four most commonly tested tendon reflexes are described here.

Biceps Reflex (C5–6)

Support the patient's partly flexed elbow with one cupped hand, thumb positioned on the biceps tendon. Strike the thumb with a percussion hammer and assess the force of flexion at the elbow.

Triceps Reflex (C7–8)

Support the patient's partly flexed arm by holding the forearm against the patient's body, or suspend the abducted arm just above the elbow so that the forearm dangles freely. Strike the triceps tendon just above the elbow and assess the force of extension at the elbow.

Quadriceps (Patellar, Knee Jerk) Reflex (L3–4)

The patient's feet can remain on the floor, but it is easier to elicit this reflex if the patient crosses one leg and lets the foot dangle. If the patient is in bed, support the leg in partial flexion with one arm under the knee. Feel for the bottom edge of the patella and strike just below it. Assess the force of extension at the knee.

Achilles (Ankle Jerk) Reflex (S1–2)

The patient's foot is passively dorsiflexed, resting its weight on the ball of the foot, or by pressing on the sole. Strike the tendon or the sole directly. Assess the force of extension at the ankle.

2. Babinski Sign

In patients over age 18 months, the normal response to stimulation of the lateral sole is plantar flexion of the toes. Extension upward of the great toe (Babinski sign) is a sensitive but nonspecific sign of central nervous system disease and can be a consequence of pyramidal tract damage or diffuse cerebral dysfunction.

The foot should be held firmly and the patient told what to expect. Place the tip of a suitable instrument, such as the bare end of a swabstick, on the lateral aspect of the sole at the heel and sweep it firmly forward to the base of the toes. Apply the least pressure necessary to evoke a response. Avoid stroking across and under the toes, a maneuver that might evoke a conflicting (foot grasp) response manifested by flexion of the toes.

3. Frontal Release Signs

Frontal release signs are primitive reflexes that can be thought of as adaptive for the infant, such as grasping or sucking, but that disappear as the brain matures. Diffuse neuronal dysfunction, especially frontal lobe damage, releases them from inhibition. The more important signs are **grasp,** or curling of the fingers in response to stimulation of the palmar surface of the hand and fingertips (it can be seen in the foot as well); **suck; snout,** or pursing of the lips; and the **glabellar sign,** or persistent blink response.

Grasp Sign

The grasp response is elicited by lightly drawing one's fingertips along the hypothenar (medial) aspect of the patient's palm and then transversely across the fingertips, gently lifting. This test is performed while the patient is distracted. In a pronounced grasp response, the patient's fingers will hook around the examiner's firmly. Even the touch of an inanimate object such as a chair arm may elicit a tenacious grasp.

Suck Sign

This sign is elicited by gently stroking the patient's lips with the fingers or with a tongue depressor. Sucking or swallowing movements constitute a positive response. The same responses may occur at the mere sight of an approaching finger.

Snout Sign

With an index finger positioned vertically over the lips, tapping the finger with the other hand or with a reflex hammer normally elicits protrusion of the lips. An abnormal response is exaggerated protrusion.

Glabellar Sign

This sign is elicited by repetitive tapping between the patient's eyebrows. The normal response is to blink a few times and then stop. The response is abnormal if the patient continues to blink with each tap as long as the stimulus continues. The glabellar sign may also be present in extrapyramidal disorders.

4. Pathologic Reflexes

Pathologic reflexes appear with upper motor neuron damage and consequent loss of inhibition. If tendon reflexes are hyperactive (particularly if asymmetric) or if spasticity is found, these pathologic reflexes need to be sought—though they are not in themselves diagnostic of disease and may in fact be present in normal individuals. Pathologic reflexes include the crossed adductor, finger flexor, jaw jerk, and clonus reflexes.

Crossed Adduction Reflex

Place a hand on the patient's thigh adductor tendon just above and medial to the knee and strike briskly. Normally, only the struck leg will adduct. With upper motor neuron lesions, both legs may adduct and the patient's legs may make a scissoring motion.

Finger Flexor Reflex

Let the patient's arm and hand relax on the bed or table. With thumb and forefinger, pick up the patient's hand so that it dangles with the wrist dorsiflexed and the fingers partly flexed. With the other hand, "snap" the nail of the patient's middle finger with the thumbnail. Alternately, suspend the hand by hooking the flexed fingertips over your extended forefinger, then strike your forefinger sharply with a reflex hammer. An abnormal response consists of adduction and flexion of the thumb and exaggerated flexion of the fingers.

Jaw Jerk Reflex

With an index finger on the patient's relaxed chin, strike the finger downward with a reflex hammer. Exaggerated contraction of the masseter suggests bilateral pathology above the mid pons.

Clonus

Clonus is repetitive, rhythmic, involuntary contraction induced by sudden passive stretching of a muscle or of its tendon. It may occasionally occur spontaneously or be induced in response to a mild stimulus such as the weight of the bedclothes. It is most often seen at the ankle after strong and sustained dorsiflexion.

To elicit ankle clonus, grasp the foot firmly, push sharply upward against the sole, and maintain the pressure. A few beats of alternating flexion and extension of the foot are occasionally seen in normal individuals, but sustained clonus (five or more beats) is abnormal.

STANCE & GAIT (CHAPTER 3)

Watching the patient walk may be the most important part of the neurologic examination. Seeing how the patient initiates a planned action, evaluating the ability to maintain balance while "repetitively hurling oneself into space"—as the act of walking has been described, and analyzing an abnormal gait for clues to the nature of the deficit all provide valuable information.

The minimal screening examination should include evaluation of the following: (1) "Normal" gait across the room. (2) "Heel-walking" with ankles dorsiflexed. (3) "Toe-walking" on the balls of the feet with heels elevated. (4) "Tandem" gait, in which the patient puts one foot directly in front of the other, heel to toe, and walks an imaginary line.

Some characteristic stances and gaits are as follows.

Steppage Gait ("Foot Drop")

Steppage gait results from an inability to dorsiflex the foot. The patient compensates by exaggerated elevation of the flexed hip and knee to allow the foot to clear the ground while walking. This abnormality is usually the consequence of a peripheral nerve disorder such as a peroneal palsy or other neuropathy, but occasionally it results from a radiculopathy or central lesion.

Cerebellar Gait

This is a wide-based, irregular, staggering, or reeling gait, as if drunk.

Sensory-Ataxic Gait

A wide-based, short, uneven gait characterized by high steps and slapping down of the feet is seen with proprioceptive loss, as in tabes dorsalis. The eyes may remain "glued" to the ground.

Hemiplegic Gait

With the affected spastic leg extended and internally rotated and the foot in inversion and plantar flexion, the leg circumducts at the hip to allow the foot to clear the floor.

Paraplegic Gait

A slow, stiff shuffling gait with the toes scraping and the legs "scissoring" because of increased adductor tone associated with spasticity is seen in myelopathy or other bilateral corticospinal tract disease.

Dystrophic Gait

Waddling and lordotic posture may result from pelvic muscle weakness.

Parkinsonian Gait

This consists of slow starting and short shuffling steps with a tendency to accelerate ("festinate") as if chasing the center of gravity. The posture is stooped, turns are "en bloc" with the feet moving only in tiny steps, and there is loss of normal associated movements, such as arm swinging, that help to maintain balance.

Apraxic Gait

Apraxia consists of an inability to execute a learned motor program. Gait apraxia is loss of the ability to walk and results from diffuse cerebral damage—more specifically, damage to the frontal lobe—despite normal strength and coordination. The gait is similar to a parkinsonian gait, but if severe the patient will simply stand, partially upright, unable to "remember" how to go about walking, the feet seeming to be "glued to the floor." Alternatively, the patient will lift and lower the feet without advancing, as if drawn to the floor by magnetic force.

Antalgic Gait

Antalgic gait is a response to pain—favoring one leg by putting as little weight as possible on it.

Choreic Gait

Choreic gait is described as lurching, "jerky twitching," and "dancing." Falls are surprisingly rare.

APPENDIX B: A BRIEF EXAMINATION OF THE NERVOUS SYSTEM

Occasionally, a screening neurologic examination briefer than that in Appendix A is needed. An approach to such a screening examination follows.

COGNITIVE FUNCTION

The level of consciousness (whether the patient is awake and alert, confused and somnolent or agitated, or comatose) should be noted and orientation to person, place, and time specifically tested. Patients with acute confusional states typically demonstrate impaired orientation to time and place; patients with psychiatric disorders may also be disoriented to person. Language function can be tested rapidly by asking the patient to repeat a phrase such as "no ifs, ands, or buts," since repetition is impaired in most aphasias. The examination of cognitive function is discussed in detail elsewhere (see Chapter 1).

GAIT

A singularly helpful test for detecting nervous system dysfunction is observation of the gait. Every patient must be observed standing and walking. Standing, starting to walk, stopping, and turning should each be assessed and the associated movements of the limbs noted with each maneuver. These actions require coordination of sensory, motor, cerebellar, visual, and vestibular function and thus provide a sensitive indication of abnormal functioning of these systems.

CRANIAL NERVES

Cranial nerve abnormalities are the hallmark of brainstem dysfunction and of some neuromuscular disorders. They can also reveal the presence of hemispheric disease or elevated intracranial pressure.

Optic disk swelling (papilledema) is the cardinal sign of increased intracranial pressure; spontaneous venous pulsations upon the disk indicate that intracranial pressure is normal.

Examination of the visual fields surveys the visual pathways of the retina, optic nerves, and chiasm; the lateral geniculate body; the temporal and parietal lobes; and the occipital cortex. A rapid screening technique consists of assessing the patient's ability to detect small movements of the examiner's finger in the temporal fields (or, in obtunded patients, the response to threat).

Unilateral facial weakness that involves especially the lower part of the face is a common sign of contralateral hemispheric lesions. Facial strength should be tested by having patients close their eyes as tightly as possible so that the eyelashes are "buried." Asymmetry of eye closure—or the examiner's ability to open one or both of a patient's eyes against resistance—is a clear sign of motor system dysfunction. Facial grimacing with retraction of the lips when patients are asked to show their teeth may also reveal facial weakness.

MOTOR SYSTEM

The most common abnormality affecting the motor system is upper motor neuron, or pyramidal weakness, such as results from hemispheric stroke. Severe hemiparesis or hemiplegia is obvious to even the inexperienced examiner, but even very mild hemiparesis can be detected by observing slowed fine finger movements or minor weakness or increased tone in a pyramidal distribution. Thus, the power of finger abductors, finger and wrist extensors, triceps, dorsiflexors of the foot, and the hamstring muscles should be compared on the two sides.

SENSORY SYSTEM

The distribution of regional or segmental sensory abnormalities can be discerned by asking patients to sketch out on their bodies the limits of the perceived sensory impairment. The peripheral nerve or nerve root to which this pattern of sensory involvement best corresponds can then be determined (see Figure 6–4). Polyneuropathy usually produces distal, symmetric sensory deficits that are especially prominent in the feet. If present, such deficits should then be differentiated according to whether large nerve fibers (mediating vibratory sense) or small nerve fibers (mediating pain and temperature appreciation) are predominantly affected. The differential diagnosis of these disorders can then be undertaken (see Chapter 6).

REFLEXES

The major issue here is whether the deep tendon reflexes are symmetric, which suggests that no lateralized impairment of upper or lower motor neuron function is present. Reflexes should be elicited by percussing the tendons on both sides with the same force and with the limbs on both sides in similar positions; if no asymmetry is found, the force of percussion should be progressively decreased until the threshold for eliciting the response can be compared from side to side. Impairment of a single reflex is most compatible with nerve root involvement at the level of the reflex (C5–6, biceps and rachioradialis reflex; C7–8, triceps reflex; L3–4, knee jerk; S1, ankle jerk). Bilateral depression or the absence of ankle jerks suggests a polyneuropathy.

In eliciting the plantar reflex, stroking the lateral border of the sole of the foot leads to plantar flexion of the great toe in normal subjects, whereas extension occurs in those with upper motor neuron disturbances (Babinski's sign).

APPENDIX C: CLINICAL EXAMINATION OF COMMON ISOLATED PERIPHERAL NERVE DISORDERS

The accompanying illustrations are a guide for examining sensory and motor function of selected peripheral nerves: radial (Figure C–1), median (Figure C–2), ulnar (Figure C–3), peroneal (Figure C–4), and femoral (Figure C–5).

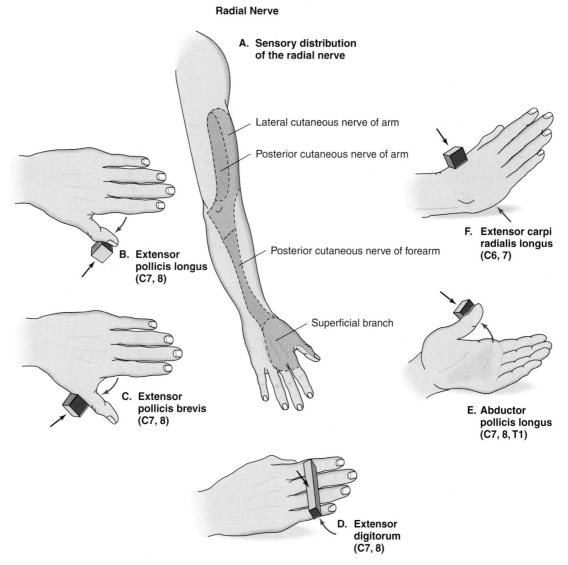

Radial Nerve

A. Sensory distribution of the radial nerve

Lateral cutaneous nerve of arm

Posterior cutaneous nerve of arm

Posterior cutaneous nerve of forearm

Superficial branch

B. Extensor pollicis longus (C7, 8)

C. Extensor pollicis brevis (C7, 8)

D. Extensor digitorum (C7, 8)

E. Abductor pollicis longus (C7, 8, T1)

F. Extensor carpi radialis longus (C6, 7)

Figure C–1. Testing the radial nerve. **A:** Sensory distribution. The radial nerve supplies the dorsolateral surface of the upper arm, forearm, wrist, and hand, the dorsal surface of the thumb, the dorsal surface of the index and middle fingers above the distal interphalangeal joints, and the lateral half of the dorsal surface of the ring finger above the distal interphalangeal joint. **B:** Extensor pollicis longus. The thumb is extended at the interphalangeal joint against resistance. **C:** Extensor pollicis brevis. The thumb is extended at the metacarpophalangeal joint against resistance. **D:** Extensor digitorum. The index finger is extended at the metacarpophalangeal joint against resistance. **E:** Abductor pollicis longus. The thumb is abducted (elevated in a plane at 90 degrees to the palm) at the carpometacarpal joint against resistance. **F:** Extensor carpi radialis longus. The wrist is extended toward the radial (thumb) side against resistance.

Median Nerve

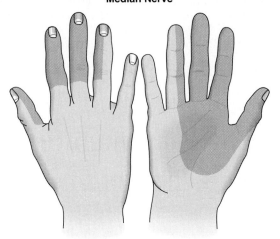

A. Sensory distribution of the median nerve

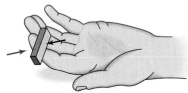

B. Flexor digitorum profundus I and II (C7, **8**, T1)

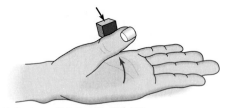

C. Abductor pollicis brevis (C8, **T1**)

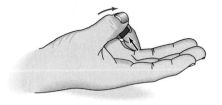

D. Opponens pollicis (C8, **T1**)

Figure C–2. Testing the median nerve. **A:** Sensory distribution. The median nerve supplies the dorsal surface of the index and middle fingers, the lateral half of the dorsal surface of the ring finger, the lateral two-thirds of the palm, the palmar surface of the thumb, index finger, middle fingers, and the lateral half of the palmar surface of the ring finger. **B:** Flexor digitorum profundus I and II. The index and middle fingers are flexed at the distal interphalangeal joints against resistance. **C:** Abductor pollicis brevis. The thumb is abducted (elevated at 90 degrees to the plane of the palm) at the metacarpophalangeal joints against resistance. **D:** Opponens pollicis. The thumb is crossed over the palm to touch the little finger against resistance.

Ulnar Nerve

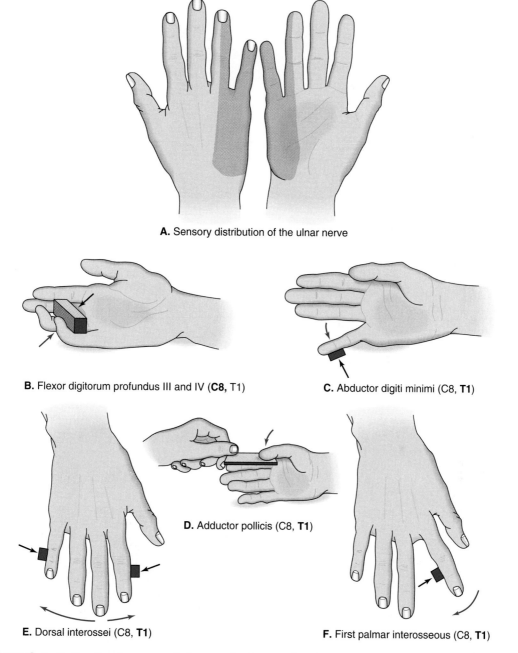

A. Sensory distribution of the ulnar nerve

B. Flexor digitorum profundus III and IV (**C8,** T1)

C. Abductor digiti minimi (C8, **T1**)

D. Adductor pollicis (C8, **T1**)

E. Dorsal interossei (C8, **T1**)

F. First palmar interosseous (C8, **T1**)

Figure C–3. Testing the ulnar nerve. **A:** Sensory distribution. The ulnar nerve supplies the dorsal and palmar surfaces of the medial one-third of the hand, the dorsal and palmar surfaces of the little finger, and the dorsal and palmar surfaces of the medial half of the ring finger. **B:** Flexor digitorum profundus III and IV. The index and middle fingers are flexed at the distal interphalangeal joints against resistance. **C:** Abductor digiti minimi. The little finger is abducted against resistance. **D:** Adductor pollicis. A piece of paper is grasped between the thumb and the palm with the thumbnail at 90 degrees to the plane of the palm while the examiner tries to pull the paper away. **E:** Dorsal interossei. The fingers are abducted against resistance. **F:** First palmar interosseous. The abducted index finger is adducted against resistance.

Peroneal Nerve

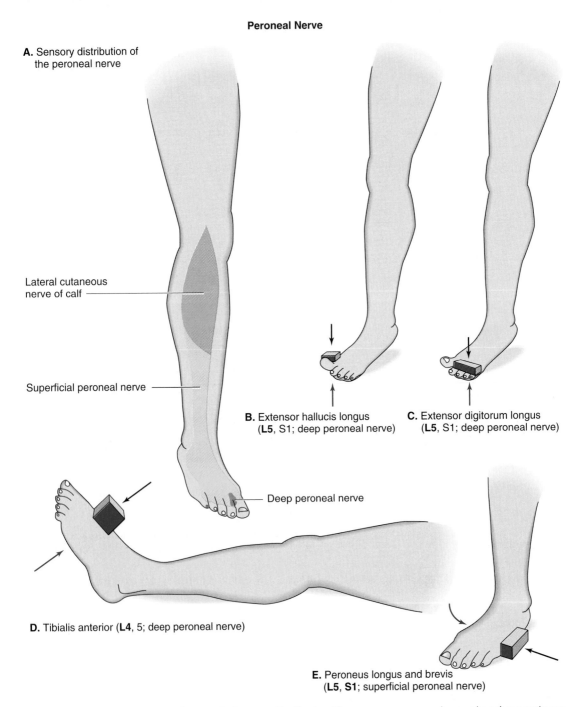

A. Sensory distribution of the peroneal nerve

Lateral cutaneous nerve of calf

Superficial peroneal nerve

B. Extensor hallucis longus (**L5**, S1; deep peroneal nerve)

C. Extensor digitorum longus (**L5**, S1; deep peroneal nerve)

Deep peroneal nerve

D. Tibialis anterior (**L4**, 5; deep peroneal nerve)

E. Peroneus longus and brevis (**L5**, **S1**; superficial peroneal nerve)

Figure C–4. Testing the peroneal nerve. **A:** Sensory distribution. The common peroneal nerve has three main sensory branches. The lateral cutaneous nerve of the calf supplies the lateral surface of the calf, the superficial peroneal nerve supplies the lateral surface of the lower leg and the dorsum of the foot, and the deep peroneal nerve supplies a roughly triangular patch of skin on the dorsum of the foot between the first and second toes. **B:** Extensor hallucis longus. The large toe is extended (dorsiflexed) against resistance. **C:** Extensor digitorum longus. The second, third, fourth, and fifth toes are extended against resistance. **D:** Tibialis anterior. The foot is dorsiflexed at the ankle against resistance. **E:** Peroneus longus and brevis. The foot is everted (rotated laterally) at the ankle against resistance.

Femoral Nerve

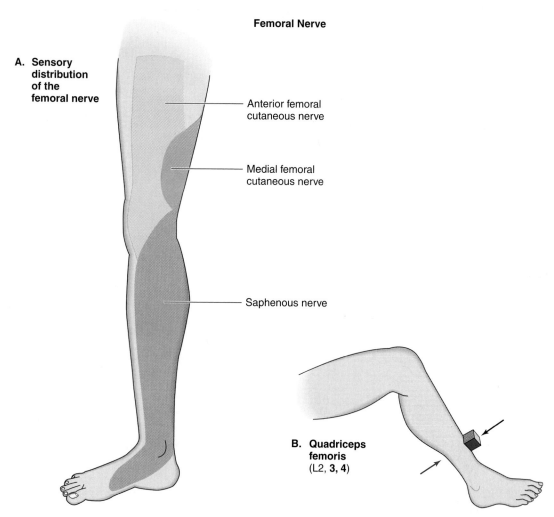

A. Sensory distribution of the femoral nerve

Anterior femoral cutaneous nerve

Medial femoral cutaneous nerve

Saphenous nerve

B. Quadriceps femoris (L2, 3, 4)

Figure C–5. Testing the femoral nerve. **A:** Sensory distribution. The femoral nerve has three main sensory branches. The anterior femoral cutaneous nerve supplies the anterior surface of the thigh, the medial femoral cutaneous nerve supplies the anteromedial surface of the thigh, and the saphenous nerve supplies the medial surface of the lower leg, ankle, and foot. **B:** Quadriceps femoris. The leg is extended at the knee against resistance.

Index

NOTE: Page numbers in **bold face** type indicate a major discussion. A "t" following a page number indicates tabular material and an "f" following a page number indicates a figure. Drugs are listed under generic names. When a drug trade name is listed, the reader is referred to the generic name.